AIDS
The Second Decade

Heather G. Miller, Charles F. Turner,
and Lincoln E. Moses, *Editors*

COMMITTEE ON AIDS RESEARCH AND THE
BEHAVIORAL, SOCIAL, AND STATISTICAL SCIENCES

COMMISSION ON THE BEHAVIORAL AND
SOCIAL SCIENCES AND EDUCATION

NATIONAL RESEARCH COUNCIL

NATIONAL ACADEMY PRESS
WASHINGTON, D.C.   1990

National Academy Press • 2101 Constitution Avenue, N.W. • Washington, D. C. • 20418

NOTICE: The project that is the subject of this report was approved by the Governing Board of the National Research Council, whose members are drawn from the councils of the National Academy of Sciences, the National Academy of Engineering, and the Institute of Medicine. The members of the committee responsible for the report were chosen for their special competences and with regard for appropriate balance.

This report has been reviewed by a group other than the authors according to procedures approved by a Report Review Committee consisting of members of the National Academy of Sciences, the National Academy of Engineering, and the Institute of Medicine.

The National Academy of Sciences is a private, nonprofit, self-perpetuating society of distinguished scholars engaged in scientific and engineering research, dedicated to the furtherance of science and technology and to their use for the general welfare. Upon the authority of the charter granted to it by the Congress in 1863, the Academy has a mandate that requires it to advise the federal government on scientific and technical matters. Dr. Frank Press is president of the National Academy of Sciences.

The National Academy of Engineering was established in 1964, under the charter of the National Academy of Sciences, as a parallel organization of outstanding engineers. It is autonomous in its administration and in the selection of its members, sharing with the National Academy of Sciences the responsibility for advising the federal government. The National Academy of Engineering also sponsors engineering programs aimed at meeting national needs, encourages education and research, and recognizes the superior achievements of engineers. Dr. Robert M. White is president of the National Academy of Engineering.

The Institute of Medicine was established in 1970 by the National Academy of Sciences to secure the services of eminent members of appropriate professions in the examination of policy matters pertaining to the health of the public. The Institute acts under the responsibility given to the National Academy of Sciences by its congressional charter to be an adviser to the federal government and upon its own initiative, to identify issues of medical care, research, and education. Dr. Samuel O. Thier is president of the Institute of Medicine.

The National Research Council was established by the National Academy of Sciences in 1916 to associate the broad community of science and technology with the Academy's purposes of furthering knowledge and of advising the federal government. Functioning in accordance with general policies determined by the Academy, the Council has become the principal operating agency of both the National Academy of Sciences and the National Academy of Engineering in providing services to the government, the public, and the scientific and engineering communities. The Council is administered jointly by both Academies and the Institute of Medicine. Dr. Frank Press and Dr. Robert M. White are chairman and vice-chairman, respectively, of the National Research Council.

The work that provided the basis for this volume was supported by a contract from the U.S. Public Health Service.

Library of Congress Catalog Card Number 90-50389

International Standard Book Number 0-309-04278-X, cloth
International Standard Book Number 0-309-04287-9, paper

Copyright ©1990 by the National Academy of Sciences

Printed in the United States of America

Committee on AIDS Research and the Behavioral, Social, and Statistical Sciences

MARSHALL H. BECKER, School of Public Health, University of Michigan

ROBERT F. BORUCH, Graduate School of Education and Department of Statistics, University of Pennsylvania

THOMAS J. COATES, Division of General Internal Medicine, and Center for AIDS Prevention Studies, University of California at San Francisco

RAMON C. CORTINES,* Superintendent of Schools, San Francisco Unified School District

ROBYN M. DAWES, Department of Social and Decision Sciences, Carnegie Mellon University

DON C. DES JARLAIS, Chemical Dependency Institute, Beth Israel Medical Center, New York, and Mount Sinai School of Medicine

JOHN H. GAGNON, Department of Sociology, State University of New York at Stony Brook

ALBERT R. JONSEN, Department of Medical History and Ethics, University of Washington at Seattle

SHIRLEY LINDENBAUM, Department of Anthropology, Graduate Center, City University of New York

JANE MENKEN *(Vice Chair),* Department of Sociology, and Population Studies Center, University of Pennsylvania

LINCOLN E. MOSES *(Chair),* Department of Statistics, Stanford University

CLADD E. STEVENS, The New York Blood Center

BAILUS WALKER, School of Public Health, State University of New York at Albany

National Research Council Staff

TRACY L. BRANDT, *Research Assistant,* Committee on AIDS Research and the Behavioral, Social, and Statistical Sciences

SUSAN L. COYLE, *Study Director,* Panel on the Evaluation of AIDS Interventions

KIRSTEN J. JOHNSON, *Sr. Project Assistant,* Panel on the Evaluation of AIDS Interventions

HEATHER G. MILLER, *Study Director,* Panel on AIDS Interventions and Research

KAREN E. ORLANDO, *Sr. Project Assistant,* Committee on AIDS Research and the Behavioral, Social, and Statistical Sciences

JEFFREY S. STRYKER, *Study Director,* Panel on Monitoring the Social Impact of the AIDS Epidemic

CHARLES F. TURNER, *Director,* Committee on AIDS Research and the Behavioral, Social, and Statistical Sciences

* *Served through September 1, 1989.*

iii

Panel on AIDS Interventions and Research

MARSHALL H. BECKER *(Chair)*, School of Public Health, University of Michigan

PHILIP W. BLUMSTEIN, Department of Sociology, University of Washington at Seattle

MARGARET A. CHESNEY, Department of Epidemiology and Biostatistics, and Center for AIDS Prevention Studies, University of California at San Francisco

ANKE A. EHRHARDT, HIV Center for Clinical and Behavioral Studies, New York State Psychiatric Institute, Columbia University

MINDY T. FULLILOVE, HIV Center for Clinical and Behavioral Studies, New York State Psychiatric Institute, Columbia University

KAREN HEIN, Division of Adolescent Medicine, Albert Einstein College of Medicine, and Montefiore Medical Center, Bronx, New York

JANE ALLYN PILIAVIN, Department of Sociology, University of Wisconsin at Madison

JAMES L. SORENSEN, Substance Abuse Services, San Francisco General Hospital, and University of California at San Francisco

REED V. TUCKSON, March of Dimes Birth Defects Foundation, White Plains, New York

JAMES A. WILEY, Survey Research Center, University of California at Berkeley

Consultants

JANE C. BALIN, Department of Sociology, University of Pennsylvania

MIMI CANTWELL, National Academy Press

WENDY CHAVKIN, School of Public Health, Columbia University, and Chemical Dependency Institute, Beth Israel Medical Center, New York

JUDITH B. COHEN, San Francisco General Hospital, and University of California at San Francisco

SUSHAMA GUNJAL, National Research Council staff

SAHR J. KPUNDEH, Department of Political Science, Howard University

ANDREW S. LONDON, Department of Sociology, and Population Studies Center, University of Pennsylvania

LEAH MAZADE, National Academy Press

BARBARA S. MENSCH, School of Public Health, Columbia University

LISA A. RATMANSKY, Department of Sociology, University of Pennsylvania

LAURA RUDKIN-MINIOT, Department of Sociology, Princeton University

PEARL T.C.Y. TOY, San Francisco General Hospital, and University of California at San Francisco

DOOLEY WORTH, Department of Epidemiology and Social Medicine, Montefiore Medical Center, Bronx, New York

Liaison Representatives, U.S. Public Health Service

LINDA ALEXANDER, Walter Reed Army Institute for Research

ZILI AMSEL, National Institute on Drug Abuse

WENDY BALDWIN, National Institute of Child Health and Human Development

G. STEPHEN BOWEN, Centers for Disease Control

DAVID F. BROWNELL, Centers for Disease Control

VIRGINIA CAIN, National Institute of Child Health and Human Development

ALLAN W. CZARRA, National Heart, Lung, and Blood Institute

WILLIAM W. DARROW, Centers for Disease Control

TIMOTHY J. DONDERO, JR., Centers for Disease Control

ANITA EICHLER, National Institute of Mental Health

JACOB A. GAYLE, Centers for Disease Control

MICHELE KIELY, National Institute of Allergy and Infectious Diseases

LLOYD J. KOLBE, Centers for Disease Control

LYNN LEVIN, Walter Reed Army Institute for Research

SAMUEL C. MATHENY, Health Resources and Services Administration

KEVIN O'REILLY, Centers for Disease Control

MARCIA ORY, National Institute on Aging

CHRISTINE PARKER, National Heart, Lung, and Blood Institute

AMY R. SHEON, National Institute of Allergy and Infectious Diseases

ELLEN STOVER, National Institute of Mental Health

MATILDA WHITE RILEY, National Institute on Aging

RONALD W. WILSON, National Center for Health Statistics, Centers for Disease Control

Preface

It is sometimes difficult today to remember that only 10 years ago the acquired immune deficiency syndrome (AIDS) was unknown. During the first decade of this epidemic, more than 65,000 people died from this disease in the United States, and many more were infected with the human immunodeficiency virus (HIV), which causes AIDS. We do not know what effects this epidemic will ultimately have. The available evidence indicates, however, that the swathe cut by this disease is widening and, despite considerable efforts to retard the spread of HIV infection, it is likely that morbidity and mortality from HIV infection will continue throughout the 1990s.

During the first decade of this epidemic our nation has faced enormous challenges. Some of those challenges have been met. The development of tests to detect antibodies to HIV, for example, led to a substantial reduction in risk associated with transfusions and blood products. Many challenges, however, remain unmet. One of the most serious and enduring obstacles arises from the thin substrate of facts pertaining to the prevalence of HIV infection in the United States and to the effectiveness of alternative strategies to prevent further spread of HIV in our population. The nation's future success in curbing the spread of the virus and reducing the toll exacted by this disease will depend to a great extent on the nation's commitment to empirical efforts that will improve this knowledge base.

With this second report, our committee continues the work it began in 1987 to monitor the AIDS epidemic and to investigate issues related to preventing the transmission of HIV. The committee's deliberations on the issues discussed in this report began in the spring of 1989 at the behest of a consortium of Public Health Service agencies that have supported the work of the committee since its inception. A specially appointed Panel on AIDS Interventions and Research assisted in this latest effort, as did many other individuals too numerous to mention here. All gave generously of their time and knowledge, for which the committee expresses its sincere gratitude.

Establishing the scope of a report such as this is always difficult. There is often tension between keeping the text concise and straightforward and providing sufficient background material to make the issues comprehensible to a broad range of readers. This report attempts to tread a fine line between satisfying the needs of readers who are expert in at least one area and those who are being introduced to new topics. The committee recognizes that it cannot meet the needs of all readers. For some, the material presented here will be too basic. For those who are less familiar with these issues, however, it is our hope that this report will provide a useful introduction.

The topics addressed in the report span a range of substantive areas, from improving the quality of survey data on behaviors associated with HIV transmission to modifying the behavior of blood donors. The report also considers two specific populations in whom much interest has been centered: adolescents and female prostitutes. The inclusion of these populations in separate chapters of this report does not signify that either group is thought to be a major source of infection. Rather, in the case of adolescents, the committee sought to highlight the opportunity to limit the spread of infection in this population and to encourage health-promoting behaviors by young people who have, in many cases, only begun to experiment with risk-associated behaviors. In the case of female prostitutes, the committee's work serves another purpose: to lay to rest concerns that have lingered since the beginning of the epidemic that prostitutes were a major bridge for HIV transmission to the larger heterosexual population. Epidemiologic evidence indicates that HIV infection is not an occupational disease for this group and that it is unlikely that prostitutes will serve as a major conduit of infection. As is the case with all women, however, their risk of becoming infected has increased over the past few years. As the patterns of HIV infection have undergone subtle shifts, there arises a need to focus more attention on the risks that women in general face.

After a decade of struggle against AIDS, the logical question is: Where do we go from here? Some individuals claim that the epidemic has peaked and no longer needs the attention—and resources—that have been directed toward it in the past. Others say that there are more pressing problems facing our nation. The committee, although recognizing the frustration that often underlies such viewpoints, finds little credible evidence that the end of this epidemic is in sight. The picture for the near future is one of a continuing toll of sickness and death. Behavioral change continues to be our primary weapon in retarding the spread of HIV. Amassing the knowledge needed to better understand and facilitate behavioral change will require a long-term commitment to rigorous scientific investigation. That commitment must be made and maintained—to forestall the bleak prospect of a third decade of this epidemic that is little different from the last.

HEATHER G. MILLER, *Study Director*

CHARLES F. TURNER, *Director*

LINCOLN E. MOSES, *Chair*

Committee on AIDS Research and the Behavioral, Social, and Statistical Sciences

Acknowledgments

During the course of this study, the committee was assisted by a number of scientists who took time to share their insights and expertise. To those who assisted us in our work, the committee extends its sincere thanks and appreciation. The committee's work has been supported by the U.S. Public Health Service, and by the Rockefeller, Russell Sage, and Sierra Foundations.

Note on Contributions

This report is the collective product of the committee, and it was prepared with the assistance of the committee's Panel on AIDS Interventions and Research. The content of this report reflects the deliberations of the committee, and the report presents the committee's recommendations. The list below identifies the persons who shared major responsibility for preparing initial drafts of materials for each chapter in this report. The committee reviewed all contributions, and they have been revised and edited in light of the committee's discussions and the comments of outside reviewers. The purpose of the following alphabetical list, therefore, is to give credit to individuals but not to assign final responsibility for the published text. It should also be noted that, although the list covers major sections of this volume, these sections frequently contain additional paragraphs or pages from other hands.

SUMMARY: Coyle, Miller, Turner

CHAPTER 1: Coates, Des Jarlais, Miller, Moses, Turner, Worth

CHAPTER 2: Chavkin, Coates, Des Jarlais, Ehrhardt, Miller, Stryker, Worth

CHAPTER 3: Des Jarlais, Ehrhardt, Fullilove, Hein, Menken, Mensch, Miller, Turner

CHAPTER 4: Cohen, Coyle

CHAPTER 5: Chesney, Miller, Piliavin, Stevens, Toy

CHAPTER 6: Blumstein, Dawes, Lindenbaum, Rudkin-Miniot, Sorensen, Turner, Wiley

Contents

AIDS
The Second Decade

Summary

More than 115,000 persons in the United States have been diagnosed with acquired immune deficiency syndrome, or AIDS, since the illness was first identified in this country almost 10 years ago. As we enter the second decade of the epidemic, residual problems from the first decade continue to compel the nation's attention. Moreover, new issues are emerging that call for immediate consideration and action. The dimensions of the epidemic are sizable and will continue to grow, presenting enormous challenges to the nation and to those individuals who must track its course, design and implement intervention programs, and provide medical care and other services. This report reviews the course of the epidemic and its current status. It also discusses prevention activities designed to curb the future spread of the human immunodeficiency virus (HIV) and offers recommendations regarding potential avenues for achieving this goal.

This report was prepared by the Committee on AIDS Research and the Behavioral, Social, and Statistical Sciences,[1] which was established in 1987. The formation of such a committee within the National Research Council reflected a growing awareness that understanding HIV transmission, facilitating behavioral change to prevent further spread of infection, and coping with the social consequences of the epidemic raise questions that properly lie within the domain of the social, behavioral, and statistical sciences. At the request of the Public Health Service (PHS) and with support from the Russell Sage and Rockefeller Foundations, the committee reviewed estimates of the extent of HIV infection in the U.S.

---

[1] This work builds on the past and ongoing work of the Institute of Medicine (IOM)/National Academy of Sciences (NAS). The IOM/NAS has produced two major reports that focused on public health, biological research, and medical care issues: *Confronting AIDS: Directions for Public Health, Health Care, and Research* (1986) and *Confronting AIDS: Update 1988* (both published by the National Academy Press, Washington, D.C.).

1

population and the patterns of sexual behavior and drug use that transmit HIV. It also reviewed intervention strategies that showed promise of producing behavioral change to slow the spread of HIV infection in the general population. In 1989 the committee issued its first report, *AIDS, Sexual Behavior, and Intravenous Drug Use.*[2]

The committee's studies during this most recent phase of its efforts have considered the evolving shape of the epidemic, focusing attention on populations and research topics that will be of increasing importance in coming years. After discussions with liaison representatives of the PHS, the committee accepted the following as its charge: to review the changing nature of the epidemic in the United States and the needs of the diverse populations being affected by it, such as adolescents and women (including female prostitutes); to describe behavioral research and intervention strategies that could assist in protecting the blood supply; and to review a selected set of methodological issues that affect the quality of data collected in surveys of drug use and sexual practices. This volume is the committee's response to its charge. In preparing it, the committee was assisted by a specially appointed Panel on AIDS Interventions and Research.[3]

In continuing to monitor the progression of the epidemic and the nation's response, the committee notes several important changes in this evolving and enduring health problem. New populations that are at risk are emerging—from populations that heretofore have not been touched directly by AIDS and from subgroups of populations that are already known to bear infection. Moreover, shifts in patterns of risk-associated behaviors are now becoming apparent. For example, although the threat of disease transmission posed by intravenous (IV) drug use has been recognized since the early years of the epidemic, there is now a growing appreciation of the indirect hazards (e.g., sexual risk taking in the context of drug use) posed by drugs that are not injected, such as the form of cocaine known as crack. There is also increasing awareness of the need to maintain risk-reducing behaviors once they have been initiated. The persistence of risk in the environment and the problem of relapse mandate a long-term commitment to prevention.

---

[2]Turner, C. F., Miller, H. G., and Moses, L. E. (1989) *AIDS, Sexual Behavior, and Intravenous Drug Use.* Report of the National Research Council Committee on AIDS Research and the Behavioral, Social, and Statistical Sciences. Washington, D.C.: National Academy Press.

[3]The committee also benefited from the work of a second panel, which reviewed methodologies for evaluating the effectiveness of AIDS prevention programs. The panel's report, *Evaluating AIDS Prevention Programs, Expanded Edition* (S. L. Coyle, R. F. Boruch, and C. F. Turner), will be published in mid-1990 by the National Academy Press.

In the second decade of the epidemic, new pockets of infection are being identified in more diverse geographical locations in the United States, and the changing distributions of AIDS cases and HIV infection indicate that the disease is becoming more a generalized American phenomenon and less a bicoastal, urban entity. Moreover, the pattern of infection is also beginning to reveal some subtle shifts in the distribution of AIDS cases across transmission categories; the proportion of cases attributable to same-gender contact has decreased slightly as the proportion ascribed to heterosexual contact has grown. Even the characteristics of the disease itself are somewhat in flux. With the development of drugs capable of decreasing morbidity associated with HIV infection and prolonging the lives of those infected with the virus, the disease takes on some of the characteristics of a long-term rather than an acute illness. The changing locus of the epidemic, the new populations at risk, and the emerging longer term nature of the disease point to the need for new outreach and intervention strategies to prevent further spread of infection, as well as services and treatment to assist those who are already infected.

The first two sections of this summary (and Chapters 1 and 2 of the full report) describe the evolving nature of the epidemic and the range of prevention activities that are being implemented to retard the spread of HIV in the U.S. population. A particular focus of these sections is the increasing burden of HIV infection and AIDS among women. The next three sections (Chapters 3, 4, and 5, respectively, of the full report) review three domains of particular interest: the ways in which HIV infection is affecting adolescents and female prostitutes, and the challenge of protecting the blood supply while simultaneously ensuring the adequacy of that supply. The final section of the report (Chapter 6) reviews factors that affect the quality of data collected in surveys of AIDS-related behaviors.

Although many of the specific issues raised in this report are persisting problems from the first decade of the epidemic, it is important to note that some predicted problems have not emerged. For example, despite considerable speculation regarding the role prostitution could play in a self-sustaining heterosexual epidemic, the data presented in Chapter 4 do not support the notion that HIV infection is an occupational disease of sex workers. Rather, the infection found among female prostitutes appears to have been acquired through IV drug use or from sexual contact with a husband or boyfriend, and, in several surveys, substantial proportions of prostitutes reported condom use with paying customers. Moreover, in a field where there have been few real successes, the story of the blood supply stands out. The development of HIV antibody tests, which when coupled with behavioral interventions to enhance appropriate blood donor deferral, has dramatically reduced the number of infections associated with the blood supply. However, as donor deferral becomes more effective, there will be fewer individuals to contribute to the blood supply, thus raising additional problems concerning adequate supplies. The committee cautions that encouraging results and promising situations should not lead to complacency. The lessons learned from the first decade of the epidemic warn us of the need for vigilance as the patterns of disease shift and new problems emerge.

THE CHANGING EPIDEMIOLOGY OF AIDS IN THE UNITED STATES

Despite the greater diversity now recognized to exist among at-risk and infected populations, gay men still account for the majority of AIDS cases in this country. Yet more and more cases are reportedly associated with IV drug use and heterosexual transmission, and this shift has resulted in a noticeable increase in the number of women who are affected by the AIDS epidemic. Among adolescents in contact with the military (either as applicants or on active duty), rates of HIV infection among females are comparable with those for males. Gender parity in seroprevalence (i.e., prevalence of HIV infection) for this population indicates that for some groups women will be bearing a larger share of the AIDS burden in the future.

Although the majority of female AIDS cases have been attributed to IV drug use, substantial numbers of infected women report heterosexual contact with an infected male IV drug user. Thus, injection of illicit substances poses direct and indirect threats to women in this country. The stabilization of infection rates seen among drug users in some cities (e.g., New York, San Francisco, Amsterdam) affords some hope that interventions directed toward this population can be effective.[4] Nevertheless, stable rates of infection in selected cities do not signify the elimination of viral transmission. Other areas of the United States, as well as foreign countries, are seeing rapid increases in the incidence of infection among IV drug users. The mobility of this population coupled with the

---

[4]For some groups at highest risk for HIV infection, stable rates signify that all vulnerable individuals are already infected, a phenomenon known as saturation. This phenomenon does not appear to explain stable rates in New York City, however, where approximately 50 percent of IV drug users are estimated to be infected. If saturation had occurred, one would expect to see higher seroprevalence rates. For example, approximately 90 percent of IV drug users in New York City have been infected with hepatitis, a virus that is transmitted in the same manner as HIV and appears to have reached saturation in this population.

persistence of the behaviors that transmit HIV (namely, sharing injection equipment) indicates that the potential for very rapid spread still exists.

Furthermore, growing awareness of the indirect threat posed by drugs such as crack and alcohol supports the notion that HIV risk related to drug use now goes beyond the use of contaminated injection equipment. Although crack and alcohol do not directly transmit HIV, researchers note that both drugs are associated with high-risk sexual practices and thus confer an indirect risk for the acquisition and transmission of the virus. The rapid emergence of new, drug-related threats highlights the need for vigilance regarding changing patterns of transmission. Thus, **the committee recommends that the Public Health Service establish mechanisms across its agencies for rapid identification and assessment of the relationship of new drug use problems to the spread of HIV.** At present it is clear that crack use and its associated unsafe sexual activity represent a potentially important new mode of HIV transmission in the United States, but it is unclear how large an impact this mode might have. **The committee recommends that the Public Health Service support additional research on crack use, including its epidemiology, its relationship to sexual behavior, strategies to reduce its occurrence (both initiation of use and continuance among low- and high-frequency users), and methods for facilitating change in the sexual behavior of persons who continue to use crack.**

Among the changing facets and aspects of the epidemic, one epidemiological trend has remained disturbingly constant. Black and Hispanic men and women continue to be overrepresented in every AIDS risk category. The committee urges a renewed commitment to providing effective AIDS prevention programs for at-risk minority individuals. Therefore, **the committee recommends that the agencies of the Public Health Service encourage and strengthen behavioral science research aimed at understanding the transmission of HIV in various black and Hispanic subpopulations, including men who have sex with men, drug users and their sexual partners, and youth. The committee further recommends that the PHS develop plans for appropriate interventions targeted toward these groups and support the implementation of intervention strategies (together with appropriate evaluation components) in both demonstration projects and larger scale efforts.**

The evolutionary, dynamic nature of this epidemic imposes additional demands on surveillance data collection. High-quality data on changing rates of risk-associated behavior and HIV infection are needed to track the course of the epidemic and to evaluate the effectiveness of intervention efforts to stop its progression. **To facilitate the Centers for Disease**

Control's (CDC) ongoing efforts to improve its AIDS-related data collection systems, the committee recommends that the agency initiate a systematic review of current programs. This effort should draw on the expertise of both CDC staff and outside experts.

PREVENTION: THE CONTINUING CHALLENGE

The first decade of the AIDS epidemic in this country brought considerable progress in solving the biological and epidemiological puzzles of AIDS and HIV infection. The causative agent was discovered, and serologic tests to detect infection were devised, produced, and implemented. In addition, drugs were developed to treat both the underlying viral infection and the opportunistic infections that are the hallmarks of the disease. Yet despite this progress, the epidemiological data reveal a steady progression of HIV-related morbidity and mortality, in part because the development of HIV prevention strategies has not kept pace with the growing dimensions of risk. Effective intervention strategies are needed to sustain healthy behavioral patterns in individuals who are not currently at risk and to facilitate change among individuals who are. The committee finds that ongoing efforts fall far short of the magnitude of intervention needed, given the current prevalence of infection and evidence of continued risk-associated behavior among many of the groups at risk for AIDS.

AIDS Prevention Challenges in the Coming Decade

At the beginning of the epidemic, interventions to prevent the spread of HIV infection focused primarily on adult gay men; subsequent prevention efforts encompassed the population of IV drug users. Today, that focus requires redefinition and expansion once again as changing epidemiological patterns reveal greater diversity among at-risk groups. A further requirement is to consolidate study findings from cohorts of gay men and to incorporate relevant findings into the design and development of prevention activities for other groups. Unfortunately, an understanding of such lessons has been hampered by a host of methodological complications that preclude meaningful cross-study comparisons. Therefore, **the committee recommends that the Public Health Service assemble and summarize data reported by gay men in PHS-funded studies regarding seroprevalence, seroconversion, and high-risk behavior and determine what conclusions can be drawn from the research.**

Of particular concern to the committee are the epidemiological data indicating that HIV infection is spreading to disparate subpopulations of women. The diversity of the at-risk female population mandates the development of multiple approaches to prevent both horizontal transmission from sexual and drug use partners and vertical transmission from a mother to her infant. In general, the best way to prevent vertical transmission is to prevent infection in women of childbearing age.

Prevention efforts focused on women during the first decade of the epidemic relied heavily on testing and counseling, but several studies have shown that the information provided to women by such a strategy did not necessarily prevent transmission. Therefore, **the committee recommends careful review of the goals of testing and counseling programs for women of childbearing age and the implementation of research efforts to ascertain the effect of such programs on future risk-taking behavior.** Additional, innovative strategies are clearly needed to prevent vertical transmission; there may be important lessons to be learned from existing programs that have sought to prevent other vertically transmitted diseases, such as genetic disorders. **The committee recommends that the Public Health Service convene a symposium of experts in genetic counseling to consider the potential contribution of this field's expertise and experience to the design and implementation of counseling programs for HIV-infected women and to identify research opportunities in this area.**

In its first report, the committee recommended that knowledge concerning the efficacy of intervention programs be built in a systematic fashion through the use of planned variations of key program elements accompanied by rigorous evaluation. This process is admittedly quite time-consuming, but unfortunately there is no shortcut to the accumulation of such critical information. Behavioral interventions are still the only available means of disease containment, and the committee anticipates that the need for well-designed, carefully implemented, and thoughtfully evaluated intervention efforts will not decrease over the course of the next 10 years. Therefore, the committee reiterates its earlier recommendations and in addition **recommends the following:**

- **that the Public Health Service encourage and support behavioral research programs that study the behaviors that transmit HIV infection and that the PHS develop and evaluate mechanisms for facilitating and sustaining change in those behaviors;**
- **that intervention programs incorporate planned variations that can be carefully evaluated to determine their relative effectiveness;**
- **that the PHS regularly summarize the data derived from currently funded behavioral and epidemiological**

research on AIDS (in terms of incidence of infection and high-risk behaviors) to determine intervention priorities for various subpopulations at risk; and

- that all agencies of the PHS that are currently funding intervention programs and evaluation research regularly summarize the data derived from these studies to determine which, if any, programs can be recommended for wider dissemination.

There is some indication that AIDS prevention activities to date have, at least in part, achieved their goal; significant risk reduction has been reported among subsets of gay adult males and IV drug users. Yet segments of every at-risk group continue to practice unsafe behaviors. Some have not yet initiated change; others have not been able to sustain changes initiated earlier. **The committee recommends that the Alcohol, Drug Abuse, and Mental Health Administration focus research efforts on AIDS-related relapse prevention, including the determinants of such relapse and the role that alcohol and other drugs play in the return to unsafe sexual and injection practices.**

The inconsistent use of condoms is a common theme that cuts across all populations associated with this epidemic. Gay men, IV drug users, and female sexual partners of infected or at-risk individuals have all reported problems in initiating or maintaining condom use, despite clear evidence of perceived risk. In its first report the committee urged widespread availability and promotion of the use of condoms (with spermicides) as a means for preventing sexually transmitted HIV infection. The epidemiological data show, however, that sexual transmission of the virus continues to be a major route of infection, and self-reported data on risk taking indicate that more research is needed to understand how to help people take preventive action against sexually transmitted HIV infection. **The committee recommends that the Public Health Service fund research on condoms to achieve the following objectives:**

- **understand the determinants of condom use for the diverse populations at risk for sexually transmitted HIV infection;**
- **improve condom design and materials to make them more acceptable to users; and**
- **develop interventions to promote their consistent use.**

Regardless of belief in the efficacy of condoms to prevent HIV transmission, not all subpopulations at risk will be able to implement this means of protection. Women in particular often find condom use problematic. Not only do condoms require the cooperation of the male partner but they may also require substantial changes in the attitudes and behaviors of some women. The gravity of the AIDS epidemic calls for other methods of protection that are more "user friendly" (i.e., more attractive, easier to purchase, and easier to use) and that can be unilaterally employed by women. **The committee recommends that the Public Health Service support research to develop protective measures other than condoms for preventing HIV transmission during sexual contact—specifically, methods that can be used unilaterally by women and methods that will be acceptable to both men and women who do not currently use condoms.** The partnership between technology and the behavioral sciences has succeeded in devising mechanisms to protect the blood supply (see Chapter 5 of the report). Similar partnerships are needed to develop innovative means for protecting individuals from sexual transmission of the disease.

Impediments to Improved Intervention

AIDS prevention programs must identify, contact, and help at-risk individuals to assess their level of risk and access appropriate services. Providing AIDS prevention also involves first facilitating and then sustaining behavioral change. Delivering programs to at-risk individuals becomes extremely difficult if people believe that seeking help may threaten their jobs, housing, and supportive relationships. During the first decade of this epidemic, effective interventions and research were compromised by difficulties in identifying and reaching those most in need. Now, it is even more crucial to reach infected individuals because there are potentially beneficial prophylactic treatments that may forestall the progression of disease. Antidiscrimination legislation has been proposed by several organizations to provide the institutional underpinnings necessary to enable individuals to redress inequities and protect those who would seek care and other AIDS-related services. The committee is gratified to see that the federal antidiscrimination measures urged in its first report and recommended by the President's Commission on the HIV Epidemic are under active consideration. It would point out, however, that this legislation alone is unlikely to ameliorate all of the conditions associated with discrimination in this country. For example, legislation may protect the rights of HIV-infected children to education but cannot prevent hostile encounters with the community. A separate panel of the committee is currently considering methods to monitor and measure the social impact of the epidemic; the panel's report is expected to be released in 1991.

The progress made in instituting antidiscrimination provisions, however, cannot obscure the fact that other hurdles remain in the path of improved intervention. The financial barriers to health care that have impeded preventive care for other health conditions also affect individuals seeking AIDS-related services. Barriers to these services may be especially daunting for women, in particular women who need prenatal care or treatment for drug use. Moreover, even delivering information to those most in need is sometimes problematic, in part because societal attitudes continue to hinder the implementation and evaluation of promising interventions. A significant controversy has surrounded the appropriate level of sexual explicitness in AIDS prevention information and the degree to which these interventions should emphasize the erotic. Political debate abounds regarding the propriety of using public monies to support the development of sexually explicit materials, despite preliminary evidence that, for some populations, they have a degree of effectiveness.

Programs to provide IV drug users with sterile needles have also been stymied. Previous reports on AIDS from the National Academy of Sciences and the Institute of Medicine recommended that the U.S. government sponsor research on syringe exchange programs as a means of reducing the spread of HIV infection in the drug-using population. Evaluation of ongoing efforts abroad have found that participation in syringe exchange programs is associated with the reduction but not the elimination of behaviors that can transmit HIV and that syringe exchanges do not lead to any detectable increase in illicit drug injection, either among current users or by new injectors. The U.S. Department of Health and Human Services has considered the types of research that would be needed to evaluate the impact of syringe exchange programs on the spread of HIV, but it has not officially determined whether it will support such research now or in the future.

There is a general fear expressed by many policy makers that explicit messages concerning sterile injection equipment and condom use will result in increased rates of IV drug use and sexual intercourse. Yet what evidence there is from various intervention programs suggests otherwise: having the information and the means to protect oneself from a deadly disease is likely to result in protective action against AIDS, as well as in generalized increases in healthy behaviors (e.g., seeking drug treatment) among people who are already engaging in risky activities. Furthermore, information and services do not appear to entice the uninitiated into risk-associated actions. The committee believes that the time has come to commit sufficient resources to the task of collecting data that would permit an assessment of whether current intervention strategies, including needle exchange programs, effectively decrease risky behaviors and the subsequent spread of HIV. To continue to rely on hunches and suspicions rather than on data gives too much credence to guesswork and may arbitrarily obstruct a promising course of action for preventing the spread of the epidemic.

ADOLESCENTS

The committee finds no credible evidence that the AIDS epidemic will cease in the foreseeable future in this country. As a result, prevention efforts remain critically important. In terms of the adolescent population, the committee believes that intervention efforts will be most effective if the programs reach teens before they begin practicing the behaviors that put them at risk. Because patterns of both health behavior and risk taking are often established during the teenage years, intervention efforts for adolescents offer the hope of protecting our youth and preventing future problems in the adult population.

It is important to note that not all teens are equally at risk for HIV infection. Some, by virtue of their low level of risky behavior or because of the absence of the virus among their potential partners, will remain uninfected. However, the available data on HIV seroprevalence indicate that there are presently localized pockets of the teen population in which the rates of infection are relatively high. Findings from CDC's neonatal surveillance activity (i.e., anonymous antibody testing of newborn infants)[5] indicate, for example, that almost 1 percent of black teenagers who delivered children in New York City during 1988 were infected with HIV. The prevalence of HIV infection among Hispanic teenage mothers is almost as high. Data from serosurveys of nonprobability samples of hospital patients and data on infection rates among applicants for military service confirm the fact that the HIV virus is seeded in the adolescent population, albeit at varying rates. Yet these sources of information are limited; consequently, there is a paucity of appropriate data available to scientists for monitoring the spread of HIV in the teen population. To provide better information about HIV infection and AIDS among adolescents, **the committee recommends that the Centers for Disease Control make available to the research community AIDS-related data that permit separate consideration of teenagers and other age groups. Specifically, the committee recommends that:**

---

[5]This testing provides unbiased estimates of the prevalence of HIV infection among childbearing women because infants circulate maternal antibody during the first months of life whether or not they are actually infected.

- data on AIDS cases be made available in a form that permits tabulation by specific ages or by narrow age groups (these data should be as complete as possible without threatening inadvertent disclosure of the identity of any individual case);

- every state that participates in the neonatal surveillance activity include the age of the mother coded in years or by narrow age group; and

- CDC provide data from its family of surveys[6] by specific ages or in narrow age groups, as well as by race, gender, and ethnicity.

Behaviors That Put Adolescents at Risk

As noted above, not all teens are at risk for HIV infection. The vast majority of very young teenagers, as well as most older adolescents who have not begun sexual intercourse and do not inject drugs, have little to worry about. But as these individuals get older, move to different geographic locations, or engage in new behaviors, their relative risk level may change. Currently, the adolescent population contains pockets of adolescents whose behavior puts them at relatively high risk for acquiring HIV infection.

Sexual Behaviors. By age 19 most teenagers—whether black or white, male or female—report that they have engaged in sexual intercourse. The proportion of teenagers who report intercourse at an early age is not small. Roughly one-third of 15-year-old boys report having engaged in sexual intercourse, and 21 percent of teenage girls report sexual intercourse by their 16th birthday. The available data, although sparse, indicate that a substantial fraction of young people engage in sex with multiple partners during their teens, and although condom use among teens increased during the 1980s, the majority of teens do not routinely

---

[6]The CDC's family of surveys collects data on HIV infection from several subpopulations, including clients attending drug treatment, STD, tuberculosis, and prenatal clinics, patients at general hospitals, and newborn infants. With the exception of the survey of infants, all of the other surveys rely on nonprobability samples. Data collected through this program are intended to provide information on the prevalence and incidence of infection in selected populations, to provide early warning of the emergence of infection in new populations, to target intervention programs and other resources, and to evaluate the effectiveness of prevention efforts.

use condoms. The number of adolescents who experiment with same-gender sex is not known with any certainty, but same-gender behavior does not appear to be rare.

Survey evidence of sexual risk taking by teens is supported by the fact that approximately 1 million teenage girls become pregnant each year and that, in the last year for which data are available, more than 7,000 cases of gonorrhea were reported among 10- to 14-year-olds and more than 180,000 cases were reported among 15- to 19-year-olds. The high incidence of sexually transmitted diseases (STDs) among sexually active adolescents is worrisome, not only because it affirms that substantial risk taking is occurring within this population but also because there is growing evidence that genital lesions increase the likelihood of HIV transmission during sexual contact.

Drug Use. Overall, rates of drug use among teens have declined since their peak in 1979, although the proportion of adolescents who use drugs remains considerable. The precise number of adolescents and young adults who inject drugs is not known; however, most persons who inject illicit drugs first do so either in late adolescence or early adulthood. Local surveys find considerable variation in the proportion of respondents who report needle use; rates approach 1 in 10 in some segments of the teen population. Many more teens report alcohol use, and an unknown number are using crack. Drug-related behaviors that put people at risk for HIV infection now go beyond injecting. Thus, risk assessment must also take into account sexual behavior associated with drugs such as alcohol or crack.

High-risk Youth. Environmental factors appear to affect the risk level of teens. Youth interviewed in detention centers and teenagers who live on the streets report high rates of drug use and sexual risk taking. Such youth are at greater risk for virtually all medical disorders of childhood than are children who live in more favorable conditions, and the scant epidemiological evidence that is available indicates that they also experience higher levels of HIV infection.

AIDS Prevention Programs for Teens

There is a consensus both within the committee and in the nation as a whole that drug use is, in itself, physiologically destructive and psychologically debilitating. Thus, AIDS prevention programs for teenagers and adults properly discourage drug use among all persons. From a public health perspective, for persons who do use drugs, AIDS prevention programs have the goals of (1) discontinuance of drug use, if possible; and

(2) if discontinuance is not possible, encouragement of precautions to reduce the risk of HIV transmission (e.g., the use of sterile needles).

With regard to premarital and same-gender sexual behaviors, there is no similar consensus. Rather, ample evidence suggests that such behaviors are an extremely controversial subject in contemporary America. Given the disjunctures in public opinion on this topic, federal AIDS education efforts have stumbled for several years over disputes about the need to offer "realistic" advice to young people about the protective value of condoms versus counterclaims that the AIDS epidemic requires moral education to promote abstinence from sex prior to marriage and sexual fidelity within marriage.

The committee believes that, in the context of a deadly, sexually transmitted epidemic, AIDS prevention programs must heed the data on risk-associated behavior reported by the adolescents themselves and not be sidetracked by wishful thinking about patterns of behavior some might hope teenagers would follow. All intervention programs should provide information, motivation, skills, and practical assistance to help these young people avoid future risks. The ultimate goal of AIDS prevention is to prevent HIV transmission, and programs should accommodate the range of challenges young people will face and the variety of choices they may make. Abstinence, delay of intercourse until marriage, and other traditional behavioral patterns are effective ways of eliminating the risk of sexual transmission of HIV. Some teens, however, will choose to begin sexual behaviors during adolescence, as noted earlier. Given the evidence of early sexual activity among some groups of teens, the committee believes that all teenagers should be educated about the protective value of condoms and spermicides. In addition, **the committee recommends that AIDS prevention programs make special efforts to reach very young teens and, in some subpopulations, to reach youth before they enter adolescence.** AIDS prevention programs for teens should also ensure that youth who engage in male-male sexual contacts have sufficient knowledge and skills to protect themselves in such encounters. Furthermore, all teens should be educated about the dangers posed by the use of illicit drugs.

The relatively small group of adolescents who engage in multiple high-risk behaviors, some of whom may already be infected with HIV, present the greatest challenges to AIDS prevention. Intervention programs for these teens should make every effort to assist them in changing the behaviors that place them at risk and should also seek to alter any social or economic conditions that support their risk taking. Teens who are using illicit drugs, especially those who inject drugs, should be encouraged to seek treatment. Such a policy in turn requires effective referral networks to treatment programs that are tailored to adolescent needs. Those who continue to use needles should be informed of the hazards associated with this practice, educated about protective measures, and urged not to share needles or other injection equipment. Adolescents who are living on the streets, engaging in prostitution, or exchanging sex for crack will require additional services, such as shelter, counseling, and medical care. Adolescents who are already infected with HIV will require a range of services as well. The resources required to provide these services are likely to be extensive, but their precise nature and quantity have not yet been determined.

Reaching Adolescents

Surveys of knowledge and attitudes indicate that many of the basic facts about AIDS appear to be reaching the nation's youth. Nevertheless, misconceptions persist, and the segments of the adolescent population that are epidemiologically most vulnerable appear to be less informed than the majority about the disease. Small surveys of minority youth, for example, find that they are less aware than white youth of the behaviors that risk HIV transmission.

The committee believes that a particularly crucial message for adolescents in the 1990s pertains to their own vulnerability. Some adolescents, as well as some adults, still view AIDS as a disease of gay, white adult males. This belief is especially widespread in areas in which the prevalence of AIDS is currently low. It is crucial that adolescents (especially those engaging in high-risk activities) recognize the extent of the epidemic and the possibility that it might affect them. In addition to information, however, adolescents may also require new skills to be able to apply what they have learned in real, day-to-day situations. Broaching difficult topics in conversations, resisting peer pressure to have unprotected sex or use drugs, and negotiating less-risky activities may be more difficult than learning the facts about HIV transmission routes.

Families and other adult social institutions have a major responsibility for educating adolescents about health risks. Yet the available evidence indicates that parent-child communication about sexual behavior is often insufficient and it frequently does not occur until after initiation of sexual activity. Such findings indicate a need for interventions to motivate and assist parents in the difficult and important task of educating their children about the dangers of HIV transmission. These findings also suggest that it would be a mistake to rely exclusively on parents as the source of AIDS education for teenagers.

The committee believes that AIDS prevention efforts targeting adolescents should involve teenagers themselves in the design and execution of these programs. Not only does this policy allow the program to benefit from the counsel of members of the targeted audience, but it empowers adolescents by including them in the processes that will affect their own lives. For many adolescents, inclusion in such activities will provide another stimulus for thinking about AIDS and planning for their futures.

There are many venues in which AIDS prevention programs for adolescents can be delivered. CDC has developed and funded prevention programs in schools and other organizations that serve youth, and it has recommended guidelines for AIDS education to help school personnel set the scope and content of their programs. As of May 1989, however, only half of the states required that students receive HIV/AIDS education. Of the AIDS education programs that have been implemented, few have undergone evaluation, making it difficult to draw conclusions about program adequacy or effectiveness. The committee, however, applauds CDC's plans to conduct systematic evaluations of its activities.

Although venues such as schools include most youth, they miss some of the teens who are at highest risk (e.g., youth who drop out of school, runaways). Other approaches that use the media or other outreach strategies for special populations can provide access to these groups. In addition, community-based organizations have some unique and important characteristics that make them promising vehicles for reaching this important segment of the adolescent population.

There are in addition a broad range of services that may be helpful to youth who participate in high-risk behaviors. Such services include family planning clinics, drug use and prevention programs, teenage pregnancy programs, STD clinics, and comprehensive service programs that target a variety of social, psychological, and physical problems of adolescents. Current demands on these programs for non-HIV-related services are considerable; the feasibility of adding responsibility for HIV-related prevention strategies, counseling, testing, and follow-up services for at-risk teens, their partners, and families is not known. It is not unreasonable to speculate, however, that substantial personnel, financial, logistical, and administrative resources will be required to provide the necessary services.

Doing Better with Adolescents in the Second Decade

It is not yet clear how best to educate the nation's youth about the behavioral changes required to retard the spread of HIV. The committee believes that much is to be gained from the systematic study of planned variations of intervention strategies, and it regrets the persisting lack of understanding regarding the types of behavioral interventions that will be most effective in containing the spread of this disease. The committee believes that the Public Health Service would realize substantial returns in practical and scientific knowledge from careful investments in research to determine the effects of planned variations of those behavioral interventions to be implemented in the future. This strategy offers hope that should the epidemic extend into the third decade, our understanding of how to curb the spread of HIV infection will be far greater than it is today.

The committee also wishes to reiterate that the diversity of the adolescent population requires a multiplicity of venues and formats to deliver AIDS prevention messages effectively. For some adolescents, intervention may be most effective if it is provided by AIDS prevention programs in the school systems at an early age—before students initiate the behaviors that can threaten their futures. However, to reach many of the adolescents at highest risk for HIV infection requires going beyond the schools. Most important, the committee notes that a small segment of the teen population is at relatively high risk for HIV infection. This segment includes runaway and "throwaway" children, teenage prostitutes, and homeless youth. The committee believes that AIDS prevention programs should focus attention on these youth in a manner commensurate with the elevated risks they face.

PROSTITUTES

In the beginning stages of the AIDS epidemic, many people feared that female prostitutes would become widely infected and spread the AIDS virus to their clients. At present, this fear appears to be unfounded, at least in the United States. Rather, the evidence suggests that the risk of transmission for this population is more closely associated with drug use than with multiple sexual clients and that the threat posed to and by prostitutes through sexual contact is greater in personal relationships than in paying ones. For these reasons, intervention efforts for this group need to focus not only on risky sexual behaviors but also on drug-related transmission.

AIDS prevention efforts for female prostitutes and their clients are hobbled by the current sparseness of studies related to these populations.

There are few data on prostitutes' clients; the limited data on prostitutes themselves come from ethnographic research and convenience samples, neither of which are representative of the diversity of the population. Lack of representativeness notwithstanding, CDC's recent multicenter study of 1,396 female prostitutes provides much valuable information. The study draws on nonprobability samples recruited from eight sites, including brothels, detention centers, methadone clinics, STD clinics, and networks of "streetwalkers" and "call girls." The total sample reflects some of the heterogeneity of the female prostitute population, which includes a spectrum of sex worker lifestyles: street and bar prostitution, brothel work, massage parlor business, outcall services, and crack-house prostitution. Each has a unique pattern of operation and of experiences with the criminal justice system, with most enforcement activity directed against street prostitution. This variety of independent, pimp controlled, and organized prostitution, as well as the exchange of sex for drugs or other commodities (which may not be conceptualized or acknowledged as prostitution), suggest that different avenues of access will be needed, and different barriers must be overcome, to implement appropriate interventions. On the one hand, independent sex workers are often clandestine and isolated, making them hard to reach. On the other hand, pimps and agents of organized sites (brothel madams, massage parlor and escort agency owners) often constitute additional hurdles to the dissemination of AIDS prevention information and training.

Risk Factors

Data from the CDC study indicate that rates of HIV infection among female prostitutes vary greatly from site to site (ranging from zero to 47.5 percent) and reflect two important factors. First, rates of HIV infection are much higher among sex workers who report a history of IV drug use than among those who show no evidence of drugs (surveys of female prostitutes from southern Nevada, Atlanta, Colorado Springs, Los Angeles, San Francisco, Miami, and northern and southern New Jersey found that, on average, 19.9 percent of women who reported injecting drugs were infected, compared with 4.8 percent of women who did not inject drugs). Second, among women who do not report IV drug use, HIV infection is associated with a large number of personal (i.e., nonpaying) sexual partners. The distribution of IV drug use among female prostitutes is not clearly understood, but it appears to be skewed toward streetwalkers and ethnic minority sex workers.

Given the evidence that HIV infection among prostitutes has occurred mainly among those who use IV drugs and that prostitutes thus appear to be at increased risk for HIV infection primarily through drug use rather than through sexual practices, **the committee recommends that the National Institute on Drug Abuse and the Centers for Disease Control continue to support and strengthen current efforts to understand and intervene in the relationship between drug use and prostitution.** An additional yet related problem has recently emerged—that of exchanging sex for crack (a noninjected drug)—and the committee believes that this new phenomenon also warrants special attention.

The other major risk factor for female prostitutes is multiple non-paying sexual partners. The available evidence indicates that prostitutes engage in unprotected intercourse more frequently with nonpaying partners than with their clients. For example, the CDC multicenter study found that only 16 percent of female prostitutes used condoms with nonpaying partners (e.g., husbands, boyfriends), compared with 78 percent who used condoms at least occasionally with clients. Other evidence has shown that women who exchange sex for crack also do not use condoms.

Yet even with clients, some prostitutes report only sporadic use of condoms, perhaps because of the client unwillingness to take protective action and the pressure this reluctance exerts on women whose livelihood depends on fulfilling clients' demands. The distribution of sexual practices—including unprotected vaginal, oral, and anal sex—offered by women and requested by their partners has implications not only for the transmission of the virus but also for the types of educational interventions needed to reduce that transmission. Thus far, the number of cases of AIDS ascribed to contact with female sex workers has been small, and the available data, although limited, suggest that there is little danger that female prostitutes will be a "bridge" of infection to the general population. Indeed, as noted earlier, it appears that female prostitutes are more at risk of *acquiring* HIV than they are of transmitting it. Therefore, given the factors that are known to distinguish the risk profile of many prostitutes (multiple unprotected sexual contacts and IV drug use), **the committee recommends that the Centers for Disease Control continue to monitor the effects of the AIDS epidemic on this population. Activities should include a continuing, systematic effort to track the incidence and prevalence of both HIV infection and sexually transmitted diseases in this group.**

There have been very few studies of prostitutes' clients, and although the committee recognizes the difficulties involved in doing research on sex workers' customers, it believes better data should be collected. Relying on information provided by prostitutes about their clients will not suffice, nor can studies rely on interviews with men who are already infected or who have AIDS to ascertain the prevalence of prostitute patronage in the larger population of men. Because so little is known about the role of prostitutes' clients in the spread of HIV infection, and because the future dynamics of the HIV epidemic are unclear, **the committee recommends that the Public Health Service undertake a series of feasibility studies to determine the best ways to gather appropriate information about prostitutes' clients and their role in the spread of HIV to the larger population.**

Interventions

Various types of AIDS prevention programs for female prostitutes have been implemented, including street outreach to teach safer drug use and safer sex techniques, similar types of outreach and workshops for organized sites, and voluntary HIV testing and counseling. Many of the outreach programs involve peer-led interventions delivered by ex-prostitutes or current sex workers to facilitate the location and recruitment of prostitutes into the programs and to improve communication between the research community and the targeted population. To a small extent, interventions have also been directed toward eliminating prostitution.

As in all areas of AIDS prevention programs, there are often obstacles to the delivery of services for female prostitutes. For example, there are too few drug treatment centers to treat prostitutes who are IV drug users; the centers, on the other hand, frequently report problems retaining individuals in treatment. In some locales, the criminal justice system has worked against the adoption of safer sex technologies by allowing the possession of condoms to be used as probative evidence of intent to solicit prostitution. Along the same lines, client demand for unprotected sex works against instituting condom use among prostitutes. The criminalization of prostitution acts as a further barrier to participant recruitment in intervention programs and thus to the implementation of AIDS prevention. Getting around these obstacles to the delivery of services to both prostitutes and their clients will require additional efforts.

In summary, researchers must consider a number of variables in prostitutes' lifestyles and risk patterns in designing appropriate interventions and overcoming barriers to their implementation. It should be reemphasized that these factors and the epidemiology of HIV among prostitutes are not well understood, in part because little research is available on this heterogeneous group. Given their current risk levels and the prevailing uncertainty regarding the future spread of the epidemic, female sex workers warrant continuing prevention efforts and focused research on patterns and prevalence of infection.

PROTECTING THE BLOOD SUPPLY

Infectious diseases have always been a major concern of those responsible for protecting the blood supply. Since the advent of the AIDS epidemic, however, the transmission of infections through contaminated blood and blood products has taken on paramount significance; measures to deal with these concerns in turn have raised additional problems related to the adequacy of the blood supply. In 1985, blood collection organizations began using a new serologic test to screen blood donations for antibody to the AIDS virus. Although this technological innovation dramatically reduced the incidence of transfusion-related infection, it was not (nor is it yet) capable of detecting all contaminated donations. For example, recently infected individuals who have not begun to produce antibodies to the AIDS virus cannot be identified by this test. Therefore, additional screening mechanisms were instituted. Donors who had engaged in risk-associated behaviors were asked to refrain from donating (self-deferral), and specific procedures were established to help donors assess their level of risk. Today, as donor eligibility requirements become even more stringent (reflecting new information about risk behaviors) and deferrals increase, the question of how to maintain an adequate supply of blood has inevitably arisen. The demand for blood in this country is substantial but not without some flexibility. Consequently, there has been renewed examination of appropriate uses of blood and blood components and of the mechanisms needed to support and encourage such uses.

Exclusionary Procedures

Over the past few years, a number of mechanisms have been developed to screen (and subsequently defer) at-risk donors to protect the safety of blood and blood products. Individuals are deferred from donation, either temporarily or permanently, for a number of reasons, including fever, anemia, a history of exposure to malaria, recent infection, signs or symptoms of HIV infection, or a history of risk-associated behavior. At the beginning of the donation process, each prospective donor is given information about donation and about infections that may be transmitted by blood, especially HIV. Individuals with signs of HIV infection or AIDS or a history of behaviors known to transmit HIV are asked not to donate and are informed that they may leave the donation site without providing an explanation to staff or others that might compromise the confidential nature of this information. Individuals who choose to continue with the donation process then provide a confidential health history that includes questions about AIDS-related symptoms and behaviors. Deferral may also occur at this point. Finally, following the health history, all donors are offered yet another opportunity to exclude their blood from the transfusion pool. Because some people feel pressured by peers or coworkers to donate blood, blood collection organizations have instituted the confidential unit exclusion, or CUE, procedure to lessen the chance that an infected individual will give blood. CUE uses a form that allows the donor to select one of two options for handling the donated unit of blood: (1) the blood may be used for transfusion, or (2) the blood should not be transfused. CUE is an important mechanism that allows these individuals to participate without the stigma of deferral for sensitive reasons and at the same time protect the safety of the blood supply.

Maintaining an Adequate Supply of Blood

Estimates of the size of the nation's potential donor population suggest that more than half the men and women in the United States are eligible to give blood. Yet less than 10 percent of men surveyed by CDC and less than 5 percent of women reported giving blood last year. Most blood is given by repeat donors, who are disproportionately white males; women, members of minorities, blue-collar workers, the very young, and older people are underrepresented in samples of blood donors. Current recruitment efforts seek to tap some of these underrepresented sources of donors to augment the blood supply, but it is likely that additional attention and research will be needed to encourage participation by individuals from these groups and, in some cases, to identify subgroups that are the least likely to report risk-associated behaviors.

The question of why some people give blood and others refuse to give is important to the development of effective strategies to recruit and retain donors. Many donors report altruistic reasons for donating. Some give in response to social pressure or to fill a perceived need in the community; others participate to receive special benefits that may accrue to donors, such as blood typing or cholesterol testing (where available). The effects on donor recruitment of offering material rewards (e.g., raffle prizes, reduced-price merchandise) are not clear. Indeed, the precise factors that motivate blood donors are poorly understood.

Donation may be inhibited by a number of other elements, some of which include medical ineligibility, fear, adverse physical reactions to the act of donation, and inconvenience. The extent to which any of these factors discourages people from donating (that is, in those cases in which they have not been deferred for medical reasons) may be lessened by a blood collection process that considers the needs of both first-time and repeat donors. The ideal experience is one involving personal attention, professional treatment, and a clear exchange of information in a setting that expresses concern for the donor's welfare and privacy. Realistically, however, the needs of donors must be reconciled with those of blood collection organizations, which must carefully balance efficiency (and economy) with the need to inform donors adequately about HIV infection and the importance of deferral for those who may be at risk.

To increase the blood supply, **the committee recommends that:**

- **blood collection organizations prepare and deliver (in cooperation with the mass media) clear and accurate information concerning both the need for donation and the absence of health risks from donation;**
- **the National Heart, Lung, and Blood Institute support research on the design, systematic testing, and implementation of new methods for attracting healthy first-time donors, retaining and encouraging repeat donations, and enlisting the aid of repeat donors in donor recruitment;**
- **blood collection organizations undertake to make the actual donation process as comfortable, friendly, and efficient as possible through changes in scheduling procedures, physical accommodations, donor processing, and staff training;**
- **blood collection agencies, Public Health Service agencies, and community leaders employ innovative recruitment approaches among populations such as minority and certain age groups that traditionally have not been represented in the donor pool; and**
- **physicians and blood banks encourage autologous donation (i.e., predeposit of an individual's own blood) in cases in which surgery is anticipated** (see later section on the appropriate use of blood).

Improving the Safety of the Blood Supply

Maintaining the safety of the blood supply depends on the use of tests to detect antibody to HIV in the donations of individuals who do not report engaging in behaviors that transmit the virus (i.e., individuals at indirect risk) and on the exclusion of individuals who are at even minimal risk. Although HIV antibody tests are sensitive enough to detect most infected donations, biomedical scientists are continuing research to improve test capacities while social and behavioral scientists continue to work on ways to improve donor recruitment and deferral strategies. To design effective strategies to recruit healthy donors, however, it is necessary to understand the characteristics of donors who have been found to be infected and those whose blood is "safe."

Surveys of HIV infection among blood donors find more infection among men than women, more infection among younger donors than older ones, and more infection among minorities than among whites. In addition, comparisons of the pattern of HIV prevalence among blood donors with that of specific risk groups show that women and bisexual men are overrepresented among infected blood donors; a substantial proportion of infected donors, moreover, report no identifiable risk factor. It is important to remember, however, that it is participation in high-risk behaviors and not membership in any particular group that confers a risk for HIV infection. Therefore, as with all recruitment efforts, blood donation drives directed toward minorities and other groups that bear disproportionate burdens of HIV-related illness should seek those individuals whose behavior predicts a low risk of HIV infection. The low prevalence of AIDS and HIV (and the presumably low prevalence of high-risk behavior) among the elderly and the late middle-aged segments of the population makes them an obvious focus for blood drives. Traditional concerns that older people will not be able to meet donor eligibility requirements seem outmoded today, considering the health and vigor displayed by many who are past retirement age.

In the past, women were considered to be at relatively low risk for HIV infection. Now, however, as the epidemic enters its second decade, the risk profile of women appears to be changing. In addition, current exclusionary mechanisms may not be sufficient to screen out all infected women. Many women are unaware of their level of risk because exposure to the virus is indirect (e.g., from an infected sexual partner as opposed to their own IV drug use). For such women, voluntary self-deferral is not possible. The ability to assess the risk posed by individuals who may have been exposed indirectly to HIV infection presents enormous challenges to the current system. Yet, considering the potential importance of women to the donor pool, it seems reasonable to pursue solutions to this problem, as well as to support research that would shed light on why women are underrepresented among blood donors and the factors that might increase their participation.

One strategy to increase participation of safe donors involves the use of members of a targeted group as role models for prospective donors and as staff for donor recruitment and blood collection. Seeing known or similar people involved in the process seems to increase the perception among potential donors that blood donation is something individuals in their community do. Ultimately, such a perception may lead to increased donation from currently underrepresented groups. Yet for a strategy to increase donor participation, it must also encompass mechanisms to enhance appropriate deferral, in part because of recent concerns regarding the effectiveness of self-exclusion procedures. It has become apparent that some donors simply do not understand the materials intended to inform them about exclusionary criteria. Others do not perceive their own risk; a lack of perceived risk has been shown even among infected donors. Finally, a worrisome subset of donors uses blood collection organizations to secure HIV testing.

These problems have obvious implications for self-deferral strategies. Providing comprehensible information is a reasonable starting point for improving the self-deferral process. Research is needed to ascertain the relative effectiveness of different forms of communication. Focusing on risk behaviors rather than membership in a risk group and including in the health history direct questions concerning intimate but risky personal behaviors are promising strategies to ameliorate the blood safety problems associated with a lack of risk perception. Attention must also be given, however, to issues of donor privacy and to staff training in the conduct of health history interviews. In addition, because there will probably continue to be some at-risk individuals who donate blood as a way of being tested, efforts must be made to reach these donors and refer them to alternative testing sites.

To improve the safety of the blood supply, **the committee recommends that:**

- **blood collection agencies strive for clearer communication of the exclusion criteria to potential and actual donors;**

- **blood collection agencies work to increase donation by those who can safely give and abstention by those who are at even minimal risk through recruitment approaches that stress altruistic appeals rather than the use of competitions, incentives, and social pressure; and**

- **the National Heart, Lung, and Blood Institute continue its support for research to investigate why some donors with identifiable risk factors continue to donate while others without risk factors inappropriately exclude themselves.**

The Appropriate Use of Blood

In recent years, blood centers have seen a shift from the practice of transfusing whole blood to the use of only the specific blood component needed. This trend reflects sound medical practice and has the added benefit that a single donation can be used to treat as many as four different patients, thus relieving some of the strain on the blood supply. A drawback of this practice, however, is that two to four patients may be exposed to blood components from one contaminated donation. There is some evidence that blood utilization in the United States has been affected by concern over the risk of HIV transmission. For example, total red blood cell transfusion rates remained constant between 1982 and 1985, after a period of increasing rates; the use of plasma stabilized in a similar manner. Total platelet transfusion rates, however, continued to increase. Thus, the use of blood and blood components continues to require monitoring, and strategies should be explored to ensure the appropriate use of transfused blood.

Under certain conditions, individuals can predeposit their own blood for transfusion during elective surgery, a practice known as autologous donation. Before 1985, autologous transfusions were rarely used, and many blood centers in the United States did not have procedures for handling predeposited blood. From the perspective of the HIV epidemic, the infrequent use of autologous transfusion is regrettable. Even today the practice is underutilized. Because transfusion with autologous blood is the safest form of transfusion, the data indicating its infrequent use warrant further consideration and, if necessary, interventions to reverse this situation.

In the absence of autologous donation, another strategy is to reduce the exposure of transfusion recipients to homologous blood (i.e., blood from a community's general donor pool). This can be accomplished in several ways. In principle, these approaches involve more appropriate use of blood by decreasing the nonessential use of blood and blood components, reducing the need for transfusion, and inactivating HIV and other viruses that may be present in blood products. Another strategy for reducing exposure to homologous blood is to shorten the patient's bleeding time and enhance his or her own red blood cell production. Promising approaches include the use of desmopressin acetate, which has been shown to reduce blood loss in patients undergoing complex cardiac surgery, and the hormone erythropoietin, which can substantially increase red blood cell production.

To implement any of these strategies, programs will be needed to educate physicians and their patients and to modify relevant behaviors.

Audits of blood use and educational programs that go beyond dissemination of pamphlets and the traditional didactic method appear to hold the most promise; however, more data are needed to specify the characteristics of programs that are likely to be effective in modifying prescribing patterns of physicians. **The committee recommends that agencies of the Public Health Service sponsor the development, systematic testing, and implementation of transfusion-related intervention and education programs to facilitate change in physicians' attitudes and behaviors with regard to:**

- **encouraging healthy patients to donate blood;**
- **encouraging autologous donation where medically appropriate;**
- **eliminating the unnecessary use of blood and blood components; and**
- **employing appropriate procedures (e.g., perioperative blood salvage, use of erythropoietin) that reduce the need for transfusion.**

Standards or criteria regarding the appropriate use of blood and blood components are currently lacking, making it difficult to determine with certainty whether transfusions are being given appropriately. As a result, **the committee recommends that the Public Health Service sponsor research to monitor trends in transfusion practices nationally to permit evaluation of the appropriateness of blood and blood component utilization and to identify targets for change. It further recommends that the PHS develop and evaluate effective strategies for informing patients about the risks and benefits of transfusion.**

SURVEY METHODS IN AIDS RESEARCH

Surveys or, more generally, the method of asking questions and recording answers from a sample of a population of interest continue to be one of the most important techniques for obtaining essential information about the epidemiology of AIDS and HIV, the behaviors that spread HIV, and the effectiveness of AIDS prevention efforts. Given the important role that this information plays in understanding the AIDS epidemic, the committee has reviewed what is known about the quality of existing data on behaviors associated with HIV transmission and provides recommendations on steps that can be taken to improve this information.

Sampling

Much of what is now known about the epidemiology of AIDS comes from small-scale, local studies targeted at subgroups thought to be at high risk of infection. Participants in these studies are recruited from a variety of sources—from the clientele of local clinics or treatment facilities, from the membership rosters of local organizations, from newspaper advertisements and physician referrals, and occasionally from "street sampling." The yield from this research has been remarkably rich. As valuable as these studies are, however, the data they provide cannot address many important public health questions that arise from the problem of AIDS, such as how large is the epidemic and what is the potential for general spread of HIV infection?

To answer questions such as these, lessons learned from local studies of special subgroups must be applied in large-scale investigations of populations that are chosen not because of convenience or ease of access but because of their importance in understanding the course of the epidemic. To review the adequacy of current survey work in the general population and in local areas, the committee reviewed 15 selected surveys. Most of these studies were initiated after the AIDS epidemic began and represent responses to the need for population-based estimates of behaviors known to be associated with HIV transmission. The committee assessed the execution of each survey's sampling plan and, in particular, the rate of participation (i.e., the response rate). The committee also considered the available evidence on nonresponse bias; that is, the disproportionate underrepresentation of identifiable segments of the population, especially those who differed on the characteristics being measured. Response rates are used as a "yardstick" for assessing the accuracy of survey estimates because high response rates reduce the influence of selective participation in surveys and hence the potential for bias in the estimates.

There was substantial variation in the response rates achieved in the surveys examined by the committee. No strong associations were observed, however, between response rates and modes of data collection (i.e., personal interviews, telephone interviews, or self-administered questionnaires given in the context of a personal interview). There were also no substantial associations between response rates and the scope of the sampling (local versus national), the number of questions on sexual behavior in the interview, or, surprisingly, whether sample persons were asked to donate blood specimens for serologic testing.

From the review conducted by the committee, it appeared that "piggybacking" a small number of questions about sexual behavior onto established large-scale surveys is a particularly feasible strategy for obtaining estimates of the prevalence of certain risk factors for sexual transmission of HIV in general populations. Relatively high rates of participation have been achieved by several established surveys. The ingredients for such success are well known to survey practitioners: prior experience with similar surveys, continuity of interviewing staff, a high "target response rate" combined with a field operation that promotes diligent follow-up of nonrespondents, and adequate resources. Under these conditions, it is possible to achieve response rates for small subsets of sex-related items that are similar to the rates achieved by well-conducted surveys that do not inquire about sensitive personal behaviors.

The collection of survey data through telephone interviews has become an increasingly popular alternative to face-to-face interviewing (telephone interviews are less expensive and easier to conduct as a result of developments in sampling and interviewing technology). Experience with surveys of sexual behavior conducted by phone is too limited, however, to determine the levels of participation that can be achieved in such surveys and whether the somewhat lower response rates in the few available cases are a generic feature of telephone surveys or simply the result of early and somewhat idiosyncratic first attempts. In view of the substantially lower cost of telephone as compared with face-to-face surveys, as well as the limited scope of current experience, carefully designed experiments should be undertaken to test the feasibility of this methodology for surveys of sexual behavior in general populations.

Seroprevalence surveys involve the application of well-established principles of probability sampling and survey methodology to the problem of collecting sample blood specimens in such a way that population prevalence can, *in theory,* be estimated with known margins of error. However, the practical difficulties involved in mounting a seroprevalence survey on a local or national basis are formidable. Not the least of these are the problems of potentially high levels of noncooperation among sample persons and possible correlations between participation and HIV serostatus.

A trade-off between streamlined designs that maximize response rates and intensive epidemiological investigations with lower response rates is apparent in the available examples of such surveys. Survey designs that limit the demands on respondents—by making participation relatively easy, anonymous, and nonthreatening—may be a wise choice. Further testing and refinement of this approach on a larger scale will establish whether it constitutes a feasible design for a national survey.

Nonresponse Bias

Nonresponse bias occurs when participation in a survey is selective with respect to a characteristic whose distribution is to be estimated from the survey responses. A high response rate tends to minimize the effects of such selectivity on survey estimates as long as the procedures used to attain it do not in fact increase the correlation between the characteristic of interest and the act of participation. Response rates in most surveys, however, usually are not sufficiently high to justify ignoring problems of selective participation.

What is presently known about the structure of nonresponse bias in sex and seroprevalence surveys comes from two kinds of comparisons: comparisons of survey estimates with census data and internal analyses of the correlates of different levels of nonresponse. There is an apparent positive correlation between years of schooling and participation in several of the surveys, but the committee could detect few other regularities in the available analyses of deviations between survey estimates and census figures. In any case, a good match between census and sample survey distributions, although encouraging in some respects, does not imply unbiased estimates of prevalence rates for sexual behavior or HIV infection.

In many surveys, it is possible to study nonresponse at a given stage of the survey by looking at information collected at a previous stage—for example, by comparing responses given by respondents and nonrespondents in the preliminary interview or comparing the characteristics of persons who agreed to give a blood specimen with those who refused. In reviewing selected surveys, the committee found many opportunities for such comparisons, few of which had been seized. The addition of a careful study of nonresponse bias to the short sexual behavior component of the 1988 National Opinion Research Center's General Social Survey (GSS) is an important exception. In the GSS, nonresponse biases were found to be quite small among those variables most closely associated with differences in sexual behavior. Although these results are informative about the nature of nonresponse in this one survey, it would be premature to generalize them to other surveys. Rather, careful studies are required of the effects of nonresponse in a wider range of sexual behavior and seroprevalence surveys. In this regard, the committee encourages further exploitation of existing data from past sex and seroprevalence surveys to learn more about the structure of nonresponse.

Validity and Reliability

Behind every n-way tabulation, logistic regression, or other analytical model used in AIDS behavioral research lies a human encounter between two individuals, an interviewer and a respondent. The situational, cognitive, social, and psychological factors that arise within that interpersonal exchange affect the answers that are given and the data that are thereby generated. To understand the sexual and drug-using behaviors that are at issue in survey research on HIV transmission, one must ultimately confront the uncertainties introduced by this question-and-answer process.

Although there is a substantial literature on the effects of nonsampling factors in survey measurements, the problems encountered in studying sexual and drug use behavior are unique in some respects—most notably, with respect to validation of responses. There is reason to believe (and empirical evidence to support such a belief) that some respondents conceal behaviors under even the most benign of survey circumstances. This possibility must be given considerable weight in the face of statutes in many states that classify some sexual behaviors (including male-female and male-male oral and anal sex) as crimes. Finally, there is the possibility that behaviors engaged in while the respondent is under the influence of drugs or alcohol may be poorly recalled, if at all. Given these considerations, lingering concern about the trustworthiness of key survey estimates is virtually inevitable. In light of such concern, the committee reviewed the available evidence on the accuracy of self-reports of sexual and drug use behaviors.

Sexual Behavior

There is only a very limited range of evidence that can be collected to provide independent corroboration of the validity of self-reported sexual behaviors. One type of evidence is the reports of sexual partners. Studies by Kinsey and several later investigators find a rather high degree of congruence between reports of sexual partners. Indeed, in some of the instances, the levels of agreement are striking.

Although partners provide the most obvious source of independent information on sexual behavior, they are not the only validation method that has been used. One investigator, for example, went to unusual lengths (including the use of a lie detector) to motivate respondents to correct "misreports" they made in completing a survey questionnaire. The "corrections" made to the original survey data provide an indication of the types of reporting biases that afflict typical survey measures. For every sexual behavior included in this study, a substantial fraction of the respondents (college men) misreported their actual behaviors. Thus, although virtually every male ultimately indicated that he had masturbated, approximately one out of every three in the initial survey denied masturbating. Similarly, although 22 percent of these college men ultimately reported some history of male-male sexual contact, the majority of these men initially denied such contact.

In two instances, analyses have been reported of measurements of sexual behavior derived from independent replications of surveys on samples of the same population. Although some deviations could be detected statistically between the measurements made in different surveys, the discrepancies found were actually quite small. Although only two behaviors were compared (age at first occurrence of heterosexual intercourse and number of partners in past year), these examples demonstrate that surveys *can* produce replicable measures of sexual behavior in well-defined populations.

A parallel approach to the replication of entire surveys on new samples from a population is the repeated measurement of a stable characteristic of the same respondent. Results of such studies indicate substantial levels of consistency between answers to questions about sexual behavior obtained at two different points in time. The observed consistency, however, is not as high as the consistency obtained for some other topics, such as smoking behaviors.

Drug-Using Behaviors

The methodological difficulties encountered in studying drug use behaviors are similar to those found in studying sexual behaviors. As in measuring sexual behaviors, a major problem in measuring injection behaviors arises from the fact that researchers usually cannot directly observe the behaviors of interest and thus must rely on self-reports. Several studies have compared reports of drug use with the results of urinalysis. Evidence from these studies suggests that there are moderate levels of underreporting of drug use. Generalizations from such studies are constrained by the fact that past research has usually examined a relatively restricted range of behaviors typically focusing on drug use *per se* in populations that were already identified as ex-drug users. In AIDS research, however, questions of particular interest include not just whether drugs are used but how they are administered, how often needles are shared or cleaned, and so forth. Little is known about the accuracy of responses to more fine-grained questions such as these, although some data suggest that respondents share needles at a rate higher than they report to researchers.

Summary of Findings

Although there is ample evidence of error and bias in existing surveys of sexual behavior and such evidence should be of concern to investigators, some important and promising conclusions can nevertheless be drawn from this body of work.

First, there appears to be little question that surveys of sexual and drug use behavior can enlist the cooperation of the vast majority of the American public.

Second, the recent literature contains two instances in which independently conducted surveys of aspects of sexual behavior (age of first intercourse and number of sexual partners in past year) produced reassuringly similar results. This similarity was achieved despite variations in survey methodology.

Third, in most sexual behavior and drug use surveys, it will be difficult (if not impossible) to obtain convincing evidence of measurement validity. The committee finds nonetheless that the research literature contains several important demonstrations of the validity of behavioral measures. These results are certainly encouraging, but there is also a variety of other evidence that suggests that some behaviors may be considerably underreported in surveys. For example, although the data are limited, it appears that male-male sexual contacts may be significantly underreported (at least by college student populations).

Finally, there is a fairly large body of research addressing the consistency of responses over short periods of time in survey reports on various aspects of sexual behaviors. These studies have generally demonstrated moderate levels of response consistency over time. It must be noted, however, that consistency in itself does not guarantee accuracy.

Improving Measurements

The above evidence leads naturally to questions regarding how to improve the reliability and validity of self-reported data on these behaviors. To begin answering those questions, **the committee recommends that the Public Health Service and other organizations supporting AIDS research provide increased support for methodological research on the measurement of behaviors that transmit HIV. Such research should consider inferential problems introduced by nonresponse and by nonsampling factors, including (but not limited to) the effects of question wording and question context, the time periods and events that respondents are asked to recall, and the effects of anonymity guarantees on survey responses.** In addition to adopting procedures that ensure that respondents can understand the questions they are being asked, it is desirable to supplement self-reports with alternative measures whenever possible. Ethnographic observations, physical evidence, skills demonstrations, and reports of "significant others" can provide important data on the biases that may affect key measurements. **The committee recommends that, whenever feasible, researchers supplement self-reports in behavioral surveys on HIV transmission with** other indicators of these behaviors that do not rely on respondent reports. Furthermore, the committee recommends that, where appropriate, researchers embed experimental studies within behavioral surveys on HIV transmission to assess the effects of key aspects of the survey measurement process.

Although it is impossible to provide firm guarantees as to the beneficial effects of any particular tactic, the committee believes that there is strong presumptive evidence to indicate that a considerably larger investment of resources needs to be made in exploratory work prior to the fielding of major survey investigations. For surveys of behaviors that risk HIV transmission, this lack of exploratory research is particularly troubling, given the underdeveloped state of research in this field. In this regard, the committee notes that some of the questionnaires it reviewed made impossible demands on the memory of respondents, an unfortunate error that would have been detected if the questionnaires had received more thorough pilot testing. The committee recommends that researchers who conduct behavioral surveys on HIV transmission make increased use of ethnographic studies, pretests, pilot studies, cognitive laboratory investigations, and other similar developmental strategies to aid in the design of large-scale surveys.

SYNOPSIS AND MAJOR RECOMMENDATIONS

Throughout the report the committee reviews a variety of issues and presents a series of recommendations. Because the material is presented in some detail, the committee wishes to highlight some of the major points here.

The committee finds that the broadening scope of the AIDS epidemic calls for increased prevention efforts to reach a variety of subpopulations at differential risk, such as adults and adolescents, men and women, homosexuals and heterosexuals. The committee is particularly concerned about the epidemiological evidence that finds a disproportionate burden of disease among minority subpopulations. Therefore, the committee recommends that the agencies of the Public Health Service encourage and strengthen behavioral science research aimed at understanding the transmission of HIV in various black and Hispanic subpopulations, including men who have sex with men, drug users and their sexual partners, and youth. The committee further recommends that the PHS develop plans for appropriate interventions targeted toward these groups and support the implementation of intervention strategies (together with appropriate evaluation components) in both demonstration projects and larger scale efforts.

Adolescents and women are other groups that present both important opportunities to prevent future disease and challenges to providing effective intervention programs. It is during the adolescent years (and sometimes earlier) that many of the behaviors that risk transmission of HIV are initiated. For programs to be most effective, however, teens must be reached before they begin the behaviors that put them at risk. Thus, **the committee recommends that AIDS prevention programs make special efforts to reach very young teens and, in some subpopulations, to reach youth before they enter adolescence.** Thus far over the course of the epidemic, a considerable proportion of the resources allocated to prevent horizontal and vertical transmission among women have been devoted to counseling and testing programs. Yet important questions remain about how this service is delivered and what impact it has on subsequent risk-associated behaviors. Therefore, **the committee recommends careful review of the goals of testing and counseling programs for women of childbearing age and the implementation of research to ascertain the effect of such programs on future risk-taking behavior.** Moreover, **the committee recommends that the Public Health Service support research to develop protective measures other than condoms for preventing HIV transmission during sexual contact—specifically, methods that can be used unilaterally by women and methods that will be acceptable to both men and women who do not currently use condoms.**

Designing and implementing relevant and effective programs requires knowledge about the targeted population and the risk-associated behaviors of concern. Thus, **the committee recommends:**

- **that the Public Health Service encourage and support behavioral research programs that study the behaviors that transmit HIV infection and that the PHS develop and evaluate mechanisms for facilitating and sustaining change in those behaviors;**
- **that intervention programs incorporate planned variations that can be carefully evaluated to determine their relative effectiveness;**
- **that the PHS regularly summarize the data derived from currently funded behavioral and epidemiological research on AIDS (in terms of incidence of infection and high-risk behaviors) to determine intervention priorities for various subpopulations at risk; and**
- **that all agencies of the PHS that are currently funding intervention programs and evaluation research regularly**

summarize the data derived from these studies to determine which, if any, programs can be recommended for wider dissemination.

Understanding the behaviors that transmit the virus depends on the availability of valid and reliable data regarding those behaviors, including the distribution and variation of the behaviors across various subpopulations. Unfortunately, the data on AIDS-related behaviors are extremely limited, and most are out of date. Moreover, these data rely for the most part on self-reported information of unknown quality. Consequently, **the committee recommends that the Public Health Service and other organizations supporting AIDS research provide increased support for methodological research on the measurement of behaviors that transmit HIV. Such research should consider inferential problems introduced by nonresponse and nonsampling factors, including (but not limited to) the effects of question wording and question context, the time periods and events that respondents are asked to recall, and the effects of anonymity guarantees on survey responses.**

In addition to the diversity of at-risk groups, the committee wishes to note the dynamic nature of the patterns of behavior that contribute to the spread of infection. The role played by IV drug use in HIV transmission has been apparent since the early years of the epidemic, but only recently has there been a growing appreciation of the role of other drugs, such as crack and cocaine, in sexual transmission of the AIDS virus. Therefore, **the committee recommends that the Public Health Service establish mechanisms across its agencies for rapid identification and assessment of the relationship of new drug use problems to the spread of HIV.** Given the continued threat of HIV and AIDS and given the lack of biomedical solutions to this serious health problem, the committee finds that sustaining behavioral change and preventing relapse are issues that require immediate and sustained attention. Thus, **the committee recommends that the Alcohol, Drug Abuse, and Mental Health Administration focus research efforts on AIDS-related relapse prevention, including the determinants of such relapse and the role that alcohol and other drugs play in the return to unsafe sexual and injection practices.**

There has been substantial progress in reducing the risks of HIV transmission associated with the blood supply, progress achieved through technological solutions, augmented by behavioral interventions. Yet, as the risk of exposure to contaminated blood and blood products diminishes, the issue of maintaining an adequate supply of blood arises. Efforts to exclude at-risk donors must take into account the need to maintain sufficient quantities of blood donated by individuals who pose no risk to the blood supply. **The committee recommends that:**

- **blood collection agencies strive for clearer communication of the exclusion criteria to potential and actual donors;**
- **blood collection agencies work to increase donation by those who can safely give and abstention by those who are at even minimal risk through recruitment approaches that stress altruistic appeals rather than the use of competitions, incentives, and social pressure;**
- **the National Heart, Lung, and Blood Institute continue its support for research to investigate why some donors with identifiable risk factors continue to donate while others without risk factors inappropriately exclude themselves; and**
- **physicians and blood banks encourage autologous donation in cases in which surgery is anticipated.**

Reducing the exposure of potential transfusion recipients to homologous blood can be accomplished in several ways, depending on the circumstances that prompt transfusion. Educating physicians and their patients, establishing guidelines for blood use, and modifying prescribing behavior are necessary to achieve this goal.

1

The AIDS Epidemic in the Second Decade

In its first report, the Committee on AIDS Research and the Social, Behavioral, and Statistical Sciences reviewed what was known about the distribution of cases of acquired immune deficiency syndrome (AIDS) in the United States and the behaviors that transmit infection by the human immunodeficiency virus (HIV). In addition, the committee looked at rational strategies for preventing further spread of infection. Since issuing that report, the committee has continued to monitor the progression of the epidemic and the nation's response to what is now clearly seen as an evolving and enduring health problem. This report identifies several important changes that point toward new and developing issues to be addressed during the second decade of the epidemic, as well as continuing problems from the first decade that compel the nation's sustained attention.

AIDS surveillance data indicate gradual changes in the loci of the epidemic in the U.S. population and the emergence of either new populations at risk or segments within already at-risk populations that appear to be at higher risk than was previously thought. Whereas AIDS case data provide a sense of the scope and nature of the current problem, however, data on HIV infection portend the future of the epidemic in the second decade. The future is likely to bring other changes as well, including decreased morbidity associated with HIV infection as new treatments become available. This change in the character of AIDS, with the beginnings of a shift away from an emphasis on the acuteness of infection toward a view of AIDS as a long-term illness, will have important implications for treatment and care and for the design of intervention strategies to facilitate behavioral change, still the only available means to prevent the spread of infection. This report considers the changing face of the epidemic and highlights recent data and research on several groups or populations whose risk for HIV transmission has emerged more clearly or changed over the past decade. It also presents an update on the implementation of prevention approaches discussed in the committee's first report and offers recommendations on directions for the future.

INTRODUCTION

In its earlier report, the committee noted that the AIDS epidemic is a social as well as a biomedical phenomenon. From a biomedical perspective, AIDS is a disease caused by a virus, HIV-1, that is transmitted by anal or vaginal intercourse, by exposure to contaminated blood (either through shared injection equipment associated with intravenous drug use or transfusion), and from mother to fetus. Once it is acquired, HIV infection appears to persist for life. The AIDS virus destroys subpopulations of white blood cells that are crucial to normal functioning of the immune system. As the immune system deteriorates, infected individuals are no longer able to ward off infections, and some develop unusual cancers and other conditions that appear rarely among individuals with uncompromised immune functioning.[1] A sizable proportion of the people who were infected have, after variable periods of time, progressed to severe disease and death. At present, there is no cure for AIDS and no vaccine to prevent infection. In fact, the only means available to prevent further spread of the epidemic are strategies to alter the behaviors that transmit the virus. From a social perspective, AIDS is, for the most part, a preventable disease that is inextricably rooted in the behaviors that transmit HIV. Halting the progression of the epidemic will require a better understanding of the distribution of risk-associated behaviors, the social settings in which they are enacted, and the mechanisms that facilitate change in these behaviors. Like other epidemics in the past, AIDS will leave its mark on many aspects of the societies in which it becomes prevalent.[2] In the United States, the primary target of the disease is the nation's most productive population—20- to 40-year-old adults. As discussed below, however, the epidemic is moving in ever-widening circles to reach more people and geographic areas across the country.

---

[1] For more information on the medical and biological aspects of AIDS and HIV infection, see *Confronting AIDS: Directions for Public Health, Health Care, and Research,* Washington, D.C.: National Academy Press, 1986; and *Confronting AIDS: Update 1988,* Washington, D.C.: National Academy Press, 1988.

[2] The committee's Panel on Monitoring the Social Impact of the AIDS Epidemic is currently examining certain social consequences of the epidemic and will be preparing recommendations on specific methods to monitor these effects. The report is expected to be published in 1991.

In this country, gay men still bear the burden of most of the illness related to AIDS. But as the epidemic progresses and the number of persons who are at risk increases, changes in disease prevalence are becoming apparent. For example, extensive studies of gay men conducted in urban epicenters of the epidemic over a period of several years have consistently shown lower incidence rates of HIV infection, but this downward trend in new infections is not uniform across the country. Moreover, young gay men report less behavioral change to prevent infection than has been reported among older gay men, a phenomenon that leaves adolescents and young adults who engage in male-male sex at potentially increased risk. Shifts in membership in the population of men who have sex with men may also produce changes in incidence as individuals enter or leave this group. Thus, the risk of HIV infection among gay men continues to be an important concern.

Other populations are also feeling the effects of the disease. Increasingly, AIDS has become a problem of intravenous (IV) drug users and heterosexuals. Indeed, the proportion of AIDS cases in the United States attributable to heterosexual contact is growing, and a significant fraction of these cases report contact with a drug user. The rise in reported AIDS cases among females—especially minority women—occasions particular concern. As more women are infected, questions concerning the horizontal spread of the virus (to sexual and drug use partners) and its vertical transmission (from an infected mother to her unborn infant) have become prominent in national discussions on AIDS. In this chapter, the committee presents data on AIDS and HIV infection among women as an example of an emerging problem that embraces a diverse subpopulation and that is likely to require new strategies for reaching the infected and for facilitating change in risky behaviors.

Other epidemiological patterns show increasing geographic diffusion of the virus. Research in the first decade of the epidemic showed pockets of high seroprevalence in such cities as New York, Newark, San Francisco, and Miami for a variety of populations. More recent data show increased numbers of AIDS cases in the central region of the country, making the epidemic less a bicoastal phenomenon and more a problem that may soon directly touch more and more individuals throughout this society. Data from U.S. military applicants support this finding of increasing geographic diffusion of HIV, showing increased rates of seroprevalence among black and white applicants from nonepidemic regions of the country.[3] Yet even though some patterns have changed, others

---

[3] Significant increases for the past 24 months are reported in California, Florida, Illinois, Ohio, and Texas (Gardner et al., 1989).

have endured. One pattern that has remained dauntingly constant is the disproportionate magnitude of HIV infection and AIDS among minority men and women, who are overrepresented in every transmission category.

Changes are also being seen in the patterns of behavior that transmit the AIDS virus. Many gay men with AIDS acquired HIV infection through unprotected sexual contact. In addition, since the earliest days of the epidemic it has been clear that sharing injection equipment posed a risk for the acquisition and spread of HIV infection. Today, there is growing appreciation of other factors that may influence risk, including the role in risk taking played by drugs such as alcohol. Indeed, the use of noninjected drugs, such as crack and alcohol, has been linked with both high-risk sexual behavior and HIV infection in a variety of populations. Another potential risk comes from recent increases in the use of drugs such as opiates and cocaine, which in many areas are taken primarily through smoking. These drugs offer the possibility of wider spread of HIV infection if the route of their administration should shift to injection.

Getting ahead of the epidemic requires foresight to prevent infection in populations and regions that currently have a low prevalence of AIDS and HIV infection. Such opportunities should not be overlooked, for, once lost, they cannot be recaptured. The third chapter of this report considers the scope of the AIDS problem among adolescents. In it, the committee notes opportunities for intervention with this group and the characteristics of this population that put adolescents at risk and that require consideration in the design of intervention strategies.

Keeping pace with the epidemic requires perseverance—an enduring, long-term commitment to surveillance, research, and improved intervention. Short-term approaches that result in one study, one report, one intervention will not suffice. The type of commitment required is one that includes a range of strategies and techniques, behavioral as well as biomedical. The response of the U.S. blood supply system to the threat of AIDS, which is discussed in Chapter 5, offers an example of such a commitment. The blood supply system has combined biomedical techniques (e.g., HIV blood screening) and behavioral approaches (e.g., self-exclusion procedures for high-risk donors, training programs for physicians to alter transfusion-related practices) to reduce dramatically the risk of transfusion-related transmission and the number of cases associated with exposure to contaminated blood products. Yet despite the success these reductions represent, problems remain. Although the current prevalence of HIV infection in the general population is believed to be low, as the virus spreads and more people become infected, some parts of the country may find that the pool of uninfected, "safe," and willing blood donors has shrunk to a point that could compromise the adequacy of the blood supply. The second decade of the epidemic thus brings continuing as well as new challenges in managing the effects of HIV infection and preventing its further spread.

In its first report, the committee commented on the need for systematic improvement of intervention strategies to facilitate change in the behaviors known to transmit HIV. It noted in particular that the intervention efforts described in that report had not resulted in data that offered a clear sense of which strategies worked best for specific subpopulations. The paucity of planned variations of intervention strategies and of information garnered through rigorous outcome evaluation that was cited by the committee has not been remedied. The gap is particularly problematic for innovative programs that have targeted groups such as IV drug users, in which infection has been shown to spread at an alarmingly fast rate in the absence of effective intervention efforts and in which potentially efficacious but politically sensitive efforts have come under attack. A year ago the committee recommended well-designed, carefully evaluated pilot tests of sterile needle exchange programs to ascertain the effectiveness of this strategy in preventing further infection among IV drug users. Although several programs were initiated, there are now crippling restrictions on the use of federal funds to support and evaluate these activities.[4]

This chapter relies extensively on counts of diagnosed AIDS cases reported to the Centers for Disease Control (CDC). In its last report, the committee noted some of the pitfalls that cause undercounting or misclassification of AIDS cases and deaths (Turner, Miller, and Moses, 1989:32–33).[5] It recommended that both vigilant quality control and special methodological studies be undertaken to improve our understanding of the errors and biases that affect the reporting of AIDS cases and deaths. The committee finds that the need for such methodological work continues, and it commends the Public Health Service for its plan to give priority to the funding of such research (PHS, 1988; CDC, 1989). As we embark on a second decade of understanding and coping with the AIDS epidemic, these efforts will provide needed attention to the quality of this key data system.

More than 115,000 cases of AIDS have been reported in the United

---

[4] See Public Law 101-166 [H.R. 3566], Title V—General Provisions, Section 520. Departments of Labor, Health and Human Services, and Education and related agencies appropriations, 1990. November 21, 1989. Washington, D.C.

[5] Other reports have also looked at completeness of reporting of AIDS cases. See, for example, the estimates of Conway and colleagues (1989) and Modesitt, Hulman, and Fleming (1990).

States, and more than half of the people reflected by this statistic have died. Moreover, AIDS has become the leading cause of death for 30- to 50-year-old males and 20- to 40-year-old females in New York City (New York State Department of Health, 1989). Despite advances in the medical treatment of AIDS and other sequellae of HIV infection,[6] it is likely that HIV and AIDS will remain significant threats to individual and public health for the foreseeable future. The persistence of risk in the environment and the potential for relapse among those who have taken protective action mean that, as we enter the 1990s and the epidemic's second decade, it is important to reaffirm the nation's commitment to preventing further spread of infection. To be more successful in future prevention endeavors than we have been in the past, we must commit talent and resources to the rigorous outcome evaluation of well-designed interventions while developing new approaches based on current understanding of the evolutionary and persistent aspects of the problem. The task of devising intervention strategies to fulfill this commitment rests on obtaining sound information about the populations at risk and the behaviors transmitting the virus to guide program planners and policy makers. The section that follows discusses the current profile of the disease in the United States on the eve of the epidemic's second decade.

THE CHANGING EPIDEMIOLOGY OF AIDS IN THE UNITED STATES

As of December 1989, the CDC reported 117,781 cases of AIDS in the United States.[7] Of the adult and adolescent cases, a significant majority (70,093) are attributed to male homosexual or bisexual contact, and an additional 8,117 are ascribed to both homosexual contact and IV drug use (CDC, 1990a). Of all men with AIDS who report same-gender sexual contact, more than one-quarter (27 percent) are black or Latino[8] (CDC, 1990a); moreover, homosexual contact is the predominant AIDS risk category among black and Latino males, accounting for 45 and 47 percent of cases, respectively (CDC, 1990a).

---

[6]Gail, Rosenberg, and Goedert (1990), for example, recently presented evidence suggesting that prophylactic use of zidovudine among seropositive homosexual and bisexual men (particularly in New York City, San Francisco, and Los Angeles) may be responsible for the lower than expected incidence of AIDS cases reported in this population since the middle of 1987.

[7]Although the degree of underreporting of AIDS cases is not known with any certainty, recent studies have judged reporting to be between 83 and 100 percent complete (Chamberland et al., 1985; Hardy et al., 1987; Lafferty et al., 1988). A recent survey of hospital discharge billing records in South Carolina, however, found that only 59.5 percent of cases meeting CDC diagnostic criteria were reported; underreporting was significantly worse among black patients than among whites (Conway et al., 1989).

[8]In this report the terms Latino and Latina are used interchangeably with Hispanic.

TABLE 1-1 Distribution of Reported AIDS Cases (percentage) by Year of Diagnosis and Exposure Category

Year of Diagnosis	Adults								Pediatric				Total	N
	Male Homo-Bisexual	IVDU[a]	Male Homosex. +IVDU	Hemo-philiac	Hetero-sexual	Pattern II[b]	Trans-fusion	Other[c]	Hemo-philiac	Risky Mother[d]	Trans-fusion	Other[c]		
1981	64.9	11.0	7.1	0.5	0.5	6.0	0.5	4.5	0.0	4.5	0.0	0.5	100	382
1982	60.7	16.9	9.4	0.6	1.1	5.1	0.8	2.9	0.2	1.7	0.4	0.3	100	1,076
1983	61.4	17.8	9.4	0.5	1.0	3.5	1.5	2.3	0.1	2.0	0.3	0.0	100	2,933
1984	64.3	16.7	8.7	0.9	1.5	2.2	1.7	2.1	0.1	1.5	0.3	0.0	100	5,926
1985	64.1	17.5	7.5	1.0	2.0	1.6	2.5	1.8	0.1	1.5	0.4	0.0	100	11,038
1986	62.9	18.2	7.8	0.9	2.5	1.4	2.7	2.1	0.1	1.3	0.2	0.0	100	17,777
1987	60.5	20.1	6.8	1.0	3.2	1.2	2.9	2.7	0.1	1.4	0.2	0.0	100	25,987
1988	56.9	22.8	6.3	1.0	4.1	1.1	2.5	3.7	0.1	1.3	0.1	0.1	100	29,761
1989[e]	55.3	23.2	5.8	0.7	5.0	1.2	1.9	5.3	0.1	1.2	0.1	0.1	100	22,901
Total	59.5	20.6	6.9	0.9	3.4	1.4	2.4	3.3	0.1	1.4	0.2	0.1	100	117,781

[a]IVDU: intravenous drug user. [b]The cases assigned to this category involve individuals from those countries in central, eastern, and southern Africa and some Caribbean countries in which the majority of AIDS cases have been ascribed to heterosexual transmission, the male-to-female case ratio is approximately 1:1, perinatal transmission is more common than in other areas, and intravenous drug use and homosexual transmission occur at a very low level. [c]This category includes cases currently under investigation for which no history of exposure has yet been reported and cases for which no exposure mode could ever be determined. [d]Mother with, or at risk for, HIV infection. [e]The 1989 figures include only those cases reported through December 31, 1989. All data shown in this table are subject to delays in reporting. Therefore, counts of cases diagnosed in a particular year may understate the number that will ultimately be reported. This type of understatement is particularly likely for cases diagnosed in 1988 and 1989.

SOURCE: Computed from CDC's AIDS Public Information Data Set for AIDS cases reported through December 31, 1989.

Data from the Multicenter AIDS Cohort Studies (MACS) and the San Francisco Men's Health Study suggest that incidence rates among gay and bisexual men have stabilized (Winkelstein et al., 1987, 1988), and there is some evidence that the number of new cases of AIDS in this population appears to be leveling off in New York City and Los Angeles (Berkelman et al., 1989). Indeed, the proportion of all AIDS cases attributed to male homosexual and bisexual contact has dropped from 64.9 percent in 1981 to 55.3 percent in 1989.[9] At the same time, the proportions of cases attributable to heterosexual contact and to IV drug use have grown. In 1981 cases attributable to heterosexual transmission and IV drug use constituted 0.5 and 11.0 percent, respectively, of all reported cases; by 1989 these rates had increased to 5.0 and 23.2 percent (Table 1-1).

Among IV drug users, after several years of progressively worsening infection statistics, there is now evidence that HIV seroprevalence has stabilized in some areas, such as New York City (Des Jarlais et al., 1989; Stoneburner et al., 1990), San Francisco (Moss et al., 1989), Detroit (Ognjan et al., 1989), Amsterdam (van Haastrecht, van den Hoek, and Coutinho, 1989), and Stockholm (Olin and Kall, 1989).[10] However, this stabilization reflects lower rates of new cases of HIV infection within a dynamic population and should not be confused with elimination of viral transmission. In fact, the evidence of stabilization in some regions is offset by data on the recent, very rapid spread of the disease in other areas. The proportion of cases attributed to drug use is increasing in Louisiana (Atkinson et al., 1989) and Maryland (Horman and Hamidi, 1989), as well as throughout cities in the northeast region of the United States (see Figure 1-1). The population of IV drug users is mobile and quite capable of carrying the virus from one geographic area to another (Comerford et al., 1989; McCoy, Chitwood, and Page, 1989). Such mobility is one factor that can contribute to the possibility of rapid rises in seroprevalence rates in various parts of the country. There is some evidence that homosexual and bisexual IV drug users may play a role in introducing HIV infection to other IV drug users in areas with

---

[9] Decreasing proportions, however, do not indicate decreasing numbers of cases. This smaller proportion of an ever-increasing whole still continues to result in increasing morbidity.

[10] For some groups at highest risk for HIV infection, stable rates may signify that all vulnerable individuals are already infected, a phenomenon known as saturation. This phenomenon does not appear to explain stable rates in New York City, however, where approximately 50 percent of IV drug users are estimated to be infected. If saturation had occurred, one would expect to see higher seroprevalence rates. For example, approximately 90 percent of IV drug users in New York City have been infected with hepatitis, a virus that is transmitted in the same manner as HIV and appears to have reached saturation in this population.

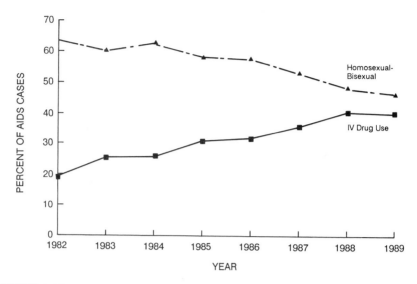

FIGURE 1-1 Percentages of reported AIDS cases among men (aged 13 and older) in northeastern cities that have been attributed to homosexual contact or IV drug use, 1982–1989. (Cases reported as both IV drug use and homosexual/bisexual contact are not shown.) NOTE: Cities in the Northeast region include the OMB Metropolitan Statistical Areas (or New England County Metropolitan Areas) of Bergen-Passaic, N.J.; Buffalo, N.Y.; Boston, Mass.; Hartford, Conn.; Nassau-Suffolk, N.J.; New York City; and Newark, N.J. SOURCE: Tabulated from CDC's AIDS Public Information Data Set for AIDS cases reported through December 31, 1989.

low prevalences of HIV infection (Battjes, Pickens, and Amsel, 1989). Although the distribution of cases in the IV drug-using population has shown considerable variation, one constant remains: the burden of AIDS related to IV drug use falls most heavily on minorities (Selik and Petersen, 1989). Nearly half (47.6 percent) of all males reporting IV drug use as their only risk factor for AIDS are black, and 32 percent are Latinos (CDC, 1990a).

Addressing the problem of IV drug use in relation to AIDS remains a high priority, but a focus solely on drug injection will no longer suffice to prevent further spread of HIV infection among individuals who use drugs. The evolving nature of the epidemic also requires a broadened perspective to encompass what appear to be new patterns of risk associated with drug use. In particular, the emergence of "crack" cocaine use as a risk factor for the transmission of HIV infection is a new and disturbing development in the epidemiology of AIDS in the United States. The risks associated with the use of crack are indirect (crack use is not in itself a mode of HIV transmission). However, the tendency of those who use crack to engage in unsafe sexual activity offers the potential for viral transmission.

Unlike other forms of cocaine that are snorted or injected, crack is smoked.[11] It can produce a rapid, intense effect that for most users is a feeling of euphoria, including an increased sense of self-worth and power. The effect of the drug wears off rapidly, however, and may be followed by a craving to use more. As a result, some users will "binge," using crack every 10 to 20 minutes until they or their supply of drug is exhausted. Thus, the intensity and transience of the crack "high" encourage the development of dependence on the drug. For many males, crack is reported to produce intensified sensations of sexual arousal and sexual pleasure; indeed, in some places crack is marketed by highlighting the sexual effects of the drug.[12] Some females who become dependent on crack show a willingness to exchange sex for the drug or for money to obtain the drug. (Chapter 4 discusses at greater length the relationship between crack use and female prostitution.) It is possible, of course, for crack users to practice safer sex, including condom use, but the effects of the drug and the perceived exigencies of repeating those effects reduce the likelihood that safer sex will be practiced consistently (Friedman et al., 1988). Small surveys of crack users have indicated an association between crack use and sexually transmitted diseases (STDs) (Fullilove et al., 1989), which supports the hypothesis that unprotected sex occurs in such settings. Because STDs appear to be cofactors in the acquisition of HIV infection, this association bodes ill for preventing the sexual transmission of HIV. Indeed, surveys of patients at STD clinics in New York have already found individuals with HIV infection whose only behavioral risk factor appears to be sexual activity associated with crack use (Chiasson et al., 1989; Hoegsberg et al., 1989).

The rapid emergence of crack as a risk factor for HIV infection highlights the need to be vigilant for signs of new patterns of risk. Thus, **the committee recommends that the Public Health Service establish mechanisms across its agencies for rapid identification and assessment of the relationship of new drug use problems to the spread of HIV.** But changes in drug use are not the only new trends that are

---

[11] Usually, cocaine is sold as a hydrochloride salt; in this form it must be either "sniffed" and absorbed through the nasal mucosa or injected. To produce crack cocaine, the hydrochloride is removed; in this form the cocaine may be vaporized and thus inhaled. Inhaling any drug into the lungs permits it to be absorbed into the blood stream rapidly and transported to the brain. Chemically, smoking crack is identical to "freebasing" the hydrochloride salt form of cocaine. Previously, persons who wanted to freebase had to purchase cocaine hydrochloride and convert it themselves to the base form through a complicated and dangerous process that involved heating volatile chemicals that could easily catch fire. The rise in the use of crack has come from the development of new and safer methods for removing the hydrochloride so that the drug can be sold in its base form.

[12] Some crack houses (the locations at which the drug is sold and used) employ women to provide sex to customers.

becoming apparent at the end of the first decade of the epidemic. There are also noticeable shifts in the groups being affected directly by the disease.

Throughout its studies, the committee has been struck by the diversity of the populations now represented in the AIDS statistics. It has chosen to look at women and the risks HIV poses to them as an example of a heterogeneous population that will require considerably more attention in the second decade of this epidemic than it received in the first. Because most of the cases of AIDS reported in the early years of the epidemic were diagnosed in men, few women appreciated their potential risk of acquiring this disease. Yet as the epidemic has progressed, women of all races have begun to account for a greater proportion of cases. The majority of women represented by these statistics have a history of intravenous drug use; a subset report no drug use themselves but indicate a sexual relationship with an intravenous drug user in their risk profile. The range of women at risk for AIDS, however, goes beyond those involved through drug use. The sections that follow discuss the profile of risk among women in the United States, noting the varied subgroups of this population that are increasingly affected by the epidemic.

A PICTURE OF EMERGING RISK:
THE AIDS EPIDEMIC AMONG WOMEN

Early in the epidemic, vertical or perinatal transmission of HIV infection (transmission from an infected pregnant woman to her offspring) was of particular concern because the majority of female AIDS cases (75.4 percent) had been diagnosed in women between the ages of 20 and 39, prime childbearing years. Today, concerns about perinatal transmission must be joined with the recognition that the risk of HIV infection among women of all ages is increasing, and more and more women are confronting the disease in their own lives or in the lives of those around them.

This increasing risk can be seen in the epidemiological data in Table 1-2, which show rising numbers of female AIDS cases over the past decade. By December 1989, a cumulative total of 10,611 cases of AIDS had been reported in women 13 years of age or older; however, this figure is likely to underestimate the scope of the problem owing to a failure to report cases and reporting delays. The upward trend shown in Table 1-2 is particularly ominous for minority women, who are disproportionately represented in almost every risk category (Table 1-3). In 1989 women also accounted for a larger proportion of all AIDS cases diagnosed in this country than they did in the early years of the epidemic, a temporal trend that is most striking in northeastern metropolitan areas (Figure 1-2).[13]

Unlike men, among whom the majority of cases have been ascribed to same-gender sexual contact, the major transmission category for women with AIDS is IV drug use (see Table 1-2) (Guinan and Hardy, 1987; CDC, 1990a). As Table 1-2 shows, there has been a slight decrease in the proportion of female cases attributed to IV drug use since 1983, but this drop is offset by the doubling of the proportion of female heterosexual cases. AIDS case data show that women are at greater risk than men of acquiring infection through heterosexual contact[14] and that the proportion of U.S. AIDS cases attributable to heterosexual contact is growing.[15] A majority of female heterosexual cases, however, are related to sexual contact with an infected intravenous drug user.[16] Thus, women are at risk for HIV infection both directly through their own drug use and indirectly through sexual exposure to partners who inject drugs.

Almost a thousand women with AIDS[17] ($N = 934$) have reported

---

[13]The proportion of all cases reported among women has grown from approximately 6 percent in 1982 to roughly 10 percent in 1989; accordingly, the male-to-female ratio of cases has dropped from 14.7:1 in 1982 to 8.6:1 in 1988. As the data in Table 1-2 show, the decline in the male-to-female ratio has been steady over the course of the epidemic and represents a statistically significant change ($p <$ .001). Data from New York City also find a significant decline in the male-to-female ratio over time (Stoneburner et al., 1990).

[14]By December 1989, almost one-third of female cases but only 2 percent of male cases were attributed to heterosexual contact with an infected partner (CDC, 1990a). Unfortunately, these data probably underestimate the risk associated with heterosexual transmission, in part because of case classification criteria. In a case in which heterosexual risk is found in combination with some other risk factor, the case will be classified in the other risk category. Moreover, unless the index partner in a case is reported to have AIDS, to be at increased risk for HIV infection, or to be infected with HIV, the case will not be ascribed to heterosexual transmission but will be categorized as having no identifiable risk factor. Castro and colleagues (1988) reported that a significant portion of AIDS cases with no identifiable risk factor are likely to be heterosexually acquired, a conclusion supported by relatively high rates of other sexually transmitted diseases among cases in this category.

[15]In 1982, only 1.1 percent of cases were associated with heterosexual contact; by December 1989 the proportion had grown to 5 percent (Curran et al., 1988; CDC, 1990a).

[16]More than 67 percent of heterosexually acquired AIDS cases in women are ascribed to unprotected intercourse with an infected male intravenous drug user (see Guinan and Hardy, 1987; Curran et al., 1988).

[17]Exposure to contaminated blood accounts for 3 percent of all AIDS cases. However, 10.3 percent of AIDS cases among women are related to transfusions, blood products, or tissue transplant whereas only 2.7 percent of cases among men are so categorized. The greater number of blood-related AIDS cases among men ($N = 2,417$) reflects both a greater burden of illness born by men to date and a greater prevalence of coagulation disorders found in males. Hemophilia, a complex of different co-agulation disorders, is a sex-linked hereditary disease that affects the body's ability to produce the various proteins needed to clot blood. Although a small subset of women have coagulation disorders, men constitute the vast majority of hemophiliacs.

TABLE 1-2 Distribution of Reported AIDS Cases (percentage) Among Males and Females Aged 13 Years and Older by Year of Diagnosis and Exposure Category

| | | | | | | Exposure Category | | | | |
Year	Homo-/ Bisexual	IVDU[a]	IVDU + Homosex.	Blood	Hetero- sexual	Pattern II[b]	Other[c]	Total	N
Male cases									
Pre-1983	68.2	13.5	9.7	1.0	0.2	5.1	2.3	100	1,322
1983	67.7	15.2	10.4	1.6	0.1	3.2	1.9	100	2,663
1984	69.9	14.4	9.5	2.1	0.4	2.0	1.8	100	5,451
1985	70.4	15.1	8.3	2.9	0.4	1.3	1.6	100	10,052
1986	69.4	15.7	8.6	2.9	0.5	1.1	1.8	100	16,109
1987	67.7	17.1	7.6	3.1	1.0	1.0	2.5	100	23,204
1988	64.5	20.0	7.2	2.8	1.3	0.8	3.5	100	26,269
1989[d]	63.0	20.3	6.7	2.2	1.9	0.9	5.0	100	20,104
All years	66.6	17.8	7.7	2.7	1.1	1.1	3.0	100	105,174

Female cases

Pre-1983	NA[e]	50.0	NA	6.7	13.3	11.1	18.9	100	90
1983	NA	60.4	NA	9.1	13.7	8.6	8.1	100	197
1984	NA	56.1	NA	12.3	18.0	6.3	7.4	100	367
1985	NA	53.3	NA	12.2	24.0	5.8	4.7	100	762
1986	NA	51.4	NA	12.5	26.0	4.4	5.6	100	1,375
1987	NA	53.1	NA	12.0	26.1	3.5	5.3	100	2,338
1988	NA	51.0	NA	10.0	29.1	3.5	6.4	100	3,016
1989[d]	NA	49.8	NA	7.1	30.4	3.9	8.9	100	2,466
All years	NA	51.7	NA	10.3	27.2	4.1	6.7	100	10,611

[a]IVDU: intravenous drug use. [b]Pattern II refers to individuals immigrating from those countries in central, eastern, and southern Africa and some Caribbean countries where the majority of cases are ascribed to heterosexual transmission. The male-to-female ratio is approximately 1:1 in these countries; perinatal transmission is more common than in other areas, and intravenous drug use and homosexual transmission occur at a very low level. [c]This category includes cases currently under investigation for which no history of exposure has yet been reported and cases for which no exposure mode could ever be determined. [d]The 1989 figures include only cases reported through December 31, 1989. All data shown in this table are subject to delays in reporting. Therefore, counts of cases diagnosed in a particular year may understate the number that will ultimately be reported. This type of understatement is particularly likely for cases diagnosed in 1988 and 1989. [e]NA: not applicable.

SOURCE: Computed from CDC's AIDS Public Information Data Set for AIDS cases reported through December 31, 1989.

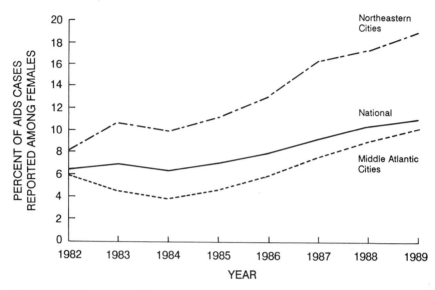

FIGURE 1-2 Percentages of reported AIDS cases diagnosed among females, 1982–1989. (Tabulation includes only cases diagnosed among persons aged 13 and older.) NOTE: Cities in the Northeast region include the OMB Metropolitan Statistical Areas (or New England County Metropolitan Areas) of Bergen-Passaic, N.J.; Buffalo, N.Y.; Boston, Mass.; Hartford, Conn.; Nassau-Suffolk, N.J.; New York City; and Newark, N.J. Cities in the Mid-Atlantic region include Baltimore, Md.; Norfolk, Va.; Philadelphia, Pa.; Pittsburgh, Pa.; and Washington, D.C. SOURCE: Tabulated from CDC's AIDS Public Information Data Set for AIDS cases reported through December 31, 1989.

exposure to contaminated blood as their only risk factor. This route of transmission accounts for only a small proportion of all AIDS cases, but it accounts for a greater proportion of AIDS cases among women than among men, a finding that is related to gender differences in the distribution of cases across transmission categories. Because all blood donors are now screened for risk factors and all donations are screened for antibodies to HIV, the decline in transfusion-related new infections that has been seen over the course of the epidemic is expected to continue. However, there remain a number of AIDS-related blood supply issues that are discussed in more detail in Chapter 5 of this report.

Although the number of new AIDS cases related to contaminated blood is expected to continue to diminish, the impact of past exposures on the immediate future is uncertain because no one knows the number of individuals who are already infected with HIV. Unfortunately, some estimates suggest that a substantial portion of the hemophiliac population is infected.[18] Women who have sexual contact with male hemophiliacs are

---

[18] Of the estimated 20,000 hemophiliacs in the United States (National Hemophilia Foundation, 1988),

thus at indirect risk of acquiring HIV infection. (Because very few women have coagulation disorders, they have little direct risk of blood-related infection.) Small surveys of female sexual partners of hemophiliac men have found between 0 and 21 percent to be infected (Kim et al., 1988; Ragni et al., 1988; Smiley et al., 1988; Lawrence et al., 1989;1990). In addition, women who have received needle-stick injuries while helping to administer clotting factor treatments to an infected male partner may also be at risk (Smiley et al., 1988).[19]

The AIDS case data thus present a picture of emerging risk for women, one that is strengthened by recently available seroprevalence data on HIV infection in this population. CDC and the National Institutes of Health (NIH) are currently conducting a neonatal survey throughout the United States that takes a small part of the dried blood samples collected from hospital-born babies for metabolic disease testing and tests them for antibodies to HIV. Because newborns carry the mother's HIV antibodies (if present), seroprevalence rates derived from this survey can be projected to the population of childbearing women.[20] Forty-four states, as well as the District of Columbia and Puerto Rico, currently participate in statewide surveys of newborns. Thus far, preliminary data have been aggregated for 18 states and territories in four regions of the country; state-specific data have also been reported for selected states.

Rates of infection are highest in the Northeast and in the southern region and approach 0.7 and 0.5 percent, respectively, of cases among childbearing women in those areas.[21] Data aggregated at this level, however, do not clearly reflect the considerable variation in rates across the country. For example, pockets of "alarming HIV infection"[22] are found

---

Jackson and colleagues (1988) speculate that 15,000 may be infected with HIV; Mason, Olson, and Parish (1988) have estimated that 92 percent of people with hemophilia A, the most common form of the disease, are infected.

[19] In a survey of 32 hemophiliac couples, one woman who seroconverted (i.e., her antibody status changed from negative to positive) reported eight needle-stick injuries she had incurred while helping her spouse with clotting factor treatments (Smiley et al., 1988).

[20] It is important to note, however, that not all infants found to have antibodies for HIV will remain antibody positive. Moreover, not all women at risk for HIV infection will be captured by this survey. Specifically, this group will not include women who choose not to have children, those who cannot have children, women who choose abortion or who miscarry prior to delivery, and postmenopausal women (Turner, Miller, and Moses, 1989).

[21] Seroprevalence rates ranged from 0.03 to 0.66 percent nationally and regionally as follows: 0.03 to 0.66 percent for different locations in the Northeast, 0.09 to 0.46 percent in the South, 0.06 to 0.09 percent in the north central region, and 0.03 to 0.04 percent in the mountain zone (Pappaioanou et al., 1989).

[22] In his article, "One in 61 Babies in New York City Has AIDS Antibodies, Study Says," Bruce

among women of childbearing age in New York City; the rate of infection among women giving birth in this city is 1.7 percent.[23] Palm Beach County, Florida, has reported rates of slightly more than 1 percent among women delivering infants, but the rate in Duval County (which includes Jacksonville, Florida) is very much lower (0.28 percent) (Withum et al., 1989).

Both AIDS case data (see Table 1-3) amd neonatal seroprevalence rates reflect the differential risk of AIDS among minority women.[24] Among births in New York City, racial and ethnic trends are striking: 2.17 percent of black, 1.46 percent of Hispanic, and 0.39 percent of white newborns were found to have antibodies to HIV (Novick et al., 1989).[25] Disproportionate rates of infection among black and Hispanic women have been seen in other parts of the country as well.[26]

An association has been noted between IV drug use and the risk of HIV infection for a substantial portion of pregnant women and their babies.[27] In New York City, the neonatal seroprevalence rate was 2.2

Lambert reviewed the New York neonatal data for the *New York Times* (January 13, 1988, pp. A1 and B4). The state health commissioner was quoted as saying "results in the first 19,157 newborn blood specimens demonstrate an alarming HIV infection rate among women of childbearing age in New York City."

[23] Data from 276,609 consecutive births that occurred in New York between November 1987 and November 1988 showed substantially higher rates of HIV infection in New York City (1.25 percent) than in upstate New York (0.16 percent) (Novick et al., 1989). Moreover, there is substantial variation in infection rates within New York City. The highest rate was found in the Bronx (1.7 percent), followed by Manhattan (1.65 percent), Brooklyn (1.31 percent), Staten Island (0.68 percent), and Queens (0.62 percent) (Novick et al., 1989). A survey of 3,556 women giving birth and having abortions in New York City in 1987 and 1988 found that rates for both groups had stabilized (i.e., the rates demonstrated statistically insignificant fluctuations over this period of time) (Araneta et al., 1989). In this study, women between the ages of 25 and 29 had seroprevalence rates of 1.89 and 2.17 percent (for 1987 and 1988, respectively). Among Medicaid recipients, the rates for the two years were 3.36 and 2.31 percent.

[24] Black women account for 51.7 percent of all AIDS cases diagnosed among women, and Hispanic women account for an additional 20.0 percent of cases. However, blacks and Hispanics constitute only 11 percent and 8 percent of the U.S. population, respectively (U.S. Bureau of the Census, 1987).

[25] Statewide rates of infection in New York show similar disproportions: 1.8 percent for black, 1.3 percent for Hispanic, and 0.13 percent for white newborns (Novick et al., 1989).

[26] Data from 65,007 infants born in Florida between July and December 1988 indicated that 1.2 percent of black babies were seropositive, whereas only 0.17 percent of white infants had circulating HIV antibody (Withum et al., 1989). In Texas, black infants accounted for 48.1 percent of all positive tests even though blacks constituted only 12.8 percent of all specimens tested (Thompson et al., 1989). Hispanics were not differentially represented among positive specimens from Texas: 14.8 percent of seropositive infants were Hispanic, but 28.3 percent of the specimens came from Hispanic babies.

[27] Among female AIDS cases attributed to heterosexual contact, 51 percent of whites, 57 percent of blacks, and 83 percent of Latinas reported unprotected sex with an IV drug user as their risk factor

TABLE 1-3 Distribution of AIDS Cases Reported Through December 31, 1989, Among Women Aged 13 Years and Older by Exposure Category and Ethnic Group

Exposure Category	White	Black	Hispanic	Other[a]	Total
IV drug use					
N	1,175	3,171	1,110	35	5,491
%	21.4	57.7	20.2	0.6	100.0
Heterosexual					
N	781	1,297	769	36	2,883
%	27.1	45.0	26.7	1.2	100.0
Blood					
N	733	213	119	25	1,090
%	67.2	19.5	10.9	2.3	100.0
Pattern II[b]					
N	1	433	2	3	439
%	0.2	98.6	0.5	0.7	100.0
Other risk[c]					
N	200	374	119	15	708
%	28.2	52.8	16.8	2.1	100.0
Total cases					
N	2,890	5,488	2,119	114	10,611
%	27.2	51.7	20.0	1.1	100.0

[a] This category includes Asians and Pacific Islanders, American Indians, Alaskan natives, and persons whose race or ethnicity is unknown. [b] Pattern II refers to individuals immigrating from those countries in central, eastern, and southern Africa and some Caribbean countries where the majority of cases are ascribed to heterosexual transmission. The male-to-female ratio is approximately 1:1 in these countries, perinatal transmission is more common than in other areas, and intravenous drug use and homosexual transmission occur at a very low level. [c] This category includes cases currently under investigation for which no history of exposure has yet been reported and cases for which no exposure mode could ever be determined.

SOURCE: Computed from CDC's AIDS Public Information Data Set for AIDS cases reported through December 31, 1989.

percent for ZIP Code areas with drug abuse rates (as determined by drug-related hospital discharge data) in the top quartile of the distribution for the city;[28] the rate in the remainder of the city's ZIP Code areas was 0.8 percent (Novick et al., 1989). In New Jersey, the rates of seropositivity

---

(CDC, 1990a). In a survey of 165 couples, black and Latina women were more likely than whites to report an intravenous drug user as their index case (Padian et al., 1989).

[28] Indeed, more than half of the seropositive newborns resided in ZIP Code areas that fell within the top quartile of the drug use statistics for the city (Novick et al., 1989).

among newborns were highest in the two counties with the highest AIDS case rates and the largest portion of cases related to IV drug use (1.58 and 1.27 percent in the two counties versus a statewide rate of 0.49 percent) (Altman et al., 1989).

Smaller serologic surveys show geographic variability in the distribution of HIV infection, a pattern that lends additional weight to the evidence provided by actual AIDS cases. Specifically, pockets of high seroprevalence rates and the strong association between HIV infection and IV drug use have been reported by large and small serologic surveys as well as national surveillance data on AIDS cases (see Table 1-4). Five of the six studies in Table 1-4 that report seroprevalence rates of 10 percent or greater are based on samples of female intravenous drug users.[29] It is difficult to draw conclusions from these studies, however, because of various methodological constraints.[30]

Seroprevalence studies of female applicants for military service and women on active and reserve duty in the U.S. Army provide another view of the pattern of infection in a large population of women.[31] Since October 1985, 383,112 women have been tested by the military for antibodies to HIV. The crude seroprevalence rates in these groups were 0.7 percent for female applicants, 0.9 percent for women on active duty, and 0.8 percent for women in the reserves (Cowan et al., 1989; Horton, Alexander, and Brundage, 1989). In each group, the seroprevalence rates among teenage females were comparable to those for teenage males. Gender parity in infection rates for this population is a very different pattern than that seen

---

[29] Johnson et al. (1987); Chandrasekar, Matthews, and Chandrasekar (1988); Brown et al. (1989); Schoenbaum et al. (1989); and Wolfe et al. (1989).

[30] For further discussion of methodological problems related to convenience samples, see Turner, Miller, and Moses (1989). Comparisons across these studies are also problematic because samples were recruited from different organizations and locations, and each sample displayed considerable heterogeneity with respect to age, race, and risk behaviors among the women enrolled in the studies. Variable participation rates and potentially significant differences between participants and nonparticipants make these results extremely difficult to interpret. For example, in a study of 7,400 women who delivered babies at a Miami hospital between July and December 1988, 93 percent consented to HIV testing, and 2.3 percent of those who consented were found to be infected (O'Sullivan et al., 1989). Of the 274 women who refused testing, blinded blood specimens were assayed, and the infection rate for this group was found to be 4.9 percent. This substantial difference in prevalence rates between consenters and nonconsenters indicates an important source of bias and calls into question the accuracy of estimates that have relied exclusively on volunteer samples. It should be noted however, that the direction of the bias has not always resulted in higher rates in blinded samples. See, for example, Chiasson and colleagues, 1990.

[31] It should be understood, however, that this population is not representative of the national female population.

TABLE 1-4 Seroprevalence Rates Among Women Derived from Samples of Convenience Drawn from Varied Settings

State/City or Area	Study Period	Setting[a]	Percent HIV+	No. HIV+/ No. Tested	Reference
California					
Orange County	3/85 to 11/88	Prison	3.0	53/1,781	Prendergast et al. (1989)
Alameda County	11/85 to 8/86	Premarital	0.53	2/377	Del Tempelis et al. (1987)
		STD	0.67	2/299	
San Diego	1/87 to 1/88	Prenatal (U.S. Navy)	0.56	3/532	Harrison and Moore (1988)[b]
San Francisco	1988	MM/DTX	10.6	32/303	Wolfe et al. (1989)
Los Angeles	3/88 to 9/88	FPC	0.13	4/2,968	Fehrs et al. (1989)
Los Angeles	9/88 to 12/88	Obstetric	0.04	3/7,186	Hill et al. (1989)
Los Angeles	Begun 1/89	Prenatal	0.6	1/170	Cozen et al. (1989)
Colorado					
Denver	1988	ATS	1.9	4/208	Cohn et al. (1989)[c]
		STD	1.9	4/212	
		MM	2.5	1/40	
		Street	1.7	1/59	
Florida					
Belle Glade	2/86 to 9/86	Community	3.0	12/403	Castro et al. (1987)
Jacksonville	12/86 to 3/87	Prenatal	0.67	2/299	Kaunitz et al. (1987)
Georgia					
Atlanta	12/85 to 7/87	Prenatal	5.7	29/513	Lindsay et al. (1989)

continued

TABLE 1-4 Continued

State/City or Area	Study Period	Setting[a]	Percent HIV+	No. HIV+/ No. Tested	Reference
Louisiana					
New Orleans	5/88 to 12/88	Prenatal	0.5	20/3,846	McFarland et al. (1989)
Maryland					
Baltimore	1986 – 1987	Prenatal	29.6	34/115	Johnson et al. (1987)[d]
Baltimore	2/87 to 4/87	STD	2.8	37/1,310	Quinn et al. (1988)
Baltimore	2/87 to 1/89	Prenatal	4.1	34/824	Barbacci et al. (1989)
Michigan					
Detroit	NA	IVDU in hospital	21.7	5/23	Chandrasekar et al. (1988)[e]
Minnesota	7/85 to 7/86	ATS	0.8	5/638	Danila et al. (1987)
New Jersey					
Newark	9/87 to 9/88	Obstetric	4.4	98/2,205	Connor et al. (1989)
New Mexico					
Albuquerque	3/87 to 5/87	STD	0	0/429	Hull et al. (1988)
New York					
New York City	10/86 to 7/87	Prenatal	16.0	4/25[f]	Krasinski et al. (1988)
		Obstetric	2.35	28/1,192	
Brooklyn	12/86 to 1/87	Obstetric	2.0	12/602	Landesman et al. (1987)
Bronx	6/85 to 4/86	MM	37.4	82/219	Schoenbaum et al. (1989)

Location	Dates	Site	Percent	Ratio	Reference
Bronx	2/88 to 10/88	Sentinel hospital[g]	4.1	70/1,695	Ernst et al. (1989)
Brooklyn and Manhattan	1987	MM	54.0	NA/78	Brown et al. (1989)
New York City	11/87 to 1/88	Obstetric	2.7	6/224	Sperling et al. (1989)
North Carolina Central	5/88 to 10/88	STD	0.5	NA[h]	Landis et al. (1989)
Pennsylvania Western	4/86 to 4/87	FPC	0	0/433	Valdiserri et al. (1988)
Philadelphia	NA	Obstetric	0	0/366	Armson, et al. (1988)
Rhode Island Providence	6/85 to 2/87	ATS	4.1	9/218	Brondum et al. (1987)

[a] ATS: alternate test site; community: community-based seroepidemiological study; DTX: detoxification program; FPC: family planning clinic; MM: methadone maintenance clinic; NA: not available; premarital: premarital screening clinic; STD: sexually transmitted disease clinic; and street: indigenous outreach to intravenous drug users (IVDUs) not in treatment. [b] The study by Harrison and Moore (1988) in San Diego was conducted at a U.S. naval hospital prenatal clinic. [c] The study by Cohn and coworkers (1989) in Colorado reports statistics for prostitutes and heterosexual women. These figures were combined in this table. [d] In this sample, 90 percent of women reported intravenous drug use and 10 percent were sexual partners of IVDUs. [e] The study by Chandrasekar and colleagues (1988) in Detroit involved IVDUs hospitalized for non-HIV-related illnesses. [f] Four of 25 women with identified risk factors. [g] The sentinel hospital is the Bronx Lebanon Hospital reported in Ernst and coworkers (1989). [h] The preliminary findings reported by Landis and coworkers (1989) are based on 1,440 blood samples collected from male and female patients attending an STD clinic. The final sample consists of blood from 3,124 consecutive patients, 55 percent of whom are males.

with AIDS case data[32] and indicates that, for some populations, women will be bearing a larger share of the AIDS burden in the future. For all age groups in the military surveillance data, the rates of HIV infection were highest for black women.

These epidemiological data outline a picture of increasing risk of HIV infection for subsets of women, in particular, minority women and women who are directly (through their own IV drug use) or indirectly (through their sexual partner's drug use) at risk because of drug-related exposure to the virus. Yet, the data on AIDS case distributions and HIV infection give only a profile of risk in this population. A more complete picture, one that provides a sense of depth and breadth, must include a sense of who these women are, how they live, and how they have come to be at risk for this disease. Unfortunately, as in many other areas of understanding related to the epidemic, information about these groups and the patterns of behavior that spread the virus—information crucial to the design of efficacious interventions—is limited, although the base of knowledge is growing. The sections below present what is now known about several subsets of the population of women at risk for HIV infection.

Women Who Inject Drugs

Of the women at risk for HIV infection, those who are exposed directly and indirectly (see the next section) to IV drug use have been shown to be particularly vulnerable. A small body of research provides some information about the women who inject drugs and the social environments in which they live. For example, a subset of women injectors report a history of physical and sexual abuse (Weiner, Kaltenbach, and Finnegan, 1989; Worth et al., 1989). Indeed, as Worth and her coworkers reported in an ethnographic study of 96 female intravenous drug users from the South Bronx, drug-related violence and illegal activities often characterize the relationships of these women with their sexual partners. Sowder, Weissman, and Young analyzed preliminary data from ongoing NIDA demonstration projects[33] targeting women at risk for HIV infection

---

[32] The ratio of male-to-female AIDS cases diagnosed among adolescents and adults was 14.7:1 in 1982 and 8.6:1 in 1988.

[33] The National AIDS Demonstration Research Project, sponsored by the National Institute on Drug Abuse (NIDA), is providing interventions at 63 sites throughout the United States and Puerto Rico, and on the U.S.-Mexican border. These interventions are designed to change risk-associated behaviors and sustain healthier lifestyles, as well as to provide referral to drug treatment and other needed health and social services. The intervention efforts also seek to collect data to evaluate the effectiveness of interventions and to understand the sociodemographic characteristics, lifestyles, and risk behaviors of targeted women (Sowder, Weissman, and Young, 1989).

and found that many women who inject drugs are poorly educated and depend on illegal sources of income or government programs for their livelihood (Sowder, Weissman, and Young, 1989).[34] In addition, several small ethnographic studies of female injectors have found high rates of unemployment, unstable housing, and homelessness (Watters, 1988; Weiner, Kaltenbach, and Finnegan, 1989). It is no surprise, therefore, that many women injectors report that they feel powerless and lack control over their lives.

Many women report that they are introduced to drug injection by a male sexual partner or family member (Chambers, Hinesley, and Moldestad, 1970; Chambers and Moffitt, 1970; Eldred and Washington, 1976; Gerstein, Judd, and Rovner, 1979; Worth and Rodriguez, 1987). Unfortunately, our understanding of the process by which women become injectors is incomplete. Regardless of how the process starts, once women begin to inject, they may engage in the behavior that puts other injectors at risk—namely, the sharing of injection equipment with drug users who may be infected with the AIDS virus.[35] Sharing may occur in a variety of contexts: with friends or family members, within a couple, with "running buddies," in "shooting galleries," or using rented "works" from the drug dealer (Turner, Miller, and Moses, 1989:Ch. 3).[36] Preliminary data from the NIDA-sponsored multisite study of female IV drug users indicate that the majority of women who report injecting drugs have shared injection equipment and rented or borrowed equipment in the past (Sowder,

---

[34] Of the women ($N = 1,229$) participating in a NIDA demonstration projects on which Sowder, Weissman, and Young (1989) reported, fewer than half graduated from high school. Among intravenous drug users in the projects ($N = 736$), 31 percent relied on illegal sources of income, and 28 percent received their major income from government programs. Among women who did not inject drugs but who were sexual partners of IV drug users ($N = 493$), 9 percent relied on illegal sources of income, and 41 percent relied on government programs (Sowder, Weissman, and Young, 1989).

[35] The degree of risk is also associated with the duration of drug use and the frequency of injection; the drug used (some drugs, such as cocaine, have a relatively short-lived effect and are therefore injected more frequently); the number of other people who have shared the injection equipment; seroprevalence rates in the local intravenous drug-using community; and the method of injection. For example, sharing injection equipment that has been used to "boot" drugs (i.e., to draw blood back into the syringe while the needle is still in the vein to pulse the amount of drug being delivered and to extract the maximum amount of drug from the syringe) is riskier than using separate, sterile injection equipment but sharing a cooker.

[36] "Running buddies" are colleagues with whom drug users may pass recreational time and share drugs and injection equipment; running buddies may also be sexual partners. "Shooting galleries" are communal injection sites that are often found in large cities. "Works" are the IV drug user's injection paraphernalia, at least five elements of which carry the potential for contamination. For a more complete discussion, see Turner, Miller, and Moses (1989:189–195).

Weissman, and Young, 1989).[37] Newcomers to intravenous drug use are unlikely to have their own equipment; therefore, they often employ the works of a more experienced user for their initial injection.[38] Women may also seek assistance with injections, depending on male partners, a female friend, or a "doc" (someone who specializes in injecting others and is often paid with part of the drug being injected) to inject them (Rosenbaum, 1981).

Sharing may be encouraged by drug withdrawal. Often as addicted injectors find themselves experiencing withdrawal symptoms, the desire to inject becomes stronger. Reducing the time between the purchase of the drug and its injection may assume great urgency; as a result, addicts in withdrawal may be unusually likely to rent a dealer's works or use a nearby shooting gallery (Mandell, Vlahov, and Cohn, 1989). Although it is difficult to estimate precisely the number of female IV drug users and the distribution of risk-associated behaviors, there appears to be sufficient evidence to state that the injection practices of most female IV drug users leave them vulnerable to HIV infection.

HIV transmission through sexual behaviors is also a risk for women who inject drugs. Small surveys that have included female injectors have found that significant proportions report risk-associated behaviors, including multiple sex partners and unprotected intercourse (Snyder and Myers, 1989; Tross et al., 1989; Whittaker et al., 1989). In interviews with 736 female injectors who are participating in the NIDA demonstration project, 38 percent reported two or more sex partners who injected drugs, and 83 percent stated that they never or rarely used condoms (Sowder, Weissman, and Young, 1989). A separate survey of IV drug users recruited from the streets of Long Beach, California (110 of whom were women), found that approximately one-third of the sample (38 percent) reported that they had engaged in prostitution or had exchanged sex for drugs (Corby, Rhodes, and Wolitski, 1989). As noted earlier, the use of crack may increase the risk for women of acquiring HIV infection through sexual behaviors; indeed, crack use may be an especially important risk

---

[37] Of the 736 women with a history of IV drug use who are participating in the National AIDS Demonstration Research Project, 93 percent have shared needles, 71 percent have shared injection equipment with two or more partners, and 76 percent have used borrowed or rented needles (Sowder, Weissman, and Young, 1989). Other studies confirm the risk these behaviors pose to women. In a small survey of 220 female IV drug users recruited from methadone and detoxification programs in the San Francisco area, sharing needles with more than 10 partners over the past year was associated with HIV infection (Wolfe et al., 1989).

[38] Des Jarlais, Friedman, and Strug (1986) note that almost all injectors share needles at some point in their drug use career.

factor among women who inject drugs.[39] Several studies have shown an association between crack use in women (injectors and noninjectors) and higher levels of both unprotected sex and seropositivity.[40] These findings, as well as the documented practice of women exchanging sex for crack, point to the need for further study of this relatively new drug-related risk pattern.

As is true for any woman of childbearing age who is at risk of becoming infected, women who inject drugs have the potential to transmit HIV vertically to their offspring. Stereotypical depictions of IV drug users do not usually include a family and children. Yet most of the female drug users who have been recruited for studies through treatment programs have children (Brown et al., 1989; Wolfe et al., 1989).[41] IV drug users are reputed to be ineffective or inconsistent users of contraception (Ralph and Spigner, 1986). However, recent data from interviews with female IV drug users indicate that women who were uncertain about wanting children tended to employ safer sex practices (Tross et al., 1989). These data suggest the possibility that behaviors usually labeled as risk taking (i.e., unprotected vaginal intercourse) may not necessarily reflect relapse from condom use in some segments of the IV drug-using population but rather a desire for children.

Vertical transmission of HIV would also appear to be an issue for the female partners of male IV drug users. Yet the parameters of the problem in this subset of women are unknown because there are few available data on many aspects of these women's lives. The next section discusses

---

[39] Intravenous drug use does not preclude the use of noninjectable substances, such as cocaine or crack. In fact, the use of multiple drugs (so-called polydrug use) is the norm rather than the exception for some samples of female injectors (Weiner, Kaltenbach, and Finnegan, 1989). In Sowder, Weissman, and Young's (1989) sample of 736 female IV drug users, almost half (46 percent) smoked or inhaled cocaine on less than a daily basis; an additional quarter (24 percent) used noninjectable cocaine daily. Sixteen percent reported daily use of marijuana, and 31 percent reported daily use of alcohol. Abramowitz and coworkers (1989) report a dramatic and statistically significant increase in crack use since 1986 among drug users seeking treatment in San Francisco.

[40] Of 303 female IV drug users recruited from drug treatment programs in San Francisco, 84 (27.7 percent) reported that they had used crack in the past 30 days, and crack use displayed a significant association with seropositivity (Wolfe et al., 1989). A separate study of New York City women seeking care for pelvic inflammatory disease (of whom approximately 8 percent injected drugs) found that more than half (51 percent) reported crack use (Hoegsberg et al., 1989). Moreover, crack users had twice as many sexual partners as nonusers and were more likely to be infected with HIV.

[41] In a study of the medical records of 593 women participating in a methadone maintenance program in Brooklyn and Manhattan in 1987, Brown and coworkers (1989) found that these women reported a total of 2,298 pregnancies, which resulted in 2.51 live births and 1.37 abortions per woman. In each age group that was studied, black and Hispanic women on average reported more pregnancies and live births and fewer abortions than white women.

the limited information available on this group and delineates, as far as is possible, the risk profile of these women.

Female Sexual Partners of IV Drug Users

The population of female sex partners of IV drug users has been a difficult population to study and reach with prevention programs because these women are not readily identifiable, they do not belong to any unifying social group, and they may have very unstable living conditions. Although there has been only limited research on this group, service providers, law enforcement officials, and the drug users themselves indicate that the population is quite diverse with respect to race, ethnicity, education, and income (Arguelles et al., 1989). Some researchers have suggested that many female sexual partners of men who inject drugs do not themselves use drugs intravenously (Des Jarlais et al., 1984; Murphy, 1987)[42] and therefore are not at direct risk of acquiring HIV from this mode of transmission. They may, however, use noninjectable drugs, such as alcohol or marijuana, which may, like crack, increase their risk of acquiring HIV through sexual transmission.

Preliminary ethnographic data on this group of women raise another disturbing possibility in relation to their increased risk of acquiring HIV through sexual transmission. Some women who do not use drugs are ignorant of their partner's injection practices;[43] others may not be able or willing to acknowledge this behavior (Weissman, 1988). Indeed, women may fear the confrontation that might ensue if such practices were openly recognized. Alternatively, male drug users may take pains to prevent their female sex partners from knowing about their drug use. Without knowledge of their partners' risky practices, these women may perceive their risk as unrealistically low, and there will be little likelihood that they will consider protective action. A survey of 62 female sexual partners of IV drug users found a positive association between the women's perception of risk for HIV infection and an awareness of the needle-sharing practices of their partners (Wermuth and Ham, 1989). In this small study, the perception of risk did not differentiate women who used condoms from those who did not (preventive action in the group was predicated instead on knowing the partner's seropositive status). Nevertheless, theories of health behavior indicate that such a perception

---

[42] Almost half (42 percent) of 325 IV drug users interviewed in Long Beach, California reported having sexual partners who did not use IV drugs (Corby, Rhodes, and Wolitski, 1989).

[43] In a survey of 325 IV drug users recruited from the streets of Long Beach, California, 18 percent indicated that their partner did not know of their drug use (Corby, Rhodes, and Wolitski, 1989).

is important in beginning to motivate the behavioral change process.[44] The findings of this study emphasize the crucial need for data on these populations to design effective interventions to fight the spread of the epidemic.

Female Sexual Partners of Male Hemophiliacs and Transfusion Recipients

Women who engage in unprotected intercourse with men who have become infected through exposure to contaminated blood are themselves at risk of acquiring HIV infection, although the exact extent of the risk is not known. As of December 1989, 48 current or former heterosexual partners of hemophilic men had been diagnosed with AIDS; an additional 59 reported cases among women were ascribed to sexual contact with a transfusion recipient (CDC, 1990a).[45] The total number of women who have acquired infection in this manner is not known with any certainty; a number of small surveys have generated widely ranging estimates of HIV prevalence in this population.[46] Methodological limitations of these studies make it difficult to interpret the findings: most have relied on small samples of volunteers, and much of the data has been gathered from limited geographic areas. Women participants in these studies have varied with respect to symptoms, infection, contraceptive methods, frequency and duration of sexual contact with an infected partner, and other risk-associated behaviors.

The factors that contribute to transmission of the AIDS virus in discordant heterosexual couples (i.e., couples in which only one partner is known to be infected) are uncertain.[47] It is clear, however, that

---

[44] For further information on motivating health behavior changes, see Chapter 4 in Turner, Miller, and Moses (1989).

[45] It is not possible to calculate prevalence rates for this population because the total number of women who have had sexual contact with hemophilic men is not known. Jackson and colleagues (1988) have estimated that 15,000 hemophiliacs in the United States received large-pool, non-heat-treated factor VIII or factor IX concentrates. This number includes individuals of all ages, but virtually all are males.

[46] CDC estimates that between 10 and 60 percent of the spouses and sexual partners of hemophiliacs may have become infected through unprotected sexual intercourse (CDC, 1987). Some researchers have speculated that women who are symptomatic may be more inclined to volunteer for research programs, thus leading to high seroprevalence rates in some studies (Lawrence et al., 1989, 1990). A national telephone survey of physicians and hemophilia treatment centers found that, among the 34 percent of female heterosexual partners of hemophiliacs who were tested for HIV infection, 10 percent were positive. A review of 11 other studies of heterosexual partners of hemophiliacs conducted in the United States found seroprevalence rates between 0 and 21 percent (Lawrence et al., 1990). Between January 1988 and September 1989, 667 partners of hemophiliacs sought testing and counseling through programs supported by CDC; 34 (5.1 percent) were seropositive (CDC, 1990b).

[47] Transmission may require active viral replication—that is, the infection must have progressed to the

risk-associated behaviors are reported by these couples to varying degrees. Few female partners of infected hemophilic men appear to be celibate,[48] and, despite the risk of sexually transmitted HIV infection, many couples do not use condoms consistently.[49] It is unclear why such risk taking has not led to a greater level of infection in this population. When the only reported risk factor is unprotected vaginal intercourse, it appears that seroconversion rates among the female sexual partners of infected hemophiliacs are generally low (Brettler et al., 1988; Kim et al., 1988; Ragni et al., 1988; Jackson et al., 1989). Yet despite the incomplete understanding of the association between risk and infection in this population, the committee would emphasize that repeated exposure through unprotected intercourse can and does lead to infection among female sex partners of infected men (Lawrence et al., 1990). With consistent protection, however, transmission among discordant couples can be avoided.[50]

---

point at which HIV can be isolated from serum (Laurian, Peynet, and Verroust, 1989)—or immunologic deficiencies in the infected partner (Smiley et al., 1988). The frequency of sexual intercourse and the appropriate and consistent use of condoms may also affect the likelihood of transmission to the uninfected partner, but there are no data supporting their contributions, if any, at least at present. In fact, the available data show no difference in either frequency of coitus or condom use between seroconverters and nonconverters (Ragni et al., 1988), nor does the rate of other genital infections differ between these two groups (Smiley et al., 1988). The lack of hard evidence on HIV prevention through condom use by such couples may also reflect their prior inconsistent use of condoms (especially during early infection), the uncertain quality of self-reported data, the small samples used in many studies, or perhaps the failure of condoms to prevent transmission (Lawrence et al., 1990). Furthermore, the evidence has been weakened by posing questions to couples that are too general to be valid or reliable or that have been worded inconsistently. The contribution of other factors is also uncertain. Anal intercourse is not required for HIV transmission in discordant heterosexual couples (Kim et al., 1988; Ragni et al., 1988; Smiley et al., 1988), nor is the co-occurrence of other sexually transmitted diseases or sex during menstrual periods (Goedert et al., 1987). However, regardless of the factors that contribute to transmission, Mason, Olson, and Parish (1988) report that the risk of infection among these couples does appear to increase with time.

[48] In two separate studies of approximately 50 female sexual partners of hemophilic men, all of the women except one individual in each study reported engaging in vaginal intercourse (anal intercourse is rarely reported in studies of hemophiliac couples) (Lawrence et al., 1990).

[49] In a study by Wilson and Wasserman (1989), for example, fewer than one-fourth (24.3 percent) of sexually active hemophilic men reported consistent condom use. A survey of 56 female sex partners of infected hemophilic men confirms this statistic. An alarming 72 percent of women whose partners were infected and symptomatic and 54 percent of women whose infected partners were asymptomatic reported that they never or rarely used condoms (Lawrence et al., 1989). Parish and colleagues (1989) also report that of 351 hemophilic men in their study, only a third reported consistent condom use. A more detailed discussion of condom use (or lack of use) appears in Chapter 2.

[50] A small cohort of women remained uninfected after five years of protected sexual contact with an infected hemophiliac partner (Goedert et al., 1987). Other studies have also demonstrated that consistent condom use can prevent infection in this population (Forsberg et al., 1989; Laurian, Peynet, and Verroust, 1989). There is no evidence that transmission occurs from intimate but nonsexual contact (Brettler et al., 1988).

The epidemiological data presented above indicate that the profile of the epidemic among women is changing. It is apparent that actual infection as well as the threat of infection is spreading to encompass wider segments of the female population. AIDS prevention efforts must now address this more diverse group in addition to the unique role of women in vertical transmission of the virus. Some of the issues related to interventions for women are discussed in the next chapter.

The epidemiological data presented earlier also indicate the dynamic, fluid quality of the epidemic among other populations and emphasize the fact that the future path of AIDS in this country is still uncertain. Despite the knowledge gained over the past decade, there are persisting gaps in understanding of the dynamics of HIV infection among all at-risk populations. The next section reviews some of the data needs for improved surveillance efforts.

TRACKING THE EPIDEMIC: DATA NEEDS

Substantial progress has been made during the first decade of the epidemic in monitoring AIDS prevalence throughout various subpopulations. A case reporting system is in place, and AIDS case data are available to researchers from CDC. As noted earlier, however, our understanding of the spread of HIV infection and the behaviors that transmit it is far from complete. The committee finds that several technical issues impinge on that understanding, including sampling techniques, completeness of reporting, data access, and standardization of items that appear in different surveys.

In general, attempts to ascertain the prevalence of HIV infection in this country have relied on small cross-sectional studies, which can provide only snapshot views of the problem in selected groups in specific locations at one point in time. Seroprevalence estimates for IV drug users, for example, often come from samples of convenience recruited through treatment programs or criminal justice agencies. Seroprevalence data for the gay male population come from a variety of sources, including smaller studies of patient populations recruited through STD clinics and HIV testing and counseling facilities. Improved data collection efforts are needed to understand the spread of HIV infection in these and other at-risk populations, including women. Such efforts should include information on the behaviors that transmit the virus as well as the prevalence of infection.

There are, however, some important exceptions to these smaller surveys. Large-scale serosurveys of military and Job Corps applicants, which are described in the chapter on adolescents, have provided information on the prevalence of infection in these special populations. In addition, large prospective studies of gay men, such as the National Institute of Allergy and Infectious Disease's Multicenter AIDS Cohort Studies (MACS), have gathered valuable data on the natural history of the disease, the prevalence of infection, and patterns of risk-associated behavior in that population.[51] (Both the military and the MACS surveys can provide additional information on the incidence of infection in their samples.) As discussed earlier, CDC's population-based serologic survey of newborn infants has generated some new and very valuable data on infection rates among childbearing women. This effort is only one of several systematic inquiries—CDC's "family" of surveys—intended to measure the prevalence of infection in potentially high-risk locations and subpopulations (e.g., clients at STD clinics, patients at certain "sentinel hospitals," college students). Unlike the neonatal survey, however, these other elements of the family of surveys were originally designed to gather data from non-population-based samples. As a result, in its earlier report, the committee recommended that the design of these surveys be augmented to use probability sampling and thus permit researchers and epidemiologists to make generalizations beyond the particular group being studied. The committee is gratified to learn that CDC has already taken steps to convert the college survey to a population-based sample and to explore similar strategies for other elements of the family of surveys.

Understanding the course of the epidemic, however, and measuring it as it moves through different populations requires attention to issues broader than sampling. Monitoring the spread of HIV and AIDS requires careful surveillance for changes both in the behaviors that transmit infection and in the manifestations of disease. As AIDS cases are diagnosed among varied subpopulations, epidemiologists have come to recognize a wide spectrum of clinical signs and symptoms that may be associated with the disease. This diversity has resulted in changes in the case definition used for surveillance purposes, which in turn has led to changes in the

---

[51] MACS cohorts of gay men were established in Chicago, Pittsburgh, Baltimore, and Los Angeles in the early years of the epidemic, as was the San Francisco Men's Health Study. Although these cohorts have provided very valuable data, they may not be representative of the larger population of men who have sex with men. For example, as Frutchey and Walsh (1989) suggest, MACS participants are volunteers who have made a long-term commitment to a research project; consequently, they may differ from the larger population in terms of motivation. In addition, the cohorts have aged and thus do not adequately represent younger men who may have different patterns of sexual behavior. The men have also been extensively counseled and studied (and as a result may have decreased their risk taking more than men who have not had similar experiences). Moreover, these cohorts provide little information about gay men living in nonurban areas or about men of different ages and cultural backgrounds.

prevalence of AIDS across risk categories. For example, the increase in AIDS cases attributed to IV drug use (noted earlier) is probably a result of an increasing number of IV drug users developing AIDS and the broader case definition established by CDC in September 1987. The original surveillance definition for AIDS was developed primarily through studies of the natural history of the disease among homosexual and bisexual men and reflected the disease as it appeared in those individuals. It is now understood that there may be very different manifestations of the underlying immune defect across risk categories, including a "wasting syndrome" and AIDS-related dementia, and these conditions are now included as criteria in the surveillance definition of AIDS.[52] Completeness of reporting is thus a complex issue in these circumstances and is likely to require continued attention as the epidemic evolves over the course of the next decade.

Monitoring changes in risk-associated behaviors that can lead to subsequent acquisition and spread of infection is also critically important. During the first decade of the epidemic, investigators who considered the risks associated with drug use focused primarily on injection practices. As the epidemic has matured, however, greater appreciation of the role of other drugs, such as crack, has emerged. At present it is not possible to predict how rapidly HIV will spread among crack users. Factors that affect the rate and extent of spread and that require monitoring include the following:

- the number of people who use crack, the frequency with which it is used, and the contexts in which it is used;
- the efficiency of heterosexual transmission of HIV from males to females and from females to males;
- the number of already-infected persons who may bring the virus to locations where sex is exchanged for crack;
- the rates of partner change among different groups of crack users;
- the extent to which syphilis and other STDs facilitate HIV

---

[52] Several studies from New York City indicate that many of the IV drug users who are dying from HIV-related illnesses have never developed Kaposi's sarcoma or an opportunistic infection, the previous criteria of the case surveillance definition of AIDS (Selwyn et al., 1988; Stoneburner et al., 1988). Recent analyses of national data find that a greater proportion of cases meeting *only* the new criteria have been reported among heterosexual IV drug users than among homosexual men and among blacks and Hispanics than among whites (Selik et al., 1990). Some researchers estimate that, if all previously unrecognized fatal illnesses associated with HIV infection were reclassified as AIDS, the number of AIDS-related deaths among IV drug users might be as much as twice the count derived from official statistics (Stoneburner et al., 1988).

transmission and the extent to which the incidence of these diseases can be controlled; and

- the extent to which crack users can adopt safer sexual practices.

It is clear that crack use and its associated unsafe sexual activity represent a potentially important new wave of HIV transmission in the United States. What is unclear is how large a wave this might be. **The committee recommends that the Public Health Service support additional research on crack use, including its epidemiology, its relationship to sexual behavior, strategies to reduce its occurrence (both initiation of use and continuance among low- and high-frequency users), and methods for facilitating change in the sexual behavior of persons who continue to use crack.** Understanding the use of crack and its role in the spread of HIV infection will require basic behavioral research, research on the social factors associated with initiating and sustaining crack use, biological research to determine effective treatment strategies, and demonstration projects to assess the effectiveness of intervention efforts.

Collecting good data regarding AIDS and HIV infection is intrinsically difficult because of the sensitivity of the subject matter and the difficulties involved in locating and studying some of the subgroups at highest risk. (The last chapter of the report is a more detailed discussion of how the quality of sensitive data can be improved.) Many researchers rely on secondary analyses of data collected by others, including agencies of the state and federal governments that are responsible for public health. Timely access to those data is sometimes constrained by policies pertaining to confidentiality as well as by other data release regulations. Moreover, it is often difficult to compare data across data sources. For example, in the CDC serologic survey of newborn infants, the data collected on the sociodemographic characteristics of the mother vary from state to state, precluding comparisons. In addition, in those states that only collect limited sociodemographic information, efforts by state and local public health agencies to design and implement programs and services may be constrained by a lack of data on the subgroups who need attention. Mathematical models hold some promise for improving our understanding of the course of the epidemic and thus for planning the delivery of programs and services. However, shortcomings in existing data on the prevalence and distribution of risk-associated behaviors and

HIV infection, on the natural history of the disease,[53] and on other factors relevant to the spread of infection currently limit the use of such models.

Improving data quality for all populations will require a wide range of additional efforts. In some instances (e.g., studies of adult gay men), improvement will demand that new and younger cohorts be recruited as part of ongoing efforts to understand the disease's natural history and changing patterns of risk. For drug users, improvements in data quality will require innovative sampling strategies, modification of existing surveillance approaches, and attention to the appearance of new drugs whose use may pose additional risk to this population. Progress is needed in several other areas as well, including improving the quality of data from sites currently collecting information on the prevalence of infection and risk behaviors (e.g., STD clinics), resolving interjurisdictional problems of confidentiality and data release, and establishing mechanisms for determining what information to obtain in each survey (e.g., how much detail to elicit concerning mothers in the neonatal surveys or patients in surveys conducted in STD clinics).

Improving data quality is vital to improving our capacity to monitor the movement of the epidemic. It is also essential for evaluating the impact of intervention efforts to halt the spread of HIV infection. As the agency within the Public Health Service with primary responsibility for collecting surveillance data, CDC instituted data collection programs in the first decade of the epidemic, targeting diverse at-risk populations. The dynamic nature of the epidemic, however, mandates continuing attention to these programs to ensure that relevant subgroups are being monitored. Thus, **to facilitate the Centers for Disease Control's (CDC) ongoing efforts to improve its AIDS-related data collection systems, the committee recommends that the agency initiate a systematic review of current programs. This effort should draw on the expertise of both CDC staff and outside experts.**

In summary, sound epidemiological data are important in developing accurate and detailed pictures of at-risk populations. The finer the grain of these pictures, the more useful they become. Depictions that can distinguish subgroups at varying levels of risk and that can detect changing risk patterns are vital in directing intervention resources to those in greatest need; they are also essential to the development of relevant intervention programs and to the evaluation of these programs.[54] Having

---

[53] As noted earlier, prospective studies of large cohorts of gay men (e.g., the MACS) have provided valuable information on the natural history of the disease—for this population. Unfortunately, less is known about the natural history of the disease in other populations, such as adolescents and women.

[54] For more information on program evaluation, see the recent report of the committee's Panel on the

identified and characterized the problem, insofar as the data permit, the committee turns to the question of what should be done. The next chapter reviews intervention strategies for populations at risk and discusses the barriers that may impede their implementation.

REFERENCES

Abramowitz, A., Guydish, J., Woods, W., and Clark, W. (1989) Increasing crack use among drug users in an AIDS epicenter: San Francisco. Presented at the Fifth International Conference on AIDS, Montreal, June 4–9.

Altman, R., Grant, C. M., Brandon, D., Shahied, S., Rappaport, E., et al. (1989) Statewide HIV-1 serologic survey of newborns with resultant changes in screening and delivery system policy. Presented at the Fifth International Conference on AIDS, Montreal, June 4–9.

Araneta, M. R. G., Thomas, P. A., Ramirez, L. L., Weisfuse, I., and Schultz, S. (1989) No change in HIV-1 seroprevalence among parturients and women having induced abortions in New York City, 1987–1988. Presented at the Fifth International Conference on AIDS, Montreal, June 4–9.

Arguelles, L., Rivero, A. M., Reback, C. J., and Corby, N. H. (1989) Female sex partners of IV drug users: A study of socio-psychological characteristics and needs. Presented at the Fifth International AIDS Conference, Montreal, June 4–9.

Armson, B. A., Mennuti, M. T., and Talbot, G. H. (1988) Seroprevalence of human immunodeficiency virus (HIV) in an obstetric population. Presented at the Fourth International Conference on AIDS, Stockholm, June 12–16.

Atkinson, W., Troxler, S., Dal Corso, M., and McFarland, L. (1989) Intravenous drug use as a risk factor for AIDS and HIV infection in Louisiana, 1981–1988. Presented at the Fifth International Conference on AIDS, Montreal, June 4–9.

Barbacci, M., Chaisson, R., Anderson, J., and Horn, J. (1989) Knowledge of HIV serostatus and pregnancy decisions. Presented at the Fifth International AIDS Conference, Montreal, June 4–9.

Battjes, R. J., Pickens, R. W., and Amsel, Z. (1989) Introduction of HIV infection among intravenous drugabusers in low prevalence areas. *Journal of Acquired Immune Deficiency Syndromes* 2:533–539.

Berkelman, R., Karon, J., Thomas, P., Kerndt, P., Rutherford, G., and Stehr-Green, J. (1989) Are AIDS cases among homosexual males leveling? Presented at the Fifth International Conferenceon AIDS, Montreal, June4–9.

Brettler, D. B., Forsberg, A. D., Levine, P. H., Andrews, C. A., Baker, S., and Sullivan, J. L. (1988) Human immunodeficiency virus isolation studies and antibody testing. *Archives of Internal Medicine* 148:1299–1301.

Brondum, J., Debuono, B., Dondero, L., Hodge, J., and Johnson, A. (1987) The alternative test site (ATS) in Rhode Island. Presented at the Third International Conference on AIDS, Washington, D.C., June 1–5.

Evaluation of AIDS Interventions (Coyle, Boruch, and Turner, 1990). In this report, the panel lays out specific strategies for assessing the effectiveness of three of CDC's major AIDS prevention programs: the national media campaign, testing and counseling, and the health education projects sponsored by its group of funded community-based organizations.

Brown, L. S., Mitchell, J. L., DeVore, S. L., and Primm, B. J. (1989) Female intravenous drug users and perinatal HIV transmission. *New England Journal of Medicine* 320:1493–1494.

Castro, K. G., Lieb, S., Calisher, C., Witte, J., and Jaffe, H. W. (1987) AIDS and HIV infection in Belle Glade, Florida. Presented at the Third International Conference on AIDS, Washington, D.C., June 1–5.

Castro, K. G., Lifson, A. R., White, C. R., Bush, T. J., Chamberland, M. E., et al. (1988) Investigations of AIDS patients with no previously identified risk factors. *Journal of the American Medical Association* 259:1338–1342.

Centers for Disease Control (CDC). (1987) Human immunodeficiency virus infection in the United States. *Morbidity and Mortality Weekly Report* 36:801–804.

Centers for Disease Control (CDC). (1989) HIV/AIDS Projections Workshop October 31–November 1, 1989: Draft Working Group Reports and Summary (December 3, 1989). Atlanta, Ga.: Centers for Disease Control.

Centers for Disease Control (CDC). (1990a) *HIV/AIDS Surveillance: U.S. AIDS Cases Reported Through December 1989.* Atlanta, Ga.: Centers for Disease Control.

Centers for Disease Control (CDC). (1990b) Publicly funded HIV counseling and testing–United States, 1985–1989. *Morbidity and Mortality Weekly Report* 39:137–140.

Chamberland, M. E., Allen, J. R., Monroe, J. M., Garcia, N., Morgan, C., et al. (1985) Acquired immunodeficiency syndrome in New York City: Evaluation of an active surveillance system. *Journal of the American Medical Association* 254:383–387.

Chambers, C. D., and Moffitt, A. (1970) Negro opiate addiction. In J. C. Ball and C. D. Chambers, eds., *The Epidemiology of Opiate Addiction in the United States.* Springfield, Ill.: Thomas.

Chambers, C. D., Hinesley, R. K., and Moldestad, M. (1970) Narcotics addiction in females: A race comparison. *International Journal of the Addictions* 5:257–278.

Chandrasekar, P. H., Matthews, M., and Chandrasekar, M. C. (1988) Risk factors for HIV infection among parenteral drug abusers (PDA) in a low-prevalence area. Presented at the Fourth International Conference on AIDS, Stockholm, June 12–16.

Chiasson, M. A., Stoneburner, R. L., Telzak, E., Hildebrandt, D., Schultz, S., et al. (1989) Risk factors for HIV-1 infection in STD clinic patients: Evidence for crack-related heterosexual transmission. Presented at the Fifth International Conference on AIDS, Montreal, June 4–9.

Chiasson, M. A., Stoneburner, R. L., Lifson, A. R., Hildebrandt, D. S., Ewing, W. E., et al. (1990) Risk factors for human immunodeficiency virus type 1 (HIV-1) infection in patients at a sexually transmitted disease clinic in New York City. *American Journal of Epidemiology* 131:208–220.

Cohn, D., Douglas, J., Koleis, J., Feeney, F., and Judson, F. (1989) Comparison of prevalence of HIV infection in IV drug users (IVDU) from four different testing and treatment programs. Presented at the Fifth International Conference on AIDS, Montreal, June 4–9.

Comerford, M., Chitwood, D. D., McCoy, C. B., and Trapido, E. J. (1989) Association between former place of residence and serostatus of IVDUs in south Florida. Presented at the Fifth International Conference on AIDS, Montreal, June 4–9.

Connor, E., Denny, T., Goode, L., Niven, P., Oxtoby, M., et al. (1989) Seroprevalence of HIV-1 and HTLV-1 among pregnant women in Newark, N.J. Presented at the Fifth International Conference on AIDS, Montreal, June 4–9.

Conway, G. A., Colley-Niemeyer, B., Pursley, C., Cruz, C., Burt, S., and Heath, C. W. (1989) Underreporting of AIDS cases in South Carolina, 1986 and 1987. *Journal of the American Medical Association* 262:2859–2863.

Corby, N. H., Rhodes, F., and Wolitski, R. J. (1989) HIV serostatus and risk behaviors of street IVDUs. Presented at the Fifth International Conference on AIDS, Montreal, June 4–9.

Cowan, D. N., Brundage, J., Miller, R., Goldenbaum, M., Pomerantz, R., and Wann, F. (1989) Prevalence of HIV infection among U.S. army reserve component personnel. Presented at the Fifth International Conference on AIDS, Montreal, June 4–9.

Coyle, S. C., Boruch, R. B., and Turner, C. F., eds. (1990) *Evaluating AIDS Prevention Programs, Expanded Edition.* Washington, D.C.: National Academy Press.

Cozen, W., Mascola, L., Giles, M., Bauch, S., Finn, M., and Heneman, C. (1989) Routine HIV antibody screening in Los Angeles county prenatal clinics: A demonstration project. Presented at the Fifth International Conference on AIDS, Montreal, June 4–9.

Curran, J. W., Jaffe, H. W., Hardy, A. M., Morgan, W. M., Selik, R. M., and Dondero, T. J. (1988) Epidemiology of HIV infection and AIDS in the United States. *Science* 239:610–616.

Danila, R. N., Shultz, J. M., Osterholm, M. T., MacDonald, K. L., Henry, K., and Simpson, M. (1987) Minnesota counseling and testing sites: Analysis of trends over time. Presented at the Third International Conference on AIDS, Washington, D.C., June 1–5.

Del Tempelis, C. D., Shell, G., Hoffman, M., Benjamin, R. A., Chandler, A., and Francis, D. (1987) Human immunodeficiency virus infection in women in the San Francisco Bay area. *Journal of the American Medical Association* 258:474–475.

Des Jarlais, D. C., Friedman, S. R., and Strug, D. (1986) AIDS and needle sharing within IV-drug use subculture. In P. A. Feldman and T. M. Johnson, eds., *The Social Dimensions of AIDS: Method and Theory.* New York: Praeger Press.

Des Jarlais, D. C., Chamberland, M. E., Yancovitz, S. R., Weinberg, P., and Friedman, S. R. (1984) Heterosexual partners: A large risk group for AIDS. *Lancet* 2(8415):1346–1347.

Des Jarlais, D. C., Friedman, S. R., Novick, D. M., Sotheran, J. L., Thomas, P., et al. (1989) HIV-1 infection among intravenous drug users in Manhattan, New York City, from 1977 through 1987. *Journal of the American Medical Association* 261:1008–1012.

Eldred, C. A., and Washington, M. N. (1976) Interpersonal relationships in heroin use by men and women and their role in treatment outcome. *International Journal of the Addictions* 17:117–130.

Ernst, J. A., Bauer, S., Amaral, L., St. Louis, M., and Falco, I. (1989) HIV seroprevalence at the Bronx Lebanon Hospital Center—A CDC sentinel hospital. Presented at the Fifth International Conference on AIDS, Montreal, June 4–9.

Fehrs, L., Hill, D., Kerndt, P., Rose, T., and Henneman, C. (1989) HIV screening program at a Los Angeles prenatal/family planning center. Presented at the Fifth International Conference on AIDS, Montreal, June 4–9.

Forsberg, A. D., Sullivan, J. L., Willitts, D. L., Kraus, E., and Brettler, D. B. (1989) Results of HIV antibody testing in sexual partners of seropositive hemophiliacs over a 5-year period. Presented at the Fifth International Conference on AIDS, Montreal, June 4–9.

Friedman, S. R., Dozier, C., Sterk, C., Williams, T., Sotheran, J. L., et al. (1988) Crack use puts women at risk for heterosexual transmission of HIV from intravenous drug users. Presented at the Fourth International Conference on AIDS, Stockholm, June 12–16.

Frutchey, C., and Walsh, K. (1989) Marginalization of gay men in AIDS funding and programs. Presented at the Fifth International Conference on AIDS, Montreal, June 4–9.

Fullilove, R. E., Fullilove, M. T., Bowser, B. P., and Gross, S. A. (1989) Crack use and risk for AIDS among black adolescents. Presented at the Fifth International Conference on AIDS, Montreal, June 4–9.

Gail, M. H., Rosenberg, P. S., and Goedert, J. L. (1990) Therapy may explain recent deficits in AIDS incidence. *Journal of Acquired Immune Deficiency Syndromes* 4:296–306.

Gardner, L. I., Brundage, J. F., Burke, D. S., McNeil, J. G., Visintine, R., and Miller, R. N. (1989) Evidence for spread of the human immunodeficiency virus epidemic into low-prevalence areas of the United States. *Journal of Acquired Immune Deficiency Syndromes* 2:521–532.

Gerstein, D. R., Judd, L. L., and Rovner, S. A. (1979) Career dynamics of female heroin addicts. *American Journal of Drug and Alcohol Abuse* 6:1–23.

Goedert, J. J., Eyster, M. E., Biggar, R. J., and Blattner, W. A. (1987) Heterosexual transmission of human immunodeficiency virus: Association with severe depletion of T-helper lymphocytes in men with hemophilia. *AIDS Research and Human Retroviruses* 3:355–361.

Guinan, M. E., and Hardy, A. (1987) Epidemiology of AIDS in women in the United States: 1981 through 1986. *Journal of the American Medical Association* 257:2039–2042.

Hardy, A. M., Starcher, E. T., Morgan, W. M., Druker, J., Kristal, A., et al. (1987) Review of death certificates to assess completeness of AIDS case reporting. *Public Health Reports* 102:386–391.

Harrison, W. O., and Moore, T. A. (1988) Prenatal HIV screening in a low-risk population. Presented at the Fourth International Conference on AIDS, Stockholm, June 13–16.

Hill, D., Kerndt, P., Frenkel, L. M., Settlage, R., Lee, M., et al. (1989) HIV seroprevalence among parturients in Los Angeles County, 1988. Presented at the Fifth International Conference on AIDS, Montreal, June 4–9.

Hoegsberg, B., Dotson, T., Abulafia, O., Tross, S., Des Jarlais, D., et al. (1989) Social, sexual and drug use profile of HIV-positive and HIV-negative women with PID. Presented at the Fifth International Conference on AIDS, Montreal, June 4–9.

Horman, J., and Hamidi, C. (1989) The epidemiology of AIDS in Maryland, 1981–1987. Presented at the Fifth International Conference on AIDS, Montreal, June 4–9.

Horton, J., Alexander, L., and Brundage, J. (1989) HIV prevalence among military women: An examination of military applicant, active duty, and reserve testing data. Presented at the Fifth International Conference on AIDS, Montreal, June 4–9.

Hull, H. F., Bettinger, C. J., Gallaher, M. M., Keller, N. M., Wilson, J., and Mertz, G. J. (1988) Comparison of HIV-antibody prevalence in patients consenting to and declining HIV-antibody testing in an STD clinic. *Journal of the American Medical Association* 260:935–938.

Jackson, J. B., Sannerud, K. J., Hopsicker, J. S., Kwok, S. Y., Edson, J. R., and Balfour, H. H. (1988) Hemophiliacs with HIV antibody are actively infected. *Journal of the American Medical Association* 260:2236–2239.

Jackson, J. B., Kwok, S. Y., Hopsicker, J. S., Sannerud, K. J., Sninsky, J. J., et al. (1989) Absence of HIV-1 infection in antibody-negative sexual partners of HIV-1 infected hemophiliacs. *Transfusion* 29:265–267.

Johnson, J. P., Alger, L., Nair, P., Watkins, S., Jett, K., and Alexander, S. (1987) HIV screening in the high-risk obstetric population and infant serologic analysis. Presented at the Third International Conference on AIDS, Washington, D.C., June 1–5.

Kaunitz, A. M., Brewer, J. L., Paryani, S. G., de Sausure, L., Sanchez-Ramos, L., et al. (1987) Prenatal care and HIV screening. *Journal of the American Medical Association* 258:2693.

Kim, H. C., Raska, K. III, Clemow, L., Eisele, J., Matts, L., et al. (1988) Human immunodeficiency virus infection in sexually active wives of infected hemophiliac men. *American Journal of Medicine* 85:472–476.

Krasinski, K., Burkowsky, W., Bebenroth, D., and Moore, T. (1988) Failure of voluntary testing for HIV to identify infected parturient women in a high-risk population. *New England Journal of Medicine* 318:185.

Lafferty, W. E., Hopkins, S. G., Honey, J., Harwell, J. D., Shoemaker, P. C., and Kobayashi, J. M. (1988) Hospital charges for people with AIDS in Washington State: Utilization of a statewide hospital discharge data base. *American Journal of Public Health* 78:949–957.

Landesman, S. H., Minkoff, H., Holman, S., McCalla, S., and Sijin, O. (1987) Serosurvey of human immunodeficiency virus infection in parturients: Implications for human immunodeficiency virus testing programs of pregnant women. *Journal of the American Medical Association* 258:2701–2703.

Landis, S., Schoenbach, V., Weber, D., Mittal, M., Koch, G., and Levine, P. (1989) HIV-1 seroprevalence in sexually transmitted disease (STD) clinic patients in central North Carolina. Presented at the Fifth International Conference on AIDS, Montreal, June 4–9.

Laurian, Y., Peynet, J., and Verroust, F. (1989) HIV infection in sexual partners of HIV seropositive patients with hemophilia. *New England Journal of Medicine* 320:183.

Lawrence, D. N., Jason, J. M., Holman, R. C., Heine, P., Evatt, B. L., and the Hemophilia Study Group. (1989) Sex practice correlates of human immunodeficiency virus transmission and acquired immunodeficiency syndrome incidence in heterosexual partners and offspring of U.S. hemophilic men. *American Journal of Hematology* 30:68–76.

Lawrence, D. N., Jason, J. M., Holman, R. C., and Murphy, J. J. (1990) Human immunodeficiency virus transmission from hemophilic men to their heterosexual partners. In N. J. Alexander, H. L. Gabelnick, and J. M. Spieler, eds., *The Heterosexual Transmission of AIDS*. New York: Alan R. Liss.

Lindsay, M. K., Peterson, H. B., Mundy, D. C., Slade, B. A., Feng, T., et al. (1989) Seroprevalence of human immunodeficiency virus infection in a prenatal population at high risk for HIV infection. *Southern Medical Journal* 82:825–828.

Mandell, W., Vlahov, D., and Cohn, S. (1989) IVDU characteristics associated with needle sharing. Presented at the Fifth International Conference on AIDS, Montreal, June 4–9.

Mason, P. J., Olson, R. A., and Parish, K. L. (1988) AIDS, hemophilia, and prevention efforts within a comprehensive care program. *American Psychologist* 43:971–976.

McCoy, C. B., Chitwood, D. D., and Page, J. B. (1989) Mobility, risk cities, risk behavior, and HIV status of IV drug users. Presented at the Fifth International Conference on AIDS, Montreal, June 4–9.

McFarland, L., Dean, H., Trahan, B., and Muirhead, L. (1989) HIV infection in pregnant women at a public hospital in New Orleans, Louisiana. Presented at the Fifth International Conference on AIDS, Montreal, June 4–9.

Modesitt, S.K., Hulman, S., and Fleming, D. (1990) Evaluation of active versus passive AIDS surveillance in Oregon. *American Journal of Public Health* 80:463–464.

Moss, A. R., Bachetti, P., Osmond, D., Meakin, R., Keffelew, A., and Gorter, R. (1989) Seroconversion for HIV in intravenous drug users in San Francisco. Presented at the Fifth International Conference on AIDS, Montreal, June 4–9.

Murphy, D. L. (1987) Heterosexual contacts of intravenous drug users: Implications for the next spread of the AIDS epidemic. *Advances in Alcohol and Substance Abuse* 7:89–97.

National Hemophilia Foundation. (1988) What you should know about hemophilia (brochure). National Hemophilia Foundation, New York.

New York State Department of Health. (1989) *AIDS in New York State through 1988.* Albany: New York State Department of Health.

Novick, L. F., Berns, D., Stricof, R., Stevens, R., Pass, K., and Wethers, J. (1989) HIV seroprevalence in newborns in New York State. *Journal of the American Medical Association* 261:1745–1750.

Ognjan, A., Markowitz, N., Pohlod, D., Lee, H., Belian, B., and Saravolatz, L. D. (1989) HIV-1 and HTLV-1 infections in intravenous drug users (IVDUs) in Detroit, 1985–1989. Presented at the Fifth International Conference on AIDS, Montreal, June 4–9.

Olin, R., and Kall, K. (1989) HIV status and changes in risk behavior among arrested and detained intravenous drug abusers in Stockholm, 1987–88. Presented at the Fifth International Conference on AIDS, Montreal, June 4–9.

O'Sullivan, M. J., Fajardo, A., Ferron, P., Efantis, J., Senk, C., and Duthely, M. (1989) Seroprevalence in a pregnant multiethnic population. Presented at the Fifth International Conference on AIDS, Montreal, June 4–9.

Padian, N., Moreno, A., Glass, S., Shiboski, S., and Maisonet, G. (1989) Ethnic differences in the heterosexual transmission of HIV in California. Presented at the Fifth International Conference on AIDS, Montreal, June 4–9.

Pappaioanou, M., George, R., Hannon, H., Hoff, R., Willoughby, A., et al. (1989) National surveys of HIV seroprevalence in women delivering live children in the United States. Presented at the Fifth International Conference on AIDS, Montreal, June 4–9.

Parish, K. L., Mandel, J., Thomas, J., and Gomperts, E. (1989) Prediction of safer sex practice and psychosocial distress in adults with hemophilia at risk for AIDS. Presented at the Fifth International Conference on AIDS, Montreal, June 4–9.

Prendergast, T. J., Maxwell, R., Greenwood, J. R., Burrell, P., and Swatzel, C. (1989) Incidence and prevalence of HIV infection during 44 months of testing prostitutes/IVDUs in the women's prison, Orange County, California. Presented at the Fifth International Conference on AIDS, Montreal, June 4–9.

Public Health Service (PHS). (1988) Report of the Second Public Health Service AIDS Prevention and Control Conference. *Public Health Reports* 103 (Supplement No. 1):1–98.

Quinn, T. C., Glasser, D., Cannon, R. O., Matuszak, D. L., Dunning, R. W., et al. (1988) Human immunodeficiency virus infection among patients attending clinics for sexually transmitted diseases. *New England Journal of Medicine* 318:197–203.

Ragni, M. V., Gupta, P., Rinaldo, C. R., Kingsley, L. A., Spero, J. A., and Lewis, J. H. (1988) HIV transmission to female sexual partners of HIV antibody-positive hemophiliacs. *Public Health Reports* 103:54–58.

Ralph, N., and Spigner, C. (1986) Contraceptive practices among female heroin addicts. *American Journal of Public Health* 76:1016–1017.

Rosenbaum, M. (1981) When drugs come into the picture, love flies out the window: Women addicts' love relationships. *International Journal of the Addictions* 16:1197–1206.

Schoenbaum, E. E., Hartel, D., Selwyn, P. A., Klein, R. S., Davenny, K., et al. (1989) Risk factors for human immunodeficiency virus infection in intravenous drug users. *New England Journal of Medicine* 321:874–879.

Selik, R., and Petersen, L. (1989) Epidemiology of AIDS associated with intravenous drug use, United States, 1979–1988. Presented at the Fifth International Conference on AIDS, Montreal, June 4–9.

Selwyn, P. A., Schoenbaum, E. E., Hartel, D., Klein, R. S., Davenny, K., et al. (1988) AIDS and HIV-related mortality in intravenous drug users (IVDUs). Presented at the Fourth International Conference on AIDS, Stockholm, June 12–16.

Smiley, M. L., White, G. C. II, Becherer, P., Macik, G., Matthews, T. J., et al. (1988) Transmission of human immunodeficiency virus to sexual partners of hemophiliacs. *American Journal of Hematology* 28:27–32.

Snyder, F., and Myers, M. (1989) Risk-taking behaviors of intravenous drug abusers. Presented at the Fifth International Conference on AIDS, Montreal, June 4–9.

Sowder, B., Weissman, G., and Young, P. (1989) Working with women at risk in a national AIDS prevention program. Photocopied materials distributed at the Fifth International Conference on AIDS, Montreal, June 4–9.

Sperling, R. S., Sacks, H. S., Mayer, L., Joyner, M., and Berkowitz, R. L. (1989) Umbilical cord blood serosurvey for human immunodeficiency virus in parturient women in a voluntary hospital in New York City. *Obstetrics and Gynecology* 73:179–181.

Stoneburner, R. L., Des Jarlais, D. C., Benezra, D., Gorelkin, L., Sotheran, J. L., et al. (1988) A larger spectrum of severe HIV-1 related disease in intravenous drug users in New York City. *Science* 242:916–919.

Stoneburner, R. L., Chiasson, M. A., Weisfuse, I. B., and Thomas, P. A. (1990) The epidemic of AIDS and HIV-1 infection among heterosexuals in New York City. *AIDS* 4:99–106.

Thompson, E. G., Suarez, L., Reed, C. M., Buchanan, B. K., and Therrell, B. L. (1989) Serosurvey of women of childbearing age in Texas, U.S.A. Presented at the Fifth International Conference on AIDS, Montreal, June 4–9.

Tross, S., Abdul-Quader, A. S., Des Jarlais, D. C., Kouzi, A. C., and Friedman, S. R. (1989) Determinants of sexual risk reduction in street-recruited female IV drug users. Presented at the Fifth International Conference on AIDS, Montreal, June 4–9.

Turner, C. F. (1989) Research on sexual behaviors that transmit HIV: Progress and problems. *AIDS* 3:S63–S71.

Turner, C. F., Miller, H. G., and Barker, L. (1989) AIDS research and the behavioral and social sciences. In R. Kulstad, ed., *AIDS, 1988: AAAS Symposium Papers.* Washington, D.C.: American Association for the Advancement of Science.

Turner, C. F., Miller, H. G., and Moses, L. E., eds. (1989) *AIDS, Sexual Behavior, and Intravenous Drug Use.* Washington, D.C.: National Academy Press.

U.S. Bureau of the Census. (1987) *Statistical Abstract of the United States: 1988.* 108th ed. Washington, D.C.: U.S. Government Printing Office.

Valdiserri, R. O., Bonati, F. A., Proctor, D., and Glaser, D. A. (1988) HIV antibody testing in a family planning clinic setting. *New York State Journal of Medicine* 88:623–625.

Valdiserri, R. O., Arena, V. C., Proctor, D., and Bonati, F. A. (1989) The relationship between women's attitudes about condoms and their use: Implications for condom promotion programs. *American Journal of Public Health* 79:499–501.

van Haastrecht, H. J. A., van den Hoek, J. A. R., and Coutinho, R. A. (1989) No trend in yearly HIV seroprevalence rates among IVDU in Amsterdam: 1986–1988. Presented at the Fifth International Conference on AIDS, Montreal, June 4–9.

Watters, J. K. (1988) Meaning and context: The social facts of intravenous drug use and HIV transmission in the inner city. *Journal of Psychoactive Drugs* 20:173–177.

Weiner, S. M., Kaltenbach, K. A., and Finnegan, L. P. (1989) Drug abuse and pregnancy: Concomitant risk factors for HIV infection. Presented at the Fifth International Conference on AIDS, Montreal, June 4–9.

Weissman, G. (1988) Community outreach and prevention: A national demonstration project. Presented at the 116th annual meeting of the American Public Health Association, Boston, November.

Wermuth, L., and Ham, J. (1989) Perception of AIDS risk among women sexual partners of intravenous drug users in San Francisco. Presented at the Fifth International Conference on AIDS, Montreal, June 4–9.

Whittaker, S., Calsyn, D., Saxon, A., and Freeman, G. (1989) Sexual behaviors of intravenous drug users. Presented at the Fifth International Conference on AIDS, Montreal, June 4–9.

Wilson, P. A., and Wasserman, K. (1989) Psychosocial responses to the threat of HIV exposure among people with bleeding disorders. *Health and Social Work* August:176–183.

Winkelstein, W., Samuel, M., Padian, N. S., Wiley, J. A., Lang, W., et al. (1987) The San Francisco Men's Health Study: III. Reduction in human immunodeficiency virus transmission among homosexual/bisexual men, 1982–1986. *American Journal of Public Health* 77(9):685–689.

Winkelstein, W., Wiley, J. A., Padian, N. S., Samuel, M., Shiboski, S., et al. (1988) The San Francisco Men's Health Study: Continued decline in HIV seroconversion rates among homosexual/bisexual men. *American Journal of Public Health* 78:1472–1474.

Withum, D. G., LaLota, M., Holtzman, D., Buff, E. E., Chan, M. S., et al. (1989) Prevalence of HIV antibodies in childbearing women in Florida. Presented at the Fifth International Conference on AIDS, Montreal, June 4–9.

Wolfe, H., Keffelew, A., Bacchetti, P., Meakin, R., Brodie, B., and Moss, A. R. (1989) HIV infection in female intravenous drug users in San Francisco. Photocopied materials distributed at the Fifth International Conference on AIDS, Montreal, June 4–9.

Worth, D., and Rodriguez, R. (1987) Latina women and AIDS. *Siecus Report* January/February:5–7.

Worth, D., Drucker, E., Eric, K., Chabon, B., Pivnick, A., and Cochrane, K. (1989) An ethnographic study of high-risk sexual behavior in 96 women using IV heroin, cocaine, and crack in the South Bronx. Presented at the Fifth International Conference on AIDS, Montreal, June 4–9.

2

Prevention: The Continuing Challenge

The epidemiological data presented in the first chapter enable researchers and program planners to identify shifts in the epidemic and in the subpopulations being affected. Although such data are vital for targeting programs to populations at risk, they say little about how to stop the spread of infection. Given that there is no convincing evidence that AIDS or HIV infection is abating and that there are no cures or vaccines on the immediate horizon, the need for effective behavioral intervention will persist into the second decade of the epidemic. Many intervention efforts of the first decade were designed and implemented quickly in response to a new health problem that in some areas took on the characteristics of a crisis. As the United States enters the second decade of efforts to contain the spread of disease, the committee believes that the time has come to view behavioral intervention from a more long-term perspective. This view of AIDS calls for a commitment to the careful and systematic accrual of information capable of identifying those strategies that will facilitate change in risk-associated behaviors, maintain safer behaviors, and thus alter the course of the epidemic.

In its first report, the committee recommended that the Public Health Service (PHS) support basic research on human sexual behavior and give high priority to research on the social contexts of IV drug use to provide the data needed to design efficacious intervention strategies to prevent the spread of HIV infection. The committee further recommended that knowledge about the efficacy of intervention programs be built systematically through the use of planned variations of key program elements with subsequent rigorous evaluation. The committee reiterates these recommendations and notes that the need for well-designed, carefully implemented, and thoughtfully evaluated intervention efforts and good behavioral research continues today. Although there are many projects currently in place whose goal is to educate people about the threat of AIDS, few of these programs have been sufficiently well designed to provide the data needed to assess the effect of their efforts—especially their effects on changing the behaviors associated with transmission. Moreover, as the first decade of the epidemic draws to a close, it is apparent that, although data have accrued from a range of behavioral research activities, those data are of varying quality. Consequently, it is often difficult to draw firm conclusions from such studies or to reach consensus about the next set of issues to be studied.

The first three sections of this chapter consider intervention-related issues pertaining to gay men (among whom the greatest share of the burden of disease continues to reside), IV drug users, and women. At the beginning of the epidemic, interventions to prevent the spread of HIV infection focused primarily on gay men, the population that showed the first evidence of disease. However, as evidence accumulated on the risks associated with other behaviors, intervention efforts began to expand, encompassing, for example, IV drug users and heterosexuals with multiple sexual partners. Today, the focus of AIDS prevention requires expansion once again to accommodate the changing epidemiological patterns noted in the previous chapter and the changing character of the disease.

· IMPACT OF INTERVENTIONS AMONG GAY MEN

Studies of gay men since the first years of the epidemic have indicated considerable behavioral change among some members of this population, especially men living in large urban areas (e.g., San Francisco, Los Angeles, New York City) (Becker and Joseph, 1988; Stall, Coates, and Hoff, 1988; Catania et al., 1989). This change is largely reflected in the decreased frequency of unprotected anal intercourse and fewer sexual partners. More recent data from the epicenters or focal points of the epidemic have shown that gay men are continuing to alter risky behaviors.[1]

---

[1] For example, at recruitment into the AIDS Behavioral Research Project in 1983 and 1984, 45.3 percent of subjects reported practicing unprotected insertive anal intercourse, and 32.8 percent reported unprotected receptive anal intercourse. However, only 12 percent of the 435 nonmonogamous men who continue to participate in this longitudinal study reported unprotected anal intercourse at their last assessment in 1988 (McKusick et al., in press). Similarly, among participants in the San Francisco Men's Health Study, prevalence rates for insertive and receptive anal intercourse dropped from 37.4 and 33.9 percent in 1985 to 1.7 and 4.2 percent, respectively, in 1988. In 1988 only 8.5 percent of participants in this study reported one or more episodes of relapse (i.e., return to risk-associated behavior after safer behavior had been initiated) during the previous year (Ekstrand and Coates, in press).

Similar change has also been reported among gay men from other communities, such as Denver (Judson, Cohn, and Douglas, 1989; O'Reilly et al., 1989), Long Beach (California) and Dallas (O'Reilly et al., 1989). Reports of behavioral change have coincided with stable HIV incidence rates and stable rates of other sexually transmitted diseases, which suggests that the intervention programs targeting these men have had some success (Lindan et al., 1989). Despite the encouragement provided by these data, however, other studies indicate that safer sex practices have not been universally instituted among gay men, and there appears to be substantial variation in the degree of behavioral change across geographic areas and across age and ethnic groups in the gay community (Office of Technology Assessment, 1988; Coates et al., 1988a, 1989b; Kelly et al., 1989c). In particular, reports of unprotected anal intercourse among men living in low-prevalence cities raise serious concerns about the future spread of the epidemic in these communities.[2]

The existing data on behavior change and HIV seroprevalence, although imperfect, are sufficient to provide a sense that a major risk for new HIV infection still exists among samples of self-identified gay men, despite the profound behavioral risk reductions that have occurred since the onset of the AIDS epidemic and despite widespread understanding of health education guidelines for the prevention of HIV infection (Stall, Coates, and Hoff, 1988). Especially in the epicenters of the AIDS epidemic, the high prevalence of infection estimated to exist among homosexually active men, combined with the increased infectivity believed to be associated with later stages of infection,[3] confers a substantial risk

---

[2]For example, about 21 percent of a sample of 270 gay men in Boston who were interviewed in 1987 (McCusker et al., 1988) reported engaging in unprotected anal intercourse in the previous month. In a study of 127 gay men in Atlanta, a high-incidence city, only 13 percent of the men reported unprotected anal intercourse in the previous two months; however, 35.4 percent of 163 men in low-prevalence cities (Birmingham, Alabama, and Tupelo, Mississippi) reported such activity, as did approximately one-quarter of 355 men interviewed in Hattiesburg and Biloxi, Mississippi, and Monroe, Louisiana (St. Lawrence et al., 1989; Kelly et al., 1990a). Among a cohort of 249 male sexual partners of HIV-seropositive men in Toronto, 43 percent reported practicing unprotected insertive anal intercourse, and 42 percent reported engaging in unprotected receptive anal intercourse in the previous month (Calzavara et al., 1989). In a study that involved four south Florida counties, half (51 percent) of the gay and bisexual men who participated (N = 586) had previously sought HIV testing and counseling (suggesting that they considered themselves to be possibly at risk for infection), but only 25 percent reported that they always used condoms during anal intercourse (Lieb et al., 1989). For reviews of changes in sexual behavior among gay men, see Becker and Joseph (1988); Coates, Stall, and Hoff (1988); Coates and coworkers (1988b); Office of Technology Assessment (1988); and Stall, Coates, and Hoff (1988).

[3]In studies of men with hemophilia and their female sexual partners, Goedert and coworkers found that the probability of HIV infection increased significantly for female partners of men with HIV p24 antigenemia or extreme immune deficiency (Dr. James Goedert, National Cancer Institute, personal communication, April 23, 1990).

of disease transmission by any single homosexual contact. Thus, notwithstanding the number of AIDS prevention programs that have already been established for gay men, continuing intervention remains a high priority.

Research to understand the distribution and determinants of behavioral change among gay men is currently in progress,[4] but certain aspects of the studies limit their usefulness. Despite the tremendous diversity among homosexual men, most research to date has involved older, white, self-identified gay men in urban areas. Relatively little is known about other subgroups of gay men who may in fact be at highest risk (e.g., younger men, black and Hispanic men, men who have sex with other men but do not self-identify as gay). In addition, piecing together the findings from different projects presents certain difficulties. First, data are collected and reported in different ways by different investigators, making it difficult to compare rates of change and prevalences of high-risk behaviors across studies. Second, the results are often reported in a piecemeal fashion, using a variety of publication channels (e.g., scientific journals, scientific conferences, government reports, technical reports, personal communications). It is an arduous and extremely time-consuming task to assemble and collate the entire set of studies to identify any patterns among the results. Third, behaviors are reported for varying time periods, ranging from 1 and 2 months to 6 and 12 months. Finally, the fragmentation of funding sources provides little opportunity or incentive to communicate with other investigators whose efforts are being supported by other funders.

Establishing standards for reporting on at least selected subsets of data would facilitate comparisons across studies. But quantifying change does not provide insight into *why* men alter their behavior. Developing a more coherent sense of what has been learned from studies of gay men supported by the PHS requires considerably more effort. Therefore, **the committee recommends that the Public Health Service assemble and summarize data reported by gay men in PHS-funded studies regarding seroprevalence, seroconversion, and high-risk behavior and determine what conclusions can be drawn from the research.**

---

[4] Studies of behavioral change among gay and bisexual men in San Francisco, Chicago, and New York are currently being supported by the National Institute of Mental Health. CDC sponsors demonstration and education projects among gay and bisexual men in six communities: Dallas, Denver, Albany and New York City, Seattle-King County, Chicago, and Long Beach, California. The National Institute of Allergy and Infectious Diseases supports research on the epidemiology and natural history of AIDS in cohorts of homosexual men as well as studies on behavioral and other risk factors associated with the acquisition of HIV infection. The Multicenter AIDS Cohort Study (MACS) has administered interviews and physical examinations to cohorts of homosexual men in Baltimore, Chicago, Los Angeles, and Pittsburgh. The University of California, Berkeley, also conducts studies of gay men.

Such a summary would be extremely useful in formulating a research agenda that could direct intervention efforts that are likely to be effective toward gay men who continue to require intensive attention.

One group of particular concern is young gay men. Numerous studies have found that young gay men engage in higher rates of risk taking than older gay men[5] (Joseph et al., 1988; Valdiserri et al., 1988; Ekstrand and Coates, in press; Kelly et al., 1990b). Indeed, according to data collected in the San Francisco Men's Health Study, young homosexual men were significantly more likely than older men to engage in unprotected anal intercourse and to do so with more partners (Ekstrand and Coates, in press).[6] These results indicate the dynamic nature of the gay population and highlight the need for continuing intervention and the identification of particular subgroups whose risk behaviors may warrant increased efforts.

Community-Level and Individual Intervention Efforts

It is clear that behavioral change has been occurring among some groups of gay males in this country. Yet there is also evidence that some sub-populations of men who have sex with other men have not initiated or maintained risk-reducing behavior. These findings argue for continuing intervention to prevent further spread of infection among men who engage in same-gender sex. However, which risk reduction strategies are most likely to be effective remains in doubt. Community-level intervention programs have been implemented in several gay communities to reach a critical mass of individuals with information, motivation, and skills training and to foster changes in the norms that stipulate appropriate behavior (Coates and Greenblatt, in press). In its first report, the committee recognized the importance of this mechanism for reaching many high-risk groups. However, additional strategies that focus on individual gay men are also needed.

Community-level strategies are based on the assumption that an individual is much more likely to initiate and maintain healthful behavior when a variety of avenues are used to inform and motivate, specific strategies are used to teach skills needed for low-risk activities, specific

---

[5]The ages that constitute the "young" male population, however, appear to vary across studies and are rarely defined.

[6]Other studies have also reported differential risk taking among younger gay men. In a survey of 526 bar patrons in Seattle, Tampa, and Mobile, young men were more likely than older men to engage in unprotected anal intercourse (Kelly et al., 1990b). In a 1989 survey of 100 homosexual men between the ages of 18 and 25 in three West Coast communities (Santa Cruz, Santa Barbara, and Eugene, Oregon), 43 reported engaging in unprotected anal intercourse in the previous two months (Hays, Kegeles, and Coates, in press).

health-diminishing behaviors become less socially accepted in a community, and social sanctions regarding unhealthy behaviors are perceived as persistent and inescapable (Coates and Greenblatt, in press). Programs conducted to date reflect a diversity in design and venues for delivery: educational sessions offered in homes and in bars, antibody testing and counseling in public health clinics and alternative test sites, newspaper coverage, pamphlets, and safer-sex videos (Catania et al., 1989). Prevention strategies that seek to influence entire communities have been widely advocated but less frequently implemented and rarely evaluated. One such program, the Stop AIDS Project, was developed in San Francisco and capitalized on community mobilization, using influential members of the local gay population to provide risk reduction information and skills to other gay men.[7] There are indications that the Stop AIDS Project met some of its objectives,[8] but data to determine its specific impact on behavior are lacking. The Stop AIDS model reportedly has been implemented in areas other than San Francisco (Beeker and Rose, 1989; Miller et al., 1989) and in one case has shown encouraging results (Miller et al., 1989). Without rigorous evaluation, however, conclusions about the effectiveness of this strategy cannot be drawn.

Activities for gay men in a variety of communities around the country are exploring variations of community-level interventions. For example, researchers at the University of Mississippi are recruiting groups of socially influential gay males in each of three medium-sized cities for a series of training sessions. The sessions provide detailed educational materials on HIV transmission and social skills training to teach participants how to communicate risk reduction information to others (Kelly et al., 1989b). A second project at the University of California, San Francisco, plans to implement and evaluate a peer-led, community-level intervention in three medium-sized West Coast cities to assist young homosexual men to reduce AIDS-related high-risk behaviors (S. Kegeles, University of California, San Francisco, personal communication, January 1990). The project's community mobilization strategy will include

---

[7] Initial analyses by the originators of this project (Puckett and Bye, 1987) indicated that gay men felt helplessly caught between the growing enormity of the AIDS epidemic and the sexual values and expectations of the gay community. The Stop AIDS program used a variety of strategies to elicit personal commitments to safer sex, encourage participation in intervention activities, empower individuals to take appropriate action, hasten the adoption of safer sex as a community norm, build peer support for safer sex activities, and create peer pressure against activities that would spread the virus. For a detailed description of this project, see Turner, Miller, and Moses (1989:Chapter 4).

[8] Following its fourth survey (in 1986) of gay men in San Francisco, Communication Technologies (1987) reported that 51 percent (as compared with 27 percent in 1985) said that they had heard of the project, and 20 percent said that they had attended a meeting. Stop AIDS records showed that more than 7,000 men in San Francisco attended at least one meeting.

three central elements: a system of peer outreach in formal and informal settings to communicate the need for safer sex; peer-led HIV risk reduction workshops to discuss and overcome barriers to safer sex; and an ongoing publicity campaign about the intervention program within the gay community to establish the legitimacy of intervention activities for this subpopulation and provide a continual reminder of the norms for safer sex.

New research directions for AIDS prevention strategies that target individual gay men include the use of clinical interventions. Clinical interventions are multisession, face-to-face strategies for individuals who require more intensive attention than can be afforded by community-level programs to achieve or sustain behavioral change. These interventions attempt to help gay men evaluate their personal risk for AIDS, generate group norms supportive of safer behaviors, and provide information, skills, and feedback on how well recommended behaviors are performed. Clinical interventions can be delivered in small group or individual sessions and have been employed in a variety of settings, including health care establishments, worksites, and drug treatment centers.

Several researchers have reported on promising variations of clinical interventions in samples of gay men. Kelly and coworkers (1989b, 1989c) recruited and randomized 104 homosexual men with a history of frequent high-risk behavior into experimental or wait-list control groups. The experimental intervention consisted of 12 weekly group sessions that provided AIDS risk education, cognitive behavioral self-management training that focused on refusing coercion (self-management and assertiveness training), and steady and self-affirming social supports. Participants in the experimental group reported fewer episodes of unprotected anal intercourse and higher rates of condom use than control subjects at a follow-up assessment.[9] An intervention conducted by Coates and colleagues (1989a) also showed risk reduction following an eight-week program. The intervention consisted of weekly meetings plus one retreat emphasizing meditation, relaxation, positive health habits, and

---

[9] After four months, men in the experimental group reported a mean of only 0.2 episodes of unprotected anal intercourse (compared with 1.2 at baseline) in the previous month. The control group reported a mean of 1.2 (compared with 0.9 at baseline). In addition, experimental subjects at follow-up reported using condoms in 70 percent of sexual contacts that involved intercourse, compared with 40 percent at baseline. Comparable rates for control subjects were 20 percent at follow-up and 32 percent at baseline.

coping with the stress of being seropositive.[10] In addition, a peer-led intervention effort by Valdiserri and coworkers (1989a) reported increased condom use following a skills training component.[11]

The results presented above point to a possible role for clinical interventions in AIDS prevention efforts for gay men. Additional research is needed, however, to determine whether clinical interventions can be modified for wider dissemination through different avenues (e.g., the media) and for other populations (e.g., minorities, IV drug users).

The Impact of Drug Use on Behavior Change

The disturbing finding that gay men who use drugs (including alcohol) are more likely to report unprotected sexual behaviors than those who do not use drugs has important implications for the development of intervention programs. Men who combine drugs with sex are less likely than those who do not to have changed the frequency of engaging in unsafe anal intercourse[12] and more likely to engage in sexual behaviors that carry a high risk of HIV transmission (Stall et al., 1986; Communication Technologies, 1987; Beeker and Zielinski, 1988; Robertson and Plant, 1988; Valdiserri et al., 1988; Stall and Ostrow, 1989; Martin, 1990; Martin and Hasin, in press).[13] Moreover, the use of noninjected drugs

---

[10] The 64 men recruited by Coates and colleagues (1989a) were evenly divided into an experimental group and a wait-list control group to study the effects of stress management on behavior and immune function. At posttreatment, the experimental group reported a mean of 0.5 sexual partners in the previous month (compared with 1.41 at baseline), whereas the control group reported 2.29 partners in the previous month compared with 1.09 at baseline.

[11] Valdiserri and coworkers (1989a) randomized participants to one of two peer-led interventions. The intervention that provided a skills training component to discuss and rehearse the art of negotiating safer sex resulted in more condom use at 6- and 12-month follow-ups than the intervention that provided information only.

[12] Kelly and coworkers (1990b) surveyed bar patrons in three cities (Seattle, Tampa, and Mobile) and found that 37 percent had engaged in unprotected anal intercourse at least once in the past three months. In addition, Stall and colleagues (in press) described the sexual risks for HIV infection reported by a convenience sample of 1,344 homosexual male and heterosexual male and female bar patrons in San Francisco. More than one-third (37.3 percent) of the homosexual males in the sample ($N = 593$) had engaged in unprotected intercourse in the previous month, but approximately twice as many heterosexuals (61 percent of 314 heterosexual males and 63.8 percent of 437 heterosexual females) reported intercourse without a condom during the same time period. The rates in this study are much higher than those found in other samples of convenience (McKusick et al., in press) or in population-based samples (Ekstrand and Coates, in press).

[13] A longitudinal study of 604 gay men from New York City (Martin, in press) found that the strength of the association between drug use and high-risk sex has diminished over the course of the epidemic. Nevertheless, cessation of drug use was associated with lower rates of both receptive and insertive anal intercourse.

ultimately may confer greater risk for gay men than IV drug use (Stall and Ostrow, 1989).

Several studies are currently under way in San Francisco to investigate the impact of drug use on risk-associated behaviors among gay men. The intervention strategies being used are designed to be implemented in bars and to deal with both drug use and sexual risk taking among adult gay men. These activities may provide much-needed insight into the connection between drug use and risk taking, as well as the connection between drug use and relapse.

INTERVENTIONS FOR INTRAVENOUS DRUG USERS

HIV infection has been present among IV drug users in the United States for more than a decade now (Des Jarlais et al., 1989a), and the number of studies investigating behavioral change in this population has increased greatly since the early years of the epidemic. Knowledge regarding the manifestation and spread of the infection within this population has been advancing incrementally. A nationwide program to reduce the spread of the virus among drug users has been in place over the past several years, and there is a general consensus among researchers in this area that IV drug users as a group have reduced their risk of acquiring HIV and AIDS by adopting safer injection practices. Indeed, recent studies presented in June 1989 at the Fifth International Conference on AIDS in Montreal[14] confirmed many of the conclusions offered by this committee in its first report:

- many IV drug users (usually a majority of those studied in any particular research project) have reported changes in their behavior to reduce their risk of contracting AIDS;

- behavioral change among IV drug users usually reflects risk reduction rather than complete risk elimination;

- there is no single "best" method for facilitating AIDS risk reduction among IV drug users, and consequently it is necessary to provide the means both to reduce drug use and to increase the use of "safer" injection practices; and

- more drug users report changes in drug injection behavior than changes in sexual behavior.

It does not appear likely that these conclusions will be contradicted by new research findings in the near future. Yet as the AIDS epidemic

---

[14] See, for example, Connors and Lewis (1989), Corby, Rhodes, and Wolitski (1989), Skidmore and Robertson (1989), Sunita and coworkers (1989), Vlahov et al. (1989), and Wolfe and colleagues (1989).

enters its second decade within the population of IV drug users, a shift in perspective is required. There is still great geographic variation in the extent to which HIV has spread among drug injectors in local communities. This variation affords both the hope of preventing a more widespread problem in communities that currently report low seroprevalence rates and the need for new approaches in communities that already have significant infection rates. Some populations in the United States appear to have moved beyond the immediate crisis phase of the AIDS epidemic to a longer term endemic phase. Because neither a vaccine nor a cure for HIV infection appears likely in the near future, planning is needed for the long term to limit the spread of HIV among drug injectors, their sexual partners, and their potential offspring. The conclusions noted above point to the need for a two-pronged approach to intervention: (1) reduce drug use in general, including preventing the initiation of injection, and (2) facilitate risk reduction behavior in both injection and sexual practices.

In designing programs to implement such a strategy, the knowledge gained from past efforts must be combined with new approaches geared to present needs. Many injectors have received basic information about AIDS and HIV infection, but there are indications that risk-associated behaviors in this population are not affected by information alone, nor can much change be expected to occur in response to a single intervention episode (Des Jarlais, Friedman, and Stoneburner, 1988). Rather, risk-associated behaviors are dynamic and are affected by a variety of factors, including new information from within the IV drug-using community, changing social norms regarding risky behaviors, and accessibility of the means for risk reduction (e.g., sterile injection equipment, drug treatment programs). Findings of past behavioral research would predict that individuals who have begun new, lower risk behavior would be less likely to revert to previous high-risk patterns if the means for risk reduction were readily available and were believed to be effective by the targeted population.[15]

Whereas most interventions (with the possible exception of "information-only" programs) have been associated with self-reported behavioral change among IV drug users, methadone maintenance treatment programs have been associated with reduced levels of HIV infection (Abdul-Quader et al., 1987; Blix and Gronbladh, 1988; Brown et al., 1989; Novick et al., 1989; Truman et al., 1989; and Schoenbaum et al.,

---

[15] Beliefs about effectiveness may serve as important cognitive reinforcement for AIDS risk reduction messages. In a study of street-recruited IV drug users in New York City (Des Jarlais et al., 1989b), an individual's belief that behavior change would successfully protect against HIV infection was one of the strongest predictors of maintaining risk-reducing behaviors. The importance of other beliefs in AIDS risk reduction is not as clear.

1989). Individuals who enter and stay in methadone treatment programs are less likely to be seropositive than those who have not chosen to seek treatment or those who sought treatment but were unable to find it. This finding points to the importance of reducing drug use as a way of curbing the spread of the epidemic.

Eliminating drug use among those who already inject drugs has so far proved very difficult. A more pragmatic and immediate approach raises another possibility for halting the spread of HIV: decrease the number of new drug injectors. Clearly, if HIV is present among IV drug users in a community, then it becomes critically important to reduce the number of new persons who might start injecting drugs, for it is during the initial period of use that individuals are most likely to share injection equipment (see the discussion on the progression of drug use in Chapter 3). Some have thought that the threat of AIDS in and of itself would be sufficient to deter individuals from using drugs, but the limited number of AIDS-era studies of persons beginning illicit drug injection suggest that fear of AIDS has not had any large-scale effect on whether individuals become IV drug users. This finding would be consistent with the limited effectiveness of fear arousal during drug prevention and safer injection campaigns of the past (Des Jarlais and Friedman, 1987; Ghodse, Tregenza, and Li, 1987).

In fact, the United States and most other nations have given relatively little attention to new injectors or potential injectors, an oversight that may be attributable in part to the need to address simultaneously the multitude of other health and social problems associated with injecting illicit drugs. Recent data from a survey of 256 IV drug users in New York City, however, have shown infection to be less frequent among those who have been injecting for less than five years than among drug users who have been injecting for longer periods (Friedman et al., 1989). Targeting new injectors for intervention thus appears to be a reasonable strategy for preventing further spread of HIV infection.

AIDS prevention efforts related to the initiation of injection have been stymied in some instances by political barriers. Much attention has focused on vague fears of creating new injectors through the information and services offered in HIV prevention strategies (e.g., syringe exchanges), and untested hypotheses linking these services to new drug use have been used to oppose innovative approaches. Yet there is no evidence that any form of "safer injection" program is associated with an increase in the number of new drug injectors. Considering the importance of the research and public health aspects of these issues, the development of strategies to reduce the number of persons who start injecting illicit drugs and to ensure that those who do start injecting will practice "safer" injection should be allowed to proceed without constraints that have little grounding in current scientific knowledge. (A more detailed discussion of these issues is presented at the end of this chapter.)

If one considers the changes made by individuals who already use drugs, the extent to which IV drug users have altered their behavior to reduce the risks of AIDS has been impressive, going well beyond what many experts in the field would have predicted.[16] To say that the problem has been solved, however, is to overlook the substantial difficulties involved in maintaining any kind of behavioral change. In the treatment of drug abuse, achieving abstinence from the use of drugs is relatively easy for at least short periods of time; the greater challenge is to maintain abstinence over longer periods, particularly in cases in which individuals must continue to live in the same social and economic environment in which the drug problem developed.[17] The problems involved in maintaining AIDS risk reduction affect all of the groups at risk for infection and are discussed later in this chapter.

AIDS PREVENTION STRATEGIES FOR WOMEN

The recent recognition of increased risk for women in this epidemic implies the need for greater attention to prevention efforts for this population. Programs designed to block the acquisition or transmission of infection include efforts to reach women at risk, help them to assess their level of susceptibility, and facilitate the process of changing risky behaviors and supporting healthy ones. Programs that focus on preventing transmission address two general transmission patterns: horizontal (transmission of the virus through sexual contact or shared injection equipment with an infected partner) and vertical (from a woman to her infant). Prevention programs addressing these patterns of transmission, as well as acquisition of the virus among women, are discussed below.

Preventing Horizontal Transmission in the Context of Drug Use

As noted earlier, women are at risk of horizontal transmission of HIV in the context of drug use through two routes: directly, through IV drug use itself (e.g., sharing injection equipment with an infected person) and

---

[16] For a review of behavioral changes reported among IV drug users since the beginning of the AIDS epidemic, see Turner, Miller, and Moses (1989:202-211).

[17] In a survey of 401 IV drug users from New York City, the majority (79 percent) reported behavioral change. However, more than a third (36 percent) of this group indicated that they were unable to maintain such changes (Des Jarlais et al., 1989b).

indirectly, through unprotected sex with a male infected IV drug user. Delivering interventions to either of these groups of women has proved difficult in the past, and such efforts loom large on the list of unresolved issues for the future. For example, female sexual partners of IV drug users may not readily identify themselves as being affiliated with an injector. (Alternatively, they may not know about their partner's drug use and thus may be unaware of their own risk.) Attempts to reach female sexual partners of IV drug users through men in treatment or through street outreach activities have met with very little success (Sterk et al., 1989).

Women who are currently in treatment for drug use are an obvious and relatively accessible subpopulation to target for AIDS prevention efforts, and encouraging women who use drugs to enter treatment is a reasonable prevention strategy.[18] Advocating treatment as a strategy, however, carries with it the requirement that policy makers confront the factors that prevent women from accessing such services and that lead to relapse and treatment failure. Many women report difficulties gaining entrance to treatment programs; moreover, surveys of existing drug programs have found that drug and alcohol services for women are lacking in their availability, in the types and quality of support services they provide, and in the adequacy of referral and follow-up facilities (Reed, 1987).[19] Therefore, because many female IV drug users are neither recruited into treatment nor served by it, the scope of outreach efforts must be widened to cover a broader spectrum of this population.

Additional outreach methods may also be needed for female sexual partners of IV drug users. Some recent approaches have used mobile vans to reach geographically diverse and mobile groups. Organizations that serve these women (e.g., community clinics, shelters for the homeless, emergency rooms of inner-city hospitals, family planning and prenatal care clinics, local churches, women's organizations, sexually transmitted disease clinics, beauty parlors, laundromats, prisons) are also potential points of contact, as are door-to-door efforts.

Upon closer scrutiny, however, it is clear that there are factors beyond the control of many women that affect access to needed services. Often,

---

[18] It should be noted, however, that one episode of treatment is generally insufficient to eliminate drug use. A survey of 220 women in drug treatment programs in San Francisco found that women reported a median of five episodes of previous treatment (Wolfe et al., 1989).

[19] Only two-thirds (67 percent) of the 736 female injectors participating in the NIDA demonstration projects (see Chapter 1) had ever been in a formal drug treatment program; less than a quarter (23 percent) of the noninjectors in those projects reported participation in any formal treatment (Sowder, Weissman, and Young, 1989).

taking advantage of AIDS prevention programs requires transportation, child care, and a program in an accessible location at an affordable cost. Strategies that propose the use of health care facilities to deliver such programs need to take into account the barriers that have inhibited women's access to other medical services, such as prenatal care.[20] Women report lack of money most frequently as an obstacle to prenatal care (Institute of Medicine, 1985). It is estimated that 17 percent of reproductive-age women lack any form of health insurance, a factor that undoubtedly affects access to prenatal, family planning, gynecologic, and abortion services (Alan Guttmacher Institute, 1987). Unfortunately, women who receive no prenatal care may be more likely to report risk behaviors (e.g., IV drug use, multiple sexual partners, sex with an IV drug user) than women who receive such care (Dattel et al., 1989).

Female drug users who are pregnant often have difficulties finding a treatment program that will accept them. Even when they are accepted for drug treatment, in many cases the program will not arrange for prenatal care (Chavkin, Driver, and Forman, 1989).[21] In the opinion of the committee, fragmentary services for high-risk populations are inconsistent with sound public health policies. All women of childbearing age who wish to cease drug use should have access to treatment without undue delay, and all pregnant women who use drugs should have access to appropriate prenatal care. At a minimum, effective referral networks should be established.

There is some evidence that intervention programs have reached particular subsets of women. For example, there are indications that female IV drug users have received AIDS prevention messages that describe the routes of HIV transmission (Selwyn et al., 1987). The evidence also suggests that these women are aware of the effectiveness of bleach for sterilizing injection equipment and that they have taken preventive action (Wolfe et al., 1989).[22] Studies performed in New York

---

[20] A report from the Institute of Medicine (1988) on prenatal care identified several significant barriers for women: inadequate third-party coverage of medical benefits, inadequate capacity of the existing maternity care system, and lack of coordination between health and social services for low-income women.

[21] A recent survey of drug treatment programs in New York City found that more than half (54 percent) categorically excluded pregnant women, 67 percent rejected pregnant Medicaid patients, and 87 percent denied service to pregnant crack addicts who were Medicaid recipients. Of the programs that did accept pregnant women, fewer than half (44 percent) made any effort to arrange for prenatal care (Chavkin, 1990).

[22] Among 220 women recruited from methadone and detoxification treatment programs in San Francisco, more than half (117) reported using bleach to sterilize their "works" (Wolfe et al., 1989). The longer the period of time for which women reported bleach sterilization, the less likely they were to be infected. Of the 18 women who reported bleach use for two or more years, none was found to be

City indicate that some women who have altered their injection practices have also altered risky sexual behaviors.[23] Nevertheless, there remain many potential barriers to change in this population, including problems with withdrawal for those women who are currently injecting drugs, the lack of sterile injection equipment, uncertainty about the risk associated with sharing injection equipment with one friend or a sexual partner, lack of confidence in the protection afforded by condoms, and general fear of HIV testing (Williams, 1989). Some studies have reported that brief but intensive counseling with IV drug users and their sexual partners has been effective in improving attitudes about AIDS risk reduction and condom use (D. R. Gibson et al., 1988); conventional teaching methods, on the other hand, have been found to have little or no effect on increasing knowledge about AIDS or changing risk-associated behaviors (Arenson and Finnegan, 1989). Several new intervention strategies that utilize lectures, videotapes, and support groups are being tested for women who use drugs. To date, no evaluation data are available on these programs.

Another potential barrier to change may be a lack of perception of being at risk.[24] The perception of being at risk, which is crucial to the initiation of behavioral change, is particularly important for women who are the sexual partners of IV drug users. Many of these women may not know about the drug use practices of their partners, practices that might affect individual attitudes toward or insistence on condom use and therefore their risk of exposure to the virus through unprotected intercourse. Even if they do know about their partner's drug use, there may still be obstacles that inhibit protective action. Studies have indicated that it may be more difficult to facilitate change in risky sexual behaviors among IV drug users than to facilitate change in risky injection behaviors (Celentano et al., 1989; Chitwood et al., 1989; Farley et al., 1989; Sunita et al., 1989). Consequently, although a number of IV drug users have

---

infected. However, 11 percent of the 47 women who said they had used bleach for one to two years and 17 percent of the 52 women who reported using bleach for less than a year were seropositive.

[23] Paid interviews with 175 female IV drug users found that those who reported a reduction in risky sexual behavior had also (1) decreased risky drug use practices (i.e., reduced or ceased injecting drugs, reduced the use of nonsterile injection equipment or needle-sharing); and (2) had friends who were sexual risk reducers (Tross et al., 1989). One explanation for this finding is that a shift in injection norms may have occurred, and norms that were supportive of safer practices had diffused through friendship networks and thus led to the adoption by individuals of a cluster of new health behaviors.

[24] For more information on motivating behavioral change, see Turner, Miller, and Moses (1989: Chapter 4).

reported changing injection practices in response to the AIDS epidemic,[25] fewer report changes in sexual behavior.[26]

One of the obstacles women confront in relation to condoms may be their lack of information regarding appropriate usage. Training to teach women the skills for proper condom use may be helpful, but there are no evaluation data to show how such programs can best be delivered. Moreover, simply learning the skills involved in condom use may not be the critical change that must be made to enable these women to protect themselves.[27] Intervention programs to help this group of women take protective action must also pay careful attention to outreach problems and to the psychosocial characteristics of the population and their partners. For women who deny their risk—either the risk attributable to their own drug use or to that of their sexual partner—additional interventions may be necessary. Programs may wish to provide information on the local prevalence of HIV infection to help women personalize the risk of infection. By focusing on the risk to the community rather than the risk to one individual, information concerning a serious health problem may be delivered in a less threatening way that can help women to begin to perceive and assess the level of personal risk they face for acquiring or transmitting the virus (Worth, in press).

Preventing Vertical Transmission

Efforts to prevent vertical transmission of the AIDS virus generally try to identify high-risk and infected women prior to or during the early stages of pregnancy and counsel them about the likelihood of transmitting HIV to the fetus. They also discuss the options related to continuing or terminating the pregnancy and the impact of HIV infection on newborns. Studies have shown that there is a 40 to 60 percent chance that an infected woman will pass on the virus (as opposed to only her antibodies) to her infant (Darrow, Jaffee, and Curran, 1988). AIDS prevention thus

---

[25] A survey of 7,660 IV drug users recruited through two detoxification clinics in the San Francisco area between April 1986 and September 1988 found significant decreases in reported needle-sharing (Guydish et al., 1989). The proportions of injectors sharing injection equipment dropped from 55 and 48 percent for the two clinic populations to 28 and 27 percent.

[26] For example, a survey of 298 IV drug users recruited from methadone programs in New York City found that 68 percent of sexually active clients reported no condom use (Magura et al., 1989).

[27] Powerlessness, low self-esteem, isolation, and a low perception of the risk of becoming infected with HIV were common characteristics found throughout a sample of 80 female sexual partners of IV drug users recruited for an ethnographic survey conducted by Arguelles and colleagues (1989). A separate ethnographic survey of sexual partners of drug users found substantial numbers of women who reported emotional and economic dependency, social isolation, and denial of their partners' drug use (Sterk et al., 1989).

depends on reaching two groups of women of childbearing age: women who are at risk of acquiring HIV but are not yet pregnant and pregnant infected women. Because a substantial portion of childbearing women seek care for gynecological and obstetrical problems at some time during the childbearing years, this segment of the health care delivery system has the potential to reach out to these groups of women with interventions to interrupt the vertical transmission of HIV (CDC, 1985; Landesman, Minkoff, and Willoughby, 1989). Some programs are already in place. HIV testing and counseling services, for example, are offered in local health departments and in clinics for sexually transmitted disease (STD), family planning, and prenatal care. Because not all women at risk will be reached through health care facilities, however,[28] other venues and mechanisms will be needed to deliver prevention services to the broader population of susceptible women.[29]

CDC is currently sponsoring a series of community demonstration projects that employ several mechanisms for improving programs to prevent perinatal transmission of HIV infection. The projects target childbearing-age women at risk who are not yet infected as well as women who are already infected and wish to avoid pregnancy (Berman, 1989). They recruit participants through a variety of sources: prenatal and family planning clinics, methadone maintenance programs, STD clinics, and hospitals, as well as through street and storefront outreach stations. Some of the projects use focus groups[30] and ethnographic interviews to elicit information from participants to incorporate into intervention strategies, which include individual and group counseling and education, safer sex parties, peer-led (versus professionally-led) HIV counseling groups, skills training, and empowerment messages. One activity of this multisite study involves an investigation of the role of counseling and testing in changing high-risk behaviors and increasing the use of condoms. Every six months, participants receive a standardized questionnaire that elicits information

---

[28]Indeed, IV drug users, the women at highest risk for acquiring and transmitting the virus, may be the least likely to seek preventive health care (Dattel et al., 1989; Sweeney et al., 1989).

[29]The committee's panel on evaluation recently recommended a process evaluation of CDC's HIV testing and counseling program to determine how well services are being provided and suggested gathering data from several sources on two important aspects of service delivery—the accessibility of services and client-centered barriers to program participation (see Chapter 5, Coyle, Boruch, and Turner [1990]). The committee believes that such research would shed light on the development of potentially effective intervention strategies to reach a diverse population of women at risk.

[30]Focus groups were developed by market researchers to improve their understanding of how consumers perceive a product. (This method is also used in social marketing tests of intervention programs.) A focus group is generally composed of 6 to 10 people plus a trained interviewer; volunteers may be paid for their participation. They are invited to discuss a product or program for a few hours. Interviewing generally moves from broad questions to more specific issues (Kotler and Roberto, 1989).

on changes in sexual and drug use behaviors, use of contraception and family planning services, referral efficacy, and pregnancy. Whereas these projects appear interesting and promising, no data have been presented as yet to indicate their impact on participating women.

The media are another means being used to reach women who are not in touch with the medical establishment. Although few media interventions have been evaluated, there are already some indications that improvement is needed in crafting more effective messages and reaching the targeted audience. Behavioral theory suggests that warnings about health threats must be accompanied by information on concrete actions that can be taken to avoid these threats (Turner, Miller, and Moses 1989). In New York City, faces of female film stars now peer down from subway placards, asking "Pregnant? Get a test for the AIDS virus." Unfortunately, such a message does not tell its audience why such information is useful, which is that infected women need to know about the potential impact of their infection on the fetus, the possible impact of disease progression on their pregnancy and their own health, and the availability of counseling, abortion services, and prenatal care.[31]

The second year of CDC's "America Responds to AIDS" media campaign has focused campaign messages on a broad range of women at risk, including women with multiple sexual partners, female partners of IV drug users, minority women, college students, single parents, and the newly divorced. The program's most visible component is a multimedia public service advertising campaign that consists of television and radio announcements, print advertisements, and public transit posters. At present, there are only limited evaluation data on this activity, which began in the summer of 1988, but they indicate that the program may have several problems.[32]

---

[31] Written materials, generally in pamphlet form, provide more detailed information for women than can be communicated through a poster. Information provided by the Michigan Department of Health, for example, describes the range of services it offers: from testing and counseling, to prenatal, abortion, and pediatric services. The materials note that the choice of the individual regarding the available options for dealing with the pregnancy will be respected (Michigan Department of Health, 1988).

[32] Data from the National Health Interview Survey (a weekly survey of 800 U.S. adults) for January through March 1989 showed that only 24 percent of female respondents could recall a radio or television public service announcement called "America Responds to AIDS" in the previous month (Dawson, 1989). However, 80 percent of women reported seeing other AIDS public service announcements on television and 40 percent reported hearing about AIDS from radio broadcasts in the month prior to interview. These data can only describe the penetration of the message within the targeted population and do not speak to the effect of such messages on women's beliefs and behaviors in response to AIDS. The need for research on the effectiveness of media campaigns was recently addressed by the committee's evaluation panel, which devoted a chapter of its report to specific guidance on assessing the outcomes of CDC's media intervention strategy (Chapter 3 in Coyle, Boruch, and Turner [1990]).

The Role of Counseling and Testing in
Women's Intervention Programs

Intervention strategies to prevent the vertical transmission of HIV have relied heavily on testing and counseling. These approaches presume that women who discover they are infected will avoid conception, either through contraception or sterilization (Kaunitz et al., 1987).[33] Most studies, however, rely on small samples of convenience of pregnant women and suffer from methodological problems that preclude drawing firm conclusions about their effectiveness. Thus, the evidence regarding whether HIV testing is likely to reduce perinatal transmission significantly is inconclusive. Research conducted by Kaplan and colleagues (1989), for example, shows that infected women do not always avoid conception. These researchers followed 134 women of childbearing age after the women were informed that they were HIV seropositive; they found that 7.5 percent became pregnant, despite the fact that the women were repeatedly counseled about the need to practice contraception and safer sex.[34] Other studies also report pregnancies among women who have been found to be infected.[35] On the other hand, a study of 24 infected women recruited from a university medical center in Rhode Island found that, although most of the women remained sexually active even after the diagnosis of AIDS was made, none became pregnant during the course of this 22-month study (Carpenter et al., 1989). It is not clear why this group is different from others that have been studied.

Often women find out that they are infected while receiving prenatal

---

[33] Kaunitz and coworkers (1987) provided HIV counseling and testing to 299 women attending a prenatal clinic in Jacksonville, Florida. Two women were found to be infected. After delivery, both women received additional counseling on contraceptive practices and pediatric care. One woman chose an injectable contraceptive (depot medroxy-progesterone acetate, 150 mg intramuscularly every three months); the other chose oral contraceptives. (This study did not provide information on condom use.)

[34] Of the 11 pregnancies that occurred among these ten women, seven were terminated, three were carried to term, and there was one miscarriage. There did not appear to be substantial differences in pregnancy rates for women who reported IV drug use as their risk factor and those who reported heterosexual contact. Of the 80 women in the study who reported IV drug use, 6 (7.5 percent) underwent one pregnancy, and 1 woman became pregnant two times. Of the 43 women who reported heterosexual contact as their risk factor, 3 (6.9 percent) became pregnant.

[35] In a study by Barbacci and colleagues (1989) that retrospectively studied the pregnancy decisions of women recruited from clinics in Baltimore, Maryland, 14 (16 percent) became pregnant after learning they were infected; none chose to terminate their pregnancy. In a subsequent pregnancy, however, one in this group chose abortion. In another study of 43 infected women in Newark, New Jersey, Schneck and coworkers (1989) found that 7 women (16 percent) became pregnant within 2 to 20 months after receiving their test results; 2 women became pregnant twice. Of the 9 pregnancies reported, 6 were terminated.

care. The rationale for using HIV testing to prevent vertical transmission once a woman has become pregnant is not clearly enunciated in Public Health Service guidelines, which may reflect the controversy that surrounds the role of abortion in managing this problem (Grimes, 1987; Gunn, 1988). There is evidence to suggest that, in some subpopulations, HIV testing during pregnancy may not significantly reduce perinatal transmission of HIV.[36] In many instances, knowledge of infection status occurs after 24 weeks' gestation, when legal abortion is no longer an option. For other women, abortion is an option they do not select.

A variety of factors affect whether infected women will choose abortion—for example, financial barriers to securing an abortion, or the religious beliefs or cultural objections of the woman, her partner, or the community. Other women may not understand the options available to them. In many current testing and counseling programs, recommendations from counselors concerning what, if anything, pregnant women should do when they are found to be seropositive are often nebulous, instead of being even-handed presentations of the range of available options, including abortion. Some testing programs apparently inform women who are found to be infected that abortion is an option (Rutherford et al., 1987; Sachs, Tuomala, and Frigoletto, 1987; Holman et al., 1989); however, because of the controversy surrounding abortion in this country (Grimes, 1987; Gunn, 1988), in some programs the option of abortion may not be offered or discussed.

---

[36]Holman and coworkers (1989) are currently following a group of 82 seropositive pregnant women and a matched seronegative control group from Brooklyn, New York, throughout their pregnancies and for four years thereafter. The women were recruited through several different kinds of obstetrical clinics (a clinic attached to a drug treatment program, one that provides services to Haitian women, and a referral network of clinics at municipal and state hospitals and HIV testing and counseling centers). Between January 1986 and July 1988, 840 pregnant women were counseled about HIV, and 625 consented to undergo testing; 82 (13 percent) were found to be seropositive. Only 27 of the seropositive women learned of their serostatus early enough in the course of their pregnancy to make legal abortion an option; of these, 4 chose to abort. One woman tried to get an abortion but could not find an outpatient clinic that would accept a methadone patient at her dosage level. (Inpatient service was not a possibility because she did not want her family to know about the abortion.) Thirteen of the seropositive women went on to become pregnant again, and of the 10 women who continued this latter pregnancy, 5 already had children with AIDS. An additional 4 women became pregnant a third time, and all chose to abort. Similar findings were reported in a retrospective review of pregnancy decisions by 89 seropositive women in Baltimore, Maryland (Barbacci et al., 1989). The sample was recruited through a prenatal clinic and an HIV clinic for women. Of the 89 women tested, 36 (40 percent) found that they were infected after they had already become pregnant. Of the 10 infected women who had been pregnant for less than 20 weeks, 2 opted to abort the pregnancy, and 1 suffered a miscarriage. In Wiznia and colleagues' (1989) study of 33 infected pregnant women from the Bronx, the option of legal abortion was available to 22 of the women; 6 chose to abort. Seven of the 33 infected women had previously delivered children with HIV infection; only 1 woman in this group chose to terminate her pregnancy.

Moreover, even if legal abortion is presented as an option, services for infected women may not be available. For example, 82 percent of counties in the United States (50 percent of those classified as metropolitan and 91 percent of those classified as nonmetropolitan) lacked a provider of abortion services in 1985 (Henshaw, Forrest, and VanVort, 1987), and only 13 states have Medicaid plans that cover abortion (Gold, 1990). Even where services are available, women who choose to terminate their pregnancy may not be able to do so. In a survey of 25 abortion clinics in New York City, 16 (64 percent) refused to schedule an abortion for a woman who identified herself as infected (Franke, 1989). Perhaps the most important reason women do not elect abortion, one that may be overlooked by strategies that do not attempt to consider the emotional factors that contribute to reproductive decision making, is the profound positive meanings many women associate with bearing children. For some women, having children is associated with self-worth and self-esteem, and it may represent one of the few creative options open to women who are or feel deprived of economic and educational opportunities. In addition, for women with AIDS, the continuation of a pregnancy may reflect the desire to replace a child lost to death or foster care. For women who are asymptomatic, not electing abortion may be a conscious or unconscious attempt to deny the reality of their infection.

Despite the inconclusiveness of the evidence noted above on reducing perinatal transmission, there may be other reasons as well to continue to offer testing to pregnant women. These include optimal medical management of the pregnancy (CDC, 1985; Minkoff and Landesman, 1988); the opportunity to avoid a subsequent pregnancy (Rutherford et al., 1987); the opportunity to begin therapeutic interventions that could benefit the mother and the fetus;[37] and the early identification of newborns who may be infected, thus speeding special medical attention following birth (Krasinski et al., 1988).[38]

It is unclear from the available data whether testing and counseling

---

[37] Recent improvements in treatment and the inclusion of pregnant women in drug trials may provide women with new incentives to seek testing and counseling before pregnancy or during the first trimester. Studies are planned to test whether early detection of infection and prompt treatment with antiretroviral agents such as AZT could lessen the chance of transmission of the virus to the fetus. However, other drugs (e.g., pentamidine) are not offered to pregnant women because of unknown consequences to the fetus.

[38] HIV infection and AIDS among children have engendered pressing problems related to medical treatment, day-to-day care, home and family life, and social support. The committee notes the serious consequences of HIV infection among children, and its Panel on Monitoring the Social Impact of the AIDS Epidemic is currently considering a range of issues that affect U.S. social structures and institutions, including the family and foster care, and the ability of these structures to respond to the needs of infected children. The panel's report is expected to be available in 1991.

are effective in reducing risky behavior, preventing vertical transmission of the virus, or assisting women to make informed decisions concerning childbearing. In part because of the dearth of sound evaluation data, some have questioned the merit of testing and counseling as a behavior-changing intervention (as opposed to a diagnostic service). Clearly, women who are offered such services need to understand the manner in which testing and counseling intervention is delivered and the information it can provide. For example, they need to understand the differences between confidential and anonymous testing,[39] the significance of positive and negative test results for both themselves and their offspring, the implication of positive test results on future reproductive choices, and the limitations of testing in predicting disease progression or outcomes. The ideal time to test for antibodies to the virus and to counsel women about the risk of passing HIV infection to a child is before conception occurs; yet many women do not seek testing prior to conception.[40] Moreover, to assume that positive test results will automatically lead a woman to forgo pregnancy either temporarily or permanently is to ignore the complex meaning that childbearing brings to the lives of women. Clearly, interventions to prevent vertical transmission of HIV must go beyond the means used during the first decade of the epidemic and employ new methods that take into account both the population to be served and the help that can realistically be offered. **The committee recommends careful review of the goals of counseling and testing programs for women of childbearing age and the implementation of efforts to ascertain the effect of such programs on future risk-taking behavior.**

In its review of CDC's counseling and testing program,[41] the committee's evaluation panel recommended strategies for assessing the relative effectiveness of various counseling approaches through well-controlled studies that compare services (1) delivered in different settings, (2) with different content, duration, and intensity, and (3) accompanied by different types of supportive services (see Chapter 5 in Coyle, Boruch, and Turner [1990]). This strategy need not be limited to CDC's program

---

[39] Confidential testing links test results to an individual but protects the individual's identity. Anonymous test results are free of all identifying information.

[40] For example, in a survey of 2,276 sexual partners of hemophilic men conducted by CDC in conjunction with the National Hemophilia Foundation and Hemophilia Treatment Centers, only one-third of the women had been tested (Nichols, 1989). Ten percent of the tested women were infected; 22 women who were seropositive reported a pregnancy in the two years prior to the study.

[41] For a description of CDC's testing and counseling program and resulting epidemiologic data, see CDC (1990).

but could also be applied to the evaluation of any counseling and testing project. As the epidemic enters its second decade, data to ascertain which testing and counseling formats are most effective are crucial to guide intervention planners in designing prevention strategies for the population of women at risk.

In reconsidering the role of testing and counseling for women of childbearing age, it might be useful to explore other similar counseling efforts. Preventing vertical transmission of a disease is not a problem unique to the AIDS epidemic; other disorders, including genetically determined conditions, are also passed from parent to child. Genetic counseling programs for adults at risk of transmitting genetic diseases to offspring have been in place for many years. In addition, ethical guidelines for genetic screening have been proposed by a variety of groups, including the former U.S. Department of Health, Education, and Welfare, the Hastings Center, the National Institute for Child Health and Human Development, and the National Academy of Sciences. All of these groups stress nondirective counseling, individual choice and autonomy, and respect for the moral ambiguities and complexities of decision making (Lappe, Gustafsen, and Roblin, 1972; Powledge and Fletcher, 1979).[42] Such programs may provide helpful information about decision making in relation to current and future pregnancies and the facts and services that might be helpful to women who must make difficult reproductive decisions.

Lessons from Genetic Counseling

Knowing that one may be capable of passing on a genetic disease to one's offspring does not inevitably result in a decision not to have children. Indeed, research shows that the factors that contribute to reproductive decision making in the face of genetic disorders show substantial variation. For example, early research on genetic counseling regarding phenylketonuria (PKU), a metabolic disorder that can result in mental retardation (Schild, 1964), found that information about health outcomes and the quality of life for the child appeared to be highly salient factors in the decisions made by families who already had a child with PKU to modify or restrict reproductive plans. In addition, other factors, such as the birth order of the child in question, the age of the parents, and the level of perceived risk to the child all showed some association with reproductive decisions related to PKU and other disorders (Carter et al., 1971; Emery, Watt, and Clack, 1972; Burns et al., 1984). Somewhat later studies found

---

[42]For a discussion of this issue specifically related to AIDS, see Bayer (in press).

a different pattern. Advances in the treatment of PKU and the diminished consequences of the disease (through such techniques as improving the diet of children with PKU to prevent retardation), together with readily available counseling, have resulted in decisions not to limit reproduction even when families know there is a 25 percent chance of having another child with the disease (Burns et al., 1984). It appears that the availability of a treatment or remedy that improves the health status of the child increases the likelihood that other children will be conceived.

For other types of genetic diseases, the impact of genetic counseling programs on reproductive decision making is unclear. Despite participation in counseling, many couples who are at high risk of producing a child with sickle-cell anemia (Neal-Cooper and Scott, 1988),[43] cystic fibrosis (Leonard, Chase, and Childs, 1972; McCrae et al., 1973), or Down's syndrome (Leonard, Chase, and Childs, 1972; Oetting and Steele, 1982)[44] go on to have children. These studies suggest either that some couples do not interpret the information provided by genetic counseling in a manner that leads to no further pregnancies or that the desire to have children outweighs the predicted risk. There also appears to be considerable variation in the effects of genetic counseling programs across the various subpopulations who seek such counseling, although the factors that account for this variability are not well understood (Evers-Kiebooms and van den Berghe, 1979; Murray et al., 1980), in part because of poor study design (Evers-Kiebooms and van den Berghe, 1979). What is clear is that information alone regarding a potential health problem in an unborn child does not necessarily result in postponement or relinquishment of child-bearing. When the disease in question is HIV infection, for which (unlike PKU, for example) there is no diagnostic procedure for the fetus and no prophylaxis for children who are born with the disease, the reproductive decision-making process is likely to be even more difficult. In addition, the substantial likelihood that an infected mother will pass on HIV infection to her newborn child (Darrow, Jaffe, and Curran, 1988) emphasizes the need to identify any factors that may make counseling an effective tool for infected women who face reproductive decisions. Therefore,

---

[43] In their review of 25 couples at risk of having a child with sickle-cell anemia, Neal-Cooper and Scott (1988) reported 16 pregnancies among 10 couples, 4 pregnancies among 4 of the 5 couples with an unaffected child, and 5 pregnancies among 4 of the 9 couples with an affected child.

[44] Oetting and Steele (1982) found no significant differences between counseled and matched uncounseled couples who already had a child with Down's syndrome in terms of knowledge of genetics or recurrent risks, initiation of subsequent pregnancies, or utilization of prenatal diagnosis. Although 18 of 35 couples initiated at least one more pregnancy after the birth of a child with Down's syndrome, only 3 couples used prenatal diagnosis by amniocentesis to determine the presence or absence of the condition.

the committee recommends that the Public Health Service convene a symposium of experts in genetic counseling to consider the potential contribution of this field's expertise and experience to the design and implementation of counseling programs for HIV-infected women and to identify research opportunities in this area. In addition, more research is needed to understand cultural, religious, sociodemographic, and regional variations in responses to programs that deal with reproductive decision making, including the effects of these factors on the interpretation of information, the counseling experience, medical interaction, and subsequent action.

AIDS Prevention Challenges in the Coming Decade

The clear indication that blacks and Hispanics are overrepresented in the AIDS epidemiological data has focused attention on the urgent need for AIDS prevention for these groups and for other minority subpopulations.[45] Several intervention efforts are already under way, most of which have been directed toward minority subpopulations within traditional risk groups.[46] For example, CDC has provided support for intervention programs that target minority youth, both those in school and those who cannot be reached through educational institutions. In addition, the National Institute of Mental Health (NIMH) is currently supporting two studies of HIV risk among black men who engage in same-gender sex.[47] Yet the committee finds that ongoing efforts fall far short of the magnitude of intervention needed, given the prevalence of disease and evidence of continued risk taking among many of the populations currently at risk

---

[45] For an overview of AIDS and Native Americans, see Tafoya (1989); Aoki and colleagues (1989) review AIDS prevention efforts for Asian-American communities.

[46] CDC currently funds a variety of community-based HIV interventions aimed at promoting behavioral change among these high-risk groups. However, there is little in the way of currently available evaluation data to identify the most promising strategies. In its recent report, the evaluation panel recommended that randomized experiments be conducted to evaluate the effectiveness of a subset of these projects (see Chapter 4, Coyle, Boruch, and Turner [1990]). This committee endorses the panel's recommendation.

[47] One of the NIMH studies is descriptive and focuses on the prevalence and determinants of risk behaviors in the group; the other implements and evaluates planned variations of "safer sex" workshops designed especially for black homosexual and bisexual men. Preliminary findings indicate that most men in the sample report high rates of risk-associated behavior. Of 50 black homosexual and 50 black bisexual men recruited in 1988 in San Francisco, Oakland, and Berkeley, California, 60 percent of homosexual and 88 percent of bisexual men had engaged in unsafe sexual practices in the previous month with a partner other than their primary partner. Unsafe sexual practices with primary partners were reported by 50 percent of homosexual and 78 percent of bisexual men (Peterson et al., 1989). Predictors of safer sexual practices were a heightened sense of self-efficacy (i.e., a perceived ability to successfully enact such behaviors), enjoyment of safer sexual activities, close association with persons with AIDS, and media awareness of AIDS.

for AIDS, including minority men and women. Effective intervention strategies are needed to sustain healthy behavioral patterns in individuals who are not currently at risk and to facilitate change among individuals who are at risk.

There is some recent evidence indicating that the basic facts about AIDS are reaching minority subpopulations. After controlling for education, data from the 1988 National Health Interview Survey (NHIS) showed no differences between Hispanics and white non-Hispanics or between black and white survey participants in patterns of AIDS knowledge (Dawson and Hardy, 1989a,b).[48] For all groups, however, misconceptions and gaps in knowledge remain, indicating that the job of delivering useful information is far from complete. One important factor that must be considered in planning further interventions for minority subpopulations is the diversity of these groups. For example, the term *Hispanic* may mask substantial cultural heterogeneity, given the groups that constitute this ethnic category (e.g., Puerto Ricans, Mexicans, Cubans, and individuals from Central and South American countries) (Amaro, 1988). The usefulness of AIDS prevention information to racial and ethnic minorities depends on the development of culturally and linguistically appropriate messages that are delivered through the venues and organizations deemed trustworthy by the targeted audience.[49]

Yet as the committee noted last year, for most at-risk individuals, regardless of their racial or ethnic background, information alone is

---

[48]Provisional data collected between May and October 1988 by the National Center for Health Statistics' NHIS were aggregated to provide sufficient numbers of respondents to examine differences in knowledge about AIDS in various subpopulations, including Hispanics (Dawson and Hardy, 1989b). Unfortunately, the resulting sample of Hispanic adults was still small ($N = 1,102$) compared with the sample of white non-Hispanic participants ($N = 19,963$), making it difficult to detect subtle differences that could be statistically significant. In separate analyses (Dawson and Hardy, 1989a), the responses of black participants ($N = 3,066$) were compared with those of whites ($N = 17,355$). Objective measures of knowledge about AIDS and HIV infection varied by education for Hispanics, white non-Hispanics, and blacks. After controlling for education, however, the responses of the groups were very similar: of respondents with more than 12 years of education, 89 percent of Hispanics, 90 percent of white non-Hispanics, and 82 percent of blacks knew that HIV could be transmitted through sexual intercourse, and 79 percent of Hispanics, 81 percent of white non-Hispanics, and 82 percent of blacks were aware of vertical transmission. However, the proportion of Hispanic participants who believed that condoms were not at all effective (10 percent) was twice as high as the proportion of white non-Hispanics holding a similar belief (5 percent); the proportion of blacks with similar beliefs about condoms (8 percent) was greater than the proportion of whites but smaller than the proportion of Hispanics. Only 60 percent of blacks and Hispanics and 66 percent of white non-Hispanics knew that a person could be infected with HIV and not have AIDS, and even fewer realized that a person with HIV infection could look and feel healthy. In a separate telephone survey of 460 Hispanics from the San Francisco area, Marin and Marin (1990) found that knowledge about AIDS was strongly associated with acculturation, even after controlling for education.

[49]See, for example, Amaro (1988); Marin (1990); Marin and Marin (in press).

unlikely to be sufficient to elicit change in risk-associated behaviors. Interventions that go beyond the provision of information—for example, drug treatment programs or skills training to promote condom use—are required and in the case of minority subpopulations must be tailored to reflect the cultures and languages of the individuals they seek to serve, as well as the socioeconomic and day-to-day realities of their lives. Without careful attention to these factors, intervention programs for minorities hold little promise of success in preventing further spread of HIV infection (Worth and Rodriguez, 1987; Amaro, 1988; Mays and Cochran, 1988; Marin, 1989; Schilling et al., 1989).

The broad base of information required to develop potentially effective interventions for diverse minority subpopulations, information concerning the variation and distribution of behaviors as well as the contexts in which they are enacted, clearly does not currently exist. Accumulating the necessary data will require a long-term commitment to behavioral research targeted specifically toward these subgroups. Previous attempts to gather high-quality data leave little doubt about the difficulty of conducting such research, and about limited information to illuminate current efforts. Careful ethnographic studies of the various minority subpopulations and the social context of risk, in conjunction with demonstration projects, may offer an appropriate starting point for building the knowledge base required to design effective interventions. Thus, **the committee recommends that the agencies of the Public Health Service encourage and strengthen behavioral science research aimed at understanding the transmission of HIV in various black and Hispanic subpopulations, including men who have sex with men, drug users and their sexual partners, and youth. The committee further recommends that the PHS develop plans for appropriate interventions targeted toward these groups and support the implementation of intervention strategies (together with appropriate evaluation components) in both demonstration projects and larger scale efforts.**

The committee anticipates that behavioral efforts to contain the epidemic will not decrease over the course of the next 10 years. Indeed, as the only available means of disease containment, interventions to facilitate change in risky behaviors must assume the lion's share of the burden to prevent further HIV infection. Therefore, **the committee recommends the following:**

- **that the Public Health Service encourage and support behavioral research programs that study the behaviors that transmit HIV infection and that the PHS develop** and evaluate mechanisms for facilitating and sustaining change in those behaviors;

- that intervention programs incorporate planned variations that can be carefully evaluated to determine their relative effectiveness;

- that the PHS regularly summarize the data derived from currently funded behavioral and epidemiological research on AIDS (in terms of incidence of infection and high-risk behaviors) to determine intervention priorities for various subpopulations at risk; and

- that all agencies of the PHS that are currently funding intervention programs and evaluation research regularly summarize the data derived from these studies to determine which, if any, programs can be recommended for wider dissemination.

These recommendations apply to the range of at-risk populations described earlier in this chapter. For most of the subgroups who are now faced with the threat of AIDS, the existing knowledge base is deplorably limited. Specifically, in the case of women, there is a tremendous need for more and better information regarding the behaviors that transmit the virus as well as the determinants of those behaviors. The gender-specific differences in the distribution of these behaviors and the social and psychological factors that contribute to the initiation and continuance of both risk-taking and health-seeking behavioral patterns among women warrant significant attention in the coming decade.

MAINTAINING RISK REDUCTION BEHAVIOR

Relapse prevention is a necessary component of any AIDS intervention program because maintaining risk reduction is often more difficult than initiating it. Given that AIDS prevention for some individuals requires life-long change, a significant challenge for the second decade lies in helping individuals who have initiated safer behaviors to maintain them. In addition, several new factors related to AIDS may make relapse prevention even more important today than in the early years of the epidemic. The treatment of early-stage infection with AZT (as well as with other antiviral agents that are now being developed or that may be developed in the future) may lengthen the asymptomatic period of the disease. It is not yet known whether individuals who are so treated remain infectious; it is also unclear how a more extended asymptomatic period will affect the initiation and maintenance of risk-reducing practices. Given the relatively high background rates of infection in some communities and the rise in infectivity that is suspected to occur in individuals who have been infected for some time, only the long-term and consistent practice of risk reduction by those who are infected will contain the further spread of HIV infection in these communities.

If this premise is accepted, the need for long-term modification of behavior becomes even more crucial. Such an emphasis on the long term, however, may require certain reorientations in already-established AIDS prevention programs. The example of gay men offers a case in point. AIDS prevention programs for gay men have focused primarily on the adoption of safer sex techniques, and many communities have reported extensive modification of high-risk behaviors. Nevertheless, seroconversions have continued among gay and bisexual men in cities such as San Francisco (Lifson et al,. 1989). A plausible explanation for at least some new cases of infection is relapse or the inability to maintain safer sexual practices that had been initiated previously. Thus, prevention campaigns for gay men must now include additional efforts to prevent relapse from established risk reduction behaviors.

After almost a decade of monitoring behavioral changes among gay men, there is some information about patterns of relapse in this population. Among participants in the San Francisco Men's Health Study, the frequency of risky sexual behaviors following the period of initial behavioral change in 1983 has dropped over the course of the study, and recent data from this sample indicate that behavioral change is remarkably stable (Ekstrand and Coates, in press). Nevertheless, a small proportion of men participating in this study continue to report high-risk behavior. Each year between 1984 and 1988, roughly 3.5 percent of the sample reported engaging in unprotected anal intercourse. Moreover, 8.5 percent of subjects reported at least one episode of relapse following initial behavioral change. Other research from San Francisco presents a similar but no less cautionary picture (Stall, et al., 1990); although only a small minority of men consistently reported unprotected anal intercourse, many more report initiating low-risk behavior only to relapse to high-risk behavior.

Factors that predict relapse among gay men include a preference for unprotected anal intercourse and social support for high-risk behavior; reasons for relapse given (retrospectively) by gay men included being in love, knowing the sexual partner was seronegative, receiving a request from the sexual partner for unprotected sex, using alcohol and drugs, and not having condoms available (Stall et al., 1990). Saltzman and colleagues (1989) reported that relapsers tended to have higher levels of unsafe sexual behavior at baseline and reported perceptions that behavioral change would not offer protection from infection.

Maintaining safer sex behavior over time is particularly problematic if people do not enjoy the physical result produced by the safer methods or find the psychological costs associated with change to be too great (Catania et al., 1989; Joseph et al., 1989). The importance of the link between safer sex and pleasure is underscored by data indicating that the frequency of condom use is more strongly predicted by its perceived enjoyment ratings than by its health ratings (Catania et al., 1989). Some researchers have proposed that the perception that safer sexual activities are less enjoyable than unsafe practices has hindered the adoption of such activities (Catania, Kegeles, and Coates, in press).[50]

Maintaining risk-reducing behavior also presents problems for IV drug users. In one study of 401 street-recruited IV drug users in New York City, almost 80 percent of the respondents reported that they had changed their drug use or sexual behavior, or both, since learning about AIDS. Yet more than one-third of those who had changed their behavior also reported that they had not been able to maintain those changes fully (Des Jarlais et al., 1989b). Given the biases expected from self-reported data (see Chapter 6), this figure must be considered a low estimate of the percentage of drug injectors who will have difficulty maintaining risk reduction over time.

A recent study of IV drug users in San Francisco reported some intriguing findings that also indicate some of the potential problems in maintaining AIDS risk reduction over long time periods. Sorenson and colleagues (1988) randomly assigned IV drug users to a six-hour "psycho-educational" experimental condition or an "information-only" control condition. Individuals who received the "psycho-educational" program scored significantly higher than those in the control group on a test of AIDS knowledge immediately following the intervention, but differences between the two groups had faded by the six-month follow-up interview. What is intriguing about the study are other program effects that were identified. Individuals who participated in the experimental group showed increases in measures of self-efficacy, indicating a complex relationship among knowledge, attitudes, and beliefs that is not fully understood but that may have implications for AIDS relapse prevention.

---

[50] Another problem is the strong preference of some individuals for behaviors that are risky, a preference predictive of continued risk taking and relapse. Men who report that unprotected anal intercourse is their favorite sexual activity are less likely to adopt safer sex practices and more likely to relapse than men who favor less risky activities (Stall et al., 1990; McKusick et al., in press).

Most research and intervention activities conducted during the first decade of the epidemic have been directed toward facilitating change in risky sexual and drug use behaviors. There is some indication that these activities have, at least in part, achieved their goal because significant change has been reported among subsets of gay adult males and IV drug users. Yet segments of every at-risk group continue to practice unsafe behaviors. In some instances, the reason for such continuance may be that certain subgroups (e.g., young gay males, female sexual partners of drug users, minority men and women) may not have been aware of their risk for HIV infection and thus may not have adopted the appropriate protective behaviors. In other instances, individuals may not have been able to sustain changes they had initiated, thus relapsing into previous patterns of risk. Because the threat of AIDS does not appear to be declining and because the only available strategies to prevent this disease involve changing behaviors—perhaps for a lifetime—the committee finds the problem of relapse prevention to be a serious concern. Therefore, **the committee recommends that the Alcohol, Drug Abuse, and Mental Health Administration focus research efforts on AIDS-related relapse prevention, including the determinants of such relapse and the role that alcohol and other drugs play in the return to unsafe sexual and injection practices.**

Maintaining risk-reducing behavioral change is also a problem for the diverse population of at-risk women. Prostitutes, female IV drug users, sexual partners of IV drug users, and sexual partners of hemophiliacs all report intermittent unprotected intercourse and thus continued exposure despite counseling and education (CDC, 1987; Cohen, 1989; Jackson et al., 1989; Sowder, Weissman, and Young, 1989; Turner, 1989:Table 1). The poor rates of condom use reported among hemophilic and other couples have prompted some investigators to call for "comprehensive education and counseling" programs (Smiley et al., 1988). Yet it appears from data reported by such couples (Jackson et al., 1989; Sotheran et al., 1989), as well as data reported by individuals from other subpopulations, that it is not yet known how best to reach the diverse female population or how to provide effective education and counseling that promote the consistent use of condoms.

As contraceptive options have become fewer,[51] many women find it increasingly difficult to identify a method of contraception they consider appropriate and effective. Now, women are being asked in addition to

---

[51] A recent report of the National Academy of Sciences, *Developing New Contraceptives: Obstacles and Opportunities* (Mastroianni, Donaldson, and Kane, 1990), considers the organizational, policy, and research constraints on the development of new contraceptives.

look beyond fertility control to disease prevention. Condoms plus the use of a spermicide, which currently appear to be the most effective means for accomplishing both functions, pose considerable problems for women. Not only does condom use require the cooperation of the male partner, but it may also require substantial changes in the attitudes and behaviors of women. A survey of 759 women attending birth control clinics found that attitudes about condoms were the best predictor of their use (Valdiserri et al., 1989b). Positive attitudes, however, must be converted into effective and appropriate action, which Valdiserri and coworkers have suggested is also predicated on a perceived need for protection or a sense of vulnerability. Therefore, additional measures are required—for example, informative messages[52] that build positive attitudes toward condoms while providing accurate information on their use or training in the skills needed to ensure proper usage. To circumvent cultural barriers to the adoption of condoms, intervention programs that stress condom use should also incorporate different ethnic and racial perspectives.

Talking about sexual practices and introducing safer methods is at the heart of a great deal of AIDS prevention. Yet traditional sex roles for women in most cultures do not encourage them to talk about sex, to initiate sexual practices, or otherwise control an intimate heterosexual encounter. Intervention efforts that rely on women to introduce condoms into a sexual union ask that women assume new roles in what is already an emotionally charged area, roles that in some cultures or among some groups may be construed as controlling men's sexuality. "Indeed, what is being asked of women could be dangerous to them since it raises the possibility of domestic, if not cultural, conflict . . . . No one knows in any systematic way what women face when they introduce condoms into a sexual scene or talk about changing sexual practices" (Schneider, 1988:99). Women who must take upon themselves the burden of both contraception and disease prevention need more options that are within their control and that do not depend for their effectiveness on the co-operation or consent of others.[53] **The committee recommends that the Public Health Service support research to develop protective measures other than condoms for preventing HIV transmission during sexual contact—specifically, methods that can be used unilaterally by**

---

[52] More than one-quarter (26 percent) of the sample in this study conducted by Valdiserri and colleagues (1989b) considered vaseline the best lubricant for condoms. A petroleum-based substance, vaseline is, in fact, a very poor choice because it can compromise the integrity of latex condoms and cause them to rupture.

[53] See, for example, Sakondhavat (1990) and Stein (1990).

women and methods that will be acceptable to both men and women who do not currently use condoms.

In fact, the inconsistent use of condoms is a common theme that cuts across all risk groups in the epidemic.[54] Gay men, IV drug users, and female sexual partners of infected or at-risk individuals have all reported inconsistent condom use despite clear evidence of perceived risk.[55] Many discordant couples, for reasons that remain unclear, choose not to use condoms consistently to protect the uninfected partner. For some women, there remain important questions concerning the impact of domestic violence on the initiation and regular use of condoms (Schneider, 1988). In its first report, the committee urged widespread availability and promotion of the use of condoms (with spermicides) as the main means to reduce the risk of sexually transmitted HIV infection. The committee supported the presentation of condom advertisements in print and broadcast media and argued for wider distribution of condoms through a variety of retail outlets. Increasing the role of condoms in AIDS prevention, however, also requires a clearer understanding of the contexts in which they are used. Sexual conduct is influenced by a variety of factors, including opportunity, customs, and cultural norms and values. Last year the committee recommended that funding be provided for longitudinal studies of sexual behavior and that high priority be given to studies of the social and societal contexts of sexual behaviors. Information on the dynamics of sexual interaction in dating and other social situations may enhance our understanding of the impediments to condom use and the potential opportunities for increasing this form of protection.

As the epidemic enters its second decade, it is clear that sexual transmission of the disease continues to be a major route of infection. Behavioral interventions focused on the consistent use of condoms are currently the most effective AIDS prevention strategy for this type of

---

[54]Problems with consistent condom use have been reported in other developed countries, including Norway (Sundet et al., 1989; Traeen, Rise, and Kraft, 1989), Denmark (Schmidt et al., 1989), and France (Moatti et al., 1989). On the other hand, national prospective surveys in Switzerland have found dramatic increases in the proportion of participants reporting consistent condom use—from 8 percent in February 1987 to 29 percent in October 1988 (Zeugin et al., 1989).

[55]One reason for inconsistent condom use may be the enjoyment problems condoms pose for some people. It is not uncommon to hear men complain that condoms decrease penile sensitivity. It should be pointed out, however, that other men may derive benefits from condom use (e.g., delayed orgasm for men who typically achieve orgasm sooner than they want). It is not impossible that solutions to sensory problems could be found (for instance, better condom materials might be developed); however, at present, considerable work is needed to enhance both the acceptability of condom use as well as their physical characteristics.

transmission. Consequently, **the committee recommends that the Public Health Service fund research on condoms to achieve the following objectives:**

- **understand the determinants of condom use for the diverse populations at risk for sexually transmitted HIV infection;**
- **improve condom design and materials to make them more acceptable to users; and**
- **develop interventions to promote their consistent use.**

IMPEDIMENTS TO IMPROVED INTERVENTION

In this chapter, and in the two chapters that follow, the committee describes an array of intervention efforts that have been implemented to prevent further spread of HIV infection. Unfortunately, it is not possible at this time to say which strategies will work best for the various subpopulations at risk for HIV infection. Without well-designed, well-implemented, and well-evaluated programs, there is no rational basis for assessing the effectiveness of intervention efforts or for directing finite resources. In its first report, the committee found that the absence of rigorous evaluations of the major interventions undertaken at that time and the absence of empirical studies that compared the efficacy of AIDS prevention strategies made it virtually impossible to identify *proven* techniques for facilitating the behavioral change needed to retard the spread of HIV. Thus, the committee relied on a more basic analysis of intervention strategies, using principles of human behavior established through empirical research and the theories of the social and behavioral sciences.[56] While a systematic review of the theories of human health behavior and the relevant research on the prevention of other, related diseases can assist efforts to design programs that hold the most promise of being successful,[57] accumulating sound evaluation data on planned variations of intervention strategies is perhaps the most important task for the next decade of this epidemic.

Reliable data on the behaviors that transmit the virus as well as on the prevalence of HIV infection in the population are needed to track the movement of the epidemic and to target intervention resources to the diverse groups at highest risk. The evolving nature of the epidemic means

---

[56] See Chapter 4 of Turner, Miller, and Moses (1989).

[57] See Mechanic and Aiken (1989) for a review of lessons to apply to AIDS from the provision of care for the mentally ill, the elderly, and people with cancer.

that different intervention strategies provided in different contexts must be utilized to reach ever-changing at-risk populations. Understanding the best way to reach different subpopulations and to provide the most effective strategies will also require carefully designed and executed comparative studies and careful evaluation.

Moreover, as the epidemic grows, there will be more groups, more programs, and more services competing for available resources. Therefore, comparative studies will need to take into account the cost-effectiveness of the most promising intervention strategies. As Russell (1986) notes, making good choices requires a sound understanding of both the positive and negative aspects of prevention programs, and, as resources become more scarce, making good choices becomes more important. Sound evaluation data can ensure that prevention efforts receive a reasonable share of available resources and that those resources are allocated to the most effective programs.

Successful AIDS prevention strategies will also need to look beyond the individual to the social forces that make it difficult to provide effective interventions to those at highest risk. The history of AIDS-related discrimination provides a promising example of social evolution compatible with public health goals. For example, when HIV antibody tests first became available, many individuals eschewed this service, fearing loss of job, insurance, housing, and even family if they were found to be infected. Now, however, antidiscrimination legislation has been put into place, thus providing a social structure to deal with this problem. Nevertheless, other impediments remain that continue to block the provision of additional intervention activities. In this final section of the chapter, the committee reviews the current status of antidiscrimination legislation to protect infected individuals and those with AIDS. It also considers the effect of restrictive social attitudes and public policies in impeding the implementation of innovative intervention programs (e.g., sexually explicit information and needle exchange programs) for those at highest risk and the collection of data on sensitive behaviors related to HIV transmission.

AIDS-Related Discrimination

Discrimination refers to the disadvantageous treatment, either overt or insidious, of individuals or groups that results in unequal treatment or the denial of opportunities afforded to others. Discrimination as a legal concept in the United States originated in the development of a body of law designed to protect the rights of blacks (Parmet, 1987). In addition to promoting equality, however, antidiscrimination laws and policies have instrumental value as a bulwark in the fight against the spread of HIV, an advantage recognized by a number of governmental and policy groups (World Health Organization, 1988; U.S. Conference of Mayors, 1989). Indeed, according to the Presidential Commission on the Human Immunodeficiency Virus Epidemic, discrimination has been one of the most significant barriers to reaching high-risk groups and implementing effective interventions. According to the Presidential Commission (1988:119), "HIV-related discrimination is impairing this nation's ability to limit the spread of the epidemic . . . . As long as discrimination occurs, and no strong national policy with rapid and effective remedies against discrimination is established, individuals who are infected with HIV will be reluctant to come forward for testing, counseling, and care."

The stigma associated with AIDS has prompted a wide spectrum of untoward reactions that are important to understand, monitor, and, ultimately, to counter.[58] During the first decade of this epidemic, effective interventions and high-quality research were compromised by difficulties in identifying and reaching those most in need. Indeed, it is not known to what extent public health strategies designed to prevent further spread of infection have been impeded by fears of disclosure and stigma—for example, strategies such as voluntary contact notification procedures to inform individuals who have had intimate contact with an HIV-infected person. Voluntary, confidential contact tracing is a prevention strategy that has provoked considerable debate and warrants further systematic study. Furthermore, the opportunities afforded by new modalities of care have conferred a new urgency on the need to reach and thus protect HIV-infected individuals from discrimination. The information now available on the potential benefits of prophylactic treatment of HIV-infected persons makes early diagnosis in asymptomatic individuals critical in attempts to forestall the progression of disease. Other critically important initiatives to halt the spread of the epidemic, such as surveillance to monitor the spread of HIV, are also affected by discriminatory policies (Fordyce, Sambula, and Stoneburner, 1989; Kegeles et al., 1989). The committee thus finds that a review of the legal factors involved may shed some light on intervention issues.

That discrimination has occurred against persons with AIDS and HIV infection is not in question, but its extent is far from clear, for there is only limited empirical evidence. Questions remain about how

---

[58]The stigma associated with AIDS and HIV infection was a principal focus of Chapter 7, "Social Barriers to Intervention," in Turner, Miller, and Moses (1989). Questions of stigma and discrimination will be taken up in greater depth by the committee's Panel on Monitoring the Social Impact of the AIDS Epidemic, which is preparing a report for release in 1991.

the burgeoning numbers of cases and the enduring nature of the epidemic are shaping individual and social reactions to persons with AIDS and HIV infection. Appropriate means for safeguarding the infected against discrimination have been the subject of continuing political debate regarding the forms such protection should take and whether responsibility should be lodged at the federal, state, or local level. One reason for the debate is that discrimination laws are not without costs. As Blendon and Donelan (1988) have observed, new antidiscrimination laws may result in more litigation and may call for increased staff efforts at monitoring and enforcement. Federal legislation may draw the government into complex litigation and negotiations with employers, landlords, state and local agencies, about the line between reasonable accommodation and justifiable discrimination.

Laws relating to AIDS, such as statutes enacted and cases reported (especially appellate cases that can set precedent), are only the most visible evidence of how U.S. society is dealing with HIV-related discrimination. Even this activity is considerable, as more than 170 state statutes specific to AIDS have been passed since the beginning of the epidemic (Gostin, 1989). Already, litigation surrounding AIDS has resulted in more cases than for any other single disease in the history of American jurisprudence (Gostin, 1990).

Federal Protections

Some protection from AIDS-related discrimination is afforded by the federal Rehabilitation Act of 1973, Public Law 93-112, Section 504. The act states that "no otherwise handicapped qualified individual . . . shall, solely by reason of his handicap, be excluded from the participation in, be denied the benefits of, or be subjected to discrimination under any program or activity receiving Federal financial assistance." In a 1987 case, *School Board of Nassau County v. Arline*,[59] the U.S. Supreme Court held that the definition of a handicapped individual under Section 504 included a person with a contagious disease (in that case, tuberculosis). The court also delineated guidelines for defining whether an individual with a contagious disease would be "otherwise qualified," in terms of the accommodations that would have to be made to prevent risk to co-workers.

A recent amendment to the Rehabilitation Act provides further clarification of this phrase by stating that a person with a contagious disease or infection is otherwise qualified if he or she does not "constitute a direct threat to the health or safety" of others and is able to perform the

---

[59] *School Board of Nassau County v. Arline*, 107 S.Ct. 1123 (1987).

duties of the job. In addition, the Justice Department, reversing an earlier pronouncement, has advised that Section 504 encompasses discrimination against infected individuals and prohibits discrimination based on unjustified fears of contagion. In recent years federal courts have used Section 504 to prohibit discrimination by employers or schools against individuals infected with HIV (e.g., *Chalk v. Orange County Department of Education; Doe v. Centinela Hospital; Ray v. School District of DeSoto County*).

As the above quotation from the Rehabilitation Act of 1973 implies, its major failing is its limited reach; it applies only to programs receiving federal financial assistance. Its scope was extended somewhat by the Fair Housing Amendment Act of 1988, Public Law 100-430 passed by the 100th Congress, which extends protections against discrimination to the private sector. (The Fair Housing Amendments make it illegal for private landlords to discriminate on the basis of HIV infection.) Notwithstanding this legislation, concerns about the limitations of extant federal antidiscrimination provisions and the patchwork of state and local laws (see below) prompted the drafting of a new federal bill known as the Americans with Disabilities Act,[60] which passed the U.S. Senate on September 7, 1989, by a vote of 76-8 (Congressional Record, 1989a).[61] Disability in the pending legislation is broadly defined as "a physical or mental impairment that substantially limits one or more of the major life activities of such individual" (Congressional Record, 1989b, S10954). The definition thus includes both persons with AIDS and those infected with HIV. The legislation would prohibit labor organizations, employment agencies, and employers in both the private and public sectors from discriminating against qualified individuals with disabilities. The bill's sponsors estimate that as many as 43 million Americans with various disabilities may be protected by its provisions.

State and Local Protections

In addition to federal protections, all 50 states and the District of Columbia have statutes that parallel the federal Rehabilitation Act prohibiting discrimination against handicapped persons.[62] In all but five jurisdictions, protection from discrimination applies to some private as

---

[60]B. Lambert, "Federal policy against discrimination is sought for AIDS victims," *New York Times*, September 22, 1988, A35.

[61]Action on this bill is pending in the U.S. House of Representatives. For Senate debate on this issue, see the Congressional Record 135(112):S10701-S10723, S10734-S10763, September 7, 1989.

[62]Unfortunately, as Lambert's *New York Times* article notes, relatively less protection from discrimination is provided in states with lower prevalences of infection, ironically, in situations in which protection may be most needed. Furthermore, although the trend has been for state governments to

well as public employees. More than half of the states have extended previously enacted laws to cover persons with HIV infection; often, there are a variety of sources of legal protection in any one state. To buttress statutory protections and avoid the delays inherent in enacting new laws, a number of states have used attorneys' general opinions and the statements of human rights commissions as vehicles for extending protection to HIV-infected individuals. In addition, many states and some municipalities have enacted AIDS-specific antidiscrimination statutes or ordinances.

A number of states have enacted HIV-specific measures to prevent discrimination in the workplace. Most of these provisions relate to information generated in the course of HIV testing and prohibit the use of that information as a precondition of employment or in a determination of continued employability. Protection from discrimination for simply taking an HIV test is increasingly important as more widespread testing is encouraged (Rhame and Maki, 1989), as more insurers screen potential policyholders, and as patients are tested with or without their knowledge.

A major shift is now emerging in the nature of AIDS lawsuits that have been brought under the statutes described above. As Gostin, Porter, and Sandomire (in press:45–46) observe:

> The early cases, still winding their way through the courts, often involve discriminatory practices by employers based upon prejudice or fears of transmission in the workplace. As CDC and OSHA guidelines continue to make clear that these fears are groundless, employers appear much less likely to exclude employees from ordinary workplaces. The new wave of cases involves workplace settings where there is likely to be some exposure to blood such as health care settings, laboratories, and forensic examiners. (pp. 45-46)

Access for HIV-infected persons to public accommodations is also of concern, and lawsuits have been filed against establishments ranging from a manicure salon to a spiritual retreat for refusing to serve HIV-infected customers or clients. The question of such access takes on special urgency when the "accommodations" are health care institutions. The general antidiscrimination laws of most states cover public accommodations, but only a few explicitly, or even arguably, define public accommodations to include health care services. At least five states have enacted specific measures to prevent AIDS-related discrimination by health care providers.

---

expand protections against AIDS-related discrimination, there have been moves in the opposite direction. Tennessee, for example, amended its disability statutes because of AIDS to exclude contagious diseases; its human rights agency no longer investigates cases of AIDS-related discrimination.

These states prohibit refusal of admission to facilities based on HIV status or the use of HIV testing as a condition for receiving unrelated care.

Enforcement of antidiscrimination provisions may vary tremendously among the states. Some larger states with significant caseloads, like New York and California, have been more aggressive than smaller, less affected states, imposing penalties, compensation, and punitive damages and providing provisions for civil suits and recovery of legal costs. In other states the remedies are more limited and procedures more protracted.

Because all states prohibit at least certain manifestations of HIV-related discrimination, enforcement of statute provisions and the availability of timely, equitable, and understandable procedures for pressing discrimination claims are critical. Persons with AIDS may not have the wherewithal to sustain lengthy processes. In most states the process begins with a civil or human rights commission, and lawsuits can be filed only after administrative relief has been sought. In at least 20 states, an agency or attorney general may file a complaint on behalf of an individual alleging discrimination—a critical procedure for people who wish to remain anonymous because of concerns about further discrimination from wider breaches in confidentiality.

A few crude barometers of AIDS discrimination have been cited in policy debates. The Presidential AIDS Commission cited testimony from officials of New York City's Commission on Human Rights that the number of complaints handled by its AIDS Discrimination Department has risen precipitously, from 3 in 1983 to more than 300 in 1986 and more than 600 in 1987 (City of New York Commission on Human Rights, 1988). It is impossible to tell how much the increase represents a growth in discriminatory incidents versus a greater awareness of their rights on behalf of victims, more vigorous enforcement, or some combination of these two factors.

It is clear that many lawyers have been enlisted in the fight against AIDS discrimination, often on a pro bono basis. Increasingly, "AIDS law" is a legal speciality, with some lawyers in cities with large numbers of cases of AIDS engaged in full-time AIDS law practices. A number of law schools now operate AIDS law clinics, and the first major casebook on AIDS and the law has been published. The American Bar Association is undertaking a study to gauge the extent of the legal resources now being used in this area.

Another possible benchmark of AIDS-related discrimination is violence against gay men and lesbians. Several studies have documented increases in reports of antigay violence. Herek (1989) reviews a number of such unpublished reports by social and behavioral scientists. A

National Institute of Justice report notes that "homosexuals are probably the most frequent victims" of hate violence (Finn and McNeil, 1987). Hate crimes, or bias crimes, are defined as threats of violence, intimidation, property crimes, or crimes of violence motivated by prejudice. Only recently have these crimes received the systematic attention of social scientists and policy makers. Several reports have attempted to document the extent of such crimes, and special units have been created within police forces to confront the problem. Legislative support for data collection efforts related to hate crimes is being sought at the state and federal level.

These violent acts indicate a continued potential in U.S. society for stigmatizing actions and AIDS-related discrimination, despite the protective measures that are currently in place. The committee is gratified to see that the antidiscrimination measures urged in its first report and recommended by the Presidential AIDS Commission are being instituted. It would point out, however, that this legislation alone is unlikely to ameliorate all of the conditions associated with discrimination in this country. For example, such legislation protects the rights of HIV-infected children for education but does not necessarily prevent hostile encounters with the community. Other issues addressed in the committee's first report, however, remain problematic, and their lack of resolution continues to impede efforts to contain the epidemic. These issues, which are discussed below, include the use of explicit sexual material in intervention programs, the implementation and evaluation of sterile needle programs, and the effects of public policies that restrict the acquisition of knowledge necessary to develop effective interventions.

Social Attitudes and Public Policy:
Obstacles to Continued Progress

Throughout this chapter, the committee has noted that effective intervention to prevent further spread of HIV infection requires knowing more about the people who are at risk, the behaviors that transmit the AIDS virus, and the conditions that have facilitated change in those behaviors. Gathering such information has been difficult; methodological problems have stymied efforts to understand these factors, and public policies and opinions have created impediments to acquiring knowledge. Drug researchers know, for example, that research that goes beyond the clinic or the jail to contact subjects in the settings in which the behaviors occur captures a crucial segment of the at-risk population. Although such efforts afford the important opportunity to observe subjects in their natural settings and to reach individuals who are not in drug treatment programs or other institutional settings, these efforts are more vulnerable to community pressure than are clinic-based programs. The committee notes, for example, that studies of syringe exchange programs in Great Britain were made more difficult than they might have been through picketing by members of the community (Stimson, 1988). In New York City, political opposition caused the syringe exchange pilot program to be operated from public health offices, a location distant (physically and psychologically) from major addict populations and drug use sites. Now, after a change in political administrations in New York City, the new mayor has announced the cancellation of the needle exchange program in that city.[63]

State and federal legislative action has afforded some protection to the populations these programs seek to reach. Nevertheless, constraints imposed by political opposition have limited the programs' ability to intervene and to collect much-needed surveillance data on risk behaviors. In the final section of this chapter, the committee reviews the public response to innovative and controversial intervention efforts.

Sexually Explicit Information

One of the significant controversies in intervention programs to prevent sexually transmitted HIV infection has surrounded the level of sexual explicitness of information and the degree to which interventions emphasize the erotic. Political debate abounds regarding the appropriateness of using public monies to support the development of such materials;[64] only now, however, are objective data accumulating on the effects of a sexually explicit approach to the prevention of sexually transmitted HIV infection.

Eroticizing safer sex messages makes considerable sense, given that adults at high risk for HIV and other sexually transmitted infections are those who engage in sex often and with multiple partners (e.g., Bell and Weinberg, 1978; Marmor et al., 1982; Jaffe et al., 1983). In Bullough's terms (1980), these individuals are highly "sex positive." To make safer sex messages appealing to such individuals, presentations of those messages must capture and hold their attention. In addition, the messages may

---

[63] See Todd S. Purdum, "Dinkins to End Needle Plan for Drug Users," *New York Times,* Feb. 14, 1990, B1, B4.

[64] Federally funded AIDS education efforts have historically had problems dealing with advice about the protective value of condoms, as well as the presentation of sexually explicit educational materials. For example, M. Gladwell reports in *The Washington Post* ("Publication of AIDS Pamphlet on Condoms Approved: FDA Sought Health and Human Services' Approval of Brochure in May 1988," April 5, 1990, A16) that a lack of consensus among federal officials on the effectiveness of condoms halted the production on an AIDS education pamphlet aimed at groups at highest risk for almost two years. (See also Chapter 6 in Turner, Miller, and Moses [1989].)

need to make cognitive-affective associations between *pleasurable* sex and *safer* sex. Programs using sex-positive messages have been shown to increase favorable attitudes toward condom use among individuals attending an STD clinic and heterosexual couples (Tanner and Pollack, 1988; Solomon and DeJong, 1989) and have facilitated the initiation of safer sex activities among gay and bisexual men (D'Eramo et al., 1988).

Early in the epidemic the Gay Men's Health Crisis in New York City developed workshops to promote the acceptance of safer sex by eroticizing these practices (Valdiserri, 1989). The workshops also used conventional psychotherapeutic techniques to teach men how to negotiate safer sexual encounters. Extensions of this approach that were designed to reach a much larger audience relied on erotic films and comic books. The comic books in particular created intense controversy because some federal legislators perceived them as promoting homosexuality (Valdiserri, 1989:152). Despite such controversy, however, this approach shows promise in changing risk-associated behavior.

Recently, D'Eramo and colleagues (1988) evaluated the efficacy of various sexually explicit materials by comparing four planned variations of an AIDS prevention education program that had been implemented in New York for 619 gay men. The variations included the following: (1) lectures and discussions about AIDS, how it is transmitted, and safer sex guidelines; (2) a program of eroticizing safer sex alternatives through verbal and print media; (3) the program described in (2) but with sexually explicit videos and slides; and (4) distribution of printed copies of safer sex guidelines (the comparison group). Investigators assessed the risk level of participant sexual behaviors before the application of the intervention and three months after the program ended. They concluded that the erotic program with audiovisuals (variation 3 above) was most effective in increasing the adoption of safer sex.

The goal of sexually explicit programs is to promote widespread and rapid acceptance of safer sexual behaviors. The strategies described above that have attempted to achieve these goals have relied on the principles of the behavioral theory of adoption and diffusion of innovation.[65] For example, existing networks of communication are employed to reach the targeted audience and to promote new ideas—in this case, by persuading individuals that new behavioral patterns are positive and pleasant. The use of a trusted communication system contributes to the perceived worthiness of the innovation and helps the adopter to overcome

---

[65] For a detailed discussion of this theory, see Chapter 4, Turner, Miller, and Moses (1989).

motivational barriers, thus accelerating the process of behavioral change (Valdiserri, 1989).

Sterile Needle Programs

Previous reports on AIDS from the National Academy of Sciences (NAS) and the Institute of Medicine (IOM) recommended that the U.S. government sponsor research on needle and syringe exchange programs as a means for reducing the spread of HIV among drug injectors (IOM/NAS, 1988; Turner, Miller, and Moses, 1989). Yet syringe exchange programs remain controversial in the United States,[66] currently operating on a very limited basis in only a few cities. Programs approved by local jurisdictions have been established in New York City; Tacoma and Seattle, Washington; and Portland, Oregon. The New York City program was cancelled in February 1990. Unofficial programs are operating publicly in San Francisco and Boston, and there may well be other such unofficial efforts.

None of these programs receive federal support for either operational or research activities, and this policy has resulted in limited evaluation of the effectiveness of these efforts. The early findings on U.S. needle exchange programs, however, are quite similar to findings from European and Australian studies (Buning et al., 1988; Hart et al., 1988, 1989; Ljungberg et al., 1988; van den Hoek et al., 1988; Des Jarlais et al., 1989c; Hartgers et al., 1989; Stimson, 1989; van den Hoek, van Haastrecht, and Coutinho, 1989). Evaluations of ongoing efforts abroad have found that participation in syringe exchange programs is associated with the reduction but not the elimination of HIV risk behavior and that syringe exchanges do not lead to any detectable increase in illicit drug injection, either among current users or new injectors. Program characteristics associated with successful risk reduction include readily accessible programs for potential participants and linkages and referral networks to drug use treatment and other health and social services required by drug injectors.

Despite these findings, many individuals making policy-level decisions on this matter express the general fear that explicit messages concerning sterile injection equipment will result in increased rates of IV drug use. As this committee previously noted (Turner, Miller, and Moses, 1989:Chapter 3), however, what evidence there is from various intervention programs suggests otherwise: having the information and the means to protect oneself from a deadly disease is likely to result in protective action against AIDS, as well as in generalized increases

---

[66] For an overview of this controversy, see Stryker (1989).

in healthy behaviors (e.g., seeking drug treatment) among people who are already engaging in risky activities.[67] Furthermore, information and services do not appear to entice the uninitiated into risk-associated actions.[68] Given the success of innovative interventions in other developed countries, the potential for spread of HIV to other subpopulations from individuals who inject drugs, and the seriousness of this disease, it makes sense to implement well-designed pilot studies of needle exchange programs and to collect the data that would establish whether these strategies are effective in decreasing risky behaviors and the spread of AIDS. Continued reliance on hunches and suspicions rather than on data regarding the impact of these programs gives too much credence to guesswork and may obstruct a promising path toward retarding the spread of HIV in the U.S. population.

The committee strongly reiterates the recommendation made in its

---

[67] Even before AIDS prevention programs were offered to IV drug users in New York City, the mass media and informal communication networks among IV drug users reportedly had provided an awareness of AIDS and knowledge of the routes of transmission (Des Jarlais, Friedman, and Strug, 1986). However, more information was needed to identify and implement self-protective measures against HIV infection, and this information was provided through more formal and targeted programs. Ethnographic studies of the New York drug scene in 1985 found a substantial expansion in the illicit market for sterile injection equipment (Des Jarlais, Friedman, and Hopkins, 1985); the demand for new injection equipment was so great that counterfeit sterile needles and syringes were being sold. Later in 1985, outreach programs began to teach IV drug users about AIDS and sterilization techniques, such as boiling injection equipment in water or soaking it in bleach or alcohol (Jackson and Neshin, 1986; Jackson and Rotkiewicz, 1987). Not only did drug users report increased use of bleach and other sterilization techniques but when offered coupons for free drug treatment, drug users accepted in such numbers that more than 85 percent of the vouchers were redeemed. A similar outreach program to provide information about AIDS and bleach sterilization techniques was started in San Francisco. More than half of the subjects in one study (Chaisson et al., 1987) and two-thirds in another (Watters, 1987) reported adopting the use of bleach. Data from Amsterdam, where a needle exchange program was initiated prior to the AIDS epidemic, found that the number of subjects reporting daily injection decreased as the distribution rate for sterile injection equipment increased (van den Hoek et al., 1988). Other researchers (Buning et al., 1986, 1988; Stimson, 1988, 1989; Hartgers et al., 1989) have found higher rates of needle sharing and more frequent injection among users who were not participating in the needle exchange programs in Amsterdam and Great Britain than were found among program participants. The pilot study of the New York City needle exchange program, although limited in scope and longevity, was found to be an effective "bridge to treatment" for IV drug users (New York City Department of Health, 1989). The data are far from perfect, but on balance they do provide some evidence indicating that individuals who participate in needle exchange programs are more amenable than individuals who do not participate in such programs to enrollment in drug treatment programs.

[68] For example, the Amsterdam syringe exchange program distributed 25,000 sterile needles and syringes in 1984; in 1987, the number distributed increased greatly. In addition, during the period of expansion, there was no decrease in the number of persons entering methadone maintenance or drug-free treatment programs, and the number of heroin users held constant at approximately 7,000 to 8,000 (van den Hoek, van Haastrecht, and Coutinho, 1989). During this time the average age of IV drug users increased, thus indicating little influx from younger age groups. More recent data find that individuals who receive sterile injection equipment from this program are no more likely to lend it to others than are individuals who do not participate in the program.

first report (Turner, Miller and Moses, 1989) that well-designed, staged trials of sterile needle programs, such as those requested in the 1986 IOM/NAS report *Confronting AIDS,* be implemented. Evaluation of these programs, if they were carefully implemented and monitored, could provide the evidence needed to resolve some of the questions regarding their impact. The committee notes, however, that the 101st Congress[69] adopted legislation requiring that "[n]one of the funds appropriated under this Act shall be used to carry out any program of distributing sterile needles for the hypodermic injection of any illegal drug unless the President of the United States certifies that such programs are effective in stopping the spread of HIV and do not encourage the use of illegal drugs."

The committee observes that the evidence needed by the President to make such determinations about the effect of domestic needle exchange programs requires research that has also been held hostage to this controversy. The committee repeats its recommendation that this research be carried forward.

The lack of current, valid, and reliable data, which provide the basis for sound public health policy decisions, appears to reflect a tendency to rely on intuition and hunches concerning sensitive issues rather than on empirically derived facts. Last year the committee recommended well-designed pilot tests of needle exchange programs accompanied by evaluation research to determine the effect of these efforts. It now appears unlikely that funds will be appropriated to evaluate the few pilot studies that have been executed over the past year. This year the committee reiterates its recommendation that the Public Health Service implement programs to collect sound data on the prevalence and distribution of behaviors that transmit HIV infection. In addition, it affirms its support for empirical tests of promising behavioral intervention strategies that may involve sexually explicit information. The committee continues in its calls for these measures in the belief that, despite an apparent lack of appreciation for empirical approaches to understanding the behavioral underpinnings of the AIDS epidemic, certain recent examples of progress offer hope for the mutability of social structures. (For example, empirical evidence of AIDS-related discrimination has resulted in changes in laws to protect HIV-infected individuals and those with AIDS.) The committee thus finds that this country must redouble its efforts to identify and remove other impediments to change and to affirm and support rational approaches to the resolution of controversial problems.

---

[69] Public Law 101-166 (H.R. 3566), Title V, Section 520, as finally approved by the House and Senate.

REFERENCES

Abdul-Quader, A. S., Friedman, S. R., Des Jarlais, D., Marmor, M. M., Maslansky, R., and Bartelme, S. (1987) Methadone maintenance and behavior by intravenous drug users that can transmit HIV. *Contemporary Drug Problems* Fall:425–434.

Abdul-Quader, A., Tross, S., Des Jarlais, D. C., Kouzi, A., and Friedman, S. R. (1989) Predictors of attempted sexual behavior change in a street sample of active male intravenous drug users in New York City. Presented at the Fifth International Conference on AIDS, Montreal, June 4–9.

Alan Guttmacher Institute. (1987) *Blessed Events and the Bottom Line: Financing Maternity Care in the United States.* New York: Alan Guttmacher Institute.

Alldritt, L., Dolan, K., Donoghoe, M., and Stimson, G. V. (1988) HIV and the injecting drug user: Clients of syringe exchange schemes in England and Scotland. Presented at the Fourth International Conference on AIDS, Stockholm, June 12–16.

Amaro, H. (1988) Considerations for prevention of HIV infection among Hispanic women. *Psychology of Women Quarterly* 12:429–443.

Aoki, B., Ngin, C. P., Mo, B., and Ja, D. Y. (1989) AIDS prevention models in Asian-American communities. In V. M. Mays, G. W. Albee, and S. F. Schneider, eds., *Primary Prevention of AIDS: Psychological Approaches.* Newbury Park, Calif.: Sage Publications.

Arenson, C., and Finnegan, L. P. (1989) Prevention methodologies for women at risk for AIDS. Presented at the Fifth International Conference on AIDS, Montreal, June 4–9.

Arguelles, L., Rivero, A. M., Rehack, C. J., and Corby, N. H. (1989) Female sex partners of IV drug users: A study of socio-psychological characteristics and needs. Presented at the Fifth International Conference on AIDS, Montreal, June 4–9.

Barbacci, M., Chaisson, R., Anderson, J., and Horn, J. (1989) Knowledge of HIV serostatus and pregnancy decisions. Presented at the Fifth International Conference on AIDS, Montreal, June 4–9.

Baskin, J. (1983) Prenatal testing for Tay-Sachs disease in the light of Jewish views regarding abortion. *Issues in Health Care of Women* 4:41–56.

Bayer, R. (In press) AIDS and the future of reproductive freedom. *Milbank Quarterly* (Special Supplement).

Bayer, R., Lumey, L. H., and Wan, L. (In press) The American, British and Dutch responses to unlinked, anonymous, HIV seroprevalence studies: An international comparison of ethical, legal and political issues. *AIDS.*

Becker, M. H., and Joseph, J. G. (1988) AIDS and behavioral change to reduce risk: A review. *American Journal of Public Health* 78:394–410.

Beeker, C., and Rose, T. (1989) The Stop AIDS model for community change: Acceptability in a low-incidence area for AIDS. Presented at the Fifth International Conference on AIDS, Montreal, June 4–9.

Beeker, C., and Zielinski, M. (1988) Drugs, alcohol and risky sex among gay and bisexual men in a low-incidence area for AIDS. Presented at the Annual Meeting of the American Public Health Association, Boston, November 13–17.

Bell, A. P., and Weinberg, M. S. (1978) *Homosexualities: A Study of Diversity Among Men and Women.* New York: Simon & Schuster.

Berman, S. (1989) Prevention of perinatal transmission of HIV. Presented at the Fifth International Conference on AIDS, Montreal, June 4–9.

Beschner, G., and Thompson, P. (1981) *Women and Drug Abuse Treatment: Needs and Services.* Service Research Monograph Series. DHHS Publication No. (ADM) 81–1057. Rockville, Md.: National Institute on Drug Abuse.

Biernacki, P., Mandel, J., and Aldrich, M. (1989) Gender differences in "maturing out" of intravenous drug use. Presented at the Fifth International Conference on AIDS, Montreal, June 4–9.

Blendon, R. J., and Donelan, K. (1988) Discrimination against people with AIDS: The public's perspective. *New England Journal of Medicine* 319:1022–1026.

Blendon, R. J., and Donelan, K. (1989) AIDS, the public, and the "NIMBY" syndrome. In D. E. Rogers, and E. Ginzberg, eds., *Public and Professional Attitudes Toward AIDS Patients: A National Dilemma.* Boulder, Colo.: Westview Press.

Blix, O., and Gronbladh, L. (1988) AIDS and IV heroin addicts: The preventive effects of methadone maintenance in Sweden. Presented at the Fourth International Conference on AIDS, Stockholm, June 12–16.

Bradford, J., and Johnson, D. (1989) AIDS-related behavior change of gay men in Richmond, Va., 1985–1988. Presented at the Fifth International Conference on AIDS, Montreal, June 4–9.

Brown, L. S., Chu, A., Nemoto, T., and Primm, B. J. (1989) Demographic, behavioral, and clinical features of HIV infection in New York City intravenous drug users (IVDUs). Presented at the Fifth International Conference on AIDS, Montreal, June 4–9.

Brundage, J. F., Burke, D. S., Gardner, L. I., Herbold, J., Voskovitch, J., and Redfield, R. R. (1987) Temporal trends of prevalence and incidence of HIV infection among civilian applicants for U.S. military service: Analysis of 18 months of serological screening. Presented at the Third International Conference on AIDS, Washington, D.C., June 1–5.

Bullough, V. (1980) *Sexual Variance in Society and History.* Chicago, Ill.: The University of Chicago Press.

Buning, E., Coutinho, R. A., and van Brussel, G. H. A. (1986) Preventing AIDS in drug addicts in Amsterdam. *Lancet* 1:1435–1436.

Buning, E., Hartgers, C., Verster, A. D., van Santen, G. W., and Coutinho, R. A. (1988) The evaluation of the needle/syringe exchange in Amsterdam. Presented at the Fourth International Conference on AIDS, Stockholm, June 12–16.

Burns, J. K., Azen, C. G., Rouse, B., and Vespa, H. (1984) Impact of PKU on the reproductive patterns in collaborative study families. *American Journal of Medical Genetics* 19:515–524.

Calzavara, L., Coates, R., Read, S., Johnson, K., Farewell, V., et al. (1989) Sexual behaviour changes among male sexual contacts of men with HIV disease: A 3-year overview. Presented at the Fifth International Conference on AIDS, Montreal, June 4–9.

Carpenter, C. J., Mayer, K. H., Fisher, A., Desai, M. B., and Durand, L. (1989) Natural history of acquired immunodeficiency syndrome in women in Rhode Island. *The American Journal of Medicine* 86:771–775.

Carter, C. O., Roberts, J. A. F., Evans, K. A., and Buck, A. R. (1971) Genetic clinic: A follow-up. *Lancet* 1:281–285.

Catania, J., Kegeles, S., and Coates, T. (In press). Toward an understanding of risk behavior: An AIDS risk reduction model (ARRM). *Health Education Quarterly.*

Catania, J. A., Coates, T. J., Kegeles, S. M., Ekstrand, M., Guydish, J. R., and Bye, L. L. (1989) Implications of the AIDS risk-reduction model for the gay community: The importance of perceived sexual enjoyment and help-seeking behaviors. In V. M. Mays, G. W. Albee, and S. F. Schneider, eds., *Primary Prevention of AIDS: Psychological Approaches.* Newbury Park, Calif.: Sage Publications.

Celentano, D. D., McQueen, D. V., and Chee, E. (1980) Substance abuse by women: A review of the epidemiologic literature. *Journal of Chronic Diseases* 33:383–384.

Celentano, D., Vlahov, D., Anthony, J. C., and Bernal, M. (1989) Is condom use an independent risk for HIV in IV drug users? Presented at the Fifth International Conference on AIDS, Montreal, June 4–9.

Centers for Disease Control (CDC). (1985) Recommendations for assisting in the prevention of perinatal transmission of human T-lymphotropic virus type III/lymphadenopathy-associated virus and acquired immunodeficiency syndrome. *Morbidity and Mortality Weekly Report* 34:721–726, 731–732.

Centers for Disease Control (CDC). (1987) Antibody to human immunodeficiency virus in female prostitutes. *Morbidity and Mortality Weekly Report* 36:157–161.

Centers for Disease Control (CDC). (1988) Relationship of syphilis to drug use and prostitution—Connecticut and Philadelphia, Pennsylvania. *Morbidity and Mortality Weekly Report* 36:755–765.

Centers for Disease Control (CDC). (1990) Publicly funded HIV counseling and testing—United States, 1985–1989. *Morbidity and Mortality Weekly Report* 39:137–140.

Chavkin, W. (1990). Drug addiction and pregnancy: Policy crossroads. *American Journal of Public Health* 80:483–487.

Chavkin, W., Driver, C. R., and Forman, P. (1989) The crisis in New York City's perinatal services. *New York State Journal of Medicine* 89:658–663.

Chetwynd, J., Horn, J., and Kelleher, J. (1989) Safer sex amongst homosexual men: Meaning and motivation. Presented at the Fifth International Conference on AIDS, Montreal, June 4–9.

Chiasson, R. E., Osmond, D., Moss, A., Feldman, H., and Biernacki, P. (1987) HIV, bleach, and needle sharing (letter). *Lancet* 1:1430.

Childs, B. (1979) Psychological consequences of genetic screening. In R. M. Goodman and A. G. Motulsky, eds., *Genetic Diseases Among Ashkenazi Jews.* New York: Raven.

Chimel, J., Detels, R., van Raden, M., Brookmeyer, R., Kingsley, L., and Kaslow, R. (1986) Prevention of LAV/HTL-III infection through modification of sexual practices. Presented at the Second International Conference on AIDS, Paris, June 25–26.

Chitwood, D. D., McCoy, C. B., Comerford, M., and Trapido, E. J. (1989) Risk behaviors of IV cocaine users: Implications for intervention. Presented at the Fifth International Conference on AIDS, Montreal, June 4–9.

City of New York Commission on Human Rights. (1988) Report on discrimination against people with AIDS and people perceived to have AIDS. Commission on Human Rights, New York.

Cleary, P. D., Barry, M. J., Mayer, K. H., Brandt, A. M., Costin, L., and Fineberg, H.V. (1987) Compulsory premarital screening for the human immunodeficiency virus. *Journal of the American Medical Association* 258:1757–1762.

Coates, T. J., and Greenblatt, R. M. (In press) Behavioral change using community-level interventions. In K. Holmes, ed., *Sexually Transmitted Diseases.* New York: McGraw-Hill.

Coates, T. J., Stall, R. D., and Hoff, C. C. (1988) Changes in sexual behavior of homosexual and bisexual men since the beginning of the AIDS epidemic. Background paper prepared for the Health Program, Office of Technology Assessment, Washington, D.C.

Coates, T. J., Stall, R. D., Catania, J. A., and Kegeles, S. M. (1988a) Behavioral factors in the spread of HIV infection. *AIDS* 2(Supplement 1):S239–S246.

Coates, T. J., Catania, J. A., Dolcini, M. M., and Hoff, C. C. (1988b) Changes in sexual behavior with the advent of the AIDS epidemic. Prepared for the Hudson Institute, Indianapolis, Ind.

Coates, T. J., McKusick, L., Kuno, R., and Stites, D. P. (1989a) Stress reduction training changed number of sexual partners but not immune function in men with HIV. *American Journal of Public Health* 79:885–887.

Coates, T. J., Stall, R., Catania, J., Dolcini, P., and Hoff, C. (1989b) Prevention of HIV infection in high-risk groups. In P. Volderding and M. Jacobson, eds., *1988 AIDS Clinical Review.* New York: Marcel-Dekker.

Coates, T. J., Ekstrand, M. L., Kegeles, S. M., and Stall, R. D. (1989c) Knowledge of HIV antibody status, behavior change, and psychological distress in two cohorts of gay men in San Francisco. Unpublished paper. Center for AIDS Prevention Studies, University of California, San Francisco.

Cohen, J. B. (1989) Condom promotion among prostitutes. In *Condoms in the Prevention of Sexually Transmitted Diseases.* Research Triangle Park, N.C.: American Social Health Association.

Cohn, D., Koleis, J., Cooper, S., Cole, V., and Judson, F. (1989) Incidence of HIV infection in gay and bisexual men attending a counseling and testing site or an AIDS prevention program. Presented at the Fifth International Conference on AIDS, Montreal, June 4–9.

Communication Technologies. (1987) A Report on Designing an Effective AIDS Prevention Campaign Strategy for San Francisco: Results From the Fourth Probability Sample of an Urban Gay Male Community. San Francisco AIDS Foundation, San Francisco.

Congressional Record. (1989a) Senate vote on Americans with Disabilities Act. *Congressional Record* 135(113):S10765–S10803, September 8.

Congressional Record. (1989b) Quote from text of proposed bill. *Congressional Record* 135(115):S10954–10961, September 12.

Connors, M. M., and Lewis, B. F. (1989) Anthropological and epidemiological observations of changes in needle use and needle sharing practices following twelve months of bleach distribution. Presented at the Fifth International Conference on AIDS, Montreal, June 4–9.

Corby, N. H., Rhodes, F., and Wolitski, R. J. (1989) HIV serostatus and risk behaviors of street IVDUs. Presented at the Fifth International Conference on AIDS, Montreal, June 4–9.

Coyle, S. C., Boruch, R. B., and Turner, C. F., eds. (1990) *Evaluating AIDS Prevention Programs, Expanded Edition.* Washington, D.C.: National Academy Press.

Cuskey, W. R., Berger, L. H., and Densen-Gerber, J. (1977) Issues in the treatment of female addiction: A review and critique of the literature. *Contemporary Drug Problems* 6:307–371.

Dalton, H. L. (1989) AIDS in blackface. *Daedalus* 118:205–228.

Darrow, W. W., Jaffe, H. W., and Curran, J. W. (1988) Behaviors associated with HIV-1 infection and the development of AIDS. In R. Kulstad, ed., *AIDS 1988.* Washington, D.C.: American Association for the Advancement of Science.

Dattel, B. J., Hauer, L. B., Crombleholme, W., Landers, D. V., Edison, R., et al. (1989) HIV-1 seroprevalence and risk behavior are increased in pregnant women receiving no prenatal care. Presented at the Fifth International Conference on AIDS, Montreal, June 4–9.

Dawson, D. A. (1989) AIDS knowledge and attitudes for January—March 1989: Provisional data from the National Health Interview Survey. In *Advance Data from Vital and Health Statistics of the National Center for Health Statistics,* No. 176. DHHS Publ. No. (PHS) 89–1250. Hyattsville, Md.: National Center for Health Statistics.

Dawson, D. A., and Hardy, A. M. (1989a) AIDS knowledge and attitudes of black Americans: Provisional data from the 1988 National Health Interview Survey. *NCHS Advance Data* 165:1–22.

Dawson, D. A., and Hardy, A. M. (1989b) AIDS knowledge and attitudes of Hispanic Americans: Provisional data from the 1988 National Health Interview Survey. *NCHS Advance Data* 166:1–22.

D'Eramo, J. E., Quadland, M. C., Shatts, W., Schuman, R., and Jacobs, R. (1988) The "800 men" project: A systematic evaluation of AIDS prevention programs demonstrating the efficacy of erotic, sexually explicit safer sex education on gay and bisexual men at risk for AIDS. Presented at the Fourth International Conference on AIDS, Stockholm, June 12–16.

De Vroome, E. M. M., Sandfort, T. G. M., Paalman, M., and Tielman, R. A. P. (1989) AIDS and condom use in the Netherlands. Presented at the Fifth International Conference on AIDS, Montreal, June 4–9.

Des Jarlais, D. C., and Friedman, S. R. (1987) HIV infection among intravenous drug users: Epidemiology and risk reduction (editorial review). *AIDS* 1:67–76.

Des Jarlais, D. C., Friedman, S. R., and Hopkins, W. (1985) Risk reduction for the acquired immunodeficiency syndrome among intravenous drug users. *Annals of Internal Medicine* 313:755–759.

Des Jarlais, D. C., Friedman, S. R., and Strug, D. (1986) AIDS and needle sharing within the IV-drug use subculture. In D. A. Feldman and T. M. Johnson, eds., *The Social Dimensions of AIDS: Method and Theory.* New York: Praeger.

Des Jarlais, D. C., Friedman, S. R., and Stoneburner, R. L. (1988) HIV infection and intravenous drug use: Critical issues in transmission dynamics, infection outcomes, and prevention. *Reviews of Infectious Disease* 10:151–158.

Des Jarlais, D. C., Friedman, S. R., Novick, D. M., Sotheran, J. L., Thomas, P., et al. (1989a) HIV-1 infection among intravenous drug users in Manhattan, New York City, from 1977 through 1987. *Journal of the American Medical Association* 261:1008–1012.

Des Jarlais, D. C., Tross, S., Abdul-Quader, A., Kouzi, A., and Friedman, S. R. (1989b) Intravenous drug users and maintenance of behavior change. Presented at the Fifth International Conference on AIDS, Montreal, June 4–9.

Des Jarlais, D. C., Hagan, H., Purchase, D., Reid, T., and Friedman, S. R. (1989c) Safer injection among participants in the first North American syringe exchange program. Presented at the Fifth International Conference on AIDS, Montreal, June 4–9.

Detels, R., English, P., Visscher, B. R., Jacobsen, L., Kingsley, L. A., et al. (1989) Seroconversion, sexual activity, and condom use among 2,915 seronegative men followed for up to two years. *Journal of Acquired Immune Deficiency Syndromes* 2:77–83.

District of Columbia Advisory Committee to the U.S. Commission on Civil Rights. (1989) Handicap protection for AIDS victims in Washington, D.C. Washington, D.C.

Ekstrand, M., and Coates, T. J. (1988) Prevalence and change in AIDS high risk behavior among gay and bisexual men. Presented at the Fourth International Conference on AIDS, Stockholm, June 12–16.

Ekstrand, M. L., and Coates, T. J. (In press) Gay men in San Francisco are maintaining low-risk behaviors but young men continue to be at risk. *American Journal of Public Health.*

Ellerbrock, T., Chamberland, M. E., Bush, T. J., and Rogers, M. F. (1989) National surveillance of AIDS in women, 1981–1988: A report from the Centers for Disease Control. Presented at the Fifth International Conference on AIDS, Montreal, June 4–9.

Emery, A. E. H., Watt, M. S., and Clack, E. R. (1972) The effects of genetic counselling in Duchenne muscular dystrophy. *Clinical Genetics* 3:147–150.

Eric, K., Drucker, E., Worth, D., Chabon, B., Pivnick, A., and Cochrane, K. (1989) The Women's Center: A model peer support program for high risk IV drug and crack using women in the Bronx. Presented at the Fifth International Conference on AIDS, Montreal, June 4–9.

Eskenazi, B., Pies, C., Newstetter, A., Shepard, C., and Pearson, K. (1989) HIV serology in artificially inseminated lesbians. *AIDS* 2:187–193.

Evers-Kiebooms, G., and van den Berghe, H. (1979) Impact of genetic counseling: A review of published follow-up studies. *Clinical Genetics* 15:465–474.

Farley, T., Peterson, L., Cartter, M., and Hadler, J. (1989) Trends in HIV prevalence and risk behavior among drug treatment program entrants. Presented at the Fifth International Conference on AIDS, Montreal, June 4–9.

Fehrs, L., Hill, D., Kerndt, P., Rose, T., and Henneman, C. (1989) HIV screening program at a Los Angeles prenatal/family planning center. Presented at the Fifth International Conference on AIDS, Montreal, June 4–9.

Fineberg, H. V. (1988) Education to prevent AIDS: Prospects and obstacles. *Science* 239:592–596.

Finn, P., and McNeil, T. (1987) *The Response of the Criminal Justice System to Bias Crime: An Exploratory Review.* Contract report submitted to the National Institute of Justice. Cambridge, Mass.: Abt Associates.

Fordyce, E. J., Sambula, S., and Stoneburner, R. (1989) Mandatory reporting of human immunodeficiency virus testing would deter blacks and Hispanics from being tested (letter). *Journal of the American Medical Association* 262:349.

Fox, R., Ostrow, D., Valdiserri, R., Van Raden, M., Visscher, B., and Polk, B. F. (1987) Changes in sexual activities among participants in the Multicenter AIDS Cohort Study. Presented at the Third International Conference on AIDS, Washington, D.C., June 1–5.

Franke, K. M. (1989) Discrimination against HIV positive women by abortion clinics in New York City. Presented at the Fifth International Conference on AIDS, Montreal, June 4–9.

Freeman, H., Lewis, C., Montgomery, K., and Corey, C. (1989) Recent changes in sexual behavior among men in Los Angeles. Presented at the Fifth International Conference on AIDS, Montreal, June 4–9.

Friedman, S. R., Rosenblum, A., Goldsmith, D., Des Jarlais, D. C., Sufian M., et al. (1989) Risk factors for HIV-1 infection among street-recruited intravenous drug users in New York City. Presented at the Fifth International Conference on AIDS, Montreal, June 4–9.

Frutchey, C., and Walsh, K. (1989) Marginalization of gay men in AIDS funding and programs. Presented at the Fifth International Conference on AIDS, Montreal, June 4–9.

Gaynor, S., Kessler, D., Andrews, S., and Berge, P. (1989) Lookback: An update on the New York experience. Presented at the Fifth International Conference on AIDS, Montreal, June 4–9.

General Accounting Office (GAO). (1989) *AIDS Forecasting: Undercount of Cases and Lack of Key Data Weaken Existing Estimates.* Washington, D.C.: General Accounting Office.

Gerbert, B. (1987) AIDS and infection control in dental practice: Dentists' attitudes, knowledge, and behavior. *Journal of the American Dental Association* 114:311–314.

Gerbert, B., and Maguire, B. (1989) Public acceptance of the Surgeon General's brochure on AIDS. *Public Health Reports* 104:130–133.

Gerbert, B., Maguire, B., and Coates, T.J. (1989) Are patients getting the AIDS education they want from their physicians? Presented at the Fifth International Conference on AIDS, Montreal, June 4–9.

Gerbert, B., Maguire, B., Badner, V., Greenspan, D., Greenspan, J., et al. (1988) Changing dentists' knowledge, attitudes, and behaviors related to AIDS: A controlled educational intervention. *Journal of the American Dental Association* 116:851–854.

Ghodse, A. H., Tregenza, G., and Li, M. (1987) Effect of fear of AIDS on sharing of injection equipment among drug abusers. *British Medical Journal* 295:698–699.

Gibson, D. R., Wermuth, L., Lovelle-Drache, J., Ergas, B., Ham, J., and Sorensen, J. L. (1988) Brief psychoeducational counseling to reduce AIDS risk in IV drug users and sexual partners. Presented at the Fourth International Conference on AIDS, Stockholm, June 12–16.

Gibson, P., Kohn, R., and Bolan, G. (1989) Drug use and sexual behavior in male patients at an STD clinic: Implications for AIDS prevention. Presented at the Fifth International Conference on AIDS, Montreal, June 4–9.

Gold, R. B. (1990) *Abortion and Women's Health: A Turning Point for America?* New York: Alan Guttmacher Institute.

Goodman, M. J., and Goodman, L. E. (1982) Overselling of genetic anxiety. *Hastings Center Report* October:20–27.

Gostin, L. O. (1989) Public health strategies for confronting AIDS: Legislative and regulatory policy in the United States. *Journal of the American Medical Association* 261:1621–1630.

Gostin, L. (1990) The AIDS litigation project, a national review of court and human rights commission decisions, Part I: The social impact of AIDS. *Journal of the American Medical Association* 263:1961–1970.

Gostin, L., Porter, L., and Sandomire, H. (In press) *Objective Description of Trends in AIDS Litigation: AIDS Litigation Project.* U.S. Public Health Service/AIDS Program Office. Washington, D.C.: U.S. Government Printing Office.

Greatbatch, W., and Holmes, W. (1989) Evidence of a 16–18 year mean time between HIV viral infection and AIDS onset. Presented at the Fifth International Conference on AIDS, Montreal, June 4–9.

Grimes, D. A. (1987) The CDC and abortion in HIV-positive women. *Journal of the American Medical Association* 258:1176.

Gunn, A. E. (1988) The CDC and abortion in HIV-positive women. *Journal of the American Medical Association* 259:217.

Guydish, J., Abramowitz, A., Woods, W., Newmeyer, J., Clark, W., and Sorensen, J. (1989) Sharing needles: Risk reduction among intravenous drug users in San Francisco. Presented at the Fifth International Conference on AIDS, Montreal, June 4–9.

Hargraves, M. A., Jason, J. M., Chorba, T. L., Holman, R. C., Dixon, G. R., et al. (1987) Hemophiliac patient's knowledge and educational needs concerning acquired immunodeficiency syndrome. *American Journal of Hematology* 26:115–124.

Harper, P. S., Tyler, A., Smith, S., and Jones, P. (1981) Decline in the predicted incidence of Huntington's Chorea associated with systematic genetic counseling and family support. *Lancet* 2:411–413.

Hart, G. J., Carvell, A., Johnson, A. M., Feinmann, C., Woodward, N., and Adler, M. W. (1988) Needle exchange in central London. Presented at the Fourth International Conference on AIDS, Stockholm, June 12–16.

Hart, G. J., Carvell, A. L. M., Woodward, N., Johnson, A. M., Williams, P., and Parry, J. V. (1989) Evaluation of needle exchange in central London: Behaviour change and anti-HIV status over one year. *AIDS* 3:261–265.

Hartgers, C., Buning, E. C., van Santen, G. W., Verster, A. D., and Coutinho, R. A. (1989) The impact of the needle and syringe-exchange programme in Amsterdam on injecting risk-behavior. *AIDS* 3:571–576.

Haverkos, H. W., and Edelman, R. (1988) The epidemiology of acquired immunodeficiency syndrome among heterosexuals. *Journal of the American Medical Association* 260:1922–1929.

Hayes, R., Kegeles, S., and Coates, T. J. (In press) AIDS risk among young gay men. *AIDS.*

Henshaw, S. K., and Wallisch, L. S. (1984) The medicaid cutoff and abortion services for the poor. *Family Planning Perspectives* 16:170–180.

Henshaw, S. K., Forrest, J. D., and Van Vort, J. (1987) Abortion services in the United States, 1984–1985. *Family Planning Perspectives* 19:63–70.

Herek, G. M. (1989) Hate crimes against lesbians and gay men: Issues for research and policy. *American Psychologist* 44:948–955.

Herek, G. M., and Glunt, E. K. (1988) An epidemic of stigma: Public reactions to AIDS. *American Psychologist* 43:886–891.

Hoff, R., Berardi, V. P., Weiblen, B. J., Mahoney-Trout, L., Mitchell, M. L., and Grady, G. F. (1988) Seroprevalence of human immunodeficiency virus among childbearing women. *New England Journal of Medicine* 318:525–530.

Holman, S., Berthaud, M., Sunderland, A., Moroso, G., Cancellieri, F., et al. (1989) Women infected with human immunodeficiency virus: Counseling and testing during pregnancy. *Seminars in Perinatology* 13:7–15.

Holt, K. S. (1958) The influence of the retarded child upon family limitation. *Journal of Mental Deficiency Research* 2:28–36.

Hunter, N. (1988) Testimony on discrimination in access to clinical trials of AIDS drugs before the Human Resources and Intergovernmental Relations Subcommittee of The Committee on Government Operations. Washington, D.C., April 28.

Institute of Medicine (IOM). (1985) *Preventing Low Birthweight*. Washington, D.C.: National Academy Press.

Institute of Medicine (IOM). (1988) *Prenatal Care: Reaching Mothers, Reaching Infants*. Washington, D.C.: National Academy Press.

Institute of Medicine/National Academy of Sciences (IOM/NAS). (1988) *Confronting AIDS: Update 1988*. Washington, D.C.: National Academy Press.

Jackson, J., and Neshin, S. (1986) New Jersey Community Health Project: Impact of using ex-addict education to disseminate information on AIDS to intravenous drug users. Presented at the Second International Conference on AIDS, Paris, June 25–26.

Jackson, J., and Rotkiewicz, L. (1987) A coupon program: AIDS education and drug treatment. Presented at the Third International Conference on AIDS, Washington, D.C., June 1–5.

Jackson, J. B., Kwok, S. Y., Hopsicker, J. S., Sannerud, K. J., Sninsky, J. J., et al. (1989) Absence of HIV-1 infection in antibody-negative sexual partners of HIV-1 infected hemophiliacs. *Transfusion* 29:265–267.

Jaffe, H. W., Choi, K., Thomas, P. A., Haverkos, H. W., Auerbach, D. M., et al. (1983) National case-control study of Kaposi's sarcoma and *Pneumocystis carinii* pneumonia in homosexual men. Part 1. Epidemiologic results. *Annals of Internal Medicine* 99:145–151.

Johnson, A.M., Petherick, A., Davidson, S.J., Brettle, R., Hooker, M., et al. (1989) Transmission of HIV to heterosexual partners of infected men and women. *AIDS* 3:367–372.

Joseph, J. G., Montgomery, S. B., Kessler, R. C., Ostrow, D. G., and Wortman, C. B. (1988) Determinants of high risk behavior and recidivism in gay men. Presented at the Fourth International Conference on AIDS, Stockholm, June 12–16.

Joseph, J. G., Kessler, R. C., Wortman, C. B., Kirscht, J. P., Tal, M., et al. (1989) Are there psychological costs associated with changes in behavior to reduce AIDS risk? In V. M. Mays, G. W. Albee, and S. F. Schneider, eds., *Primary Prevention of AIDS: Psychological Approaches*. Newbury Park, Calif.: Sage Publications.

Judson, F. N. (1989) What do we really know about AIDS control? *American Journal of Public Health* 79:878–882.

Judson, F., Cohn, D., and Douglas, J. (1989) Fear of AIDS and incidence of gonorrhea, syphilis, and hepatitis B. Presented at the Fifth International Conference on AIDS, Montreal, June 4–9.

Kaback, M. M., Nathan, T. J., and Greenwald, S. (1977) Tay-Sachs disease: Heterozygote screening and prenatal diagnosis—U.S. experience and world perspective. In M. M. Kaback, ed., *Tay-Sachs Disease: Screening and Prevention.* New York: Alan Liss.

Kamenga, M., Jihgu, K., Hassig, S., Ndilu, M., Behets, F., et al. (1989) Condom use and associated seroconversion following intensive HIV counseling of 122 married couples in Zaire with discordant HIV serology. Presented at the Fifth International Conference on AIDS, Montreal, June 4–9.

Kamps, B. S., Niese, D., Brackmann, H. H., Euler, P., van Loo, B., and Kamradt, T. (1989) No more seroconversions among spouses of patients of the Bonn hemophiliac cohort study. Presented at the Fifth International Conference on AIDS, Montreal, June 4–9.

Kanoff, A. B., Kietner, B., and Gordon, B. (1962) The impact of infantile amaurotic idiocy (Tay-Sachs disease) on the family. *Pediatrics* 9:37–46.

Kaplan, M. H., Farber, B., Hall, W. H., Mallow, C., O'Keefe, C., and Harper, R. G. (1989) Pregnancy arising in HIV infected women while being repetitively counseled about "safe sex." Presented at the Fifth International Conference on AIDS, Montreal, June 4–9.

Kaunitz, A. M., Brewer, J. L., Paryani, S. G., de Sausure, L., Sanchez-Ramos, L., and Harrington, P. (1987) Prenatal care and HIV screening. *Journal of the American Medical Association* 258:2693.

Kegeles, S. M., Coates, T. J., Lo, B., and Catania, J. A. (1989) Mandatory reporting of HIV testing would deter men from being tested (letter). *Journal of the American Medical Association* 261:1275–1276.

Kelly, J. A., St. Lawrence, J. S., Smith, S., Hood, H. V., and Cook, D. J. (1987) Stigmatization of AIDS patients by physicians. *American Journal of Public Health* 77:789–791.

Kelly, J. A., St. Lawrence, J. S., Hood, H. V., and Brasfield, T. L. (1989a) Behavioral intervention to reduce AIDS risk activities. *Journal of Consulting and Clinical Psychology* 57:60–67.

Kelly, J. A., St. Lawrence, J. S., Stevenson, Y. L., Diaz, Y. E., Brasfield, T. L., and Hauth, A. C. (1989b) Changing peer norms to promote AIDS precautionary behavior: Training popular people to impact on the knowledge, attitudes, and behavior of their acquaintances. Presented at a symposium on Factors Influencing AIDS-Risk Behavior Reduction: Implications for Primary Prevention at the Annual Meeting of the Association for the Advancement of Behavior Therapy, Washington, D.C., November.

Kelly, J. A., St. Lawrence, J. S., Brasfield, T. L., and Hood, H. V. (1989c) Group intervention to reduce AIDS risk behaviors in gay men: Applications of behavioral principles. In V. M. Mays, G. W. Albee, and S. F. Schneider, eds., *Primary Prevention of AIDS: Psychological Approaches.* Newbury Park, Calif.: Sage Publications.

Kelly, J. A., St. Lawrence, J. S., Brasfield, T. L., Stevenson, L. Y., Diaz, Y. Y., and Hauth, A. C. (1990a) AIDS risk behavior patterns among gay men in small southern cities. *American Journal of Public Health* 80:416–418.

Kelly, J. A., St. Lawrence, J. S., Brasfield, T. L., Lemke, A., Amidei T., et al. (1990b) Psychological factors that predict AIDS high-risk versus AIDS precautionary behavior. *Journal of Consulting and Clinical Psychology* 58:117–120.

Kenen, R. H., and Schmidt, R. M. (1978) Stigmatization of carrier status: Social implications of heterozygote genetic screening programs. *American Journal of Public Health* 68:1116–1120.

Kirp, D. L. (1989) *Learning by Heart: AIDS and Schoolchildren in America's Communities.* New Brunswick, N.J.: Rutgers University Press.

Kotler, P., and Roberto, E. L. (1989) *Social Marketing: Strategies for Changing Public Behavior.* New York: The Free Press.

Krasinski, K., Borkowsky, W., Bebenroth, D., and Moore, T. (1988) Failure of voluntary testing for human immunodeficiency virus to identify infected parturient women in a high-risk population. *New England Journal of Medicine* 318:185.

Landesman, S. H., Minkoff, H. L., and Willoughby, A. (1989) HIV disease in reproductive age women: A problem of the present. *Journal of the American Medical Association* 261:1326–1327.

Lappe, M., Gustafson, J. M., and Roblin, R. (1972) Ethical and social issues in screening for genetic disease. *New England Journal of Medicine* 286:1129–1132.

Leonard, C. O., Chase, G. A., and Childs, B. (1972) Genetic counseling: A consumer's view. *New England Journal of Medicine* 287:433–439.

Lewis, C., and Freeman, H. (1987) The sexual history-taking in counseling practices of primary care physicians. *Western Journal of Medicine* 147:165–167.

Lieb, S., Zimmerman, R. S., Kuechler, M., Langer, L. M., Sims, J., and Witte, J. J. (1989) Trends in AIDS knowledge, attitudes and behaviors (KAB) in heterogeneous, high-risk groups, Florida. Presented at the Fifth International Conference on AIDS, Montreal, June 4–9.

Lifson, A., O'Malley, P. M., Hessol, N. A., Doll, L. S., Cannon, L., and Rutherford, G. W. (1989) Recent HIV seroconverters (SC) in a San Francisco cohort of homosexual/bisexual men: Risk factors for new infection. Presented at the Fifth International Conference on AIDS, Montreal, June 4–9.

Lindan, C., Rutherford, G.W., Payne, S., Hearst, N., and Lemp, G. (1989) Decline in rate of new AIDS cases among homosexual and bisexual men in San Francisco. Presented at the Fifth International Conference on AIDS, Montreal, June 4–9.

Ljungberg, B., Andersson, B., Christensson, B., Hugo-Persson, M., Tunving, K., and Ursing, B. (1988) Distribution of sterile equipment to IV drug abusers as part of an HIV prevention program. Presented at the Fourth International Conference on AIDS, Stockholm, June 12–16.

Lowden, J. A., and Davidson, J. (1977) Tay-Sachs screening and prevention: The Canadian experience. In M. M. Kaback, ed., *Tay-Sachs Disease: Screening and Prevention.* New York: Alan Liss.

Magura, S., Shapiro, J. L., Siddiqi, Q., and Lipton, D. S. (1989) Variables influencing condom use among intravenous drug users. Presented at the Fifth International Conference on AIDS, Montreal, June 4–9.

Marin, B. V. (1990) AIDS prevention for non-Puerto Rican Hispanics. In C. G. Leukefeld, R. J. Battjes, and Z. Amsel, eds., *AIDS and Intravenous Drug Use: Future Directions for Community-Based Prevention Research.* NIDA Research Monograph 93. Rockville, Md.: National Institute on Drug Abuse.

Marin, B., and Marin, G. (1990) Effects of acculturation on knowledge of AIDS and HIV among Hispanics. *Hispanic Journal of Behavioral Sciences* 12:110–121.

Marin, G. (1989) AIDS prevention among Hispanics: Needs, risk behaviors, and cultural values. *Public Health Reports* 104:411–415.

Marin, G., and Marin, B. V. (In press) Perceived credibility of channels and sources of AIDS information among Hispanics. *AIDS Education and Prevention.*

Marmor, M., Friedman-Kien, A. E., Laubenstein, L., Byrum, R. D., William, D. C., et al. (1982) Risk factors for Kaposi's sarcoma in homosexual men. *Lancet* 1:1083–1087.

Marsh, J. C., and Miller, N. A. (1985) Female clients in substance abuse treatment. *International Journal of the Addictions* 20:995–1019.

Martin, J. L. (1987) The impact of AIDS on gay male sexual behavior patterns in New York City. *American Journal of Public Health* 77:578–581.

Martin, J. L. (1990) Drug use and unprotected anal intercourse among gay men. *Health Psychology* 9:450–465.

Martin, J. L. (In press) Drug use and unprotected anal intercourse among gay men. *Health Psychology.*

Martin, J. L., and Hasin, D. (In press) Alcohol use and sexual behavior in a cohort of New York City gay men. *Drugs and Society.*

Mastroianni, L., Donaldson, P., and Kane, T., eds. (1990) *Developing New Contraceptives: Obstacles and Opportunities.* Washington, D.C.: National Academy Press.

May, R. M., and Anderson, R. M. (1987) Transmission dynamics of HIV infection. *Nature* 326:137–142.

Mays, V. M., and Cochran, S. D. (1988) Issues in the perception of AIDS risk and risk reduction activities by black and Hispanic/Latina women. *American Psychologist* 43:949–957.

McCrae, W. M., Cull, A. M., Burton, L., and Dodge, J. (1973) Cystic Fibrosis: Parents' response to the genetic basis of the disease. *Lancet* 2:141–143.

McCusker, J., Stoddard, A. M., Mayer, K. H., Zapka, J., Morrison, C., and Saltzman, S. P. (1988) Effects of antibody test knowledge on subsequent sexual behaviors in a cohort of homosexually active men. *American Journal of Public Health* 78:462–467.

McFarland, L., Dean, H., Trahan, B., and Muirhead, L. (1989) HIV infection in pregnant women at a public hospital in New Orleans, Louisiana. Presented at the Fifth International Conference on AIDS, Montreal, June 4–9.

McKusick, L., Conant, M., and Coates, T. J. (1985) The AIDS epidemic: A model for developing intervention strategies for reducing high-risk behavior in gay men. *Sexually Transmitted Diseases* 12:229–234.

McKusick, L., Coates, T. J., Morin, S., Pollack, L., and Hoff, C. (In press) Longitudinal predictors of unprotected anal intercourse in San Francisco gay men 1984–1988: The AIDS Behavioral Research Project. *American Journal of Public Health.*

Mechanic, D., and Aiken, L. (1989) Lessons from the past: Responding to the AIDS crisis. *Health Affairs* Fall:17–32.

Michigan Department of Public Health. (1988) Perinatal AIDS in Michigan. A report of the Maternal and Infant Task Force, June.

Miller, T., Booraem, C., Flowers, J., and Iversen, I. (1989) Short- and long-term results of an AIDS prevention program. Presented at the Fifth International Conference on AIDS, Montreal, June 4–9.

Minkoff, H. L., and Landesman, S. H. (1988) The case for routinely offering prenatal testing for human immunodeficiency virus. *American Journal of Obstetrics and Gynecology* 159:793–796.

Moatti, J. P., Tavares, J., Durbec, J. P., Bajos, N., Menard, C., and Serrand, L. (1989) Modifications of sexual behavior due to AIDS in French heterosexual "at risk" population. Presented at the Fifth International Conference on AIDS, Montreal, June 4–9.

Mondanaro, J. (1989) *Chemically Dependent Women: Assessment and Treatment.* Lexington, Mass.: Lexington Press.

Moody, R., Foss, L. A., Parker, J., Callan, W., and Williamson, D. (1989) Seroprevalence of antibodies to the human immunodeficiency virus (HIV) in applicants for marriage licenses in Alabama. Presented at the Fifth International Conference on AIDS, Montreal, June 4–9.

Murray, R. F., Chamberlain, N., Fletcher, J., Hopkins, E., Jackson, R., King, P. A., and Powledge, T. M. (1980) Special considerations for minority participation in prenatal diagnosis. *Journal of the American Medical Association* 243:1254–1256.

Neal-Cooper, F., and Scott, R.B. (1988) Genetic counseling in sickle cell anemia: Experiences with couples at risk. *Public Health Reports* 103:174–178.

New York City Department of Health. (1989) The Pilot Needle Exchange Study in New York City: A Bridge to Treatment. Department of Health, New York City.

New York State Department of Health. (1989) AIDS in New York State Through 1988. Public Affairs Group, New York State Department of Health, Albany, N.Y.

Nichols, E. K. (1989) *Mobilizing Against AIDS.* Cambridge, Mass.: Harvard University Press.

NOVA Research Company. (1989) Conference Proceedings: NIDA Conference on AIDS Intervention Strategies for Female Sexual Partners. Vol. 1. Berkeley, Calif., March 19–22.

Novick, D. M., Joseph, H., Croxson, T. S., Salsitz, E. A., Wang, G., et al. (1989) Absence of antibody to HIV in long-term, socially rehabilitated methadone maintenance patients. Presented at the Fifth International Conference on AIDS, Montreal, June 4–9.

Nzila, N., Laga, M., Kivuvu, M., Mokwa, K., Manoka, A. T., et al. (1989) Evaluation of condom utilization and acceptability of spermicides among prostitutes in Kinshasa, Zaire. Presented at the Fifth International Conference on AIDS, Montreal, June 4–9.

Oetting, L. A., and Steele, M. W. (1982) A controlled retrospective follow-up study of the impact of genetic counseling on parental reproduction following the birth of a Down syndrome child. *Clinical Genetics* 21:7–13.

Office of Technology Assessment (OTA). (1988) *How Effective is AIDS Education?* Washington, D.C.: Office of Technology Assessment.

O'Reilly, K., Higgins, D. L., Galavotti, C., Sheridan, J., Wood, R., and Cohn, D. (1989) Perceived community norms and risk reduction: Behavior change in a cohort of gay men. Photocopied materials distributed at the Fifth International Conference on AIDS, Montreal, June 4–9.

Padian, N., Marquis, L., Francis, D. P., Anderson, R. E., Rutherford, G. W., et al. (1987) Male-to-female transmission of human immunodeficiency virus. *Journal of the American Medical Association* 258:788–790.

Parish, K. L., Mandel, J., Thomas, J., and Gomperts, E. (1989) Prediction of safer sex practice and psychosocial distress in adults with hemophilia at risk for AIDS. Presented at the Fifth International Conference on AIDS, Montreal, June 4–9.

Parmet, W. E. (1987) AIDS and the limits of discrimination law. *Law, Medicine & Health Care* 15:61–72.

Paul, J., Stall, R., and Davis, F. (1989) Sexual risk for HIV transmission in a gay male substance-abusing population. Presented at the Fifth International Conference on AIDS, Montreal, June 4–9.

Peterson, J. L., and Marin, G. (1988) Issues in the prevention of AIDS among Black and Hispanic men. *American Psychologist* 43:871–877.

Peterson, J. L., Fullilove, R. E., Catania, J. A., and Coates, T. J. (1989) Close encounters of an unsafe kind: Risky sexual behaviors and predictors among black gay and bisexual men. Presented at the Fifth International Conference on AIDS, Montreal, June 4–9.

Pindyck, J. (1988) Transfusion-associated HIV infection: Epidemiology, prevention, and public policy (editorial review). *AIDS* 2:239–248.

Potterat, J. J., Spencer, N. E., Woodhouse, D. E. and Muth, J. B. (1989) Partner notification in the control of human immunodeficiency virus infection. *American Journal of Public Health* 79:874–876.

Powledge, T. M., and Fletcher, J. (1979) Guidelines for the ethical, social, and legal issues in prenatal diagnosis: A report from the Genetics Research Group of the Hastings Center, Institute of Society, Ethics, and the Life Sciences. *New England Journal of Medicine* 300:168–172.

Presidential Commission on the Human Immunodeficiency Virus Epidemic. (1988) *Final Report of the Presidential Commission on the Human Immunodeficiency Virus Epidemic.* Washington, D.C.: Government Printing Office.

Price, W., Merigan, T., and Peterman, T. (1989) Condom usage reported by female sexual partners of asymptomatic HIV seropositive hemophiliac men. Presented at the Fifth International Conference on AIDS, Montreal, June 4–9.

Puckett, S. B., and Bye, L. L. (1987) The stop AIDS project: An interpersonal AIDS-prevention program. The Stop AIDS Project, Inc., San Francisco, Calif.

Reed, B. G. (1987) Intervention strategies for drug dependent women: An introduction. In G. M. Beschner, B. G. Reed, and J. Mondanaro, eds., *Treatment Services for Drug Dependent Women.* Vol. 1. Rockville, Md.: National Institute on Drug Abuse.

Reed, B. G., Lovach, J., Bellows, N., and Mosie, R. (1981) The many faces of addicted women: Implications for treatment and future research. In A. J. Schecter, ed., *Drug Dependence and Alcoholism,* Vol. 1. New York: Plenum Press.

Remafedi, G. (1987). Homosexual youth: A challenge to contemporary society. *Journal of the American Medical Association* 258:222–225.

Remien, R., Rabkin, J., Williams, J., Gorman, J., and Ehrhardt, A. A. (1989). Cessation of alcohol and drug use disorders in an HIV sample. Presented at the Fifth International Conference on AIDS, Montreal, June 4–9.

Rhame, F. S., and Maki, D. G. (1989) The case for wider use of testing for HIV infection. *New England Journal of Medicine* 320:1248–1254.

Robertson, J. A., and Plant, M. A. (1988) Alcohol, sex and risks of HIV infection. *Drug and Alcohol Dependence* 22:75–78.

Rowe, M., and Bridgham, B. (1989) *Executive Summary and Analysis: AIDS and Discrimination—A Review of State Laws That Affect HIV Infection (1983 to 1988).* Washington, D.C.: George Washington University Intergovernmental Health Policy Project.

Rubinstein, A., Sicklick, M., Gupta, A., Bernstein, L., Klein, N., et al. (1983) Acquired immunodeficiency with reversed T4/T8 ratios in infants born to promiscuous and drug-addicted mothers. *Journal of the American Medical Association* 249:2350–2356.

Rucknagel, D. L. (1983) A decade of screening in the hemoglobinopathies: Is a national program to prevent sickle cell anemia possible? *The American Journal of Pediatric Hematology and Oncology* 5:373–377.

Russell, L. B. (1986) *Is Prevention Better Than Cure?* Washington, D.C.: The Brookings Institute.

Rutherford, G. W., Oliva, G. E., Grossman, M., Green, J. R., Wara, D. W., et al. (1987) Guidelines for the control of perinatally transmitted HIV infection and care of infected mothers, infants, and children. *Western Journal of Medicine* 147:104–108.

Sachs, B. P., Tuomala, R., and Frigoletto, F. (1987) AIDS: Suggested protocol for counseling and screening in pregnancy. *Obstetrics and Gynecology* 70:408–411.

Saint Cyr-Delpe, M. (1989) Update to the community response on women and AIDS. Presented at the Fifth International Conference on AIDS, Montreal, June 4–9.

Sakondhavat, C. (1990) The female condom (letter). *American Journal of Public Health* 80:498–499.

Saltzman, S., Stoddard, A., McCusker, J., and Mayer, K. (1989) Factors associated with recurrence of unsafe sexual practices in a cohort of gay men previously engaging in "safer" sexual practices. Presented at the Fifth International Conference on AIDS, Montreal, June 4–9.

San Francisco AIDS Foundation. (1987) *Designing an Effective AIDS Risk Prevention Campaign Strategy for San Francisco: Results from the Fourth Probability Sample of an Urban Gay Male Community.* San Francisco, Calif.: Research and Decision Corporation, Communication Technologies.

Schechter, M. T., Craib, K. J. P., Willoughby, B., Douglas, B., McLeod, W. A., et al. (1988) Patterns of sexual behavior and condom use in a cohort of homosexual men. *American Journal of Public Health* 78:1535–1538.

Schild, S. (1964) Parents of children with phenylketonuria. *Children* 11:92–96.

Schilling, R. F., Schinke, S. P. Nichols, S. E., Zayas, L. H., Muller, S. O., et al. (1989) Developing strategies for AIDS prevention research with black and Hispanic drug users. *Public Health Reports* 104:2–11.

Schmidt, K. W., Krasnik, A., Bendstrup, E., Zoffman, H., and Larson, S. O. (1989) Occurrence of sexual behavior related to the risk of HIV-infection. *Danish Medical Bulletin* 36:84–88.

Schneck, M., Goode, L., Connor, E., Holland, B., Oxtoby, M., and Oleske, J. (1989) Reproductive history (HX) of HIV antibody positive (HIV+) women followed in a prospective study in Newark, N.J. Presented at the Fifth International Conference on AIDS, Montreal, June 4–9.

Schneider, B. E. (1988) Gender and AIDS. In R. Kulstad, ed., *AIDS 1988: AAAS Symposia Papers.* Washington, D.C.: American Association for the Advancement of Science.

Schoenbaum, E. E., Hartel, D., Selwyn, P. A., Klein, R. S., Davenny, K., et al. (1989) Risk factors for human immunodeficiency virus infection in intravenous drug users. *New England Journal of Medicine* 321:874–879.

Seidlin, M., Dugan, T., Vogler, M., Bebenroth, D., Krasinski, K., and Holzman, R. (1989) Risk factors for HIV transmission in steady heterosexual couples. Presented at the Fifth International Conference on AIDS, Montreal, June 4–9.

Selwyn, P. A., Feiner, C., Cox, C. P., Lipshutz, C., and Cohen, R. L. (1987) Knowledge about AIDS and high-risk behavior among intravenous drug users in New York City. *AIDS* 1:247–254.

Selwyn, P. A., Schoenbaum, E. E., Davenny, K., Robertson, V. J., Feingold, A. R., et al. (1989) Prospective study of human immunodeficiency virus infection and pregnancy outcomes in intravenous drug users. *Journal of the American Medical Association* 261:1289–1294.

Serrano, Y., and Goldsmith, D. (1989) Street outreach strategies for intravenous drug and crack users, their sexual partners, and addicted prostitutes at risk for AIDS. Presented at the Fifth International Conference on AIDS, Montreal, June 4–9.

Serrano, Y., and Johnson, P. (1989) Women injection drug users: Issues and strategies, experiences in New York City and ADAPT. Presented at the Fifth International Conference on AIDS, Montreal, June 4–9.

Shaw, M. W. (1987) Invited editorial comment: Testing for the Huntington gene: A right to know, a right not to know, or a duty to know. *American Journal of Medical Genetics* 26:243–246.

Shaw, N., and Paleo, L. (1986) Women and AIDS. In L. McKusick, ed., *What To Do About AIDS*. Berkeley, Calif.: University of California Press.

Skidmore, C., and Robertson, J. R. (1989) Long term follow-up and assessment of HIV serostatus and risk taking in a cohort of 203 intravenous drug users. Presented at the Fifth International Conference on AIDS, Montreal, June 4–9.

Smiley, M. L., White, G. C. II, Becherer, P., Macik, G., Matthews, T. J., et al. (1988) Transmission of human immunodeficiency virus to sexual partners of hemophiliacs. *American Journal of Hematology* 28:27–32.

Solnick, R. (1978) Sexual responsiveness, age and change: Facts and potentials. In R. Solnick, ed., *Sexuality and Aging*. Los Angeles, Calif.: University of Southern California Press.

Solnick, R., and Birren, J. (1977) Age and male erectile response and sexual behavior. *Archives of Sexual Behavior* 6:1–9.

Solomon, M. Z., and DeJong, W. (1986) Recent sexually transmitted disease prevention efforts and their implications for AIDS health education. *Health Education Quarterly* 13:310–316.

Solomon, M. Z., and DeJong, W. (1989) Preventing AIDS and other STDs through condom promotion: A patient education intervention. *American Journal of Public Health* 179:453–458.

Sorenson, J., Gibson, D., Heitzmann, C., Calvillo, A., Dumontet, R., et al. (1988) Pilot trial of small group AIDS education with intravenous drug abusers (abstract). In L. S. Harris, ed., *Problems of Drug Dependence, 1988: Proceedings of the Committee on the Problems of Drug Dependence*. National Institute on Drug Abuse Research Monograph 90. Washington, D.C.: U.S. Government Printing Office.

Sotheran, J. L., Friedman, S. R., Des Jarlais, D. C., Engel, S. D., Weber, J., et al. (1989) Condom use among heterosexual male IV drug users is affected by the nature of the social relationships. Presented at the Fifth International Conference on AIDS, Montreal, June 4–9.

Sowder, B., Weissman, G., and Young, P. (1989) Working with women at risk in a national AIDS prevention program. Photocopied materials distributed at the Fifth International Conference on AIDS, Montreal, June 4–9.

St. Lawrence, J. S., Hood, H. V., Brasfield, T. L., and Kelly, J. A. (1988) Patterns and predictors of risk knowledge and risk behavior across high-, medium-, and low-AIDS prevalence cities. Presented at the Fourth International Conference on AIDS, Stockholm, June 12–16.

St. Lawrence, J. S., Hood, H. V., Brasfield, T. L., and Kelly, J. A. (1989) Differences in gay men's AIDS risk knowledge and behavior patterns in high and low AIDS prevalence cities. *Public Health Reports* 104:391–395.

Stall, R. D., and Ostrow, D. (1989) Intravenous drug use, the combination of drugs and sexual activity and HIV infection among gay and bisexual men: The San Francisco Men's Health Study. *Journal of Drug Issues* 19:57–73.

Stall, R. D., Catania, J., and Pollack, L. (1988) AIDS as an age-defined epidemic. Report to the National Institute of Aging, April.

Stall, R. D., Coates, T. J., and Hoff, C. (1988) Behavioral risk reduction for HIV infection among gay and bisexual men: A review of results from the United States. *American Psychologist* 43:878–885.

Stall, R. D., McKusick, L., Wiley, J., Coates, T. J., and Ostrow, D. G. (1986) Alcohol and drug use during sexual activity and compliance with safe sex guidelines for AIDS: The AIDS Behavioral Research Project. *Health Education Quarterly* 13:359–371.

Stall, R. D., McKusick, L., Hoff, C., Lang, S., and Coates, T. J. (1989) Sexual risk for HIV infection among bar patrons in San Francisco. Presented at the Fifth International Conference on AIDS, Montreal, June 4–9.

Stall, R. D., Ekstrand, M., Pollack, L., McKusick, L., and Coates, T. J. (1990) Relapse from safer sex: The next challenge for AIDS prevention efforts. Unpublished manuscript. Center for AIDS Prevention Studies, University of California, San Francisco.

Stall, R. D., Heurtun-Roberts, S., McKusick, L., Hoff, C., and Lange, S. (In press) Sexual risk for HIV transmission among singles-bar patrons in San Francisco. *Medical Anthropology Quarterly.*

Steele, M. W. (1980) Lessons from the American Tay-Sachs experience. *Lancet* 2:914.

Stein, Z. (1990) HIV prevention: The need for methods women can use (commentary). *American Journal of Public Health* 80:460–462.

Sterk, C. E., Friedman, S. R., Sufian, M., Stepherson, B., and Des Jarlais, D. C. (1989) Barriers to AIDS interventions among sexual partners of IV drug users. Presented at the Fifth International Conference on AIDS, Montreal, June 4–9.

Stevens, R., Wethers, J., Berns, D., and Pass, K. (1989) Human immunodeficiency (HIV) and human T-lymphotropic (HTLV-1/2) viruses in childbearing women: Tests of 24,569 consecutive newborns. Presented at the Fifth International Conference on AIDS, Montreal, June 4–9.

Stimson, G. V. (1988) Injecting equipment exchange schemes: Final report. London: Monitoring Research Group, Sociology Department, Goldsmith's College.

Stimson, G. V. (1989) Syringe exchange programmes for injecting drug users. *AIDS* 3:253–260.

Stryker, J. (1989) IV drug use and AIDS: Public policy and dirty needles. *Journal of Health Politics, Policy and Law* 14:719–740.

Sundet, J. M., Kvalem, I. L., Magnus, P., Gronnesby, J. K., Stigum, H., and Bakketeig, L. S. (1989) The relationship between condom use and sexual behavior. Presented at the Fifth International Conference on AIDS, Montreal, June 4–9.

Sunita, J., Flynn, N., Bailey, V., Sweha, A., Ding, D., and Sloan, W. (1989) IVDU and AIDS: More resistance to changing their sexual than their needle-sharing practices. Presented at the Fifth International Conference on AIDS, Montreal, June 4–9.

Sweeney, P., Allan, D., and Onorato, I., and State and Local Health Departments. (1989) HIV infection among women attending women's health clinics in the United States, 1988–1989. Presented at the Fifth International Conference on AIDS, Montreal, June 4–9.

Tafoya, T. (1989) Pulling coyote's tale: Native American sexuality and AIDS. In V. M. Mays, G. W. Albee, and S. F. Schneider, eds., *Primary Prevention of AIDS: Psychological Approaches.* Newbury Park, Calif.: Sage Publications.

Tanner, W. M., and Pollack, R. H. (1988) The effect of condom use and erotic instructions on attitudes towards condoms. *The Journal of Sex Research* 25:537–541.

Traeen, B., Rise, J., and Kraft, P. (1989) Condom behavior in 17, 18, and 19 year-old Norwegians. Presented at the Fifth International Conference on AIDS, Montreal, June 4–9.

Truman B., Lehman, J. S., Brown, L., Peyser, N., Peters, D., et al. (1989) HIV infection among intravenous drug users (IVDUs) in NYC. Presented at the Fifth International Conference on AIDS, Montreal, June 4–9.

Turner, C. (1989) Research on sexual behaviors that transmit HIV: Progress and problems. *AIDS* 3:S63–S70.

Turner, C. F., Miller, H. G., and Moses, L. M., eds. (1989) *AIDS, Sexual Behavior, and Intravenous Drug Use.* Washington, D.C.: National Academy Press.

Turnock, B. J., and Kelly, C. J. (1989) Premarital testing for human immunodeficiency virus. *Journal of the American Medical Association* 261:3415–3418.

U.S. Conference of Mayors. (1989) AIDS/HIV anti-discrimination initiatives. *AIDS Information Exchange* 6:2.

Valdiserri, R. O. (1989) *Preventing AIDS: The Design of Effective Programs.* New Brunswick, N.J.: Rutgers University Press.

Valdiserri, R., Lyter, D., Callahan, C., Kingsley, L., and Rinaldo, C. (1987) Condom use in a cohort of gay and bisexual men. Presented at the Third International Conference on AIDS, Washington, D.C., June 1–5.

Valdiserri, R., Lyter, D., Leviton, L. C., Callahan, C. M., Kingsley, L. A., et al. (1988) Variables influencing condom use in a cohort of gay and bisexual men. *American Journal of Public Health* 78:801–805.

Valdiserri, R. O., Lyter, D. W., Leviton, L. C., Callahan, C. M., Kingsley, L. A., and Rinaldo, C. R. (1989a) AIDS prevention in homosexual and bisexual men: Results of a randomized trial evaluating two risk reduction interventions. *AIDS* 3:21–26.

Valdiserri, R. O., Arena, V. C., Proctor, D., and Bonati, F. A. (1989b) The relationship between women's attitudes about condoms and their use: Implications for condom promotion programs. *American Journal of Public Health* 79:499–501.

van den Hoek, J. A. R., Coutinho, R. A., van Haastrecht, H. J. A., van Zadelhoff, A. W., and Goudsmit, J. (1988) Prevalence and risk factors of HIV infections among drug users and drug-using prostitutes in Amsterdam. *AIDS* 2:55–60.

van den Hoek, J. A. R., van Haastrecht, H. J. A., and Coutinho, R. A. (1989) Risk reduction among intravenous drug users in Amsterdam under the influence of AIDS. *American Journal of Public Health* 79:1355–1357.

VanRaden, M., Kaslow, R., Kingsley, L., Detels, R., Jacobson, L., et al. (1988) Incidence and nonsexual risk factors for recent HIV risk infection in homosexual men. Presented at the Fourth International Conference on AIDS, Stockholm, June 12–16.

Vlahov, D., Anthony, J. C., Celentano, D. D., Solomon, L., Choudhury, N., and Mandell, W. (1989) Trends of risk reduction among initiates into intravenous drug use 1982–1987. Presented at the Fifth International Conference on AIDS, Montreal, June 4–9.

Watters, J. K. (1987) Preventing human immunodeficiency virus contagion among intravenous drug users: The impact of street-based education on risk-behavior. Presented at the 3rd International Conference on AIDS, Washington, D.C., June 1–5.

Weiss, R., and Thier, S. O. (1988) HIV testing is the answer—What's the question? *New England Journal of Medicine* 319:1010–1012.

Wells, J., Wilensky, G. R., Valleron, A. J., Bond, G., Sell, R. L., and DeFilippes, P. (1989) Population prevalence of AIDS high risk behaviors in France, the United Kingdom and the United States. Presented at the Fifth International Conference on AIDS, Montreal, June 4–9.

Williams, A. B. (1989) Educational needs assessment for women at risk for HIV through intravenous drug abuse. Presented at the Fifth International Conference on AIDS, Montreal, June 4–9.

Williamson, M., Dobson, J.C., and Koch, R. (1977) Collaborative study of children treated for phenylketonuria: Study design. *Pediatrics* 60:815–821.

Willoughby, B., Schechter, M. T., Douglas, B., Craib, K. J. P., Constance, P., et al. (1989) Self-reported sexual behavior in a cohort of homosexual men: Cross-sectional analysis at six years. Presented at the Fifth International Conference on AIDS, Montreal, June 4–9.

Wiznia, A., Bueti, C., Douglas, C., Cabat, T., and Rubinstein, A. (1989) Factors influencing maternal decision making regarding pregnancy outcome in HIV infected women. Presented at the Fifth International Conference on AIDS, Montreal, June 4–9.

Wolfe, H., Keffelew, A., Bacchetti, P., Meakin, R., Brodie, B., and Moss, A. R. (1989) HIV infection in female intravenous drug users in San Francisco. Presented at the Fifth International Conference on AIDS, Montreal, June 4–9.

World Health Organization (WHO). (1988) AIDS: Avoidance of discrimination in relation to HIV-infected people and people with AIDS. Forty-first World Health Assembly, World Health Organization, Geneva, May.

Worth, D., and Rodriguez, R. (1987) Latina women and AIDS. *Siecus Report* January–February:5–7.

Zeugin, P., Dubois-Arber, F., Hausser, D., and Lehmann, Ph. (1989) Sexual behavior of young adults and the effects of AIDS-prevention campaigns in Switzerland. Presented at the Fifth International Conference on AIDS, Montreal, June 4–9.

3

AIDS and Adolescents

The committee finds no credible evidence that the threat of HIV infection or AIDS will cease in the near future in the United States, as noted in Chapter 1. Therefore, the committee believes it important to sustain effective HIV prevention programs for young people at or before the age at which they begin practicing behaviors that risk transmission of this deadly virus.

Serological studies of HIV infection, surveys of sexual and drug use behaviors, and reports from clinics for the treatment of drug use and sexually transmitted diseases (STDs) all indicate that some young people begin practicing behaviors that risk HIV transmission during and in some cases before their early teens. By the end of the teenage years, the majority of young persons in America report having begun sexual intercourse, and one-half report some experience with illicit drugs.[1] Evidence from HIV seroprevalence studies conducted among patients admitted to 37 metropolitan hospitals during 1988–1989 suggests that the HIV prevalence rate is vanishingly small among 11-year-olds but begins rising at age 12 and continues to rise throughout the teenage years.[2]

These behavioral and epidemiological facts suggest that HIV prevention efforts should begin at least by early adolescence[3] and that they

---

[1] See, for example, Tables 3-7 and 3-11.

[2] Dr. Michael E. St. Louis, HIV Seroepidemiology Branch, Center for Infectious Diseases, CDC, personal communication, April 4, 1990.

[3] Adolescence, as treated in the psychological literature, is not synonymous with the teenage years. It is generally said to begin between 10 and 13 years of age and to end between 18 and 21 years (Santrock, 1981). This stage of life is characterized by significant physical, psychological, and social

should continue throughout this period. Federal funding of such programs has ample precedent in that this country has supported programs to prevent other health problems of adolescents (e.g., unintended teenage pregnancy, drug use). The committee believes that the nation must recognize the importance of and unique opportunities for preventing the spread of HIV in the teenage population and that federal agencies must intervene accordingly. Adolescents deserve special attention because patterns of health behavior and risk taking are often established during the teenage years. By targeting prevention programs to adolescents, the United States may not only be protecting its youth but also preventing future problems in the adult population.

Despite the obvious benefits associated with reaching adolescents, less is known about effective interventions for this age group than for adults. Much of the accumulated knowledge about AIDS prevention has been gained from adult programs, primarily programs for adult gay men. Adolescent health behavior is likely to be different from that of adults, however, and programs designed for adults require modification to accommodate the behavioral, social, and developmental diversity found in the adolescent population.

In this chapter, the committee describes the scope of the AIDS problem among adolescents, insofar as data on AIDS cases and HIV infection are available for this population. Subsequently, it reviews what is known about the distribution of risk-associated behaviors in the adolescent population, as well as the prevalence of sexual intercourse, condom use, and drug use and the confluence of these high-risk behaviors. Finally, the committee considers what should be done to prevent further spread of HIV infection in this population.

THE EPIDEMIOLOGY OF
AIDS AND HIV AMONG ADOLESCENTS

Before reviewing available data on the scope of the HIV/AIDS problem among adolescents, the committee notes the inadequacies of those data, a deficiency leading the committee to the conclusion that the precise degree of infiltration of HIV infection into the adolescent population is presently unknown. The relatively few cases reported to date among 13- to 19-year olds (see Table 3-1) do not accurately reflect the scope of the problem, nor should these data be taken as grounds for complacency.

---

changes. Definitions of the exact time of entry into and exit from adolescence vary from study to study, depending on such factors as the theoretical view that has been adopted, the cultural context of the adolescent, and biological and social development factors, as well as the issue or problem of interest. (See Gold and Petronio [1980] for further elaboration of varying definitions of adolescence.)

Rather, the pattern of the epidemic in the adolescent population described below should be viewed as an opportunity for primary prevention that should not be overlooked.

AIDS case statistics are probably the most reliable epidemiological data base currently available. Yet the counts of current AIDS cases represent HIV infections that were acquired several years before the diagnosis of AIDS was made. The current best estimates of the mean incubation period of the disease (i.e., the mean time between HIV infection and the onset of clinically diagnosable AIDS) are eight to ten years, but as data spanning more time become available and as more effective prophylactic treatments become available, it seems likely that this estimate will increase.[4] Furthermore, it is possible that the median incubation period for teenagers may be longer than eight years. Natural history studies of hemophiliacs infected with HIV suggest that the incubation period may be longer for children (not newborns) and adolescents than it is for adults (Goedert et al., 1989).[5]

Yet even assuming that the incubation periods for adolescents and adults are equivalent, it is likely that few persons that were infected during their teenage years would also be diagnosed as AIDS cases during their teens. Even with the assumption of a median incubation period of eight years, fewer than one-half of persons infected with HIV at age 13 would be expected to develop AIDS during their teenage years,[6] and even fewer of those *infected* in the late teens would develop AIDS before age

---

[4]The current estimate is that the majority of HIV-seropositive individuals will go on to develop AIDS, and it is not impossible that 100 percent of seropositive individuals may eventually develop full-blown disease (IOM/NAS, 1988:35-36); see also the projections of Lui, Darrow, and Rutherford (1988) and Longini et al. (1989). However, new evidence suggests that the incubation distribution of the disease may be quite different for children, adolescents, and adults, as discussed in footnote 5.

[5]Goedert and colleagues (1989:1144, Table 3) report estimated *annual* incidence rates for AIDS after HIV infection as 0.83 per hundred for 1- to 11-year-old children; 1.49 per hundred for 12- to 17-year-old adolescents; 2.39 per hundred for 18- to 25-year-old adults; 3.40 per hundred for 26- to 34-year-old adults; and 5.66 per hundred for 35- to 70-year-old adults. The ages cited are the age of the person at the time of HIV infection. It should be noted that annual AIDS incidence rates are not uniformly distributed over time following infection. Thus, for example, rates are close to zero during the first two years following infection, and they rise during the next four to six years. It should also be noted that incubation periods may vary across transmission categories for adolescents. Indeed, some teens may progress from infection to disease more quickly than others. According to case reports, teens who acquired HIV infection through drug use or sexual behavior have progressed more rapidly than adults from infection to AIDS (K. Hein, Adolescent AIDS Program, Montefiore Medical Center, Bronx, N.Y., personal communication, 1989). Other data indicate that the median survival period is shorter for patients less than 20 years of age (9.0 months) than for patients between the ages of 20 and 29 years (13.0 months) or 30 to 39 years (13.2 months) (Lemp et al., 1990).

[6]It should be realized, of course, that both the cumulative risk of infection and the rate of risky behaviors can be expected to increase with age during adolescence (see the evidence presented below).

20. Those persons who are diagnosed with AIDS during their teens will be drawn mainly from the group of persons whose incubation periods were markedly shorter than the median and who were infected during their early teens.

Seroprevalence data for probability samples of individuals drawn from well-defined populations of epidemiological interest would provide a more reliable basis for inferring the prevalence of infection among teenagers. Unfortunately, with few exceptions, seroprevalence surveys conducted in this country have relied on samples of convenience, and most have not included teenagers. The largest samples that provide information on adolescents are derived from the routine HIV screening of applicants for military service and the Job Corps. These data cannot be generalized with knowable margins of error to other populations, but they can provide some insight into segments of the teenage population in which the infection may be established.

HIV prevalence estimates derived from blinded testing of newborns for HIV antibody (i.e., CDC's neonatal surveillance activity, which is described in Chapter 1) provide a reliable indicator of the prevalence of infection among women delivering children. (Infants, whether infected or not, carry the maternal antibodies to HIV at birth if the mother is infected with the virus.) Analysis of these data by the age of the mother could provide important information about HIV infection among teenage women who bear children. Unfortunately, tabulations of HIV seroprevalence by mother's age are not presently available for most states. Indeed, the committee notes that, in some states, data on the age of the mother are not being collected.

To provide better information about HIV infection and AIDS among adolescents, **the committee recommends that the Centers for Disease Control make available to the research community AIDS-related data that permit separate consideration of teenagers and other age groups. Specifically, the committee recommends that:**

- **data on AIDS cases be made available in a form that permits tabulation by specific ages or by narrow age groups (these data should be as complete as possible without threatening inadvertent disclosure of the identity of any individual case);[7]**
- **every state that participates in the neonatal surveillance**

---

[7]The Committee on National Statistics at the National Research Council and the Social Science Research Council have jointly convened a panel to study the broad issues of confidentiality and data access in research. Their report will be available in approximately two years.

activity include the age of the mother coded in years or by narrow age group; and

- **CDC provide data from its family of surveys[8] by specific ages or in narrow age groups, as well as by race, gender, and ethnicity.**

The Scope of the Problem

AIDS Cases. As noted above, the small percentage of AIDS cases diagnosed in the adolescent population does not imply that AIDS and HIV are not a problem for teenagers. Indeed, as Vermund and colleagues (1989) argue, a substantial fraction of the AIDS cases diagnosed among persons in their twenties reflect infections contracted during the teenage years. As of December 31, 1989, approximately 24,000 cases of AIDS had been reported among teenagers and young adults (ages 13–29). Table 3-1 shows the distribution of reported AIDS cases by age at diagnosis, using the broad age categories into which CDC has coded the data released to the public. It can be seen that roughly one case in five is diagnosed among persons under the age of 30. The proportion of cases actually diagnosed among teenagers, however, is small.

Figure 3-1 displays the case counts by age at diagnosis for persons diagnosed with AIDS between the ages of 13 and 29. Allowing, as noted earlier, for an incubation period that is rarely less than two years and a mean incubation period that may be eight years or longer, one would expect that nearly all of the AIDS cases diagnosed among persons in their very early twenties would reflect HIV infections contracted during adolescence.[9] The overall impact of AIDS on teenagers and young adults is reflected in the fact that AIDS was the tenth leading cause of death among 15- to 24-year-olds as early as 1984; it had risen to the seventh leading cause of death for this age group in 1986 and the sixth in 1987 (Kilbourne, Buehler, and Rogers, 1990).

---

[8]The CDC's family of surveys collects data on HIV infection from several subpopulations, including clients attending drug treatment, STD, tuberculosis, and prenatal clinics, patients at general hospitals, and newborn infants. With the exception of the survey of infants, all of the other surveys rely on samples of convenience. Data collected through this program are intended to provide information on the prevalence and incidence of infection in selected populations, to provide early warning of the emergence of infection in new populations, and to target intervention programs and other resources.

[9]It may seem intuitively appealing to argue that at least one-half of the 4,268 cases diagnosed at age 28 reflect infections contracted during the teens. This argument is not, however, logically required. Because there is a non-zero probability of an AIDS diagnosis being recorded in each year from roughly two years after HIV infection, it would be theoretically possible (with a suitably large number of HIV infections among persons in their early twenties) to observe 4,000 cases of AIDS among 28-year-olds, none of which had been contracted by teenagers.

TABLE 3-1 Distribution of AIDS Cases Reported Through December 31, 1989, by Age at Diagnosis

Diagnosis (years)	No. of Cases	Percentage
<1	785	0.7
1–12	1,210	1.0
13–19	461	0.4
20–24	5,090	4.3
25–29	18,966	16.1
30–39	54,334	46.1
40–49	24,951	21.2
50+	11,984	10.2
Total	117,781	100.0[a]

[a]Percentages may not sum to 100.0 because of rounding.

SOURCE: Special tabulation provided by the Statistics and Data Processing Branch of the AIDS Program, Centers for Disease Control.

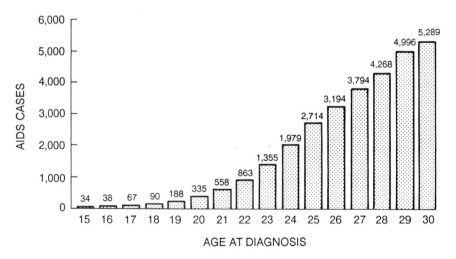

FIGURE 3-1 Number of AIDS cases reported among 15- to 30-year-olds through December 31, 1989, by single years of age at diagnosis. SOURCE: Special tabulation provided by the Statistics and Data Processing Branch of the AIDS Program, Centers for Disease Control.

HIV Seroprevalence. Since October 1985, the Department of Defense has tested applicants[10] for military service for evidence of HIV infection; in January 1986 the armed forces began screening all active-duty personnel. The crude prevalence rate for 17- to 19-year-old applicants screened between October 15, 1985 and March 31, 1989 was 0.34 per 1,000 (Burke et al., 1990). HIV prevalence rates among military applicants[11] from October 1985 to March 1986 increased directly and linearly with age from 0.25 per thousand among 18-year-olds to 4.9 per thousand among 27-year-olds (Burke et al., 1987:132).[12] Among active-duty personnel during the period October 1985 to July 1989, prevalence rates were found to have a similar distribution by age. The observed rates were lowest among soldiers less than 20 years old (0.5 per thousand), peaked at 3.4 per thousand among 30- to 34-year-olds, and gradually declined among older military personnel (Kelley et al., 1990).

Figures 3-2a and 3-2b plot these age-specific prevalence rates for military applicants and active-duty personnel. The plots demonstrate that roughly parallel age trends are found for the two groups. Data tabulated separately for applicants from the New York-New Jersey metropolitan area suggest a similar trend. The prevalence of HIV among applicants from the New York-New Jersey metropolitan area is several times higher than the rate among applicants from the rest of the nation (see Figure 3-2c). In this case, prevalence rates among military applicants 30 years of age and older are somewhat higher than those of applicants aged 26-30.

The other large group of young people who are routinely screened for HIV are persons applying to participate in the Job Corps. The Job Corps is a federal program that provides training and employment for socioeconomically and educationally disadvantaged youths. Of the 69,233 applicants between the ages of 16 and 21 years who were screened between October 1987 and November 1988, 3.9 per thousand were infected (St. Louis et al., 1989). This rate is much higher than the prevalence

---

[10] Among military applicants who had been screened between October 1985 and March 1986, 86 percent were male and 76 percent were white; 46 percent were less than 20 years old, and only 5 percent reported education beyond a high school diploma (Burke et al., 1987).

[11] The observed age-specific prevalence estimates largely reflect the rates among older males (434 seropositive among a total of 263,572 men). Overall, HIV prevalence was lower among women, and fewer were tested (26 seropositive among 42,489 women). However, among 17- and 18-year-olds, the prevalence rates for males and females were approximately equal (Burke et al., 1987). Other analyses of military data find prevalence rates among teenage females to be comparable to those among teenage males (Horton, Alexander, and Brundage, 1989; Kelley et al., 1990).

[12] The authors concluded that HIV prevalence increased linearly with age between 18 and 27 years (Burke et al., 1987:132). Estimated prevalence among males over the age of 27 was lower, however, than the prevalence rates observed among male applicants between 25 and 27 years old.

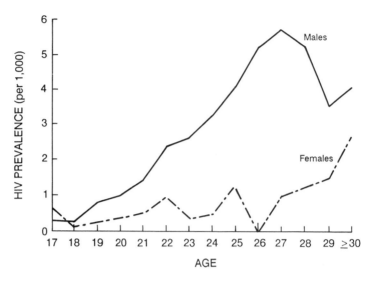

FIGURE 3-2A Prevalence of HIV (rate per 1,000 persons), by age, among male and female applicants for military service [*N* = 306,061] (October 1985 through March 1986). SOURCE: Burke et al., 1987.

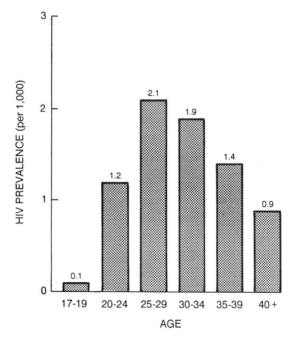

FIGURE 3-2B Prevalence of HIV (rate per 1,000 persons), by age, among active duty military personnel [*N* = 1,752,191] (January 1987 through April 1988). SOURCE: Peterson et al., 1988.

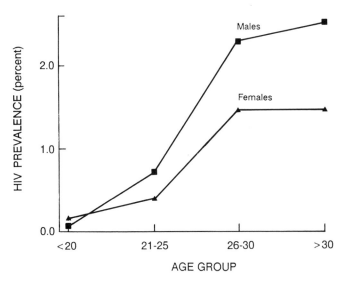

FIGURE 3-2C Prevalence of HIV (percent), by age, among male and female applicants for military service from New York-New Jersey metropolitan area [N = 44,139] (October 1985 through June 1987). SOURCE: Brundage et al., 1988.

rates found among the youngest groups of applicants for military service, which may reflect differences in the populations represented in applications to these two organizations.

HIV Seroprevalence in Childbearing Women. Anonymous antibody testing of newborn infants provides information on the prevalence of HIV infection among childbearing women (because infants circulate maternal antibody during the first months of life). As noted earlier, data are not available for every state, and some states do not provide information on the age of the mother. Data have been published for New York City and the rest of New York State (Novick et al., 1989a). Among babies born in New York State between November 1987 and November 1988, the seroprevalence rate was 1.6 per thousand outside New York City and 12.5 per thousand for births in New York City. Figure 3-3 plots the age-specific rates of infection found in New York City. Although these data show an age trend similar to that found in other studies, the rates of infection—even among teenage mothers—are substantial.[13] Almost 10 per thousand or 1 percent of black teenagers who delivered children in New York City during this period were infected with HIV.

---

[13] Analyses of ZIP Code-specific areas with high rates of drug use (determined by comparing rates of drug-related hospital discharges) found rates as high as 40 per thousand or 4 percent in some ZIP Codes areas of New York City (Novick et al., 1989a).

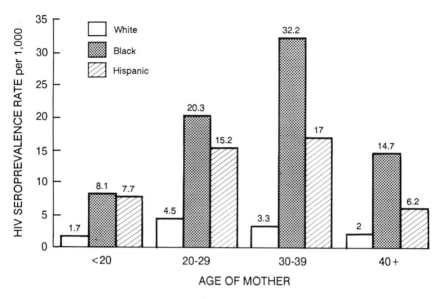

FIGURE 3-3 HIV seroprevalence rates (per 1,000 persons) among New York City women giving birth between November 30, 1987, and November 30, 1988. Of 125,120 New York City women tested, race/ethnicity was unknown for 2,461, and age was unknown for 2,334. SOURCE: Novick et al., 1989a:Table 4.

The prevalence of HIV infection among Hispanic teenage mothers was almost as high. In considering Figure 3-3, the committee would note that it is only the contrast with rates of almost 30 per thousand found among 30- to 39-year-old black mothers that make the observed teenage prevalence rates appear *relatively* low.

HIV Seroprevalence in Other Studies. The seroprevalence rates provided above on women bearing children in New York City are buttressed by emerging data from serosurveys of nonprobability samples of hospital patients. Ernst and colleagues (1989), for example, recently reported that, among patients aged 15 to 24 at the Bronx Lebanon Hospital, 36 per thousand or 3.6 percent of males and 25 per thousand or 2.5 percent of females were infected with HIV. Table 3-2 summarizes selected results of this and other small-scale seroprevalence studies among teenagers and young adults. Although the observed prevalence of HIV infection varies from population to population and from study to study, one finding is clear: the AIDS virus is substantially seeded in some segments of the adolescent population. Moreover, although the variation in estimates argues for more comprehensive and standardized monitoring of the spread of infection in this population, the lesson for prevention is nonetheless apparent. HIV infection is already spreading in the teenage population, and in some locales and population subgroups, the spread has been substantial.

Variation of AIDS and HIV Prevalence by Gender. Just as more AIDS cases are seen among adult males than among adult females, so too are there more cases of AIDS among teenage boys than among teenage girls.[14] Of all AIDS cases reported as of December 31, 1989, males outnumbered females by a 9:1 ratio.[15] As the first row of Table 3-3 shows, however, the ratio of male to female cases is much lower among teenagers than among adults in the United States. Thus, it can be seen that the male-to-female ratio, which is roughly 1:1 among cases diagnosed in infants (younger than 1 year), increases to 4:1 among teenagers, to 6:1 among 20- to 24-year-olds, and ultimately to 16:1 for cases diagnosed among persons in their forties.

In addition to variations by age, the ratio of male-to-female cases of AIDS and HIV infection varies substantially among populations. Eleven percent of AIDS cases among teenagers have been diagnosed in the New York metropolitan area,[16] and the male-to-female ratio for those cases is approximately 2:1 (Table 3-3). The size of this ratio indicates that girls in the New York area are supporting a greater burden of disease than girls nationally.[17] HIV infection rates calculated for military applicants

---

[14]As of July 1, 1986, there were more than 35 million individuals in this country between the ages of 10 and 19 years, constituting approximately 14.6 percent of the total population. The ratio of males to females is essentially 1:1 (1.044:1) (U.S. Bureau of the Census, 1987:17).

[15]As of December 31, 1989, females of all ages accounted for 11,524 cases of AIDS out of a total of 117,781 reported cases.

[16]As of December 31, 1989, a total of 461 AIDS cases had been reported among 13- to 19-year-olds; 50 of these cases were from the New York Primary Metropolitan Statistical Area. In 1983, the Office of Management and Budget changed the classification system used to define metropolitan areas in federal statistical reports. The basic term for such areas, formerly known as Standard Metropolitan Statistical Areas or SMSAs, was changed to Metropolitan Statistical Areas or MSAs. The basic concept of a metropolitan area, however, remained that of an area with a large population nucleus and the adjacent communities, e.g., suburbs, that have a high degree of economic and social integration with that nucleus. Within metropolitan complexes of one million or more population, separate Primary Statistical Areas (PMSA) may be designated under the new classification system. Any metropolitan area containing one or more PMSAs was, in turn, designated a Consolidated Metropolitan Statistical Area (CMSA). The New York PMSA, for example, includes the five counties that comprise the City of New York, plus the suburban counties of Westchester, Rockland, and Putnam. Adjacent areas include other PMSAs, e.g., the Nassau-Suffolk (Long Island) PMSA. The New York PMSA and the Nassau-Suffolk PMSA are 2 of the 12 PMSAs that constitute the Consolidated Metropolitan Statistical Area that bears the awkward name: "New York-Northern New Jersey-Long Island, NY-NJ-CT CMSA." (U.S. Bureau of the Census, 1985, Appendix 2).

[17]The higher proportion of cases among females of all ages in New York reflects the greater relative proportion of cases attributable to IV drug use and heterosexual transmission in the Northeast than other areas. (See for example, Figure 1-1 in Chapter 1.)

TABLE 3-2 Prevalence Rate of HIV Infection (per 1,000) Among Adolescents Found in Selected Studies Based on Nonprobability Samples

Study Period	Site	Sample	N	Reference	HIV Prevalence
1988–1989	17 U.S. college campuses	Students using college health units	13,810	Gayle et al. (1989)	2[a]
Feb.–April 1987	Baltimore	15- to 19-year-olds using an STD clinic	943	T.C. Quinn et al. (1988)	22
Feb.–August 1987	Los Angeles	16- to 18-year-olds in juvenile detention	1,878	Baker et al. (1989)	2[b]
Oct. 1987–Jan. 1989	Washington, D.C.	Patients at an adolescent clinic	3,520	D'Angelo et al. (1989)	4[c]
Sept. 1987–Nov. 1988	New York City	Homeless youths aged 13–18	620	N.Y. State Dept. of Health (1989)	36
Sept. 1987–Nov. 1988	New York City	Homeless youths aged 19–23	725	N.Y. State Dept. of Health (1989)	88
Feb. 1988–Oct. 1988	Bronx Lebanon Hospital	Hospital patients aged 15–24 Males Females	245 630	Ernst et al. (1989)	36 25

[a]Rate rounded up from 1.7. [b]Rate rounded up from 1.6. [c]Rate rounded up from 3.7.

TABLE 3-3 Percentage of AIDS Cases Reported Through December 31, 1989, Diagnosed Among Males and Male-to-Female Case Ratios, by Age at Diagnosis, for All Cases Diagnosed in the United States and in the New York Metropolitan Statistical Area (MSA)

Population, Statistic	Age at Diagnosis (years)							
	< 1	1–12	13–19	20–24	25–29	30–39	40–49	50+
United States								
% Male	49	57	80	85	88	91	94	91
M:F Ratio	1.0:1	1.3:1	4.0:1	5.7:1	7.3:1	10.1:1	15.7:1	10.1:1
(Base *N*)	(785)	(1,210)	(461)	(5,090)	(18,966)	(54,334)	(24,951)	(11,984)
New York MSA								
% Male	52	54	70	76	79	85	92	92
M:F Ratio	1.1:1	1.2:1	2.3:1	3.2:1	3.8:1	5.7:1	11.5:1	11.5:1
(Base *N*)	(229)	(311)	(50)	(716)	(3,077)	(10,799)	(5,209)	(2,274)

SOURCE: Special tabulation provided by the Statistics and Data Processing Branch of the AIDS Program, Centers for Disease Control.

from the New York City area yield male-to-female ratios of roughly 1.4:1 (Brundage et al., 1988; Horton, Alexander, and Brundage, 1989). Among Job Corps applicants, the male-to-female ratio nationally is approximately 1:1 among 16- to 18-year-olds, but for applicants between the ages of 19 and 21, the ratio climbs to approximately 4:1 (St. Louis et al., 1989). Overall, the number of infected men is approximately equal to the number of infected women among 17- to 19-year-old military applicants (1.09:1), but among 17- and 18-year-old applicants, fewer men than women were found to be seropositive (0.9:1) (Burke et al., 1990).

Surveys of clinic populations have found roughly equivalent rates of infection among teenage males and females. T. C. Quinn and coworkers (1988), for example, screened anonymous blood samples from 943 consecutive patients at STD clinics in Baltimore; among 15- to 19-year-old patients, 2.5 percent of 434 female patients tested positive for HIV, compared with 2 percent of 509 males in this age group. Among young adults (aged 20 to 24) attending the same clinics, the prevalence of HIV infection was higher but remained roughly equal for males and females (3.4 percent of 385 females versus 3.8 percent of 840 males). Among older patients, males were two to three times more likely than females to be infected.[18] Among college students in a blinded serosurvey of a

---

[18] Among 25- to 29-year-olds, Quinn and coworkers (1988) found that 2.9 percent of 239 females and 6.9 percent of 598 males were infected with HIV. Among patients 30 years of age and older, the Quinn team found that 4.3 percent of 185 females and 11.4 percent of 636 males were infected with HIV.

TABLE 3-4 Distribution of AIDS Cases (percentage) Reported Through December 31, 1989, by Race/Ethnicity

Age Group (years)	Race/Ethnicity				Total	N
	White	Black	Hispanic	Other[a]		
0–12	21.9%	52.6%	24.6%	0.9%	100%	1,995
13–19	43.4	35.8	18.4	2.4	100	461
20–24	48.9	31.6	18.5	1.0	100	5,090
25–29	53.4	28.6	17.1	0.9	100	18,966
30 +	57.9	26.3	14.8	1.0	100	91,269
All ages	56.1	27.4	15.5	1.0	100	117,781

[a] This category includes persons of unknown ethnicity ($N = 226$), Asians/Pacific Islanders ($N = 596$), and American Indians/Alaskan natives ($N = 121$).

SOURCE: Special tabulation provided by the Statistics and Data Processing Branch of the AIDS Program, Centers for Disease Control.

nonprobability sample of persons visiting clinics at 17 colleges, the vast majority of HIV infections (87 percent) were found among males (Gayle et al., 1989).[19]

Variation by Race/Ethnicity in AIDS and HIV Prevalence. A disproportionate share of the burden of adolescent AIDS cases is borne by minority youth. Table 3-4 displays the racial composition of AIDS cases for various age groups. As shown, 36 percent of teenage cases have been diagnosed among black teenagers, who make up only 15.3 percent of the population; 18 percent of cases are found among Hispanics, who constitute less than 10 percent of the national teenage population.[20] The table also shows that, compared with adult cases, a larger proportion of adolescent cases have been diagnosed among blacks and Hispanics (54 percent of teen cases versus 41 percent of cases among persons 30 years of age and older).

Data on HIV infection also indicate a greater prevalence of HIV infection among blacks and Hispanics than among whites. Among teenage military applicants, seroprevalence rates are highest among blacks; the prevalence rate for black females (0.77 per 1,000) was four times greater

[19] Of 13,810 specimens tested, 23 were positive for HIV, for a prevalence rate of 0.17 percent or 1.7 per thousand. Twenty of these 23 specimens were from males.

[20] The racial distribution of the teenage population is similar to that found among adults: 81 percent of 10- to 19-year-olds in the United States are white, 15.3 percent are black, and slightly less than 10 percent (9.5 percent) are Hispanic (U.S. Bureau of the Census, 1987:16-17). Because Hispanic persons may be of any race, the percentages noted here reflect overlapping groups (and thus in total exceed 100 percent). The Hispanic category includes anyone self-identified as Mexican, Puerto Rican, Cuban, Central or South American, or of other Spanish/Hispanic origin.

than that for white males (0.18 per 1,000) (Burke et al., 1990).[21] Sero-prevalence surveys of teenage mothers of newborns in New York City found that 0.77 percent of Hispanics, 0.81 percent of blacks, and 0.17 percent of whites were infected (Novick et al., 1989a) (see Figure 3-3). Among female military recruits, seroprevalence rates were highest among black, non-Hispanic women (Horton, Alexander, and Brundage, 1989; Burke et al., 1990). Among male applicants, the relative excess of cases among blacks is greatest for those men from the Northeast and north central regions of the country (Sharp et al., 1989). Among Job Corps applicants, the rate of infection among blacks was approximately five times higher than that for whites (0.7 versus 0.14 percent), and the ratio of male-to-female cases was much closer to unity for blacks (1.2:1) than for whites (7.8:1) (St. Louis et al., 1989).

Mode of Transmission for AIDS Cases. Table 3-5 shows the distribution of all AIDS cases by gender and risk category. These data suggest that a substantial proportion of cases among adolescent boys and young men are related to homosexual contact: 37 percent of teen cases and 68 percent of cases among 20- to 24-year-olds. Yet the largest risk category for teenage boys is exposure to contaminated blood and blood products, which accounts for 44 percent of diagnosed cases among 13- to 19-year-olds. The relatively high rate of cases among teenage boys resulting from transmission through blood products is explained in part by hemophilia, a sex-linked genetic disorder that is almost exclusively a problem of males.

The distribution across risk categories of AIDS cases diagnosed in teenage girls is different from that seen among teenage boys. Heterosexual contact accounts for 37 percent of cases among teenage females and 41 percent of cases among women 20 to 24 years of age; 28 and 40 percent of cases, respectively, are ascribed to IV drug use. Among women who have been diagnosed with AIDS, females between the ages of 13 and 24 years are more likely than older women to report exposure through heterosexual contact.

Geographic Variation in AIDS and HIV Prevalence. The geographic distribution of AIDS cases among teenagers and young adults is shown in Table 3-6. Teenage and young adult AIDS cases are found throughout the country, and the overall distribution of young adult AIDS cases does not show marked deviations from the distribution of adult

---

[21] Of the 1,141,164 military applicants aged 17 to 19 screened for HIV infection between October 15, 1985, and March 31, 1989, 393 were found to be infected, giving an overall prevalence rate of 0.34 per 1,000 (Burke et al., 1990). Crude seroprevalence rates (per 1,000 applicants) were 1.00 for blacks, 0.29 for Hispanics, and 0.17 for whites.

TABLE 3-5 Distribution of AIDS Cases (percentage) Reported Through December 31, 1989, Among Persons 13 Years of Age and Older (at diagnosis), by Transmission Category, Gender, and Age

Age at Diagnosis	Homosex (1)	IVDU (2)	Homo-IVDU (3)	Blood (4)	Hetero (5)	Pattern II (6)	Other (7)	Total	N
MALES									
13–19	37.1%	7.1%	6.3%	43.6%	1.1%	1.4%	3.5%	100%	367
20–24	68.2	11.2	11.2	4.0	1.1	1.2	3.3	100	4,346
25–29	68.6	14.4	10.2	1.5	1.0	1.8	2.4	100	16,744
30 +	66.3	18.9	7.0	2.7	1.1	1.0	3.1	100	83,718
All Males 13+	66.6	17.8	7.7	2.7	1.1	1.1	3.0	100	105,175
FEMALES									
13–19	na	27.7%	na	18.1%	37.2%	6.4%	10.6%	100%	94
20–24	na	40.3	na	5.4	40.6	5.2	8.5	100	744
25–29	na	52.3	na	4.1	32.8	4.8	6.0	100	2,222
30 +	na	53.0	na	12.5	24.1	3.8	6.6	100	7,551
All Females 13+	na	51.7	na	10.3	27.2	4.1	6.7	100	10,611

Transmission Category

NOTE: Transmission categories are as follows: (1) male homosexual/bisexual contact; (2) intravenous (IV) drug use; (3) male homosexual/bisexual contact and IV drug use; (4) hemophilia/coagulation disorder; receipt of transfusion of blood; (5) heterosexual contact; (6) born in a Pattern II country (e.g., individuals from those countries in central, eastern, and southern Africa and some Caribbean countries in which the majority of AIDS cases has been ascribed to heterosexual transmission, the male-to-female ratio is approximately 1:1, and perinatal transmission is more common than in other areas); and (7) other/undetermined. Pediatric exposure categories (all cases under the age of 13 years) are separately defined and are not included in this table.

SOURCE: Special tabulation provided by the Statistics and Data Processing Branch of the AIDS Program, Centers for Disease Control.

AIDS cases. There is more geographic variation in the distribution of teenage cases, but the total number of cases diagnosed in adolescents (461) is still quite small. The largest observed deviation between the adult and teenage distributions is for cases outside metropolitan areas (43 percent of teenage cases versus 27 percent of cases among adults aged 30 and older.[22]

Behind the statistics presented in Table 3-6 are localized areas with very high prevalence rates of AIDS. Gayle, Manoff, and Rogers (1989) report, for example, that more than one-half of the AIDS cases among 13- to 19-year-olds came from five states and Puerto Rico.[23] Similarly, as noted earlier, only 3.6 percent[24] of the U.S. population lives in the New York metropolitan area, but 11 percent of teenage AIDS cases were from New York.

The AIDS case data indicating a concentration of adolescent AIDS cases in urban areas, especially New York City, are paralleled by screening data on infection rates among applicants for military service.[25] Figure 3-4 shows the distribution of the prevalence of infection among individuals who applied to enter the military between October 1985 and September 1989. The elevated peaks indicate pockets of infection, largely around the coastal areas of the country. However, cases of HIV infection have been identified among 17- to 19-year-old military applicants from 200 counties in 41 states and the District of Columbia (Burke et al., 1990).

HIV prevalence among Job Corps applicants also shows considerable geographic variation, although the variation appears to be race specific (St. Louis et al., 1989). Seroprevalence rates among black and Hispanic Job Corps applicants were highest in the Northeast (10.2 and 7.7 per

---

[22]Hemophilia- and transfusion-associated AIDS cases comprise a larger proportion of the cases reported among teens than among older persons. Hemophilia- and transfusion-associated AIDS cases are also more geographically dispersed than those associated with sexual and IV drug-using behaviors. To examine whether these factors might account for the smaller proportion of AIDS cases reported in nonmetropolitan areas by adults (versus teens), Table 3-6 was recomputed excluding these cases. The result is only slightly attenuated: 37 percent of *teen* AIDS cases (excluding hemophilia- and transfusion-associated cases) were reported in nonmetropolitan areas versus 27 percent of cases reported among persons aged 30 and older.

[23]This includes both the metropolitan and nonmetropolitan areas of these states.

[24]In the 1980 Census of the Population, slightly more than 8 million people were counted in the New York, New York, primary metropolitan statistical area (PMSA) out of a total U.S. population of 226 million. (The New York PMSA includes the city of New York plus the counties of Westchester, Rockland, and Putnam).

[25]Because these rates include applicants of all ages, caution must be exercised in generalizing from them. Although it is known, for example, that teenagers and young adults constitute the vast majority of military applicants, HIV prevalence rates in this population are highest among persons in their late twenties.

TABLE 3-6 Distribution of AIDS Cases (percentages) Reported Through December 31, 1989, by Region and Age at Diagnosis

Age at Diagnosis	Metropolitan Areas in					Non-Metropolitan Areas	Total	N
	Northeast[a]	Mid-Atlantic[b]	Central[c]	West[d]	South[e]			
13–19	16.5%	6.7%	9.3%	9.5%	15.2%	42.7%	100%	461
20–24	19.0	7.2	8.0	13.7	16.9	35.2	100	5,090
25–29	21.6	6.6	7.3	16.5	16.3	31.7	100	18,966
30 +	25.9	6.2	6.9	20.1	13.9	27.0	100	91,269
All ages, 13+	24.8	6.3	7.1	19.2	14.5	28.2	100	115,786

NOTE: Region of residence is defined only for persons residing in Metropolitan Statistical Areas that have populations of 1 million or more. Other cases are classified into the category "nonmetropolitan," which includes persons in all regions who reside in such nonmetropolitan areas. The metropolitan areas included in the regions shown in the table are listed below.

[a]Northeast: Bergen-Passaic, N.J.; Buffalo, N.Y.; Boston, Mass.; Hartford, Conn.; Nassau-Suffolk, N.J.; New York, N.Y.; or Newark, N.J. [b]Mid-Atlantic: Baltimore, Md.; Norfolk, Va.; Philadelphia, Pa.; Pittsburgh, Pa.; or Washington, D.C. [c]Central: Chicago, Ill.; Cincinnati, Ohio; Cleveland, Ohio; Columbus, Ohio; Denver, Colo.; Detroit, Mich.; Indianapolis, Ind.; Kansas City, Mo.; Milwaukee, Wis.; Minneapolis-St. Paul, Minn.; or St. Louis, Mo. [d]West: Anaheim, Calif.; Los Angeles, Calif.; Oakland, Calif.; Phoenix, Ariz.; Portland, Oreg.; Riverside-San Bernardino, Calif.; Sacramento, Calif.; Salt Lake City, Utah; San Diego, Calif.; San Francisco, Calif.; San Jose, Calif.; or Seattle, Wash. [e]South: Atlanta, Ga.; Charlotte, N.C.; Dallas, Tex.; Fort Lauderdale, Fla.; Fort Worth, Tex.; Houston, Tex.; Miami, Fla.; New Orleans, La.; San Antonio, Tex.; San Juan, P.R.; or Tampa, Fla.

SOURCE: Special tabulation provided by the Statistics and Data Processing Branch of the AIDS Program, Centers for Disease Control.

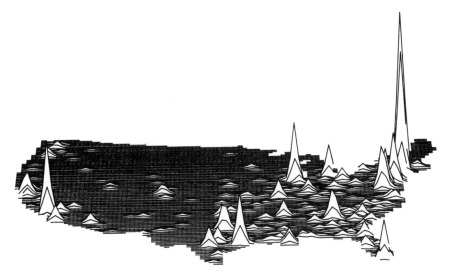

FIGURE 3-4 Map of number of HIV-infected applicants for military service ages 17 to 25 by county, October 1985 through September 1989. Counts are plotted by county, but they were not plotted for counties with 10 or fewer seropositive military applicants. SOURCE: John Brundage, Division of Preventive Medicine, Walter Reed Army Institute for Research.

thousand, respectively), whereas rates for white applicants were highest in the West (1.9 per thousand).[26]

Pockets of High-Risk Youth. As implied by the data presented earlier, not all teenagers are equally likely to come into contact with the AIDS virus. Urban-dwelling adolescents, particularly minority youths and disadvantaged teens, appear to be at increased risk for this health threat. The limited HIV seroprevalence data available suggest that runaway youth appear to be particularly at risk. A survey of more than 1,300 homeless youth seeking medical services in New York City, for example, found that 6.37 percent were infected with HIV (New York State Department of Health, 1989). Rates were higher among older youth and young adults; 8.83 percent of the 19- to 23-year-olds surveyed tested positive for HIV. The evidence regarding runaway and "problem" youths, however, is not uniform. Thus, a seroprevalence study of 1,878 16- to 18-year-olds admitted to two Los Angeles County juvenile detention facilities between February and August 1987 found that the prevalence of HIV infection (0.16 percent) was much lower than that found among runaway youth

---

[26] Although rates for black and Hispanic Job Corps applicants varied geographically over a relatively wide range (4.9 to 10.2 and 0.5 to 7.7 per thousand, respectively), rates for whites evidenced less regional variability (range 1.2 to 1.9 per thousand).

in New York City despite high rates of reported IV drug use (10 percent), needle-sharing among injectors (approximately 48 percent of male injectors and 55 percent of female injectors), and intercourse with an IV drug user (16 percent of males and 10 percent of females reported this behavior) (Baker et al., 1989).[27] The relatively low prevalence of HIV infection in this population may be related to the lower seroprevalence rates in the Los Angeles population in general (compared with New York). Nonetheless, these data indicate that, even among groups that might be expected to have high rates of infection (i.e., 16- to 18-year-old runaway and "problem" youths), there is ample reason for hoping that HIV infection can still be prevented before it makes more substantial inroads into these vulnerable populations.

Conclusion

The available data indicate that HIV infection has established itself in the teenage population, and some segments of this population report substantial infection rates. For example, the committee notes with great concern that almost 1 percent of black teenage mothers who delivered babies in New York City in 1988 were infected with HIV. Even though the available evidence is sufficient to conclude that HIV is present in the adolescent population, there are relatively few data available for accurately monitoring the spread of HIV in this group.

One of the major difficulties in presenting a clear picture of the scope of the AIDS and HIV problem among adolescents is the paucity of available data for narrowly defined age groups. Often, researchers are left to patch together data from different sources that use inconsistent age groupings. This problem is exacerbated by the fact that the AIDS case data file available for public use defines two overly broad categories spanning adolescence (ages 13 to 19) and young adulthood (ages 20 to 29).[28] In trying to compose a picture of the epidemic among adolescents, the committee has found this grouping less than optimal. Similarly, seroprevalence studies that have included adolescents provide only enough information to determine that the virus is already seeded in this population and that it appears to affect minority youth from large urban areas

---

[27] Baker and colleagues (1989) report that anonymous HIV antibody testing was done on 1,878 consecutive admissions to the juvenile facility. Self-reported data on behaviors were obtained from a random subsample of 417 of these 1,878 juveniles; 11 individuals in this subsample refused to participate in the survey.

[28] Tabulations in this chapter requiring special breakdowns were provided by the CDC at the special request of the committee. The data file that is publicly available does not provide data by finer age categories.

differentially. To understand the dimensions of AIDS and HIV infection among adolescents and to plan and target intervention programs, more detailed surveillance data are needed (see the previous recommendation).

BEHAVIORS THAT PUT ADOLESCENTS AT RISK

Not all teens are at risk for HIV infection. Some, by virtue of their low level of risky behavior or because of the absence of the virus among their potential partners, will remain uninfected. The vast majority of very young teenagers, as well as older adolescents who have not begun sexual intercourse and do not inject drugs, have little to worry about.[29] But as these individuals get older, move to different geographic locations, or engage in new behaviors, their risk level will change. Sexually active teens and those who inject drugs are certainly more vulnerable to infection than adolescents who do not engage in these behaviors, but there may be considerable fluidity in adolescent risk taking. This variation in risk taking will affect who is at risk and how many are vulnerable at a particular point in time.

The adolescent population contains pockets of teenagers whose behavior puts them at relatively high risk of acquiring HIV infection. Sexually active teens and those who share injection equipment are especially vulnerable if the virus is present within the population from which their sexual and drug use partners are selected. Some teens are already infected and thus may be capable of transmitting the AIDS virus to other adolescents. Furthermore, some teens have sex or share drug injection equipment with adults and thereby run an even greater risk of acquiring HIV infection.

Even among the youngest of teens, a subset is engaging in unprotected intercourse and drug use. (Indeed, unprotected intercourse is more common among younger teens than among older ones.) The consequences of these behaviors appear to be more serious for very young teenagers than for older adolescents. As the data presented later in this section indicate, the earlier an individual initiates one type of risk behavior, the more likely it is that he or she will initiate others. And when intercourse begins at an early age, it is less likely to involve the use of contraceptives and more likely to result in sexually transmitted diseases

---

[29] A small number of teenagers who received blood transfusions or blood products prior to the implementation of mandatory screening in 1985 were infected by contaminated blood. Since the implementation of screening programs, however, the number of persons (of all ages) who become infected through the contaminated blood transmission mode has declined dramatically (see Chapter 5).

than if it were begun later (Zelnik, Kantner, and Ford, 1981; Zelnik and Shah, 1983; Brooks-Gunn and Furstenberg, 1989; Hein, 1989a).[30]

Describing the distribution of risk-associated behaviors among adolescents is not a simple task. No single statistic captures the complex dimensions of risk, and there is considerable variation in the prevalence of sexual and drug use behaviors across ages, genders, and racial subgroups. Furthermore, the difficulty of the task is increased by the uneven quality of the available data. In the following sections the committee reviews the evidence available on sexual and drug use behaviors among adolescents. Although the review permits some relatively firm conclusions, it also highlights the need for more and better data to understand both the behaviors themselves and the individual and social factors that motivate and shape those behaviors.

Sexual Behavior

Data Sources

Previous research on unintended adolescent pregnancy has provided valuable data on adolescent sexual behavior. Three national surveys using probability samples of adolescents offer estimates of several important aspects of adolescent sexual behavior: (1) the National Longitudinal Survey of the Labor Market Experience of Youth,[31] (2) the National Survey of Young Men and Women,[32] and (3) the National Survey of Family Growth (NSFG).[33] In addition to these efforts, the 1988 National Survey of Adolescent Males (NSAM) provides information on the sexual behavior of teenage boys.[34]

---

[30] Leaving aside developmental immaturity, which affects planning and decision making among young teens, some researchers suggest that adolescent girls may be more susceptible to gonococcal and chlamydial infections because of the anatomy and physiology of the adolescent cervix (Bell and Hein, 1984; Duncan et al., 1990).

[31] The National Longitudinal Survey of the Labor Market Experience of Youth is an ongoing national probability sample of some 12,000 young people who were between 14 and 21 years of age when first interviewed in 1979.

[32] The National Surveys of Young Men and Women (frequently referred to as the Kantner and Zelnik surveys) were conducted in three waves in 1971, 1976, and 1979, using independent samples. The 1979 survey used a national probability sample of approximately 1,700 females between the ages of 15 and 19, and approximately 900 males between the ages of 17 and 21, all of whom resided in metropolitan areas. Only the 1979 survey sampled young men.

[33] The National Survey of Family Growth is a periodic survey of probability samples of women between the ages of 15 and 44 years. The survey was first conducted in 1973 and later in 1976. In 1982, the sample of 7,969 women was designed to represent all women in this age group and not just those who had been married at least once or those with children, as had been the case in earlier cycles.

[34] The 1988 National Survey of Adolescent Males used a probability sample of 1,880 boys between the ages of 15 and 19 years from the noninstitutionalized, never-married U.S. male population.

Differences in design, substantive focus, population that was sampled, and time at which data were collected preclude making precise comparisons of the estimates derived from each survey.[35] Nevertheless, reports of sexual behaviors do not stand in isolation. As discussed in a later section, the rates for adolescent pregnancies and STDs confirm the general sense provided by the above surveys of behavior that a substantial

---

[35]The National Longitudinal Survey of Youth is a panel study with annual follow-up comprising a nationally representative probability sample of 5,700 young women and 5,700 young men who were between the ages of 14 and 21 as of January 1, 1979. Individuals were selected from stratified area probability samples of dwelling units. Blacks, Hispanics, and disadvantaged whites are oversampled. Sampling criteria excluded young people who did not live within the 50 states and those who were institutionalized. Earlier waves focused primarily on labor market experiences, but information pertaining to education, marriage and fertility events, income and assets, family background, attitudes, and aspirations was also collected. Later waves have also collected data on drug and alcohol use as well as on family planning, child care, and maternal care. This survey attempts to retain the same interviewers from wave to wave; 78 percent of the 368 individuals who administered interviews in the 1984 survey reported participating in earlier waves (Campbell, 1984). Although the selection bias that has resulted from differential sample attrition does not appear to account for the lower level of sexual activity reported in this survey versus the level reported in others, the use of the same interviewers from wave to wave may affect a respondent's likelihood of being candid about reporting sensitive behaviors (Kahn, Kalsbek, and Hofferth, 1988). Reporting of drug use behavior in the 1984 wave is lowest among those who had the same interviewer in all prior waves (Mensch and Kandel, 1988b).

The design of the National Survey of Young Men and Women has varied over the different waves conducted to date. This survey includes information on contraceptive use, pregnancies, pregnancy intention, and sex education experiences. For example, the 1971 wave interviewed 15- to 19-year-old women living in households in the continental United States; women who lived in college dormitories were sampled separately. In 1979, both young women and men living in households in standard metropolitan statistical areas in the continental United States were eligible, but female participants were between the ages of 15 and 19 and males were between the ages of 13 and 17 years. Each wave includes different respondents. Because a larger fraction of female respondents in the 1979 wave had not completed their teen years, there may have been underestimation of the proportion of sexually active girls at each age.

The National Survey of Family Growth (NSFG) collects data on fertility patterns, infertility, reproductive health, contraception, fertility intentions, childbearing, adoption, adolescent pregnancy, and unwed motherhood, pre- and postnatal care, and infant health along with information on social, economic, and family characteristics. Surveys of this type began in 1955, and data were collected in 1960, 1965, 1970, 1973, 1976, 1982, and 1988; the last four years are cycles of the NSFG. This survey has used nationally representative samples of women between the ages of 15 and 44 years, although separate questionnaires have been designed for women under 25 years of age. Cycle III, which began in 1982, was the first to include all women regardless of their marital status. The NSFG (in contrast to other surveys that have included missing data codes) imputes values on variables for which the respondent did not provide an answer typically using so-called hot-deck imputation. This method is a commonly used nonresponse imputation procedure in which a sample is divided into two categories: those who respond to an item and those who fail to respond. The assumption is made that individuals who respond to several items in the same fashion (e.g., age and education) would also have similar characteristics as an item to which some subjects failed to respond (e.g., fertility intentions). Data files for respondents who provided information on each item of interest are aggregated (making a deck) and then randomized (shuffling the deck) and stacked. When the investigator encounters a data file with a missing item, he or she turns to the group or deck of complete data files and selects the next one that matches on a preselected set of items. The response for the missing item is then taken from the response provided on its matched counterpart. This process permits the calculation of both means and variances for both groups.

portion of the youth of this country are sexually active and that many of these youths do not engage in protective behaviors that prevent HIV transmission (as well as unwanted pregnancies or STDs).[36]

Vaginal Intercourse

Tables 3-7a and 3-7b present findings from the two most recent national surveys that provide estimates of the age of initiation of intercourse for teens. These tables indicate that males are more likely than females to report intercourse at any age;[37] by age 19, however, the majority of teenagers—whether black or white, male or female—report intercourse. Among 19-year-old males, 96 percent of blacks, 85 percent of whites, and 82 percent of Hispanics report having engaged in sexual intercourse. The proportions of females reporting intercourse are lower but still substantial. Among females (born between 1964 and 1972),[38] 81 percent of blacks and 62 percent of whites reported that they had engaged in sexual intercourse before their 19th birthday. In addition, the proportion of teenagers reporting intercourse at an early age is not small. Roughly one-third of 15-year-old boys report having engaged in sexual intercourse, and 21 percent of teenage girls report sexual intercourse by their 16th birthday.

In its last report, the committee noted that the proportion of persons of all ages who reported engaging in premarital intercourse had increased steadily since the early 1900s (Turner, Miller, Moses, 1989:91-98). Newly available data from the 1988 NSFG evidence a continuing trend over recent decades for more females to begin intercourse during their teens (see Figure 3-5). Thus, although roughly 30 percent of women born during the period 1944-1949 reported intercourse before age 18, more than half of the women born between 1965 and 1971 reported beginning intercourse before this age.

The racial differences found in the proportions of sexually active

---

[36] For an overview of the sexual behavior of adolescents and unintended pregnancy, see C. D. Hayes, ed., *Risking the Future: Adolescent Sexuality, Pregnancy, and Childbearing.* Washington, D.C.: National Academy Press, 1987.

[37] There is some speculation that boys are more likely than girls to exaggerate their sexual activity. Although responses from the surveys appear to be internally consistent, it is not possible to determine their validity. That is, it is not possible to say whether the responses are consistently biased toward overreporting of sexual behavior among males (see Zelnik and Kantner, 1980; Sonenstein, Pleck, and Ku, 1989a,b). See Chapter 6 for a review of the validity and reliability of survey measurements of sexual behaviors.

[38] Age definitions used for males and females differ slightly; see notes to Tables 3-7a and 3-7b.

TABLE 3-7a Percentage of Teenage Males Who Report Engaging in Premarital Sexual Intercourse, by Age and by Race/Ethnicity

| Age[a] | Males, born 1968–1973 | | | |
	All	White	Black	Hispanic
15	32.6%	25.6%	68.6%	32.8%
16	49.9	46.7	70.1	47.2
17	65.6	59.1	89.6	87.6
18	71.6	71.4	82.5	52.8
19	85.7	84.5	95.9	82.2
N	1,880	752	676	385

NOTE: The National Survey of Adolescent Males (NSAM) was conducted during 1988 using a cohort of males born 1968–1973 who were 15 to 19 years of age at the time of the interview.

[a] Estimates are the percentage of males at a given age (e.g., 16-year-olds) who have engaged in premarital intercourse. Thus, the estimates for 16-year-olds, for example, reflect the experiences of boys where ages ranged from 16.00 to 16.99.

SOURCE: Sonenstein, Pleck, and Ku (1989b:Table 1).

TABLE 3-7b Percentage of Never Married Teenage Females Who Report Engaging in Sexual Intercourse, by Age and by Race/Ethnicity

| Age | Females, born 1964–1972 | | | |
	All[a]	White	Black	Hispanic
Before 14	4.1%	2.8%	8.0%	b
Before 15	10.3	8.2	17.4	b
Before 16	20.9	18.9	31.2	b
Before 17	35.2	33.0	50.4	b
Before 18	49.7	48.8	65.8	b
Before 19	62.7	62.0	80.7	b
Before 20	68.2	66.5	87.7	b
N[c]	727	326	317	59[b]

NOTE: Estimates are the percentage of females who reported first intercourse before a given age among all females born 1964–1972 who had reached that age at the time of the interview. Thus, in calculating the percent of women who had their first intercourse before age 20, women whose age at the time of interview was younger than 20 were excluded from the calculation.

[a] Includes persons whose race was listed as other. [b] Percentages not shown for Hispanic females because of small sample size. [c] Ns shown are *minimum* unweighted sample counts. Ns for calculation of estimates of percent having intercourse at early ages are somewhat higher.

SOURCE: Tabulated from 1988 National Survey of Family Growth Public Use Data tape.

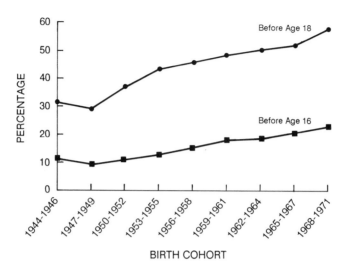

FIGURE 3-5 Percentage of women reporting first sexual intercourse before ages 16 and 18 by birth cohort. NOTE: Percentages reporting intercourse before age 18 in 1968–1971 birth cohort calculated using only women aged 18 and over at the time of the interview (unweighted n = 587). SOURCE: Tabulated from 1988 NSFG Public Use Data Tape using weighted data.

teens and age at first intercourse appear real but remain largely unexplained.[39] Multivariate analysis of the predicted probability of having premarital sexual intercourse at specific ages indicates that even controlling for a number of possibly confounding factors (e.g., age at menarche, mother's education, religious affiliation, family stability during adolescence) does not eliminate racial differences (Hofferth, Kahn, and Baldwin, 1987). One study of approximately 1,400 students from four urban junior high schools in Florida found racial differences in the progression of intimate relationships that would be consistent with the racial differences seen in the age at first coitus (Billy and Udry, 1985; Smith and Udry, 1985). The sequencing of heterosexual behaviors was more gradual and more clearly defined for white teens than for blacks who more often proceeded to intercourse without first engaging in noncoital sexual activities.[40] Although the results from this study cannot be generalized to the national population, they have important implications for AIDS

---

[39]There are a number of theories in the demographic literature that address racial differences in adolescent intercourse. Some explanations rely on biosocial factors (see, for example, Udry and Billy's 1987 discussion of pubertal development). Others look to sociological, economic, and sociocultural factors (Furstenberg et al., 1987). Empirical analyses have not led to any consensus on the most appropriate theoretical model or the most significant factors with which to explain such differences.

[40]For example, genital fondling, oral-genital contact, and so forth.

prevention strategies. The researchers suggest that those who counsel teens need "to be sensitive to cultural and ethnic differences in sexual patterns. The lack of black adolescent involvement in precoital petting behaviors places increased importance on reaching these teens very early in their heterosexual relationships" (Smith and Udry, 1985:1203).

Abstinent Teenagers

In reviewing the tables that summarize the numbers of teens who report engaging in sexual intercourse, it is important to remember that there are teens who are reporting no coitus. Issues that claim the attention of researchers tend to cluster around problems. Thus, psychologists and sociologists who have studied adolescent sexual development have generally looked at the behaviors that have resulted in unintended pregnancy and STDs. This emphasis has resulted in a more extensive data base on teens who have reported intercourse than on those who have not. It is important to note, however, that roughly one-third of females and one-fifth of males remain virgins as they enter their twenties. These teenagers are more likely than nonvirgins to be white or Hispanic[41] and to report higher levels of religiosity; they are also more likely to score higher on intelligence tests, report higher expectations for academic achievement, and live in an intact family (Hayes, 1987; Rosenbaum and Kandel, in press; see Table 3-8).

Data from the two youngest birth cohorts of the National Longitudinal Survey of Youth show that, among males born between 1963 and 1964, white teenage boys are most likely and black teenage boys are least likely to report no coital experiences. Among females, Hispanic teenage girls are most likely and blacks least likely to report no coital experience before age 19. Parental education is positively correlated and delinquency in the teenagers themselves is negatively correlated with self-reported abstinence. Yet although the demographic characteristics of teens who report no intercourse can be described, much less can be said with any certainty about the factors that encourage abstinence. Programs that have attempted to delay the onset of intercourse among teens have in general not been evaluated.

Patterns of Heterosexual Behavior

The age of initiation of heterosexual intercourse among adolescents indicates the beginning of the period of risk for HIV infection. Information on patterns of sexual intercourse, including frequency, number of sexual

---

[41] Racial differences in virginity persist even in analyses that control for the effect of socioeconomic factors.

TABLE 3-8 Estimated Percentage of Males and Females (born 1963–1964) Who Had *Not* Engaged in Sexual Intercourse Before Their 19th Birthday by Selected Social and Demographic Characteristics

Characteristic	Males		Females	
	Percentage	N	Percentage	N
Mother's education				
< High school diploma	16%	519	25%	531
High school diploma	20	638	35	589
Some college	27	296	47	259
Father's education				
< High school diploma	15	604	26	557
High school diploma	19	468	31	462
Some college	29	101	47	361
Race/ethnicity				
White	23	1,145	34	1,082
Black	5	207	19	203
Hispanic	17	381	50	95
Household structure at age 14				
Intact	23	1,024	39	967
Nonintact	12	428	20	412
1980 Delinquent acts				
None	40	231	45	484
1 or 2	24	428	29	531
3 or more	12	745	27	325
Total Sample	20	1,453	33	1,380

NOTE: Data are from the 1963 and 1964 birth cohorts of the National Longitudinal Survey of Youth. Virginity is measured by self-reports in the 1984 wave of the survey when the sample was aged 19 to 21. Delinquent acts were measured when the sample was 16 to 17 years old.

SOURCE: Derived from Rosenbaum and Kandel (in press:Table 1).

partners, and the likelihood of using condoms, provides an indication of the degree of risk. Available data on these variables are summarized below, as is the limited information collected to date on adolescent heterosexual anal intercourse.

Frequency. Data from the 1982 National Survey of Family Growth indicate that a substantial subset of sexually active adolescents have intercourse frequently. Among 15- to 19-year-old unmarried sexually experienced females, 25 percent reported intercourse two to three times per month, 20.9 percent reported intercourse once a week, and 16.3

percent reported it more than twice a week (see K.A. Moore et al., 1987:Table 1.7). Moreover, once women initiate sexual intercourse, they usually continue sexual activity. In surveys of approximately 1,800 never-married women conducted in 1976, Zelnik and Kantner (1977) found that only 14.3 percent of sexually experienced white females and 12.7 percent of sexually experienced black females between the ages of 15 and 19 reported a single episode of intercourse. More than 10 percent (11.7 percent of 15- to 17-year-olds and 25 percent of 18- to 19-year-olds) reported engaging in intercourse at least twice a week (K. A. Moore et al., 1987). In addition, in the 1982 National Survey of Family Growth, 40.5 percent of sexually experienced, single, 15- to 19-year-old females who had had intercourse during the three months prior to the interview indicated that they had done so more than four times a month (K. A. Moore et al., 1987).

Number of Partners. Although the data on numbers of sexual partners of teenagers are limited, they indicate that a substantial fraction of teens have multiple sexual partners. Figure 3-6a displays the distribution of the number of sexual partners reported by young women in the 1988 National Survey of Family Growth and by young men in the 1988 National Survey of Adolescent Males. These figures show that, although roughly one-quarter of the 18- to 19-year-olds were sexually inexperienced (i.e., they reported having no partners), a substantial fraction reported having several sexual partners. For example, among 18- and 19-year-old women, 11 percent reported 6 or more sexual partners, and 5 percent reported 10 or more partners. For young women in their early 20s, the reported numbers are considerably higher; 20 percent of 20- to 24-year olds report 6 or more partners and 10 percent report 10 or more partners.

In its previous report (Turner, Miller, and Moses, 1989:98-100), the committee contrasted parallel findings for teenage women born during the 1960s with data collected in 1970 on the number of premarital partners reported by adult women born during earlier periods of this century. The increasing number of premarital sexual partners reported by women in more recent birth cohorts suggest a major shift in the social norms governing nonmarital heterosexual sexual behavior among young women.

Unmarried young men in these surveys declared many more sexual partners than unmarried young women of the same age. As Figure 3-6b shows, 26 percent of 18- and 19-year-olds reported 6 or more partners

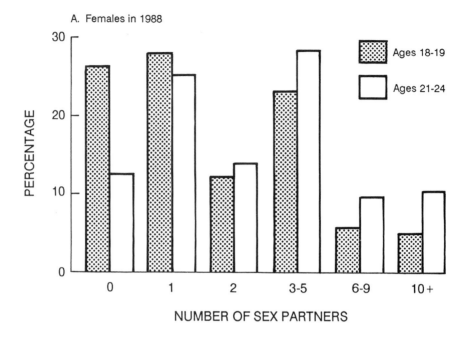

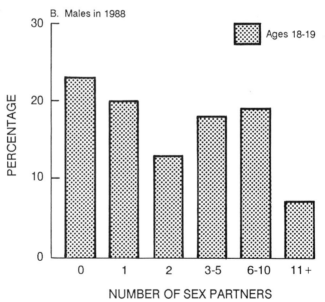

FIGURE 3-6 Number of lifetime sexual partners reported by: (a) females aged 18–19 and 20–24 in 1988, and (b) males aged 18–19 in 1988. SOURCES: 1988 National Survey of Adolescent Males, unpublished tabulation provided by F. Sonenstein (Urban Institute), J. Pleck, and L. Ku; and 1988 National Survey of Family Growth, unpublished tabulation provided by A. Campbell (National Institute of Child Health and Human Development).

and 7 percent reported 11 or more. Nonetheless, more than half of the males of this age reported two or fewer sexual partners.[42]

Contraception and Condom Use. Condoms have been shown to provide protection against AIDS and other sexually transmitted diseases (Wigersma and Oud, 1987; Feldblum and Fortney, 1988; Darrow, 1989; Perlman et al., 1990).[43] However, the fact that a significant number of adolescents report a history of STDs indicates that many sexually active teens are not using condoms or are not using them properly (Bell and Hein, 1984). The prevalence of STDs among adolescents is especially worrisome given that rates of HIV transmission are thought to increase when genital lesions are present (Nahmias et al., 1989; Telzak et al., 1989; Zewdie et al., 1989).

Although contraceptive use among teens has increased, at least through the 1970s (K. A. Moore et al., 1987:Table 2.1, 390), the fraction of U.S. teens who use birth control at first intercourse and regularly thereafter is still small in comparison with teens from other developed countries (Jones et al., 1985).[44] Among 15- to 24-year-old women who were interviewed in the 1982 National Survey of Family Growth and who reported premarital intercourse during their teens, approximately one-half (47 percent) of white females and two-thirds (66 percent) of black females did not use any contraception at first intercourse (Kahn, Rindfuss, and Guilkey, in press). Moreover, young teens are less likely to use contraception than older adolescents and more likely to delay the use of birth control until after intercourse has been initiated. This tendency has resulted in probabilities of unintended pregnancy within six months of onset of intercourse that are nearly twice as high for teenage girls who are younger than 16 years of age than for those who wait until age 18 or 19 to initiate intercourse (Zabin, Kantner, and Zelnick, 1979). Among women reporting adolescent intercourse in the 1982 National Survey of Family Growth, less than one-third of those who reported intercourse

---

[42] It should be noted that different rates of virginity reported in Figure 3-6 and Table 3-8 reflect data that are derived from separate surveys of different age groups.

[43] In vitro studies of condoms (i.e., conducted under laboratory conditions) show that HIV does not pass through latex condoms. In vivo studies of the effectiveness of condoms (i.e., data collected from actual use) are confounded by problems associated with improper and inconsistent use (see Feldblum and Fortney, 1988).

[44] For example, of the 15- to 20-year-old females interviewed in the United States in 1979, 70 percent reported using contraception at their last coitus. More than 80 percent of 16- to 17-year-old Swedish girls surveyed in 1978 reported contraception at last coitus, as did 89 percent of 16- to 18-year-old females from the Netherlands interviewed in 1981 (Jones et al., 1985).

prior to the age of 15 used some method of birth control at first premarital intercourse compared with half of those who initiated intercourse at age 17 or 18 (Mosher and Bachrach, 1987).[45]

Condoms were the method of contraception at first intercourse reported most often by 15- to 24-year-old sexually active females interviewed in the 1982 National Survey of Family Growth (Kahn, Rindfuss and Guilkey, in press). Yet despite the popularity of condoms, only a minority of respondents (21.7 percent of white teens and 13.7 percent of nonwhite teens) reported condom use at first intercourse. After first intercourse, when it appears that sex is more likely to be planned, teenagers are considerably less likely to use condoms and more likely to use birth control pills.[46] Only 12.2 percent of white sexually active 15- to 19-year-old female adolescents reported current use of condoms during the 1982 wave of the National Survey of Family Growth (Pratt et al., 1984).

Changes in teenage contraceptive practices during the 1980s have been reported in the last year for teenage males, and preliminary analyses of the 1988 NSFG suggest that parallel changes have occurred among teenage females. Sonenstein and colleagues (1989b), for example, found higher rates of reported condom use in the 1988 NSAM than had ever been found before. More than half of 15- to 19-year-old males (58 percent) claimed that they had used a condom during their last episode of intercourse. This rate of reported condom use is more than double (58 versus 21 percent) the rate reported in the 1979 National Survey of Young Men and Women (Sonenstein, Pleck, and Ku, 1989b).[47] Furthermore, the proportion of teenage males reporting condom use in 1988 did not appear to vary greatly with age (59.5 percent for 15-year-olds versus 55.2 percent for 19-year-olds). Finally, contrary to previous patterns of reported condom use, blacks were more likely (65.5 percent) than whites (54.4 percent) to report condom use.

It is not possible to be certain that boys are not exaggerating their use of condoms. Given the onset of the AIDS epidemic, the socially

---

[45] A similar pattern of findings is reported from the 1982 National Survey of Family Growth (see K. A. Moore et al., 1987, Table 2.6:400). Slightly less than half (42 percent) of the teens who participated in this survey and who reported intercourse by age 15 waited more than 12 months after first coitus to use birth control. Only 15 percent of those who started intercourse by ages 18 to 19 waited that long to take preventive action.

[46] In the 1982 National Survey of Family Growth, almost two-thirds (63.9 percent) of 15- to 19-year-old females reported the pill as their current method of birth control (Pratt et al., 1984).

[47] Although there are no available data specifying the age of purchasers, condom sales reportedly increased by more than 60 percent between 1987 and 1989 (Consumer Reports, 1989). Between 1985 and 1988, retail sales of condoms increased from approximately $180 million to $360 million (R. Rothenberg, "Condom makers change approach," *New York Times,* August 8, 1988, D-1).

responsible answer to this survey question in 1988 is clear. (See Chapter 6 for further discussion of the validity of such survey measurements.) Observed declines over this same time period in the use of female methods (e.g., intrauterine devices or IUDs, the pill, diaphragms, foam, jelly, or suppositories)[48] lend some, albeit weak, support to the inference that condom use may actually have increased substantially among sexually active adolescents.

Preliminary analyses of the 1988 wave of the National Survey of Family Growth, however, indicate a parallel trend for a greater proportion of sexually active teenage girls to report using condoms. Among sexually experienced 15- to 19-year-old females, 19.7 percent reported currently using condoms, compared with 11.4 percent in 1982.[49] Other analyses[50] of the methods used at first and last intercourse evidence a similar rise in the rates of reported condom use. Of sexually experienced females aged 15 to 19 in 1988, 47 percent reported using condoms at their first intercourse and 29 percent reported using condoms at their last intercourse.[51]

These recent indications of increased condom use raise hopeful prospects for protecting this nation's youth from HIV infection and may be evidence of the effectiveness of programs to promote greater condom use among sexually active teens. Nevertheless, the need for caution and concern remains. Half of all teenage boys in the 1988 NSAM and one-third of teenage females in the 1988 NSFG did not use *any* contraception at first intercourse. Although the rates of condom use appear to have increased substantially during the 1980s, a substantial proportion of sexually active teenagers are not using condoms. Indeed, only half of the teenage males at highest risk for infection[52] in the 1988 NSAM sample had used a condom at last intercourse (see Table 3-9).

Heterosexual Anal Intercourse. Although anal intercourse appears to be more likely than vaginal intercourse to transmit HIV (IOM/NAS,

---

[48] In 1979, 28.0 percent of 17- to 19-year-olds reported the use of a female method of contraception compared with 21.7 percent in 1988 (Sonenstein, Pleck, and Ku, 1989b).

[49] W.F. Pratt, National Center for Health Statistics, personal communication, March 7, 1990.

[50] C. F. Turner, National Research Council, unpublished tabulations, May 2, 1990.

[51] As in earlier studies, the pill was the most frequently reported contraceptive used at last intercourse; 38 percent of sexually experienced 15- to 19- year olds reported using the pill at last intercourse versus 8 percent at first intercourse.

[52] Those teens considered to have the greatest chance of becoming infected reported either same-gender sex, the use of IV drugs or a sexual partner who injected drugs, a history of other STDs, or sex with a prostitute. This high-risk group constituted 8.7 percent of the sample (Sonenstein, Pleck, and Ku, 1989a).

TABLE 3-9 Risk Behaviors and Condom Use at Last Intercourse Among Sexually Active, Never-Married Males Aged 15 to 19 Years in the United States, 1988

Risk Behavior[a]	Percent of Active Males in Category[b]	Percent Used Condoms Last Time
Group 1: Any of the following	8.7	51.2
Ever had male-male sex[c]	3.0	65.7
Ever used IV drugs or was sex partner of an IVDU	1.8	20.8
Ever had a sexually transmitted disease[d]	2.9	66.4
Ever had sex with a prostitute	1.2	16.8
Group 2: Any of the following unless in Group 1	37.7	44.5
Ever had sex with a stranger	20.0	39.9
Ever had sex with someone with many partners	31.1	40.6
Five or more sex partners in last year	7.8	36.8
Group 3: None of the above behaviors	53.6	65.9

[a] In the three composite AIDS risk categories, 5.7 percent of categorical data were missing. [b] Among those with valid responses. [c] Male-male sexual activity includes mutual masturbation, or insertive or receptive orogenital or anogenital intercourse. [d] Sexually transmitted diseases include gonorrhea, syphilis, herpes, or venereal warts.

SOURCE: Sonenstein, Pleck, and Ku (1989a).

1988:45), little is known about the number of teenage girls who have experienced anal intercourse. Small surveys of clinic populations indicate that some girls are engaging in this risky behavior and that condoms are rarely used. Jaffe and colleagues (1988) found that anal intercourse was reported by approximately one-quarter (25.2 percent) of the teenage girls attending an adolescent outpatient clinic in New York City. In addition, Kegeles and coworkers (1989) found that, of 104 girls aged 15 to 21 interviewed in a family planning clinic, 12 percent reported that they had engaged in anal intercourse. Given the potential risk for HIV infection associated with this practice, the committee believes that surveys of adolescent sexual activity should gather data on this behavior.

Same-Gender Sexual Behavior Among Adolescents

For some young people, sexual experimentation will include same-gender sexual behavior. The precise number of adolescents who experiment with same-gender sex is not known with any certainty. Using data from a 1970 survey of sexual behavior in a national probability sample, Fay and colleagues (1989) concluded that a minimum of 20 percent of American men have had sexual contact to orgasm with another male at some point in their lives, and a minimum of 6 percent have had such contact at least once during adulthood. The overwhelming majority of men who reported such contacts reported that their first male-male contact to orgasm occurred during their teenage years or earlier.[53] In the 1988 National Survey of Adolescent Males, Sonenstein, Pleck, and Ku (1989a) note that 3 percent of respondents (aged 15 to 19) reported same-gender sexual activity (mutual masturbation, oral or anal sex).

There have been other surveys of adolescent homosexual behavior, but these efforts have not relied on probability sampling techniques and thus provide estimates that cannot be generalized to the broader adolescent population. The consensus among such studies nonetheless is that adolescent homosexual activity is not rare. An anonymous, self-administered questionnaire given to 512 high school students in the Bronx, for example, found that 10 percent of female students and 9 percent of male students reported same-gender sex (Reuben et al., 1988). Among 279 homosexual and bisexual men who were interviewed by CDC in 1981 and 1982 about their medical history and lifestyle, more than half reported the initiation of same-gender sex by age 16; 20 percent reported initiation of same-gender sex by the age of 10 (Haverkos, Bukoski, and Amsel, 1989). As noted by Fay and colleagues (1989), however, much of the same-gender sexual activity during adolescence does not appear to be the first stage in the development of an exclusively homosexual identity or lifestyle. Rather, the role of same-gender sexual contact in the sexual development of heterosexual or bisexual youth has yet to be defined.

Sexually Transmitted Diseases

Different state requirements for reporting STDs and differential reporting by public versus private health care delivery systems make it difficult to estimate national STD incidence and prevalence rates. Moreover, rates that present the number of cases per 100,000 10- to 19-year-olds will underestimate the size of the problem because not all teens are sexually active.[54] There are data available, however, indicating that STDs are a public health problem for teenagers in this country. In 1987, there were 7,041 cases of gonorrhea reported to CDC among 10- to 14-year-olds and 188,233 cases among 15- to 19-year-olds, giving unadjusted rates of 42.7 per 100,000 and 1,028.1 per 100,000 for the two respective age groups

---

[53] Of those reporting age at first contact, approximately one-half reported male-male sexual contact to orgasm before age 15; approximately 90 percent reported that their first contact occurred before age 22 (C. F. Turner, National Research Council, personal communication based on unpublished tabulations from 1970 Kinsey/National Opinion Research Center [NORC] survey, January 20, 1990).

[54] Age-specific rates of various diseases are calculated by dividing the number of cases within an age group by the number of susceptible individuals in the group. Adolescents who do not report intercourse are not susceptible to STDs; therefore, including *all* 10- to 19-year-olds in the denominator of such a calculation will underestimate the rate.

(CDC, 1988e). Compared with the gonorrhea caseload, there were fewer primary and secondary syphilis cases reported for 1987; 229 cases were identified among 10- to 14-year-olds (1.4 per 100,000). Still the number of cases of syphilis increased and 4,331 cases were diagnosed among 15- to 19-year-olds, a dramatic increase that yielded a rate of 23.7 cases per 100,000. The incidence of both gonorrhea and syphilis was 1.4 to 3.1 times higher among females in these age groups than among males. In addition, although STD rates for adolescent males are substantial, teenage boys do not account for as large a proportion of male gonorrhea cases as do teenage girls for cases among women. In 1979, 38 percent of gonorrhea cases reported by females were diagnosed in adolescent girls, but only 17 percent of cases among males were in teenage boys (Bell and Hein, 1984).

There is some evidence to suggest that STDs are a greater problem in younger populations than in older ones. When the denominator for national STD rates is corrected to include only the sexually active portion of the adolescent and young adult populations, 10- to 19-year-olds have the highest rates of gonorrhea and syphilis. In 1976 the rates for gonorrhea among sexually active females 10 to 19 years old were approximately 3,500 per 100,000 (Bell and Hein, 1984). Gonorrhea rates dropped precipitously as age increased; among 20- to 24-year-old women, the rate was approximately 1,800 per 100,000, and among 25- to 29-year-old women it was approximately 700 per 100,000.

Rates that decline with age may be attributable in part to the differential use of health care facilities. Younger women may be more likely than older women to use public facilities (as opposed to private ones), and therefore may be more likely to have their case reported to the health department. Yet even within the population of clients who use public clinics, rates of STDs decrease as age increases. This trend is also reflected in lower incidence rates of hospitalized cases of pelvic inflammatory disease among older females (Bell and Hein, 1984).

Conclusion

The specter of AIDS has not stopped teens from engaging in unprotected sexual intercourse. Furthermore, continued risk taking does not appear to be related to a lack of awareness of the threat posed by unprotected sexual contacts.[55] It is clear that as long as the sexual behaviors that transmit

---

[55] CDC-assisted surveys conducted in 1988 found that the majority of students between the ages of 13 and 18 were well aware that sexual intercourse is a risk factor for HIV transmission (CDC, 1988a). Between 88.3 and 98.1 percent of the sample, which included students from areas with the highest cumulative incidence of AIDS, correctly identified sexual intercourse as a risk factor, and between 83.8 and 98.4 percent knew that IV drug use could spread HIV infection.

HIV infection are found in the adolescent population, there remains the possibility that teenagers can acquire or transmit the AIDS virus. It is therefore important to heed the empirical data, note the populations and geographic areas in which the risky behaviors tend to occur, and direct intervention resources toward those areas to prevent AIDS. Such actions will not only improve the chances for preventing the further spread of HIV infection but may also help to deal with other long-standing problems of the adolescent population, namely, STDs and unintended pregnancies.

Drug Use

As noted earlier, adolescence is a time of experimentation with a variety of behaviors that may include sex and the use of drugs. Much drug use, even though it is considered to be a significant health threat to the individual as well as to society at large, does not constitute a direct risk factor for AIDS. IV drug use,[56] on the other hand, can play a direct role in HIV transmission if drug injection equipment is shared. Moreover, the use of drugs that are not injected may pose an indirect threat. Even alcohol, for example, can play an indirect role in transmission by lowering inhibitions and perhaps clouding the judgment of those who are drinking, thereby facilitating unsafe sexual practices (Stall et al., 1986; Faltz and Madoover, 1987; Flavin and Frances, 1987). Another drug that has the potential to affect transmission of the virus is crack, a smokable and potent form of cocaine that is believed to heighten sensations of sexual arousal among males. Ethnographic studies indicate that some women exchange sex for crack (or for cash to buy crack) (Fullilove et al., 1990; Turner, Miller, and Moses, 1989:Chapter 3). In a study of 13- to 19-year-old black male and female crack users in the San Francisco area ($N = 222$), virtually all (96 percent) were found to be sexually active, slightly more than half (51 percent) reported that they had combined sex with drug use, and one-quarter of both boys (25 percent) and girls (24 percent) had exchanged sexual favors for drugs or money (Fullilove et al., 1989; 1990). The potential for unsafe sexual practices under such conditions is considerable; crack users are unlikely to know the serostatus, sexual history, or drug habits of their partners, and there is small likelihood that condoms will be used. Indeed, Fullilove and colleagues (1990) found that 41 percent of teenage crack users in their sample reported a history of an STD, and only 26 percent of boys and 18 percent of girls reported condom use during their last episode of sexual intercourse. Thus, the

---

[56]Illicit drugs that are administered through intravenous injection include heroin, cocaine, amphetamines, and so-called speedballs, a combination of heroin and cocaine.

combination of sex and drugs in the adolescent population may be a potent mixture that bolsters risky behaviors and contributes to the spread of HIV. The next section examines the prevalence of drug use in the adolescent population.

Data Sources and Limitations

The preponderance of the data presented in this section comes from three national survey programs. Monitoring the Future is an annual survey of approximately 17,000 high school seniors.[57] The National Household Survey on Drug Abuse collects data from approximately 8,000 individuals who are 12 years of age or older; slightly more than one-quarter (2,246 persons or 28 percent) of the sample are between the ages of 12 and 17. The 1987 National Adolescent Student Health Survey examined the health-related knowledge, attitudes, and behavior of 11,419 eighth and tenth grade students.

National drug use surveys that include teenagers are likely to underestimate the number of teens using drugs. School-based surveys, such as Monitoring the Future or the National Adolescent Student Health Survey,[58] do not capture adolescents who have dropped out of school or those who are chronic absentees. Thus, survey efforts may miss an important and sizable segment of the at-risk adolescent population. (Johnston and colleagues [1989] report that high school dropouts constituted 15 percent of the age group surveyed by the National Adolescent Student Health Survey, and Mensch and Kandel [1988a] found that approximately 22 percent of the 12,000 young people interviewed in the National Longitudinal Survey of Youth had dropped out of school at least once.) In 1984, there were more than a half million 14- to 17-year-olds who had dropped out of high school prior to graduation (Hayes, 1987, Table 2.3:38). Moreover, Hispanic adolescents were more likely than other youth to have dropped out of school by age 15, and 14.3 percent of Hispanic teens had dropped out of school by age 16 or 17.

Household surveys, such as the National Household Survey on Drug Abuse,[59] also have limitations in that they miss the transient, the homeless, and the incarcerated. At the time the 1980 census was taken, 0.8 percent

---

[57]Monitoring the Future, an ongoing annual survey, began in 1975. Each year, 125 to 135 schools are selected to provide a representative cross-section of U.S. high school seniors. The survey also has a longitudinal component that follows approximately 2,400 students in each class.

[58]The 1987 National Adolescent Student Health Survey included students from randomly selected classrooms chosen from a national probability sample of 217 schools in 20 states.

[59]The National Household Survey on Drug Abuse is an ongoing survey of individuals aged 12 and older who live in households in the United States. Samples have ranged from approximately 3,000 in

of all 15- to 24-year-olds were confined to institutions. Males incarcerated in prisons, jails, or juvenile detention/corrections facilities constituted the majority (83 percent) of the 360,000 individuals in this group (Wetzel, 1987). All of the groups omitted from household or school surveys are known to have higher drug use rates than the general population (Shaffer and Caton, 1984; Rothman and David, 1985; Mensch and Kandel, 1988a; Yates et al., 1988; Baker et al., 1989; Rolf et al., in press).

Inevitably, questions also arise regarding the validity of self-reported data on illegal activities, including the use of illicit drugs, that are collected in surveys. Comparisons of drug-related data from the 1984 waves of the National Longitudinal Survey of Youth with data from Monitoring the Future and the National Household Survey on Drug Abuse suggest that there is underreporting of illicit drug use (other than marijuana) in the National Longitudinal Survey. Moreover, youth who report limited involvement with a particular drug are more likely to deny such use (Mensch and Kandel, 1988b), a finding that is supported by another, more geographically circumscribed study (Single, Kandel, and Johnson, 1975). Moreover, data from the Monitoring the Future survey showed proportionately more drug use reported in the month prior to the interview than in the preceding 12 months, reflecting, perhaps, a telescoping of recall (Bachman, Johnston, and O'Malley, 1981). Given that there is some degree of underreporting of drug use and some underrepresentation of the heaviest users, these surveys may be providing lower-bound estimates of adolescent drug use in the United States.

Initiation of Drug Use

Adolescent drug users do not suddenly issue forth as full-blown addicts. Rather, there is an empirically observed progression in stages of drug use, beginning with licit drugs, such as beer and wine; continuing with cigarettes or hard liquor, or both, with some teens going on to marijuana use; and fewer finishing the progression with other illicit drugs, such as stimulants, inhalants, hallucinogens, sedatives, and nonprescription tranquilizers. Cocaine use is frequently preceded by or coincides with the use of other illicit drugs (B. A. Hamburg, Kraemer, and Jahnke, 1975; Yamaguchi and Kandel, 1984a; O'Donnell, 1985; Newcomb and Bentler, 1989; Kandel and Davies, in press). Indeed, data from the 1984 wave of the National Longitudinal Survey of the Labor Market Experience of

---

1972 to more than 8,000 in 1985. Individuals are selected using a multistage area probability design (National Institute on Drug Abuse [NIDA], 1988).

Youth found that cocaine use is almost always preceded by marijuana use (Kandel and Davies, in press).[60]

Not all drug users participate in every step of the sequence outlined above, nor does the use of a drug at a lower level inevitably lead to a higher stage of drug use (Newcomb and Bentler, 1989). When progression to the next level of drug use does occur, however, the use of drugs from the previous stages generally continues; indeed, heavy or frequent use of a familiar drug is characteristic of the transition to the next step (Kandel, 1984; Rosenbaum and Kandel, in press).

Injection Practices Among Adolescents

The sharing of injection equipment to administer illicit drugs is one of the major modes of transmission of HIV in the United States and Europe. Approximately 30 percent of AIDS cases in the United States report the use of injected illicit drugs as a risk factor for infection (see Chapter 1). Most persons who inject illicit drugs, such as heroin, first do so either in late adolescence or in early adulthood (Gerstein, Judd, and Rovner, 1979; Newcomb and Bentler, 1988). If a person has not initiated illicit drug injection by the age of 25, it is unlikely that he or she will do so. Consequently, any examination of the risk of acquiring HIV infection among adolescents and young adults should consider exposure to the virus through shared injection equipment.

Progression through the various stages of drug use does not inevitably lead to injection; as the drugs become increasingly "harder," fewer and fewer adolescents progress to the next stage of the drug use sequence, leaving only a small number who will move to the later stage of injection. This progression raises important issues concerning the economy of structuring intervention efforts that are meant to deal with the hazards associated with the end point of this sequence. There is no pharmacologic inevitability that leads adolescents to seek stronger or more powerful psychoactive drugs, although there appear to be psychosocial factors associated with progressive drug use that may be helpful in identifying individuals for early intervention. These factors include having peers who are heavily involved in drug use, beginning drug use at a relatively early age, and reporting a variety of social and developmental problems, including poor relationships with parents, peers, and authority systems (Kandell, Kessler, and Margulies, 1978).

The precise number of adolescents and young adults who inject drugs

---

[60] Among individuals who participated in that survey and reported the use of alcohol or cigarettes, marijuana, or other illicit substances, less than 1 percent reported experimentation with cocaine before the initiation of marijuana use (Kandel and Davies, in press).

is not known. However, data from the Treatment Outcome Prospective Study (TOPS)[61] have shown that, of individuals in treatment in this country, a not insignificant percentage are teenagers. Of the 8,795 TOPS participants who reported IV drug use in the year before entering treatment, 0.2 percent or 17 individuals were less than 16 years old, 1.6 percent or 140 were 16 to 18 years old, and 7.3 percent or 642 were 19 to 21 years old (Ginzburg, 1988). The impact of AIDS on the number of drug users who inject, the frequency of injection, and the use of shared injection equipment is also unknown. Of cause for concern, however, are reports such as the anecdotal information supplied by Mata and Jorquez (1988). These investigators reported that, where needle-sharing persists among Mexican Americans who inject drugs, young users are the most likely age group to participate in this hazardous practice.

Prevalence of Drug Use

The number of adolescents who use specific drugs, such as cocaine or heroin, is not known.[62] Estimates of the percentage of adolescents who report drug use rely on surveys that may provide a sense of the lower bound on these numbers. As discussed earlier, the degree of underreporting and underrepresentation in these surveys is not known, making it difficult to interpret differences in the rates of drug use found across studies. What is clear is that prevalence rates are higher in school surveys than in household surveys (compare for example, Tables 3-10 and 3-11). It is thought that these differences in estimates may be attributable to the different methods used to collect the data (i.e., a face-to-face interview in the home versus a self-administered questionnaire).[63]

Although drug use among high school students has declined since

---

[61] TOPS data were collected from three annual cohorts (1979, 1980, and 1981) of individuals admitted to more than 40 drug abuse treatment programs in this country. The survey seeks to understand the natural history of drug use before, during, and after treatment. More than 11,000 subjects who entered treatment between 1979 and 1981 were interviewed at the point of intake into treatment; a subset of 4,600 was followed after discharge from treatment through 1986.

[62] See Turner, Miller, and Moses (1989:Chapter 3); and Spencer (1989) for a review of national estimates.

[63] Differences in anonymity and privacy are likely to affect responses. In the National Household Survey of Drug Abuse noted above, drug questions were asked aloud, and responses were marked on the answer sheet by the interviewer. This procedure raises questions about protecting the privacy of the respondent and the validity of the response given the presence of parents or others in nearby proximity. In the school surveys, questionnaires were entirely self-administered. In addition, subjects' ages vary across studies. The National Adolescent Student Health Survey was conducted in the fall when eighth graders were, for the most part, 13 years old and tenth graders were 15 years old. The Monitoring the Future survey was conducted in the spring when seniors were 17 and 18. The National Household Survey of Drug Abuse covers the same aggregate population as the student surveys except for the inclusion of 12-year-olds and the exclusion of 18-year-olds.

its peak in 1979 (see Table 3-10), the proportion of adolescents who use drugs remains considerable (Johnston, Bachman, and O'Malley, 1989). The proportions of teens who report the use of specific drugs vary by drug type and route of administration. Considerably more adolescents report the use of licit than illicit substances, and drugs that are swallowed, smoked, or inhaled are more popular than drugs that are injected. Alcohol use, for example, is extremely common, with more than three-quarters of eighth graders (74 percent) having had at least one drink (see Table 3-11). From a health perspective, however, quantity and frequency of consumption are more significant than whether an individual has ever used alcohol. The data indicate that there are significant numbers of young teenagers who report drinking levels that may pose potential threats to their health. More than one-quarter (26 percent) of eighth graders and 38 percent of tenth graders reported having had five or more drinks on at least one occasion in the two weeks prior to the National Household Survey (NIDA, 1988). It is clear from these data that many adolescents not only drink but do so frequently and excessively. Heavy drinking, moreover, is known to be combined with increased sexual activity and decreased use of contraception (Ensminger, 1987). AIDS-related studies of adults also indicate that alcohol use is associated with unsafe sexual behavior (Stall et al., 1986); however, much less is known about adolescent risk taking under the influence of alcohol.

According to adolescent surveys, marijuana is the most popular illicit drug for this population.[64] In 1985, nearly one-quarter (23.6 percent) of 12- to 17-year-olds reported experimentation with marijuana, and the majority (19.7 percent) reported using the drug during the past 12 months (see Table 3-10). Among eighth graders surveyed in 1987, 14 percent had used marijuana; a third (34 percent) of tenth graders and half (50 percent) of a group of high school seniors had also smoked marijuana (see Table 3-11).

The use of marijuana, hashish, and hallucinogens decreased between 1979 and 1985, but the use of cocaine has fluctuated. Rates now appear to be approximately stable (see Table 3-10). In 1985, 5 percent of 12- to 17-year-olds reported experimentation with cocaine. In 1987, even among eighth graders, rates for cocaine use were substantial: 5 percent reported that they had used cocaine at least once (see Table 3-11). By the twelfth grade, the lifetime prevalence of cocaine use had increased threefold to 15 percent.

---

[64] Alcohol is not classified as an illicit substance here, despite the fact that it is illegal for adolescents under the age of 18 to purchase alcoholic beverages.

TABLE 3-10 Trends Between 1979 and 1985 in Percentage of 12- to 17-year-olds Reporting Use of Selected Drugs During Lifetime and During Previous Year

Drug	Reported Ever Using the Drug			Reported Using the Drug in Last 12 Months		
	1979	1982	1985	1979	1982	1985
Marijuana and hashish	30.9%	26.7%	23.6%	24.1%	20.6%	19.7%
Inhalants	9.8	NA[a]	9.2	4.6	NA	5.1
Hallucinogens	7.1	5.2	3.3	4.7	3.6	2.7
Cocaine	5.4	6.5	4.9	4.2	4.1	4.0
Heroin	0.5	b	b	b	b	b
Nonmedical use of any psychotherapeutic[c]	7.3	10.3	12.1	5.6	8.3	8.5
Cigarettes	54.1	49.5	45.2	13.3	24.8	25.8
Alcohol	70.3	65.2	55.5	53.6	52.4	51.7
N	2,165	1,581	2,246	2,165	1,581	2,246

[a] Not available. [b] Less than 0.5 percent. [c] Includes stimulants, sedatives, tranquilizers, and illicit use of analgesics or painkillers that are generally available only by prescription.

SOURCE: NIDA National Household Survey on Drug Abuse (1988:Tables 6 and 10).

Heroin use is rare among the adolescents whose responses are captured by surveys. The NIDA household surveys found that 0.5 percent of respondents indicated that they had used heroin at least once. Twelfth graders who participated in Monitoring the Future reported somewhat higher lifetime prevalence rates, with 1 percent of seniors indicating heroin use (see Table 3-11).[65]

Although national heroin use data indicate that drug injection is relatively rare among adolescents, local surveys find considerable variation in the proportion of respondents who report needle use. Surveys of students in Massachusetts and in the Bronx found that roughly 1 to 2 percent reported IV drug use (Strunin and Hingson, 1987; Reuben et al., 1988). Yet among 213 adolescent runaways between the ages of 11 and 16 who were interviewed in Texas, 7 percent had injected drugs (Hudson et al., 1989). Furthermore, the percentage of students in a CDC-assisted school survey who reported IV drug use (see Table 3-12) ranged from 2.8 percent for Michigan to 6.3 percent for Washington, D.C. (CDC, 1988a). Among male students, however, almost 9 percent (i.e., 8.7 percent) of

---

[65] Among high school seniors who participated in Monitoring the Future, 2 percent of males and 1 percent of females reported heroin use.

TABLE 3-11 Percentage of Schoolchildren Who Reported Ever Using Selected Drugs, by Grade in School Between 1985 and 1989

Drug	Those Who Reported Using the Drug at Least Once		
	8th Graders	10th Graders	12th Graders
Marijuana	14%	34%	50%
Inhalants	21	21	19
Cocaine	5	9	15
Crack	2	3	5
Heroin	NA[a]	NA	1
Other opiates	NA	NA	9
Stimulants	NA	NA	22
Sedatives	NA	NA	9
Tranquilizers	NA	NA	11
Cigarettes	NA	NA	67
Alcohol	74	85	92

NOTES: Data on 8th and 10th grade students are drawn from the National Adolescent Student Health Survey ($N \geq 4,400$ for all drugs). Data on 12th grade students are taken from the Monitoring the Future survey (N = approximately 16,800 for marijuana, cocaine, cigarettes, and alcohol; N is approximately 13,440 for inhalants and 6,720 for crack because only four fifths of students were asked about inhalant use and only two-fifths were asked about crack use). [a] Not available.

SOURCES: Association for the Advancement of Health Education, Appendix B (Sampling and Weighting Procedures); University of Michigan, press release of February 9, 1990.

the students from Washington, D.C., reported that they had injected illicit drugs.

Differential Patterns of Drug Use

Gender differences in drug use appear to be substance specific, and the gap between male and female use has declined over time (Kandel, 1980). Drug use is generally higher among teenage boys; girls, however, are more likely to smoke cigarettes and to use stimulants.

The magnitude and direction of racial and ethnic differences in drug use present a complex and sometimes contradictory picture.[66] Unlike surveys of sexual behavior, almost all national drug use surveys report that illicit drug use is lower among black youths than among whites, with Hispanics falling in between (Bachman, Johnston, and O'Malley, 1981; NIDA, 1988; Kandel and Davies, in press). Surveys that report high levels of drug use among blacks are generally restricted to poor

---

[66]Unfortunately, not all surveys collect race- or ethnicity-specific data. For example, the Monitoring the Future survey, although reporting on the prevalence of use by region, rural-urban location, college plans, and gender, does not provide specific rates for racial or ethnic groups.

TABLE 3-12 Percentage of Secondary School Students Reporting IV Drug Use, by Sex and by Age for Selected Cities and States, 1988

Site	Total	Gender		Age		
		Female	Male	13–14	15–16	17–18
California[a]	4.1%	2.6%	5.7%	2.8%	3.9%	4.3%
(N = 7,013; RR = 64%)						
Michigan	2.8	2.1	3.4	3.2	3.2	1.3
(N = 991; RR = 100%)						
Washington, D.C.	6.3	4.6	8.7	b	4.0	8.9
(N = 1,275; RR = 100%)						
San Francisco	3.7	2.4	5.1	1.4	3.9	2.4
(N = 802; RR = 88%)						

NOTES: The Ns indicate the size of the total sample, and they do not account for item nonresponse. RR refers to the school response rate, that is, the number of schools participating in the survey divided by the number of schools selected in the sample design.

[a] The sample from California excludes students in San Francisco and Los Angeles. [b] Not shown because sample size was less than 40.

SOURCE: CDC(1988a:Tables 1 and 3).

black communities (Brunswick, Merzel, and Messeri, 1985); yet even, for example, in a survey of inner-city Baltimore youth, blacks reported less drug involvement than whites (Zabin et al., 1986).

The reasons why white teens report greater involvement with drugs than blacks are not clear. Kandel and Davies (in press) suggest several possible explanations, including differential underreporting, differential levels of drug involvement, and differential use of publicly funded treatment centers and emergency rooms, which are important sources of drug-related data. There are also some preliminary findings that indicate differential validity in reported data. An analysis of two waves of the National Longitudinal Survey of the Labor Market Experience of Youth found that blacks were more likely than whites to provide internally discrepant responses to questions on illicit drug use. Among those who admitted using illicit drugs in the past year in a self-administered form in the 1980 survey, blacks were more likely than whites to deny in a subsequent interviewer-administered survey that they had ever used illicit substances (Mensch and Kandel, 1988b).[67] That blacks may be more inclined to provide socially desirable responses is supported by findings

---

[67] Inconsistent responses were twice as common among blacks and Hispanics than among whites. Approximately 13 percent of black and Hispanic males and 22 percent of black and Hispanic females who reported marijuana use in 1980 claimed never to have used this drug upon reinterview in 1984. Seven percent of white males and 10 percent of white females provided similar inconsistent responses.

from Monitoring the Future. In the 1983 wave of that survey, non-drug-using black teens were twice as likely as white teens to indicate that they would not report drug use even if they had been involved in it (Johnston, Bachman, and O'Malley, 1984).

Age appears to play an important role in the initiation of use of most drugs.[68] Surveys have shown that, for most substances, drug initiation rates peak in the late teens (Kandel, 1980). Analyses based on complete drug history data for the 1980 wave of a longitudinal study of a probability sample of tenth and eleventh grade New York State students in 1971 (a total of 1,325 students) indicated that the risk of initiating marijuana use begins at age 10 and reaches its height at age 18, declining substantially thereafter. Participants in this retrospective survey were between 24 and 25 years of age when the 1980 data were collected; of those who had used marijuana by the time they were interviewed, 90 percent had done so by age 20. Thus, if initiation did not begin by the end of the teenage years, it was unlikely to occur. A similar pattern was observed for the use of psychedelics, which peaks at age 21 (Kandel and Logan, 1984). However, the risk of initiating cocaine use does not terminate by age 20 but continues for a number of years thereafter (Kandel and Logan, 1984; Johnston, O'Malley, and Bachman, 1988).[69]

A similar pattern has been found in the Monitoring the Future surveys. Two-fifths of that sample (approximately 6,000 high school seniors) were asked to name the grade level at which they began using particular drugs.[70] As Table 3-13 shows, 2.9 percent of teens began experimenting with marijuana in the sixth grade, and nearly 13 percent[71] had initiated marijuana use by the end of the ninth grade. However, only 4 percent initiated marijuana use in the twelfth grade. Initiation of cocaine use, in contrast, was more common in the later high school grades.

Research indicates that early initiators of marijuana use are at much greater risk of becoming involved with other illicit drugs (Yamaguchi and

---

[68] For example, a recent survey of 3,454 secondary school students found age-related differences in the context of marijuana initiation (Bailey and Hubbard, 1990). The authors suggest that developmental factors may influence the context of initiation of this drug.

[69] The use of prescribed psychoactives also continues to rise beyond adolescence, particularly for females (Kandel and Logan, 1984).

[70] The figures for the twelfth grade are somewhat misleading because the survey was conducted before the school year was finished. Rates of initiation are thus low, not only because the period of risk is truncated by the survey but also because recent initiators, who are undoubtedly light users, may be less likely than more practiced users to admit involvement.

[71] Table 3-13 shows percent initiating drug use in particular grades. For marijuana, 2.9 percent reported first use in 6th grade and a further 10 percent report first use during 7th-8th grades.

TABLE 3-13 Percentage of Students in the High School Class of 1987 Reporting Initiation of Use of Selected Drugs, by Grade of First Use

Drug	Grade						Never Used the Drug
	6th	7th–8th	9th	10th	11th	12th	
Marijuana	2.9%	10.0%	12.3%	12.3%	8.2%	4.4%	49.8%
Inhalants	2.5	3.3	3.6	2.7	3.4	1.4	83.0
Hallucinogens	0.3	0.9	1.9	2.5	3.3	1.5	89.7
Cocaine	0.2	0.6	2.2	3.7	5.4	3.0	84.8
Heroin	0.1	0.1	0.3	0.4	0.2	0.1	98.8
Opiates other than heroin	0.6	1.0	2.0	2.0	2.5	1.0	90.8
Stimulants	0.6	3.8	5.7	5.4	3.8	2.4	78.4
Sedatives	0.4	1.5	2.5	1.9	1.5	0.8	91.3
Tranquilizers	0.4	1.6	2.6	2.6	2.4	1.4	89.1
Alcohol	8.8	22.6	24.5	19.3	11.5	5.5	7.8
Getting drunk	3.3	13.8	20.3	17.8	11.9	5.7	27.1
Cigarettes	21.0	19.4	10.9	7.2	5.7	2.9	32.8
Cigarettes (daily use)	1.6	5.2	5.3	4.4	3.3	1.6	78.7

NOTE: The entries in this table show percent reporting that their *first use* occurred in particular grades. The sample size for all percentages is approximately 6,000 persons.

SOURCE: Johnston, O'Malley, and Bachman (1988:Table 15).

Kandel, 1984b). Among white males in the 1984 National Longitudinal Survey of Youth who used marijuana, other illicit drugs, and cocaine (N = 926), the mean age of onset of marijuana use was 14.9 years compared with 16.9 years for those who only used marijuana (N = 1,690). The mean age of onset of marijuana use for white females (N = 583) who reported that they used alcohol (or cigarettes), marijuana, and other illicit substances was 14.8 years, compared with 17.2 years for those who restricted their drug use to marijuana (N = 1,645) (Kandel and Davies, in press).[72]

---

[72]Respondents in the 1984 National Longitudinal Survey of the Labor Market Experience of Youth, who were between the ages of 19 and 27, were by virtue of their age at very low risk of initiating marijuana use. The same is not true for cocaine. As a result, the differences reported here may be attenuated as the sample ages and some of the "marijuana only" group are transferred into the "multiple drug" group. However, data for an older sample (the 1980 New York State follow-up cohort) found the age differences in marijuana initiation for the two groups to be similar in magnitude to those seen in the national survey. Among males, the multiple drug users (N = 189) initiated marijuana use at 15.6 years of age compared with 18.3 years for the "marijuana only" users (N = 165). Among females the

Although the vast majority of teens who experiment with marijuana will not go on to inject drugs, early initiators of drug use are nevertheless at increased risk of turning to crack and IV drugs in later years, thus also increasing their risk for HIV infection. Research on adolescent drug use has provided a sense of the behavioral characteristics that distinguish adolescents who use drugs from their abstemious peers; it has also, with the help of longitudinal surveys, separated the antecedents from the consequences of use (Kandel, 1980). Unfortunately, there has been little systematic research on the predictors of early drug initiation. Identifying and reaching early initiators of drug use will be important in preventing or remolding behaviors that confer risk for a variety of health problems, including AIDS.

Clustering of Risk Behaviors

Research on adolescents has provided compelling evidence of covariation among sexual activity, alcohol use, drug use, and delinquency (Miller and Simon, 1974; Hayes, 1987). The early onset of sexual intercourse does not appear to be an isolated behavior, nor does drug use. Rather, each is part of a complex pattern of interrelated activities. R. Jessor and coworkers (1980) surmise that the co-occurrence of problem behaviors (e.g., the use of alcohol or illicit drugs, criminal acts) may reflect for some adolescents a choice of lifestyle rather than a choice of particular behaviors; the co-occurrence of these behaviors may thus reflect a single underlying tendency. This concept of a lifestyle or syndrome has found some support in the literature on adolescent problem behavior.[73] The confluence of risk-associated behaviors argues for pursuing an understanding of sexual and drug use behaviors within the larger social context of adolescence. Just as there are developmental stages of drug use, there may be a predictable sequence of problem behaviors in which one behavior, rather than being functionally equivalent to another, may actually constitute a risk factor for subsequent behaviors (Robins and Wish, 1977; Rosenbaum and Kandel, in press).

A number of recent studies have examined the association between drug use and sexual activity. Elliott and Morse (1989) reanalyzed data from the 1976–1980 waves of the National Youth Survey, a household probability sample of 2,360 adolescents aged 11 to 17 at the time of the first interview. At the time of the initial survey in 1976, the proportion of

---

mean age of marijuana initiation for multiple drug users ($N = 132$) was 15.9 years, compared with 18.9 years for the "marijuana only" users ($N = 224$) (Kandel, Murphy, and Karus, 1985).

[73] For an overview of this literature and its problems, see Osgood and coworkers (1988).

boys reporting sexual activity in the previous year ranged from 10 percent for those who had not used drugs to 23 percent for users of alcohol only, 48.3 percent for combined alcohol and marijuana users, and 72 percent for those using multiple illicit drugs.

In 1975–1976, Ensminger and Kane (1985) conducted a follow-up study of students from a poor, inner-city Chicago neighborhood who had been in the first grade in 1966–1967 when they were first interviewed. Slightly more than half of the original subjects (705 of the original 1,242 children, or 56.7 percent) participated in the follow-up survey. The investigators found that those who drank were two to three times more likely to be sexually active than those who abstained from alcohol. Similarly, males who had used marijuana at least once were ten times more likely to be sexually active than those who had not used it, and females who had used marijuana were seven times more likely to report initiation of sexual intercourse than girls who were not involved with marijuana.

There are also data on the reverse of this phenomenon showing higher rates of drug use among sexually active teens. A 1981 study of 2,557 inner-city adolescents aged 12 to 18 in four Baltimore junior and senior high schools found that, regardless of race or gender, drug use scores (which reflected the type of substance and frequency of use) were higher for sexually active adolescents than for virgins (Zabin et al., 1986). Elliott and Morse (1989), having established a relationship between sexual activity and drug use, attempted to determine the temporal order. They found that 2.25 times as many males and nearly 5 times as many females initiated drug use before sex rather than initiating sex prior to drug use. It should be noted, however, that their definition of drug use in this study was fairly comprehensive and included alcohol. Because the average age of initiation for alcohol use is very low, including alcohol in the definition of drug use tended to lower the age of initiation of drug use in the Elliott and Morse study.

Using data from the National Longitudinal Survey of the Labor Market Experience of Youth, Kandel and coworkers (Kandel and Davies, in press; Rosenbaum and Kandel, in press) investigated the association between prior drug use[74] and sexual initiation by age 16. This study controlled for such covariates as race, religion, parental education, family structure, and personality (including delinquency and school characteristics). Retrospective data from the two youngest cohorts (i.e., the 2,711 individuals who were 19 to 20 years old in 1984) showed that, for both

---

[74]Drug use was broken down into the following categories: (1) alcohol or cigarettes, or both, (2) marijuana, and (3) other illicit drugs.

males and females, the association of drug use and sexual behavior is considerable, even after the covariates above are entered into the prediction equation. Early sex is 1.4 times more frequent for boys who have used alcohol or cigarettes, or both, than for boys who did not report any prior drug use; it is 2.7 times more frequent for boys who have used marijuana, and 3.4 times more frequent for boys who have used other illicit drugs. The association is even stronger for females. Early sex is 1.8, 3.5, and 4.9 times more frequent, respectively, for female users of the three categories of drugs than for nonusers. The association is also stronger for whites and Hispanics than for blacks, which may reflect the earlier age of initiation of sexual intercourse for blacks and the relatively limited time for drug initiation to occur prior to the initiation of sexual activity.

Kandel and Davies (in press) also examined the degree to which early sexual activity is associated with an increase in subsequent drug use. Using the entire National Longitudinal Survey of the Labor Market Experience of Youth sample from 1984[75] and controlling for a number of potentially shared selection factors, Kandel and Davies found that early sexual activity was the most important predictor of cocaine involvement. In addition, among the 93 percent of males and 86 percent of females who were sexually experienced, the earlier sex was initiated, the greater the incidence of subsequent cocaine use. The predicted probability of using cocaine was 20 percent for males who waited until age 17 to initiate sexual intercourse and 12 percent for females who waited until age 18. Moreover, the frequency of intercourse in the 30 days prior to the survey was higher for cocaine users, especially males.[76]

The association of sexual activity and substance use was also shown in Mott and Haurin's (1988) analysis of retrospective data from the National Longitudinal Survey of Labor Market Experience of Youth. Their work indicated that, at a given age, teenagers who use alcohol or marijuana at least once a month are more likely than nonusers to begin sexual intercourse in the following year. Similarly, those who are sexually active are more likely than virgins to report subsequent drug use. Yet although Mott and Haurin note that sexual activity and drug use are statistically related, they point out that the majority of young

---

[75] In 1984, the 12,069 respondents in the sample were between 19 and 27 years old.

[76] The frequency of intercourse applied to young adults between the ages of 19 and 27; there were no data to indicate the frequency among teens younger than 19 years of age. It is possible, however, that the same pattern of sexual behavior may also be seen among younger teens.

adolescents (i.e., those under 16) were abstinent and had never used alcohol or marijuana.[77]

Thus, drug use and early sexual activity are, indeed, related. Prior use of drugs, both licit and illicit, significantly increases the risk of early sexual activity among adolescents. Furthermore, early sexual activity increases the likelihood of involvement with cocaine, a drug for which the age of initiation is typically later than that reported for initiation of sexual intercourse. The studies described above clearly document that sexual activity and drug use are associated; however, research has not yet revealed whether the association is a simple function of shared antecedents. Are early sexual activity and drug use in adolescents determined by a common set of behavioral attributes? Does one behavior constitute a unique risk for the other? Additional research will be needed to answer these and other important questions. Therefore, **the committee recommends that the Public Health Service give high priority to studies of the early initiation of risk-associated behaviors, including drug use and sexual behaviors, and of progression to the practice of multiple high-risk behaviors.**

Before proceeding, one further point should be emphasized. Although the committee recognizes the need for further research, it would reiterate that there is already sufficient information to conclude that early initiation of sexual behaviors or drug use carries the risk of HIV transmission for some fraction of American youth. This finding motivates the committee's call for AIDS interventions that target teenagers *before* they begin practicing risky sexual and drug-using behaviors.

Subpopulations of Teens at Higher Risk

As discussed earlier, national surveys are unlikely to reach youths who have dropped out of school or those who are not living in households. This latter group, which may be fairly sizable, includes adolescents who live on the street or in residential institutions (e.g., youth detention centers) or who have joined the Job Corps. Reaching these teenagers may be particularly important in that some of these youths may currently be at higher risk of acquiring HIV infection than the general population of adolescents.

There are several studies that support this perception of increased risk. A recent national survey of juveniles in custody, for example, found that 63 percent of these youths used drugs regularly (Bureau of

---

[77] That is, any use of marijuana, or monthly use of alcohol, or any history of sexual intercourse.

At six in the evening, four nights a week, a small white van loads up with passengers at a garage on Jerome Avenue in the Bronx. The van belongs to Project Streetbeat, a program of Planned Parenthood. The passengers are counselors. On this chilly Thursday night, as always, the van speeds downtown on the Bronx River Parkway, towards the heart of the South Bronx in search of teenage prostitutes. Loose packets of condoms, bleach kits and comic books about AIDS prevention, clutter the front seat . . .

Social worker Larry Bilick is director of Project Streetbeat, and tonight he is driving the van.

"This is an unreported life on the whole; and unreported conditions that these young people are living under. We don't hear almost anything about them. These young people are not runaways that come from other areas. They are mostly from the Bronx, they are mostly throwaways, it is not like they have some place else to go to, if only they wanted to go back home. Many of them have been victims of physical abuse and/or sexual abuse when growing up. Many of them have come out of the social service system of the city of New York; are casualties of that system. And, the circumstances of their lives have led them to these streets . . . "

The outreach workers hand out condoms, bleach kits to sterilize needles, and to new clients, a comic book explaining safe sex in the language of the streets. Because most of the teenagers are homeless, living in abandoned buildings or in cars, they also give away donated clothing and dignity packs: plastic bags filled with basic necessities like a toothbrush, a comb and a bar of soap . . .

The staff, most of whom are bilingual, don't preach or lecture, but they do gently urge these young people to come to Project Streetbeat's office where the staff can work to connect them with medical services, drug treatment programs, and shelter.

Casanova Street is the busiest prostitution block in the neighborhood, mainly because so many of these young people live in the abandoned cars in the junk yard at the top of the road. Froggy is 20 years old and has been working Hunt's Point for the last five years. She gets her name from a voice that has been gnarled by years of crack smoking and began using Project Streetbeats's condoms a year ago.

"You must see people coming round giving protections, clothes, that makes me feel good, cuz it makes me feel like they care. You know, like I'm somebody for them, you know?"

In the year and a half since Project Streetbeat began, the staff has had more than 3,000 different encounters with hundreds of prostitutes aged 13-21. One counselor has taken it upon himself to meticulously research and record the deaths of the different young people who he has worked with in the streets. Since the program began, he knows of 10 teenagers who have died; some from AIDS, some brutally murdered by pimps or johns. The deaths of these teenagers are not the stuff of newspaper obituaries, but for the counselors, it's the motivation that keeps the van driving through these streets, night after night.

EXHIBIT 3-1 Edited News Report on Teenage Prostitutes in the Bronx by David Isay. SOURCE: Crossroads, National Public Radio Network, broadcast on WAMU, Washington, D.C., January 12, 1990.

Justice Statistics, cited in the AMA Council of Scientific Affairs [AMA-CSA], 1990). It is estimated that more than 500,000 juveniles are taken into custody through public detention or correctional facilities each year (AMA-CSA, 1990:987). Smaller surveys of institutionalized adolescents provide insight into the problems of youths who reside in such settings, although the findings may not be generalizable. For example, interviews with 378 female adolescents aged 12 to 17[78] residing in detention centers in the Bronx in the late 1970s found that the average age of initiation of sexual intercourse in this sample was 12 years. Virtually all (99 percent) of this sample were sexually active (Hein et al., 1978).

STDs have been reported as problems for both teenage boys and girls in detention situations.[79] Almost one-fifth (17 percent) of 262 respondents to a survey of 16- to 17-year-olds incarcerated in the Los Angeles area reported a history of STDs (Morris et al., 1989), and almost half (47 percent) reported drinking alcohol in situations that led to intercourse. Among 184 juvenile offenders recruited through the San Francisco Youth Guidance Center, 35 percent reported exchanging sex for drugs or money, and almost half (46 percent) agreed that "sex without condoms is worth the risk of getting AIDS" (Temoshok et al., 1989).

Comparing 802 high school students with 14- to 18-year-old juvenile offenders ($N = 113$) residing in a detention facility in the San Francisco area, DiClemente and DuNah (1989) found significant differences in the prevalence of risk-associated behaviors. Youths in detention were significantly more likely than students to report ever injecting drugs (12.9 percent versus 3.7 percent); they were also more likely to report more than three sexual partners (86.4 percent versus 15.1 percent) and an earlier age of initiation of sexual intercourse.

Street youth are at greater risk than children who live in more favorable conditions for virtually all medical disorders of childhood (IOM, 1988). Consequently, it is likely that they would also be at higher risk for such health threats as drug dependency, HIV infection, and other STDs. A major contributor to higher risk for these adolescents may be prostitution, which is one method teens employ to survive. For any youngster,

---

[78] The mean age was 14.8 years.

[79] Between July 1983 and June 1984, 285 teenage girls and 2,236 teenage boys between the ages of 9 and 18 residing in a New York City detention center participated in screening for STDs (Alexander-Rodriguez and Vermund, 1987). Fewer boys than girls (3 percent versus 18.3 percent) were found to have gonorrhea, and prevalence rates for syphilis were also lower for the boys (0.63 percent versus 2.5 percent). Most of those infected had no clinical signs. In a separate survey of 2,672 youths in temporary detention in New York City (Hein, Marks, and Cohen, 1977), 2,064 boys and 374 girls were asymptomatic for venereal disease. Following culture, however, 1.9 percent of asymptomatic males and 6.9 percent of asymptomatic females were found to have gonorrhea.

prostitution can be a particularly hazardous survival tool, given the limited negotiation skills of young teens compared to those of their older patrons.

It is important to note that an understanding of the prevalence of risk-associated behaviors among street youths is compromised by difficulties in reaching and engaging this population in surveys and research. Studies of this population have necessarily used small samples of convenience, relying on volunteers recruited from shelters and the streets. Although it is not possible to provide an accurate demographic and risk profile for street youths from these studies, the available research does offer a clear sense of the problems associated with living on the streets, and several findings are consistently reported across such studies. Interviews with street youths indicate that this group is, indeed, at risk for HIV infection, and the epidemiological evidence suggests that the prevalence of HIV infection is higher among street youths—at least in New York City (see Table 3-2)—than among adolescents in general. Moreover, although the precise number of homeless youths who use drugs is not known, small surveys of this population have consistently found that the majority report drug use (Shaffer and Caton, 1984; Rothman and David, 1985; Yates et al., 1988). Most street youths who have participated in studies also report that they are sexually active, but few report the regular use of condoms (Shaffer and Caton, 1984; Yates et al., 1988; Hudson et al., 1989; Rotheram-Borus et al., 1989).

Another subpopulation of teens who are at higher risk for HIV infection comprises adolescents who are raped or sexually abused (Gellert and Durfee, 1990). Data from the 1987 wave of the National Survey of Children[80] found that 7 percent of 18- to 22-year-olds in this country report experiencing at least one episode of nonvoluntary intercourse; approximately half of the experiences reported by women occurred before the age of 14 (K. A. Moore, Nord, and Peterson, 1989).

Conclusion

In assessing adolescents' risk of acquiring HIV infection, it is clear that some teens are more likely than others to engage in the behaviors that are known to transmit HIV. In addition, the number of adolescents at risk because of a specific behavior varies in part according to the behavior. Although many teens experiment with alcohol, relatively few report the use of crack or injection of illicit drugs. Nevertheless, a substantial

---

[80] The 1987 wave of the National Survey of Children followed up on experiences reported by subjects during the first two waves. Telephone interviews resulted in an 82 percent response rate from persons interviewed in the second wave. Analyses reported above are based on 1,121 respondents aged 18-22.

proportion of teens are sexually active, and although recent data indicate that more teens than ever are using condoms, there remains a sizable subpopulation who are still engaging in unprotected intercourse. As is discussed at the end of this chapter, the differential distribution of risk-associated behaviors has important implications for intervention efforts. It is clear, however, that early onset of risky behaviors can have grave consequences, and it is therefore necessary to reach these youth before such behaviors begin. For youth who are already engaging in risky behaviors, it will be necessary to intervene as quickly and as effectively as possible to facilitate protective change in these behaviors.

INTERVENING TO PREVENT
FURTHER SPREAD OF INFECTION

The section that follows considers intervention strategies to retard the spread of HIV infection among teens. These interventions are motivated by the risky behaviors detailed in the preceding section. An examination of the contentious question of appropriate goals for AIDS prevention efforts aimed at teenagers is followed by a description of interventions to reach different segments of the teenage population. The section concludes with a discussion of the resources needed to serve the segments of the teenage population who are at relatively high risk for HIV infection.

Of paramount importance, however, is the continuing need for coupling careful evaluation research to future intervention programs.

Role of Evaluation Research

The committee strongly believes that progress in the development of successful intervention programs will depend on an iterative process in which programs are implemented and their effects assessed, following which new and better interventions are designed and tested. Toward this end, the committee recommended in its first report that **"planned variations of key program elements be systematically and actively incorporated into the design of intervention programs at an early stage"** (Turner, Miller, and Moses, 1989:307). The committee reiterates this recommendation, noting that such designs can provide invaluable evidence of the effectiveness (or ineffectiveness) of different intervention strategies. It is the committee's firm opinion that this strategy—coupling AIDS prevention programs with rigorous research efforts to determine the effects of those programs—offers the best hope of producing effective behavioral interventions for the diverse subgroups that constitute the adolescent population. Such efforts are the key to improving the inadequate knowledge base that presently hobbles efforts to design effective interventions. To further encourage the use of such designs, an evaluation panel of the committee has issued a review of research and intervention strategies that can be used to evaluate mass media campaigns, testing and counseling programs, and interventions designed by community-based organizations (Coyle, Boruch, and Turner, 1990).

In the following section, the committee offers, to the extent possible, suggestions for AIDS prevention strategies that currently appear promising for retarding the future spread of HIV among teenagers. Owing to the lack of adequate scientific evidence, readers will note that, although the committee was able to describe with *relative* confidence the various patterns of adolescent behavior that place young people at risk of acquiring or transmitting HIV, there is much less certainty about the types of programs that can help adolescents modify those risky behaviors to avoid infection. Thus, all suggestions for intervention programs carry a concomitant recommendation that the interventions be carried out in a manner that permits the collection of evidence of their effectiveness.[81] It is only through such efforts that effective interventions will be designed.

Goals of Intervention Programs for Teens

Within the adolescent population, there is tremendous variation with respect to risk taking and potential exposure to the AIDS virus. Similarly, the committee notes that considerable controversy surrounds some of the adolescent behaviors that transmit HIV infection. This section considers, in turn, the controversy concerning the general goals of AIDS prevention programs for teenagers and specific goals for three segments of the teenage population.

General Goals

With regard to the use of drugs that are associated with HIV transmission, there is a consensus both within our committee and in the nation as a whole that such drug use is, in itself, physiologically destructive and psychologically debilitating. Thus, AIDS prevention programs for teenagers and adults properly discourage drug use among all persons. For persons who do use drugs, AIDS prevention programs have the goals of (1) discontinuance of drug use, if possible; and (2) if discontinuance is not possible, implementation of practices to reduce the risk of HIV transmission (e.g., by using sterile needles). In its previous report, the committee concluded that, regardless of the availability of treatment opportunities

---

[81] As discussed by Turner, Miller, and Moses (1989:Chapter 5) and Coyle, Boruch, and Turner (1990), an optimal research strategy is likely to involve rigorous evaluations of *selected* AIDS prevention programs rather than routine evaluation of all interventions.

and programs intended to prevent drug use, a substantial number of people in the United States would continue to inject drugs, at least in the short run. Some of these persons will be teenagers and young adults. Consequently, the committee believes that AIDS prevention programs should encourage these drug users to seek treatment; they should also ensure that these young people are made aware of all effective methods for reducing their risk of contracting or transmitting HIV. The committee wishes to emphasize that the goals of prevention and risk reduction are not contradictory. None of the current studies on "safer injection" programs[82] have shown an increase in IV drug use as a result of making sterile needles available or promoting injection equipment sterilization using bleach. Indeed, it appears that safer injection programs may indirectly encourage IV drug users to seek treatment. Furthermore, although results are still preliminary, many studies indicate that such programs do reduce the risk of HIV transmission among IV drug users (Buning, Coutinho, and van Brussel, 1986; Jackson and Neshin, 1986; Jackson and Rotkiewicz, 1987; Chiasson et al., 1987; Watters, 1987; Buning et al., 1988; Stimson, 1988, 1989; Hartgers et al., 1989; van den Hoek, van Haastrecht, and Coutinho, 1989).

With regard to premarital and same-gender sexual behaviors, there is no similar consensus in this country. There is instead ample evidence that these behaviors are extremely controversial subjects. It will be seen from Table 3-14, for example, that there is a substantial divergence in the opinion of American adults about sexual intercourse among persons who are not married. Although there was some increase in tolerance of sexual intercourse among unmarried persons over the last two decades, roughly one-third of Americans report that they believe premarital sexual intercourse is "always wrong," whereas another one-third report that they believe it is "not wrong at all."[83]

Given these divisions in public opinion, it is not surprising that federal AIDS education efforts have stumbled for several years over this issue. Much of the controversy involves disputes about the need to offer "realistic" advice regarding the protective value of condoms versus counterclaims that the AIDS epidemic requires moral education to promote abstinence from sexual activity prior to marriage and fidelity within

---

[82] See Chapter 2 of this report and Turner, Miller, and Moses (1989:Chapter 3) for a detailed review of research in this area.

[83] Estimates are derived from surveys of probability samples of the noninstitutional adult population of the continental United States conducted by the General Social Survey program of the National Opinion Research Center (University of Chicago; see Davis and Smith, 1989). The estimates have been weighted to reflect the varying probabilities of selection for persons in households with different numbers of eligible adults.

TABLE 3-14 Distributions of Responses (percentage) to a Question About Premarital Sexual Relations Tabulated from Surveys of Probability Samples of U.S. Adults, 1972–1989

	Attitude Toward Premarital Sex				
Year	Always Wrong	Almost Always Wrong	Sometimes Wrong	Not At All Wrong	N
1972	35.7%	11.4%	25.2%	27.7%	1,537
1974	33.4	13.0	23.9	29.7	1,492
1975	30.6	12.4	25.2	31.7	1,427
1977	30.7	9.9	23.1	36.3	1,481
1978	29.1	12.3	20.4	38.2	1,494
1982	28.4	9.1	21.7	40.7	1,794
1983	28.1	10.7	24.6	36.6	1,561
1985	28.1	9.0	20.0	43.0	1,482
1986	28.2	8.8	22.8	40.2	1,425
1988	26.2	10.2	22.2	41.4	955
1989	27.7	8.8	23.1	40.4	971
All years	30.0	10.6	23.0	36.5	15,556

NOTE: The question was as follows: If a man and a woman have sex relations before marriage, do you think it is always wrong, almost always wrong, wrong only sometimes, or not wrong at all? Tabulations were weighted by the number of adults in the household to correct for different probabilities of within-household selection in households of different size. The Ns shown in the table are unweighted.

SOURCE: Tabulated from the General Social Survey conducted by the National Opinion Research Center, University of Chicago (Davis and Smith, 1989).

marriage.[84] Not surprisingly, this controversy has been most intense with regard to AIDS education for teenagers and young adults.

In 1987, for example, the U.S. Senate voted 94 to 2 in support of an amendment to the Department of Health and Human Services appropriations bill that required all AIDS educational materials and activities for young adults and school-aged children to emphasize "abstinence from sexual activity outside of a monogamous marriage."[85] The impact of such legislation can be seen in the constraints that have been incorporated in AIDS prevention programs mounted by the Public Health Service. CDC's "Guidelines for Effective School Health Education to Prevent the Spread of AIDS," for example, propose that, for young people who have already begun to engage in sexual intercourse, "school programs should enable

---

[84] See, for example, Turner, Miller, and Moses (1989:Chapter 7) from which this discussion is adapted.

[85] *Congressional Record,* October 14, 1987, S-14217.

and encourage them to stop engaging in sexual intercourse until they are ready to establish a mutually monogamous relationship within the context of marriage" (CDC, 1988d:4). The CDC guidelines do recognize, however, that some young people will not follow this advice, and they recommend that school systems, in consultation with parents and health officials, provide information on other strategies to prevent HIV transmission.

Guidelines such as these for teenagers and young adults do not reflect the pluralistic nature of beliefs in this country but attempt to impose a particular set of values on all adolescents. They also fly in the face of the data presented earlier in this chapter, which indicate that most contemporary teenagers in the United States begin sexual relations during their teens, that a sizable fraction begin intercourse in the early teens, and that a substantial portion of sexually active teens report having intercourse at least once a month. Indeed, more than 1 million teenagers become pregnant each year,[86] and more than 400,000 of these pregnancies occurred in young women 15 to 17 years of age (Hayes, 1987:54–55, 261).

In the context of a deadly, sexually transmitted epidemic, the committee believes that AIDS prevention programs must heed the data on risk-associated behaviors reported by the adolescents themselves and not be sidetracked by wishful thinking about patterns of behavior some might hope teenagers would follow. In 1986, Surgeon General C. Everett Koop set a high standard for rational discourse on AIDS prevention for adolescents. On release of his report on AIDS, which dealt frankly with the behaviors that transmit HIV, the surgeon general observed:[87]

> Controversial and sensitive issues are inherent in the subject of AIDS, and these issues are addressed in my report. Value judgments are absent. This is an objective health and medical report, which I would like every adult and adolescent to read . . . .
>
> Many people—especially our youth—are not receiving information that is vital to their future health and well-being because of our reticence in

[86]In 1984, it is estimated that just over 400,000 teenage girls obtained abortions (Hayes, 1987:261). More recently, Trussell (1988:262) has estimated that "One out of every 10 women aged 15-19 in the United States becomes pregnant each year, a proportion that has changed little during the past 15 years." Trussell's calculations yielded an estimate of roughly 860,000 pregnancies (837,000 pregnancies among 15- to 19-year-olds and 23,000 among girls aged 14 or younger); however, he notes that these "are underestimates of pregnancies because spontaneous abortions are ignored and because data are tabulated by age at the resolution of pregnancy instead of age at conception" (p. 262). (Hayes [1987:54-55] estimated that 134,000 teenage pregnancies ended in miscarriages in 1984.)

[87]C. Everett Koop, public statement made at press conference upon release of Surgeon General's Report on Acquired Immune Deficiency Syndrome, Washington, D.C., October 22, 1986.

dealing with the subjects of sex, sexual practices, and homosexuality. This silence must end. We can no longer afford to sidestep frank, open discussions about sexual practices—homosexual and heterosexual . . . .

As parents, educators, and community leaders we must assume our responsibility to educate our young. The need is critical and the price of neglect is high. AIDS education must start at the lowest grade possible as part of any health and hygiene program. There is now no doubt that we need sex education in school and that it should include information on sexual practices that may put our children at risk for AIDS. Teenagers often think themselves immortal, and these young people may be putting themselves at great risk as they begin to explore their own sexuality and perhaps experiment with drugs. The threat of AIDS should be sufficient to permit a sex education curriculum with a heavy emphasis on prevention of AIDS and other sexually transmitted diseases.

This committee concurs wholeheartedly with these objectives.

Specific Program Goals

As noted previously, there is tremendous variation in the behaviors of different segments of the adolescent population and in the risk of HIV infection faced by these subgroups. The committee believes that intervention programs must reflect this diversity of risk and thus proposes specific goals for three groups of teens.

Program Goals for Adolescents Who Are Not Engaging in Risk-Associated Behaviors. Intervention programs should seek to provide information, motivation, skills, and practical assistance to help these young people avoid future risks and to involve them in current AIDS prevention activities. The ultimate goal of AIDS prevention is to block HIV transmission, and programs should accommodate the range of challenges young people will face and the variety of choices they may make. Abstinence, delay of intercourse until marriage, and other traditional behavioral patterns are effective ways of eliminating the risk of sexually transmitted HIV infection if in fact these patterns are enacted. Because some teens, however, will choose to begin sexual activity, all teenagers should be educated about the protective value of condoms and spermicides. In addition, all teens should be educated about the dangers posed by the use of illicit drugs.

Intervention programs must reach youth in their very early teen or preteen years. In this regard, it is worth remembering that 23 percent of young women in the United States report that they have engaged in sexual intercourse by their 16th birthday, and 4 percent report engaging in sexual intercourse by their 14th birthday.[88] Given the serious consequences often associated with such early initiation of intercourse, **the committee**

---

[88] For the birth cohort ($N = 897$) born 1962–1964, the National Survey of Family Growth found that

recommends that AIDS prevention programs make special efforts to reach very young teens and, in some subpopulations, to reach youth before they enter adolescence.

The committee also believes that interventions should ensure that youth who engage in male-male sexual contacts have sufficient knowledge to protect themselves in such encounters. As noted earlier in this chapter, estimates derived from a probability sample of American men in 1970 (Fay et al., 1989)[89] suggest that a minimum of 20 percent of American males have male-male sexual contact to orgasm at some point in their lives and that most of these men have their first such experiences during adolescence.[90]

Program Goals for Adolescents Who Are Engaging in Sexual Intercourse but Who Are Not Using Illicit Drugs. Intervention programs for these young people should educate them about the dangers of drug use and seek to facilitate protective changes in their sexual behaviors. Although education about abstinence may be valuable, clear advice concerning the protections offered by condoms and spermicides should also be offered. In this regard, the committee wishes to draw attention to the parallel approach recommended by another National Research Council committee that addressed a more common and less deadly consequence of adolescent sexual behaviors: unwanted pregnancy. In recommending policies for dealing with adolescent pregnancy, that committee struggled with many of the same controversies that surround AIDS-related discussions. After two years of deliberations they concluded the following:

> Sexually active teenagers, both boys and girls, need the ability to avoid pregnancy and the motivation to do so. Early, regular, and effective contraceptive use results in fewer unintended pregnancies. Delaying the initiation of sexual activity will also reduce the incidence of pregnancy, but we currently know very little about how to effectively discourage unmarried teenagers from initiating intercourse. Most young people do become sexually active during their teenage years. Therefore making contraceptive methods available and accessible to those who are sexually active and encouraging them to

---

23.1 percent of women reported that they had had intercourse by their 16th birthday, and 4 percent reported intercourse by their 14th birthday (Hofferth, Kahn, and Baldwin, 1987:Table 3).

[89] These estimates are based on a national sample of the adult male population of the United States in 1970.

[90] There are only a few research efforts now under way to study gay youth. Several of the projects now being conducted (one in New York as part of the HIV Center for Clinical and Behavioral Studies funded by the National Institute of Mental Health; others directed toward street youth in Baltimore, Maryland, and Belo Horizonte, Brazil [Rolf et al., 1989]) are promising but are unlikely by themselves to be sufficient. Clearly, more research will be needed to understand the determinants of same-gender sex among adolescents and to identify the most effective mechanisms for reducing AIDS-associated risk in that age group.

diligently use these methods is the surest strategy for pregnancy prevention. (Hayes, 1987:262)

Program Goals for the Small Groups of Adolescents Engaging in Multiple High-Risk Behaviors and Those Adolescents Who May Already Be Infected with HIV. Intervention programs for these teens should make every effort to assist them in altering the behaviors that place them at risk and should seek to alter any social or economic conditions that support their risk taking. Teens who are using illicit drugs, especially those who inject drugs, should be encouraged to seek treatment. Such a policy in turn requires effective referral networks to treatment programs that are tailored to adolescent needs. For example, residential drug treatment programs have been designed to alter teen lifestyles, recreational activities, patterns of association, and other factors relevant to their drug use. It should be noted, however, that for the most part methadone treatment programs are not available to adolescents.

Those adolescents who continue to use needles should be urged not to share them or other injection equipment. Adolescents who are living on the streets, engaging in prostitution, or exchanging sex for crack will require additional services, such as shelter, counseling, and medical care. These adolescents who are at highest risk of infection should also be made aware of the availability of HIV testing and counseling, how this service is delivered (confidential versus anonymous testing), and the significance of the information provided. Teenagers known to be infected with HIV will require information and counseling regarding the potential consequences of their infection, including its possible effects on future childbearing and on sexual and drug use partners. They should also be given advice about securing the medical and social services they may need in the future.

The difficulties manifested by this last group of teens present the greatest challenges to AIDS prevention and arise from some of the nation's most severe social problems. They also highlight the lack of success previous efforts have had in dealing with these problems prior to the onset of the AIDS epidemic. These problems remain equally difficult to solve today, but AIDS has increased the price that will be paid for failing to deal with them.

WHAT DO TEENS KNOW ABOUT AIDS?

National surveys of high school students sponsored by the CDC (1988a)[91]

---

[91] In 1987 CDC (1988a) began collecting data from a national sample of high school students in grades 9 through 12. These data are intended to help local departments of education assess local knowledge,

together with local surveys[92] have found that virtually all students have heard of AIDS and the majority know about the routes of transmission. Fewer teens, however, are aware of actions that can be taken to prevent the acquisition of infection (DiClemente, Zorn, and Temoshok, 1986; Strunin and Hingson, 1987). (See Tables 3-15, 3-16, and 3-17 below.) Moreover, misconceptions remain among adolescents concerning the role of casual contact in the transmission of HIV (DiClemente, Zorn, and Temoshok, 1986; Strunin and Hingson, 1987; CDC, 1988a; DiClemente, Boyer, and Morales, 1988; DiClemente, 1989; Siegel et al., 1989).

Findings from a national sample of students in the eighth and tenth grades (the National Adolescent Student Health Survey) indicate that approximately 90 percent of these teens knew that the AIDS virus could be transmitted by sexual intercourse or by sharing needles (see Table 3-15). Similarly, results of a 1988 survey of a probability sample of 16- to 19-year-olds in Massachusetts (Table 3-16) indicate that virtually every young person in this sample was aware that AIDS could be transmitted by sexual contact or injection of drugs. Yet approximately half of teenagers in the national sample thought that AIDS could be contracted from donating blood (see Table 3-17), and substantial fractions of teenagers in the 1988 Massachusetts sample believed that AIDS could be transmitted by saliva (39 percent) or giving blood (51 percent). Even more disturbing is the number of teens who report misperceptions about ways to reduce the risk of contracting AIDS (see Table 3-17). For example, 27 percent of white males and more than 40 percent of black and Hispanic males in the national sample said that they believed that the risk of AIDS could be reduced by washing after sex. Similarly, 30 percent of males and 21 percent of females thought that "making sure your partner looks healthy" would help protect them from AIDS. Perhaps most telling, however, are

---

beliefs, and behaviors; the findings can inform the content and planning of education programs and can be used to monitor changes over time. In the survey, students completed a self-administered, anonymous questionnaire that was developed collaboratively by CDC and 24 state and local departments of education. Core questions provide information on demographic characteristics, HIV beliefs and knowledge, and behaviors associated with transmission. Most sites used a geographically stratified cluster sample, randomly selecting schools within strata, then selecting classes within schools. Other sites used a random sample of schools, then randomly selected students at each school. Response rates of schools varied from 52 to 100 percent.

[92]There have been many surveys of adolescents' knowledge, attitudes, and beliefs about AIDS, but these "KAB" surveys are of variable scope and quality. Some have surveyed national populations; others have relied on small, local samples. Some surveys have used probability sampling techniques; others have relied on samples of convenience. Variation in the wording of questions and the manner in which questions are posed complicates comparisons of different surveys. In reviewing different KAB instruments, it is important to keep in mind that the populations sampled, the recruitment process, and the methods for collecting data vary. Such variation means that caution is called for in making generalizations and looking for trends.

TABLE 3-15 Percentage of Adolescent Students (grades 8 and 10) Correctly Reporting AIDS Risk Factors, by Race/Ethnicity, 1987–1988

Transmission of the AIDS Virus	Females				Males			
	All	White	Black	Hispanic	All	White	Black	Hispanic
More likely if sexual intercourse with someone who has the AIDS virus[a]	96.2%	97.6%	93.5%	90.7%	93.5%	96.1%	87.0%	85.1%
More likely if more than one partner[a]	85.1	86.9	80.6	80.7	79.3	83.3	67.3	71.2
More likely with shared needles[a]	93.8	95.5	90.8	87.2	89.9	92.2	82.7	84.8
Less likely if condoms used[b]	84.9	86.8	85.5	67.8	87.8	89.6	83.1	81.8
Less likely if abstain from sex[b]	79.0	82.7	71.4	66.0	72.4	76.8	61.4	59.1
Possible from pregnant woman to her baby[c]	83.3	81.7	86.6	89.9	80.4	80.0	82.0	80.5
Unweighted Ns[d]	1,689	1,308	230	151	1,692	1,323	224	145

[a]Question wording: Will the following behaviors make it MORE likely for a person to become infected with the AIDS virus? (d) Having sexual intercourse (sex) with someone who has the AIDS virus; (e) Having more than one partner; (i) Sharing drug needles. [b]Question wording: Will the following behaviors make it LESS likely for a person to become infected with the AIDS virus? (b) Not having sex; (d) Using condoms (rubbers) during sex. [c]Question wording: Mark whether you think each sentence is true or false. (g) A pregnant woman who has the AIDS virus can give AIDS to her baby. [d]In estimating percentages, sampling weights supplied with the data set were used to project the results to the national student population. The unweighted Ns shown in the last row of the table are minimum base Ns on which the percentages were calculated. Because of variability across items in the amount of missing data, the actual Ns for specific items in this table may be larger than the minimums shown here by 5 to 10 persons.

SOURCE: Tabulated from the 1987–1988 National Adolescent Student Health Survey.

TABLE 3-16 Percentage of 16- to 19-Year-Olds in 1988 Survey of Probability Sample of Massachusetts Teens Who Reported Believing That the AIDS Virus Could be Transmitted by Various Means

| | Percentage Who Believed It Was HIV Transmission Route | |
Means	1986	1988
Sex between two males	99%	98%
Sex between a male and female	91	99
Injecting drugs	91	99
Vaginal fluids	69	88
Semen	76	93
Getting a blood transfusion	93	89
Kissing someone on the mouth	58	25
Giving blood	61	51
Tears	19	17
Saliva	60	39
Sharing eating or drinking utensils	38	11
Toilet seats	15	5
N	829	1,762

SOURCE: Hingson, Strunin, and Berlin (1990:Table 2).

the results presented in Table 3-17, which indicate that one teenager in every five believed that persons infected with the AIDS virus could only spread the virus if they were sick with AIDS. This substantial disbelief in the risk posed by asymptomatic but infected individuals and the misperception of protection afforded by washing are cause for concern.

Furthermore, although many of the basic facts about AIDS appear to be reaching teens, the segments of the adolescent population that are epidemiologically most vulnerable appear to be less well informed about this disease than the majority of youths.[93] The data in Table 3-15 provide evidence, for example, that minority youth are less aware than white youth of the behaviors that risk HIV transmission. Other studies have found racial differences with respect to beliefs about the benefits afforded

---

[93] For example, a survey of 1,869 students from a community college located in the South Bronx, an epicenter of the epidemic, found that only 69 percent recognized that sexual intercourse without a condom increased risk for HIV infection, and slightly more than half (55 percent) were aware of the risk of vertical transmission if a pregnant woman reported sexual contact with an IV drug user within the past five years (Lesnick and Pace, 1990).

TABLE 3-17 Percentage of Adolescent Students (grades 8 and 10) Reporting Misperceptions About AIDS by Race/ Ethnicity, 1987–1988

Misperception	Females				Males			
	All	White	Black	Hispanic	All	White	Black	Hispanic
Only people sick with AIDS can spread the virus[a]	21.6	18.2	32.3	25.2	21.7	20.1	22.1	33.9
There is a vaccine for AIDS[a]	9.9	7.4	18.8	10.4	11.5	9.5	16.2	17.7
Less likely to get AIDS from partner who looks healthy[b]	21.0	15.3	38.2	29.5	30.0	26.2	38.1	45.2
Less likely to get AIDS if you wash after sex[b]	18.7	12.7	38.7	24.8	31.2	27.0	43.3	41.6
You can get AIDS from donating blood[c]	47.8	43.3	58.3	61.5	44.8	42.7	51.5	48.3
Unweighted Ns[d]	1,678	1,299	229	150	1,689	1,319	226	144

[a]Question wording: Mark whether you think each sentence is true or false. (a) People who have the AIDS virus cannot spread AIDS unless they are sick with AIDS themselves; (f) A vaccine that protects people from getting the AIDS virus is now available. [b]Question wording: Will the following behaviors make it LESS likely for a person to become infected with the AIDS virus? Will the following behaviors make it MORE likely for a person to become infected with the AIDS virus? [c]Question wording: Will the following behaviors make it MORE likely for a person to become infected with the AIDS virus? (e) Washing after having sex; (f) Making sure that a sex partner looks healthy. [d]In estimating percentages, sampling weights supplied with the data set were used to project the results to the national student population. The unweighted Ns shown in the last row of the table are minimum base Ns on which percentages were calculated. Because of variability across items in the amount of missing data, the actual Ns for specific items in this table may be larger than the minimums shown here by 5 to 10 persons.

SOURCE: Tabulated from the 1987–1988 National Adolescent Student Health Survey.

by condom use.[94] However, it should be noted that misconceptions can be corrected. The Massachusetts survey shows considerable improvement of teens' assessment of transmission risks between the 1986 and 1988 cycles (see Table 3-16). There is a relative abundance of survey data on what adolescents know about HIV transmission, but there is very little information about the numbers of teens who may be participating in risk-associated behaviors. Thus, future information efforts might best be targeted to young teens not yet exposed to information campaigns. More important, these efforts should collect behavioral data. Finally, given the evidence reviewed in earlier sections of this chapter, all intervention programs should seek to *motivate* teenagers to avoid the use of drugs and to protect themselves against the risks of sexually transmitted HIV infections.

REACHING ADOLESCENTS

Aspects of Prevention Programs

Fear

The committee has previously noted[95] that STD prevention programs have relied to varying extents on threatening messages that evoke high levels of fear. Similar tactics have been used in programs to prevent AIDS. (For example, such messages as "Bang Bang You're Dead" have been used to call attention to the fatal consequences of sexually trans- mitted HIV infection.) Whether such messages have been effective in changing behavior is not known because there have been no controlled studies or evaluations of their impact. Research suggests, however, that the usefulness of frightening and uninformative messages has particular limitations.

Messages designed to evoke high levels of fear or those that rely ex- clusively on threats may be intuitively appealing in the case of preventing a deadly disease, but usually they have been shown to be effective for most people only if coupled with advice about how behavioral change

---

[94]DiClemente, Boyer, and Morales (1988) found that minority adolescents were less knowledgeable about protective measures than their white peers. Using data from a 1985 survey of 628 students in the San Francisco school district, they found that 71.7 percent of white students versus 59.9 percent of blacks and 58.3 percent of Hispanic students believed that condoms could reduce the risk of acquiring AIDS. There may be some inconsistency in findings across studies. Siegel and colleagues (1989), for example, reported little variation in factual knowledge of AIDS across racial or ethnic groups in a survey of 1,940 junior high school students in Oakland, California; however, only 5 percent of the Oakland students were white.

[95]See Turner, Miller, and Moses (1989:266-268). The text in this section is adapted from that treat- ment.

can reduce the threat (Sutton, 1982; Becker, 1985). For example, educational messages in the syphilis prevention campaigns undertaken by the military early in this century sought to arouse fear in the troops by using STD prevention films (e.g., "Fit to Fight" and "Fit to Win") (Brandt, 1987). Premovie and postmovie measurements of knowledge about STDs revealed that these strategies changed general impressions (e.g., horror and fear were increased and persisted for weeks after the viewing), but knowledge and behavioral changes did not persist (Lashley and Watson, 1922). In contrast, during World War II, a prophylaxis program based on condoms and treatment was initiated, and soldiers responded favorably. As many as 50 million condoms were accepted by soldiers each month, and rates of syphilis declined in this population over that time (Brandt, 1987). Nevertheless, the lack of systematic evaluation (a shortcoming of most STD programs) of the message and of prophylaxis programs foils any attempt to draw conclusions as to what factor or factors did or did not work in reducing syphilis in this population.

Like the military STD prevention programs, early drug prevention programs for adolescents and young adults were largely aimed at providing information and evoking fear (Polich et al., 1984). It is difficult to compare the relative effectiveness of these programs because of variability in the content of their messages and the time devoted to their presentation. Nevertheless, general trends in their findings indicate that increased knowledge alone does not accomplish lasting or widespread change in drug-associated behaviors; neither do messages that are solely dependent on high threat content. School-based programs that rely heavily on fear have not been successful, apparently because the fear is associated with a low-probability event and because there is a substantial time lag between risk-associated behavior and adverse outcomes (Des Jarlais and Friedman, 1987). The assumption of these programs that teenagers will not use drugs if they are simply informed about the inherent dangers of drug use does not take into account the social factors involved in initiating and sustaining drug use behavior.

Ideally, health promotion messages should heighten an individual's perception of threat and his or her capacity to respond to that threat, thus modulating the level of fear. Job (1988) has proposed five prescriptions for the role of fear in health education messages:

1. Messages containing elements of fear should be introduced before discussing the desired behavior.
2. The audience targeted for a message should perceive the negative behavior or event that is associated with the risk as real and likely to occur.

3. A reasonable, desirable alternative behavior that protects the individual against the undesired health problem should be offered. Attention to short-term benefits is desirable and can reinforce long-term behavioral change.

4. The level of fear invoked by the message should be sufficient to create awareness of a potential problem but not so high as to evoke denial. Similarly, the fear level should be low enough that it can be effectively managed by the adoption of the desired behavior.

5. The resulting reduction in fear should be of such magnitude that it will reinforce the desired behavior and confirm its effectiveness.

What is not yet known is how to introduce fear in the right way in a particular message intended for a particular audience. Acquiring that knowledge will require planned variations of AIDS education programs that are first carefully executed and then carefully evaluated (see Coyle, Boruch, and Turner, 1990).[96]

Personal Vulnerability

The committee believes that a particularly crucial message for adolescents in the 1990s pertains to their vulnerability. As discussed in Chapter 1, the segments of the American population being touched by this epidemic are changing. Some adolescents, as well as some adults, still view AIDS as a disease of gay white males (Mays and Cochran, 1987). This belief appears to be especially widespread in areas in which the prevalence of AIDS is currently low.[97] It is crucial that adolescents (especially those

---

[96] In its previous report, the committee recommended that AIDS prevention messages strike a balance in the level of threat they convey. The level should be sufficiently high that it motivates individuals to take action but not so high that it paralyzes them with fear or causes them to deny their susceptibility. The committee also recommended that fear-arousing health promotion messages provide specific information on steps to be taken to protect the individual from the threat to his or her well-being. In that vein, the committee notes that a recent community demonstration project in Dallas, Texas, coupled fear-arousing messages concerning HIV transmission with specific instructions on how individuals can reduce their vulnerability. This project developed a series of AIDS prevention posters for young adults that depicted images related to death: a tombstone, a hearse containing a casket, a body on a stretcher covered by a shroud. Each poster included a slogan and specific instructions about methods for minimizing one's risk of HIV infection (Valdiserri, 1989). Rigorous evaluation research is needed, however, to assess the actual effects of such interventions.

[97] Similarly, a study of Mexican-American IV drug users from the American Southwest reports that young people in this population who were beginning to inject drugs tended to deny or minimize the threat posed by AIDS (Mata and Jorquez, 1988). Although similar types of denial occur in adults (see Turner, Miller, and Barker, 1989:Table 4), efforts to dispel these misconceptions would be appropriate wherever they occur (as would research to understand the effectiveness of any such efforts).

engaging in high-risk activities) recognize the extent of the epidemic and how it might affect them.

Facts and Beliefs

Although Tables 3-15 and 3-17 indicate that many of the facts about HIV transmission are reaching most high school students, it cannot be safely assumed that providing information will change behaviors.[98] Nonetheless, there is an association between some types of knowledge and beliefs and the likelihood that teens will report engaging in behaviors that reduce the risk of HIV transmission. For example, in a 1988 survey of a probability sample of Massachusetts teenagers,[99] those teens who believed condoms were effective in preventing AIDS were more likely to report using them; those teens who reported that condom use was embarrassing to discuss were less likely to report using them (Hingson and Strunin, 1989). Such associations do not provide the strongest of evidence, but it would seem reasonable that pilot studies to change knowledge about condom effectiveness and decrease embarrassment about discussing condom use would be worth exploring in small-scale interventions. These interventions should be designed in a manner that allows strong conclusions to be drawn about the effectiveness of this technique in inducing sexually active teens to increase their use of condoms.

In this regard, the committee also wishes to emphasize the need for a long-term commitment to prevention efforts for adolescents. It is highly unlikely that one lecture, one public service announcement, or exposure to a few brochures will be sufficient to induce and sustain the behavioral changes needed to reduce the risk of HIV transmission among adolescents. AIDS prevention programs should take advantage of multiple venues and formats of communication to deliver clear, consistent messages about behaviors that risk HIV transmission and the ways in which those risks may be reduced or eliminated. Furthermore, the committee would point out that the long-term odds of mounting successful

---

[98]Empirical examination of the relationships among knowledge, attitudes, beliefs, and behavior relevant to HIV/AIDS has provided mixed evidence. A 1987 survey of California high school students (McKusick, Coates, and Babcock, 1988) found that students with higher AIDS knowledge scores also reported higher rates of unsafe sex, but a survey of high school students from the Bronx (Reuben, Hein, and Drucker, 1988) found that those less knowledgeable about AIDS were more likely to participate in high-risk behaviors, regardless of age, grade, grade point average, race, or gender. In looking at the relationship among knowledge, attitudes, and behavior of gay adolescents, Rotheram-Borus and colleagues (1989) found that attitudes were more highly correlated with condom use than knowledge. A survey of adolescents in detention found a similar relationship (Temoshok et al., 1989). Among college students, perceived susceptibility was associated more strongly with condom use than was knowledge (DiClemente, Forrest, and Mickler, 1989).

[99]These teens were 16 to 19 years of age ($N = 1,762$).

prevention programs will be enhanced by prudent investments in the research required to identify successful (and unsuccessful) strategies for inducing behavioral change.

Skills

In addition to information, adolescents may require new skills to apply what they have learned to actual situations. Broaching difficult topics in conversations, resisting peer pressures to have unprotected sex or to use drugs, and negotiating less risky activities may be more difficult than learning the facts about transmission routes of HIV.

More must be known about providing effective skills training for adolescents and how to combine this effort with the delivery of information. Selected sex education programs have included skills training, and some programs were able to increase knowledge about sex and contraception and change attitudes while demonstrably improving the participants' ability to use contraceptives (Gilchrist and Schinke, 1983; Schinke, 1984). The number of school-based sex education programs that have included skills training in their curriculum is small, however, and students generally graduate from these programs with little change in their ability to use contraceptives effectively or to resist pressure to have unprotected sex (Flora and Thoresen, 1988).

The available data indicate that, for the most part, drug use is learned and practiced in the context of friendship groups.[100] The social nature of early drug use points to the need for broad-scale interventions that take into account the social network of the adolescent and peer influences that may support the initiation and continuation of drug use. Thus, recent efforts to prevent adolescent drug use have gone beyond traditional didactic methods to include strategies that develop social skills and skills to resist peer pressure; other efforts include approaches that correct misperceptions of social norms and values (Severson, 1984). These programs show some promise, but they have not been uniformly successful (Howard et al., 1988; Ellickson and Bell, 1990). Teaching students skills to resist peer pressure and the lure of unhealthy models has had some success in smoking intervention efforts (Battjes, 1985),[101] and assertiveness training for early adolescents has been associated with decreased use of alcohol

---

[100] An exception to this generalization involves alcohol use, which adolescents often report they tried for the first time at home with parents or with other relatives (Severson, 1984).

[101] It is important to note, however, that success rates for smoking programs have not been the same for all subgroups of adolescents, and much of the available research involves studies of adolescents who are enrolled in school. Furthermore, these programs have been more effective among females than among males and more effective among white students than among Asian Americans, native Americans, or black students. The programs also appear to be more effective in *preventing smoking*

and marijuana (Horan and Williams, 1982). Finally, programs that combine assertiveness training plus social skills training have reported some success in decreasing rates of cigarette smoking among some young teens and pre-teens (e.g., Botvin and Eng, 1982).

Community Norms

In its recent report,[102] the committee noted the powerful role that social norms may play in modifying behaviors that risk HIV transmission. This phenomenon follows from the fact that the individual actions that risk HIV transmission (sexual behaviors and sharing of injection equipment) occur in a social environment. Thus, if AIDS prevention programs are to be successful, they must take into account several important aspects of the social factors that affect individual change. For example, people are less likely to behave in ways that will incur the disapproval of others in their social group; people tend to conform to the "shoulds" and "oughts" of behavior specified in the norms of their community. Behavioral change reported by homosexual men has been influenced by changes in the accepted standards and expectations for sexual behavior (i.e., normative shifts) in this group. Identifying the social factors that support behavioral change among adolescent social groups could lead to the development of important components of AIDS prevention programs. Furthermore, programs that seek to change behavior must inevitably confront the diverse and complex social forces that motivate and shape the behaviors at issue.

There is increasing evidence that social support has an effect on the health status of individuals. Such support appears to be especially important in the management of chronic disease or in situations in which long-term behavioral change is required to prevent or ameliorate disease (Becker, 1985). For example, family support has been shown to be important in cuing and reinforcing appropriate behaviors for the control of obesity, hypertension, arthritis, and coronary heart disease (Becker, 1985; Morisky et al., 1985). Families and other groups can affect an individual's adherence to prescribed behaviors by providing material, cognitive, and psychological support. The greater the compatibility of family roles and beliefs, the greater the support for health behaviors and the greater the likelihood that the individual will initiate and sustain them.

Furthermore, it is possible that modifying social norms to make risk-associated behavior inconsistent with the prevailing social norms in the

---

among adolescents who have not yet begun to smoke than they are in helping those who already use cigarettes to stop smoking.

[102] Turner, Miller, and Moses (1989:290-291). The following text is adapted from this source.

adolescent community may be an efficient and effective strategy for AIDS prevention in the long term. In this regard, the committee notes two small surveys of high school students in California. These studies found that the strongest predictor of a teenager's use of condoms during intercourse was the perception that the norms of his or her peers supported safer sex practices and condom use (McKusick, Coates, and Babcock, 1988; Greenblatt et al., 1989).

If norms in the adolescent community could be shifted, the probability that any given individual would indulge in high-risk behavior is likely to be reduced (Turner, Miller, and Moses, 1989:Chapter 4). If, for example, new norms specified the use of condoms for sexual intercourse, individuals might anticipate that their partners would expect them to behave accordingly. For adolescents who have reported difficulties discussing AIDS prevention measures with their sexual partners (Fisher, 1988), such changes in expectations may relieve some of the pressure of negotiating the use of safer sexual practices during difficult situations.

It should also be noted that the norms that shape gender and sex roles may have profound influences on sexual behavior. "Macho" gender roles for males, for example, may be at odds with risk reduction (Fisher, 1988), and female gender roles may be inconsistent with the assertive behaviors needed to negotiate sexual behavior or condom use. It may be possible, nonetheless, to design messages that would be consistent with both male roles and risk reduction. The committee notes, for example, attempts to disseminate the message that "real men wear condoms." The success of these efforts remains to be measured.

Sources of Messages

An important principle of human health behavior indicates that people are more likely to act on information if they perceive the source of the message to be credible (Office of Technology Assessment, 1988; Turner, Miller, and Moses, 1989:Chapter 4). Therefore, the individuals chosen to deliver AIDS messages should be determined in part by who has credibility with the targeted population. In the case of adolescents, adherence to this principle may mean using peers to present risk reduction interventions.

Indeed, although one often hears about the barriers to risk reduction posed by peer pressure, peer pressure can have a positive influence on adolescent risk taking. Positive effects of peer influence have been noted in a variety of studies of health problems such as smoking (Evans et al., 1979; Banks, Bewley, and Bland, 1981), and alcohol use (R. Jessor, Chase, and Donovan, 1980). Moreover, peer-led intervention programs have shown some promise in smoking prevention programs for adolescents. However, because many smoking prevention programs have also included other important elements—for example, skills training to resist peer pressure—it is difficult to isolate the effects of peer leadership (Flay, 1985; McCaul and Glasgow, 1985).

Another potential benefit of a peer-led strategy is that it is quite possible that teenagers will be more comfortable discussing sexual experiences with peers rather than with adults. Peer counselors have often been used in sex education programs on the assumption that teens are less embarrassed about discussing sensitive issues among themselves and that they are more likely to follow the advice of other teens (Hayes, 1987). Because these programs have not been evaluated, however, it is not possible to determine whether they have been effective in achieving their goals.

Encouraging teen participation as counselors and program leaders may also be beneficial in that it includes adolescents in the development and execution of prevention programs and makes them part of the solution to a problem rather than mere targets of interventions.[103] A program at the University of Illinois at Chicago, for example, seeks to promote adolescent health behavior and to increase teenagers' involvement in the community by training inner-city high school students as peer counselors. Teens have also created audio and visual materials to communicate the facts of HIV transmission and the impact of AIDS on their community. Similarly, in Bethesda, Maryland, specially trained high school student volunteers staff an AIDS hotline for teens, answering questions and making referrals to other sources of information. Hotlines set up and staffed by teens can also be found in Kansas City and Baltimore. In addition, peer counselors have been used on a variety of college campuses (Hein, 1989a). Unfortunately, there is little clear evidence on which to judge the overall effectiveness of such programs although it does appear that at a minimum the peer counselors benefit from participating (Hayes, 1987).

Although peer counseling has attractive features, families and other adult social institutions have a major responsibility for educating adolescents about health risks. For most adolescents, the family in particular is the social group from which they seek care when they are ill; it is also the source of insurance or money for professional medical help. As part of its information campaign, "America Responds to AIDS," CDC has produced and distributed a brochure to assist parents in discussing

---

[103] Program descriptions were provided by the National AIDS Information Clearinghouse.

HIV and AIDS-related issues with their children.[104] Indeed, more than half (62 percent) of participants in the April–June 1988 wave of the National Health Interview Survey who had children between the ages of 10 and 17 reported discussing AIDS with their children (Hardy, 1989). Yet very little is known about the amount of time spent on this issue or the precise nature of the information delivered to children by parents. Surveys indicate that most parents feel responsible for providing sex education to their children, but few actually offer specific information (Alan Guttmacher Institute, 1981; Roberts, Kline, and Gagnon, 1981). Indeed, as another National Research Council committee noted, there are many reasons to worry about the effectiveness of parents' efforts at sex education, given the fact that more than 400,000 pregnancies occur each year among teenage girls aged 15 to 17 (Hayes, 1987). That committee noted:

> First, in many cases, less parent-child communication takes place than is commonly assumed; second, such communication, whether to provide information or to prescribe behavior, may not be fully heard by the child; and third, communication about sexual behavior frequently does not occur until after initiation of sexual activity (Newcomer and Udry, 1983; Inazu and Fox, 1980). Fox (1981) points out that parents' (especially mothers') roles in sex education are relatively minor, and that the more traditionally oriented mothers are on matters of sexual morality, sex roles, etc., the less likely they are to initiate discussions of these topics with their children. Unfortunately, however, as Hofferth (1987, Vol. II:Ch. 1) points out, there is little research to specify the context of communication or to distinguish the effects of communication before and after initiation of sexual activity. (Hayes, 1987:103)

Such findings may indicate a need for interventions to motivate and assist parents in the difficult and important task of educating their children about the dangers of HIV transmission. These findings also suggest that it would be a mistake to rely exclusively on parents as the source of AIDS education for teenagers.

Venues for Program Delivery

There are many venues through which AIDS prevention programs for adolescents can be delivered. Some venues (e.g., schools) include most youth, but they miss some of the teens who are at highest risk of becoming infected (e.g., runaways). Other approaches, however, such as use of the media or outreach to special populations, can provide access to

---

[104]This element of CDC's AIDS information campaign targets 10- to 20-year-old youths and their parents. It also provides information through workshops, lectures, conferences, and various media events.

these groups. In the following sections the committee reviews four types of efforts to reach adolescents with AIDS prevention information: media and other programs designed for all adolescents, school-based programs, programs that target out-of-school youth, and interventions directed toward teenage IV drug users—a group at particularly high risk for HIV infection.

Programs for All Adolescents

Since 1983 CDC has operated a toll-free AIDS hotline (1-800-342-AIDS) whose capacity to deal with requests for information and to answer specific questions has quadrupled since the service began; contractors responsible for the hotline can now handle up to 8,000 calls per day (Mason et al., 1988), and in late 1988 and early 1989 the hotline was responding to approximately 90,000 calls per month (Coyle, Boruch, and Turner, 1990:Chapter 3). This service is available to anyone who has access to a telephone, but there are no data on the extent to which adolescents use this program. In its recent report (Coyle, Boruch, and Turner, 1990:Chapter 3), the committee's Panel on the Evaluation of AIDS Interventions recommended that a variety of data be collected on users of the national AIDS hotline—including caller age and a small number of other demographic statistics, as well as the services provided to the caller. Such data would allow estimates of the extent of teen use of this program in the future.

Limited survey data indicate that the media are an important source of information on AIDS prevention and contraception for teens (Pearl, Bouthilet, and Lazar, 1982; Price, Desmond, and Kukulka, 1985; Ziffer et al., 1989). Adolescents are estimated to spend an average of 17 hours per week watching television (Lawrence et al., 1986), and television thus represents an efficient medium for reaching teens, perhaps before risk-associated behaviors begin. Several media-based activities have been initiated for the adolescent population, including AIDS education and public service announcements. CDC has also provided support for the development of AIDS public service announcements for the national adolescent Hispanic population.[105] Research designs to assess the effects of these programs are described elsewhere (Coyle, Boruch, and Turner, 1990).

In addition, less conventional venues have also been used to reach

---

[105] See, for example, the description of the CDC-supported efforts of Hispanic Designers, Incorporated (Organization No. S–07896) and Hispanic AIDS Forum (Organization No. S–04611) in the Resource Database, National AIDS Information Clearinghouse.

out to teens with information about AIDS.[106] In such cities as Cincinnati, Los Angeles, New York, and Washington, D.C., teenagers participate in AIDS theater groups and rap sessions, performing for peer audiences. Performances are given in English and Spanish in some communities, and in many instances presentations are followed by a question-and-answer period, distribution of educational materials, and occasionally one-on-one conversations with members of the audience. Various sites are used to reach teens with dramatized presentations of AIDS-related information, including public schools, community centers, and even Job Corps sites. Although these activities are imaginative and intuitively appealing, their impact has not yet been ascertained. The committee finds that carefully designed and implemented research efforts are needed to determine which venues and formats are most effective in reaching teens and informing them about the AIDS epidemic in their communities.

Printed materials have been developed in several languages for the different age groups that constitute the adolescent population. Reading skills may vary considerably in this population, however, and very young teens and adolescents who have dropped out of school may be at a disadvantage when information is provided in written form. Small surveys of adolescents in detention centers (Rolf et al., in press) find that poor reading skills compromise the use of written AIDS prevention information (as well as questionnaires for evaluation activities). Indeed, problems in understanding written AIDS information are not confined to the adolescent population. An analysis of 16 AIDS prevention brochures for the general population found that, on average, they were written at a fourteenth grade (second year of college) reading level (Hochhauser, 1987).

Many intervention activities rely at least in part on printed matter to deliver the facts about AIDS, yet very little is known about how the adolescent and young adult populations perceive these materials. A survey of 37 universities found that providing brochures was the extent of the action most universities took regarding AIDS prevention (Caruso and Haig, 1987). With such an emphasis on this avenue of information delivery, it will be necessary to find out more about the opinions and problems of the audience to be reached by such materials, and to incorporate these findings into new editions of the brochures as a way to make them appeal to specific audiences. One comparison of two brochures using a sample of 223 undergraduate university students, for example, found significant gender differences in the evaluation of the materials. Women placed a higher value than did men on information

---

[106]Program descriptions were provided by the National AIDS Information Clearinghouse.

about specific safer sex practices and descriptions of strategies that might be used to discuss AIDS and sex with dating partners (D'Augelli and Kennedy, 1989). Further research—including experimental studies—on differences in the needs of various segments of younger populations will be crucial in developing more effective brochures in the future.

School-Based Programs

Because schools have the potential to reach 45.5 million students annually (Allensworth and Symons, 1989) and because most adolescents under the age of 18 are enrolled in school,[107] school-based programs are an efficient way to reach a substantial portion of the adolescent population. Schools are long-standing agents of socialization for American youth, and they have played important roles in trying to solve other health problems of adolescents through school-based clinics and health education classes. It is thus logical that schools should become involved in AIDS education and prevention efforts.

CDC has developed and funded a multimillion-dollar project for prevention programs in schools and other organizations that serve youth.[108] With input from a wide range of governmental and private-sector organizations, the agency has also recommended guidelines for AIDS education (CDC, 1988d) to help school personnel set the scope and content of their programs. The specifics of such programs, however, are determined locally in consultation with the health department, parent groups, and community leaders to ensure that programs are consistent with community values and needs (Mason et al., 1988).

There are very few descriptions in the scientific literature of precisely how schools are implementing CDC's guidelines on AIDS program content. As of May 1989, only half (25) of the states required that students receive HIV/AIDS education, and 22 states had no HIV/AIDS education requirements (Voelker, 1989). For states that have implemented AIDS education programs, process and outcome evaluations are limited, making it difficult to draw conclusions about the adequacy or effectiveness

---

[107] In 1984, virtually all U.S. 14- and 15-year-olds (98 percent) and 92 percent of 16- and 17-year-olds were in school, although by ages 18 and 19 the proportion of students fell to approximately 50 percent (Hayes, 1987). Although there appears to be no difference in male and female enrollment for any age group, Hispanic adolescents are less likely than white or black teens to be enrolled in school; among 16- to 17-year-olds, 91.2 percent of whites, 92.4 percent of blacks, and 85.7 percent of Hispanics are in school (Hayes, 1987).

[108] In 1987, $11.1 million was allocated to the program; in 1988, this amount increased to $29.9 million (Tolsma, 1988). In 1987, CDC set up cooperative agreements with several organizations that serve schools and youth. Five of the agreements involve organizations that will address the specific needs of black and Hispanic youth, and seven involve organizations that target out-of-school teens (Mason et al., 1988).

of the programs. Workers in the field have suggested that some adolescent AIDS prevention programs are not given sufficient classroom time and are not viewed as part of an ongoing educational activity but rather one-time events.[109] The committee cautions that the time and resources currently being devoted to adolescent AIDS prevention efforts may be insufficient to effectively block or alter risk-associated patterns of behavior before they become established.

The committee is also concerned that the subset of very young teens who report intercourse and drug use may be initiating these behaviors before they receive information about the hazards associated with them and the means to protect themselves against these hazards. For example, CDC guidelines for AIDS curricula targeting late elementary and middle school youth (i.e., early adolescence) recommend providing the following information on HIV transmission: "The AIDS virus can be transmitted by sexual contact with an infected person; by using needles and other injection equipment that an infected person has used; and from an infected mother to her infant before or during birth" (CDC, 1988d:6). The committee notes that no information is offered on protective measures that can be taken to reduce the risks of HIV transmission. Although it is true that a majority of young teens will not have initiated risk-associated behaviors during elementary or middle school (see the preceding sections), a small and particularly vulnerable group will have done so. Indeed, it appears that by the age at which most communities are prepared to accept the notion of providing explicit AIDS education for their youth, a substantial portion of their teens may already be engaging in the behaviors that transmit the virus.

If school-based programs are to reach and educate students effectively, an informed and supportive group of adults must be developed in local communities to implement these programs.[110] The CDC guidelines (1988d:3) recommend that "a team of representatives, including the local school board members, parent-teacher associations, school administrators, school physicians, school nurses, teachers, educational support personnel, school counselors, and other relevant school personnel should receive general training about:

---

[109] An AIDS education program in a medium-sized metropolitan area involved a "minimum of two hours" of instruction by trained health teachers (Copello et al., 1989). A separate educational activity for runaway youth who were admitted into a school system constituted "3 to 4 instructional classes about AIDS and prevention information" (Hudson et al., 1989).

[110] In addition to schools, there are a variety of other community-based organizations that serve the adolescent population. Organizations as diverse as the Girls Clubs, Boys Clubs, Girl Scouts, Boy Scouts, Camp Fire, 4-H, the YWCA, and the YMCA report reaching 25 million youths each year (J. Quinn, 1988).

- the nature of the AIDS epidemic and means for controlling its spread,
- the role of the school in providing education to prevent transmission of HIV,
- methods and materials to accomplish effective programs of school health education about AIDS, and
- school policies for students and staff who may be infected."

Among programs that have been implemented in schools to date, the quality varies greatly from place to place. Commentators on these programs (e.g., Valdiserri, 1989; Mantell and Schinke, in press) have pointed to the limited amounts of time and resources dedicated to them, the lack of consensus on program content and degree of explicitness of teaching materials, disagreements over the age at which AIDS education should begin, undue emphasis on lectures rather than skills training, and inadequate coordination with community organizations. At present, the effectiveness of school-based programs is unknown, but the committee applauds CDC's efforts to mount systematic evaluations of these activities (Kolbe et al., 1988).

Programs for Out-of-School Youth

Some of the youth who are at highest risk for HIV infection drop out of school before receiving any AIDS education. In 1984, there were more than half a million 14- to 17-year-olds who had dropped out of high school prior to graduation (Hayes, 1987). Hispanics who were 14 to 15 years old were twice as likely as blacks or whites to have dropped out of school; 13.2 percent of Hispanics between the ages of 16 and 17 had dropped out of school. Indeed, some risk behaviors, such as injecting illicit substances, are likely to cause teenagers to have increasing problems with absenteeism and to hasten their exit from the school system.

Obviously, efforts to reach such youth need to go beyond the schools. Community-based organizations have some unique and important characteristics that make them particularly promising vehicles for reaching this important segment of the adolescent population. These characteristics include credibility within their community, knowledge of local cultural values and beliefs, and knowledge of local channels of communication. A subset of these organizations are now involved in prevention activities for AIDS, developing and disseminating educational materials, sharing expertise, and establishing referral systems. For example, the National Coalition of Hispanic Health and Human Services Organizations (COSSMHO), with support from CDC and the Metropolitan Life

Insurance Foundation, has begun a major AIDS education initiative for out-of-school Hispanic youths (COSSMHO, 1989).

Blacks and Latinos have a tradition of using community-based and other local organizations to address social problems. The organization Hispanos Unidos Contra el SIDA/AIDS has taken responsibility for training trainers in the Hispanic community and is developing AIDS education curricula for outreach workers and educators who work with Hispanics in churches and teen and community centers in New Haven, Connecticut.

For those teens who cannot be reached through the institutions mentioned above, other mechanisms will be needed to deliver both prevention and social services. Particularly vulnerable teens, some of whom live without families or homes, can often be found on the streets.[111] The precise number of homeless youth is not known, but the dimensions of the adolescent runaway and homeless problem exceed available resources. In one year, for example, 210 programs provided at least one night of shelter to teens on 50,354 occasions, and thousands of teens were turned away from shelters because they were filled to capacity (Bucy, 1985:11).

During 1984, Congress appropriated $23.25 million to support 260 shelters for this population run by community-based organizations, as well as other selected services. Some of these monies were used to support a toll-free hotline and communication channel for youth who were either thinking about running away or were already on the street and looking for counseling or referral services. Other support went to family reunification strategies, independent living programs for older homeless teens, suicide prevention, training and employment services, programs to rehabilitate teenage prostitutes, and drug and alcohol counseling. Similarly, in September 1987, the National Network of Runaway and Youth Services, Inc., with support from CDC, began a five-year Safe Choices Program, which includes outreach and intervention activities to prevent the spread of HIV infection. Although the effects of such programs have not been rigorously assessed, the recent report of the committee's Panel on the Evaluation of AIDS Interventions describes strategies that can be used to conduct such evaluation (Coyle, Boruch, and Turner, 1990:Chapter 4).

Reaching Teenage Drug Users

Clearly, the most desirable and efficacious goal for AIDS intervention

---

[111] A pilot study of 11- to 18-year-olds contacted on the streets of Newark, New Jersey, between 10 p.m. and 2 a.m. resulted in 27 interviews with 14 males and 13 females (Hummel et al., 1989). Seven did not live with their parents, and four already had children of their own. Half (13 of 27) had dropped out of school, 11 (of 27) reported a history of STDs, and 7 (of 27) said they had a history of drug use.

efforts related to drug use is to prevent the initial use of drugs. However, given the questionable success of programs to prevent drug use among teens and the fact that a subset of youth already report drug use, the serious public health threat posed by HIV infection requires that additional strategies be explored.

One strategy for decreasing the likelihood that teens will use the "harder" illicit drugs, including injectable drugs, attempts to postpone experimentation with so-called gateway drugs (alcohol, cigarettes, and marijuana). The use of gateway drugs typically precedes the use of more dangerous substances, and recent studies have demonstrated that it is in fact possible to reduce or postpone initial experimentation with such substances (Botvin et al., 1984; Botvin, 1986; Pentz et al., 1989a,b). Successful drug prevention programs, such as the STAR program in Kansas City,[112] have reduced the percentage of adolescents who drink alcohol or smoke marijuana.[113] The design of this and similar programs uses a "comprehensive" approach, that is, one that goes beyond information delivery on the hazards of drug use and fear arousal to teach the social skills needed to refuse offers of drugs and to find sources of personal satisfaction that do not involve drug use. Such programs often reach beyond the individual adolescent to involve teachers, parents, and the community.

Unfortunately, these interventions have not been followed for sufficiently long periods to know what effects, if any, they will ultimately have on injection practices. Although decreasing the number of teens who use "soft" drugs such as marijuana seems consistent with the notion of fewer individuals injecting drugs, it is possible that even the most successful programs will have only a small effect in deterring those youths who are at highest risk for progression to injection. Furthermore, because many drug prevention programs work through local social systems, they may miss youths who are at greatest risk for injecting drugs because this

---

[112] Project STAR (Students Taught Awareness and Resistance) is a comprehensive, community-based drug and alcohol abuse prevention program that has been implemented in 15 contiguous communities that together constitute Kansas City. The program is implemented through a school-based curriculum that teaches resistance skills to middle and junior high school students and includes expanded media and community program elements that target parents, community organizations, and health policy groups (Pentz et al., 1986).

[113] Data from schools one year after the initiation of Project STAR found that prevalence rates for the use of gateway drugs were significantly lower than rates reported by a delayed intervention cohort: 17 versus 24 percent for cigarette use, 11 versus 16 percent for alcohol use, and 7 versus 10 percent for marijuana use in the previous month (Pentz et al., 1989a). The net increase in drug use prevalence in STAR schools was half that of the delayed intervention schools.

highest risk segment of the adolescent population is not well integrated into youth-oriented institutions (e.g., schools).

To conduct the research needed to determine whether a program that reduces experimentation with gateway drugs during early or middle adolescence will also reduce the number of late adolescents and young adults who inject drugs would require a very complex research design and considerable resources. It would also require following participants (who may not wish to stay in contact with any authorities) for a long period of time. Furthermore, a range of factors would need to be measured to determine the effects of any particular type of program on the rate of drug injection. In the absence of such research, it is probably safe to say that it is overly pessimistic to assume that there is *no* effect of such programs on the progression to injection, and it is overly optimistic to assume that such programs will be *sufficient* to reduce the likelihood of injection to zero.

One extreme of the range of strategies to prevent injection by reducing experimentation with gateway drugs in the broad teenage population comprises programs that focus attention on youths who are at greatest risk for the use of injectable drugs. A New York City research project (Des Jarlais et al., 1989) has attempted to determine the impact of intervening during latter stages of drug use progression. The study recruited persons who were using heroin intranasally (so-called sniffing) and paid them to participate in a four-session AIDS intervention program. One-half of the subjects were randomly assigned to an intervention that taught skills needed to refuse offers of injectable drugs, negotiate safer sex, and negotiate entry into drug abuse treatment. The other half were assigned to a control group that did not receive the four-session intervention but was otherwise treated identically. At the end of the follow-up period, the rate of injection among subjects who had received the intervention was half that reported by the control group. (Approximately 15 percent of those who received the intervention injected an illicit drug during the nine-month period.)[114] There remains, however, the question of whether less seasoned, less practiced youths would respond as favorably to such an intervention effort.

IV drug use prevention among adolescents must also take into account the diverse social factors that may affect needle use. One study from Baltimore (see Vlahov et al., 1989), for example, found evidence of less risk taking among new injectors. Yet studies conducted in the New York area present a more complex picture. New injectors, who were not

---

[114] Don C. Des Jarlais, Chemical Dependency Institute, Beth Israel Medical Center, personal communication, May 9, 1990.

fully integrated into the drug subculture, were less likely to engage in very high risk behavior, such as the use of shooting galleries (Friedman et al., 1989). Unfortunately, they were also less likely to practice deliberate AIDS risk reduction (Kleinman et al., in press).

New injectors may also be influenced by older, more practiced users. Studies of heroin use among Mexican-American adolescents found that punitive attitudes toward these youths resulted in their arrest and incarceration in jails, forestry camps, and prisons (Mata and Jorquez, 1988). This policy led to the unfortunate and unintended consequence of putting these youth in direct contact with older and more practiced users of IV drugs. One outcome of this experience was the development of a common perspective and code of conduct among the youths and older addicts, which in turn fostered norms that supported the sharing of drugs, injection equipment, and even sexual partners.

Intervening to prevent the spread of HIV infection among drug-using adolescents presents considerable challenges. Some have hoped that the fear of contracting AIDS would serve as a "natural" intervention tool, preventing would-be injectors from progressing to more hazardous patterns of behavior. (The hope for such a spontaneous event underlies much of the opposition to such controversial AIDS prevention programs as syringe exchanges, which are misperceived as encouraging drug injection.) It has also been hypothesized that the fear of a deadly disease might lead some people who were predisposed to intensive drug use to choose routes of administration other than injection. Heroin, cocaine, and amphetamines, the most commonly injected drugs in this country, can all be "smoked" to provide a drug effect that approximates the effect achieved by injecting.[115] Indeed, there has been a dramatic increase in the smoking of cocaine (as "crack") since the beginning of the AIDS epidemic, but there does not appear to be a concomitant decrease in the amount of cocaine that is injected (Des Jarlais and Friedman, 1988). Rather than substituting for cocaine injection, smoking cocaine appears to occur in addition to existing drug use; frequently, it is also associated with increased sexual risk taking (see Chapter 1). Moreover, interviews with heroin users who report intranasal administration of this drug indicate that few cite concern about AIDS as affecting their drug use.[116]

Teens who have already begun to inject drugs and who resist the notion of treatment or cessation of use require other strategies to protect

---

[115] Users report that snorting or intranasal administration of heroin and cocaine produces a less intense effect than intravenous administration.

[116] A small study of 102 persons who were using heroin intranasally found that only one person was sufficiently concerned about AIDS to report that it affected his drug use (Des Jarlais et al., 1989).

them from HIV infection. Strategies to deliver information and teach skills related to safer injection practices have been developed for adults; modifications of these approaches may be useful for adolescents. For example, older peers (e.g., more experienced injectors who no longer use drugs) may be credible sources for information about drug use. Street outreach efforts in New York, Chicago, and San Francisco have trained ex-addicts to reach out to current users to disseminate information on the risk reduction options available to injectors: treatment for those who wish it and bleach sterilization techniques for those who are unable to accept or locate available treatment, and condom use to prevent sexually transmitted HIV infection (Des Jarlais et al., 1988). Unfortunately, many drug treatment programs are not well adapted to help adolescent users, and some are not even open to individuals younger than 18 years of age (Polich et al., 1984).

Preventing AIDS by preventing the initiation of injection of illicit drugs is an appropriate public health goal whose achievement would not only reduce the transmission of HIV infection but would also reduce many of the other significant health and social problems associated with injection. The level and extent of prevention needed, however, could consume extensive resources. Implementing effective interventions is likely to require a combination of expensive programs: programs that focus on the individual and on the psychological and social problems that make individuals likely to inject illicit drugs, and programs that address social problems that have supported risky behaviors and prevented the establishment of effective intervention strategies.

Program Needs for
High-Risk and HIV-Seropositive Youth

The range of services that may be helpful to youth who participate in risk-associated behaviors is extensive. Such services include family planning clinics, drug use and prevention programs, teenage pregnancy programs, STD clinics, and comprehensive service programs that target a variety of social and physical problems of adolescents. The current demands on these programs, most of which involve non-HIV-related problems, are considerable; the feasibility of adding responsibility for HIV-related prevention strategies, testing, counseling, and follow-up services for at-risk teens, their partners, and families is not known.

As the epidemic continues, there may well be more infected teens who will require a wide range of services for their care. Three basic strategies can be used to address the needs of infected adolescents: (1) expand existing services for other adolescent health problems to include

HIV infection and AIDS, (2) expand adult HIV and AIDS programs to include adolescents, or (3) develop new programs specifically designed to treat HIV-infected teens. As an example of the first strategy, regional hemophilia centers have expanded their services to include HIV- and AIDS-related diagnosis, treatment, and care, and a few hospital-based clinics have developed the capacity to evaluate and care for infected adolescents. In the New York City area, examples of all three strategies have appeared over the past several years. For example, the Adolescent Health Service at Mt. Sinai Hospital has integrated HIV services into preexisting comprehensive health care clinics for teenagers. Similarly, the Adolescent AIDS Program at Montefiore Medical Center comprises a multidisciplinary team of professionals who have established protocols for counseling and testing teens, evaluating and caring for infected adolescents, and conducting research on the epidemiology of HIV infection and behavioral prevention strategies in this population.

Preexisting models for providing multiple services for adolescents include such comprehensive service programs as El Puente and The Door in New York City, programs for Hispanic youth and their families (Henricks, 1985; Paget, 1988). These programs have a tradition of dealing with a spectrum of adolescent problems and offer a wide range of services: family planning and sex counseling, medical services, psychiatric counseling, drug and alcohol treatment, workshops, and other social services. In addition, El Puente pairs successful members of the community with teens to provide role models and a bridge to more successful and empowered lifestyles (Paget, 1988).

The resources required to provide necessary services are likely to be extensive, but the precise nature and quantity of these resources have not been determined. It is likely, however, that staffing and training needs for prevention, as well as care for at-risk and infected teens, will be substantial.

DOING BETTER IN THE SECOND DECADE

In considering how to improve future efforts to retard the spread of HIV among teenagers and young adults, the committee returns to several issues that are discussed in the opening pages of this chapter. As previously noted, the diversity of opinion in this country concerning matters of sexual behavior has contributed to a lack of consensus on appropriate educational messages. This lack of consensus, in turn, presents substantial barriers to AIDS prevention activities. The committee recognizes the difficulties posed for some individuals by frank discussions of sensitive issues such as sexual behavior, contraceptive use, and prevention of STDs. It believes, however, that clear, appropriate, and effective educational programs can and must be crafted and delivered. Such a task is likely to be discomfiting and controversial. Yet for the sake of the nation's 35 million teens,[117] national and community leaders must shoulder the responsibility for such education and be held accountable for any failure to provide it. As former Surgeon General C. Everett Koop noted, "many young people in the United States are not receiving information that is vital to their future health because of our reticence in dealing with the subjects of sex, sexual practices, and homosexuality. As parents, educators, and community leaders we must assume our responsibility to educate our young. The need is critical and the price of neglect is high."[118]

In the task of AIDS education, the committee believes that prevention efforts should involve adolescents themselves in the design and execution of these programs. This policy not only allows the program to benefit from the counsel of members of the targeted audience but it empowers adolescents by including them in the processes that will affect their lives. For many adolescents, inclusion in such activities will provide another stimulus for thinking about AIDS and planning for their futures.

It is clear, nonetheless, that it is not yet known how best to educate adolescents about the behavioral changes required to retard the spread of HIV. The committee believes that much is to be gained from the systematic study of planned variations of intervention strategies, and it regrets the persisting lack of understanding regarding the types of behavioral interventions that will be most effective in containing the spread of this disease. The committee believes that the Public Health Service would realize substantial returns in practical and scientific knowledge from careful investments in research to determine the effects of planned variations of those behavioral interventions to be implemented in the future. This strategy offers hope that, if the epidemic enters a third decade, our understanding of how to curb the spread of HIV infection will be far greater than it is today.

Finally, the committee wishes to reiterate that the diversity of the adolescent population means that a multiplicity of venues and formats will be needed to deliver AIDS prevention messages, and a variety of strategies will be required to intervene effectively. For some adolescents, effective intervention may be provided by AIDS prevention programs in

---

[117] The U.S. Bureau of the Census estimates that in 1980 there were 37,174,000 individuals between the ages of 10 and 19 years residing in the United States (U.S. Bureau of the Census, 1987:17).

[118] C. Everett Koop, public statement at press conference on release of Surgeon General's Report on AIDS, Washington, D.C., October 22, 1986.

the school systems at an early age—before students initiate the behaviors that can threaten their future. Yet reaching many of the adolescents at highest risk for HIV infection will require going beyond the schools. Most important, the committee notes that there is a small segment of the teen population that *at this moment* is at relatively high risk for HIV infection.[119] This segment includes runaway and "throwaway" children, teens who exchange sex for survival needs, and out-of-home and homeless youths. The committee believes that AIDS prevention programs should focus attention on these youths in a manner commensurate with the elevated risks they face. In addition, although programs to prevent HIV transmission can and should be deployed for this segment of the teen population, the needs of these high-risk youth extend far beyond the scope of AIDS prevention and include shelter, medical care, education, and a reason to believe that the future will be better than the present. The committee believes that efforts to prevent HIV transmission should be complemented by interventions that seek to satisfy the broader needs of these youth.

At a time when the AIDS virus has been introduced into the adolescent population but is not evenly distributed throughout it, the near-term future presents unique and important opportunities to prevent the acquisition of infection. As stated in the first chapter of this report, the greatest opportunities for getting ahead of the AIDS epidemic lie in geographic areas or populations that currently have a low prevalence of AIDS and HIV infection. These opportunities must not be overlooked or squandered, for once lost, they are gone forever. The future course of the epidemic will be determined by actions that are taken now. If the youth of this nation are taught how to engage in healthy behaviors and protect themselves against HIV infection, these efforts may not only prevent further spread of the AIDS epidemic but may also prevent future health problems in their adult years.

REFERENCES

Alan Guttmacher Institute. (1981) *Teenage Pregnancy: The Problem That Hasn't Gone Away.* New York: Alan Guttmacher Institute.

Alexander-Rodriguez, T., and Vermund, S. H. (1987) Gonorrhea and syphilis in incarcerated urban adolescents: Prevalence and physical signs. *Pediatrics* 80:561–564.

Allensworth, D. D., and Symons, C. W. (1989) A theoretical approach to school-based HIV prevention. *Journal of School Health* 59:59–65.

---

[119] It is important to remember, however, that relative risk is a function of the prevalence of the virus and the behaviors that transmit it. Thus, as the epidemic evolves, so the relative risk for adolescents will change.

American Medical Association Council on Scientific Affairs (AMA-CSA). (1990) Health status of detained and incarcerated youth. *Journal of the American Medical Association* 263:987–991.

American School Health Association, Association for the Advancement of Health Education, and the Society for Public Health Education, Inc. (ASHA, AAHE, and SPHE). (1989) *The National Adolescent Student Health Survey*. Oakland, Calif.: Third Party Publishing Company.

Austin, G. A., and Prendergast, M. L., eds. (1984) *Drug Use and Drug Abuse: A Guide to Research Findings.* Vol. 2: *Adolescents.* Denver: ABC-Clio Information Services.

Bachman, J. G., and O'Malley, P. M. (1981) When four months equal a year: Inconsistencies in student reports of drug use. *Public Opinion Quarterly* 45:536–548.

Bachman, J. G., Johnston, L. D., and O'Malley, P. M. (1981) Smoking, drinking and drug use among American high school students: Correlates and trends, 1975–1979. *American Journal of Public Health* 71:59–69.

Bailey, S. L., and Hubbard, R. L. (1990) Developmental variation in the context of marijuana initiation among adolescents. *Journal of Health and Social Behavior* 31:58–70.

Baker, C. J., Huscroft, S., Morris, R., Re, O., Roseman, J., and Shultz, B. (1989) HIV seroprevalence and behavior survey of incarcerated adolescents. Unpublished paper. Los Angeles County Department of Health Services, Juvenile Court Health Services.

Banks, M. H., Bewley, B. R., and Bland, J. M. (1981) Adolescent attitudes to smoking: Their influence on behavior. *International Journal of Health Education* 24:39–44.

Battjes, R. J. (1985) Prevention of adolescent drug abuse. *The International Journal of the Addictions* 20:1113–1134.

Becker, M. H. (1985) Patient adherence to prescribed therapies. *Medical Care* 23:539–555.

Bell, T. A., and Hein, K. (1984) Adolescents and sexually transmitted diseases. In K. Holmes, P. Mardh, P. F. Sparling, and P. J. Wiesner, eds., *Sexually Transmitted Diseases.* New York: McGraw Hill.

Billy, J. O. G., and Udry, J. R. (1985) The influence of male and female best friends on adolescent sexual behavior. *Adolescence* 20:21–32.

Billy, J. O. G., Rodgers, J. L., and Udry, J. R. (1984) Adolescent sexual behavior and friendship choice. *Social Forces* 62:653–678.

Blum, R. W. and Resnick, J. F. (1982) Adolescent decision making: Contraception, pregnancy, abortion and motherhood. *Pediatric Annals* 11:797–805.

Botvin, G. J. (1986) Substance abuse prevention research: Recent developments and future directions. *Journal of School Health* 56:369–374.

Botvin, G. J., and Eng, A. (1982) The efficacy of a multicomponent approach to the prevention of cigarette smoking. *Preventive Medicine* 11:199–211.

Botvin, G. J., Baker, E., Renick, N. L., Filazzola, A. D., and Botvin, E. M. (1984) A cognitive-behavioral approach to substance abuse prevention. *Addictive Behaviors* 9:137–147.

Brandt, A. M. (1987) *No Magic Bullet.* New York: Oxford University Press.

Brooks-Gunn, J., and Furstenberg, F. F., Jr. (1989) Adolescent sexual behavior. *American Psychologist* 44:249–257.

Brooks-Gunn, J., Boyer, C., and Hein, K. (1988) Preventing HIV infection and AIDS in children and adolescents: Behavioral research and intervention strategies. *American Psychologist* 43:958–964.

Brundage, J. F., Burke, D. S., Gardner, L. I., Visintine, R., Peterson, M., and Redfield, R. R. (1988) HIV infection among young adults in the New York City area: Prevalence and incidence estimates based on antibody screening among civilian applicants for military service. *New York State Journal of Medicine* 88:232–235.

Brunswick, A. F. (1969) Health needs of adolescents: How the adolescent sees them. *American Journal of Public Health* 59:1736–1745.

Brunswick, A. F. (1988) Young black males and substance use. In J. T. Gibbs, ed., *Young, Black, and Male in America: An Endangered Species.* Dover, Mass.: Auburn House.

Brunswick, A. F., Merzel, C. R., and Messeri, P. A. (1985) Drug use initiation among urban black youth: A seven-year follow-up of developmental and secular influences. *Youth and Society* 17:189–216.

Bucy, J. (1985) *To Whom Do They Belong? A Profile of America's Runaway and Homeless Youth and the Programs That Help Them.* Washington, D.C.: The National Network of Runaway and Youth Services, Inc.

Buning, E., Coutinho, R. A., and van Brussell, G. H. A. (1986) Preventing AIDS in drug addicts in Amsterdam. *Lancet* 1:1435–1436.

Buning, E., Hartgers, C., Verster, A. D., van Santen, G. W., and Coutinho, R. A. (1988) The evaluation of the needle/syringe exchange in Amsterdam. Presented at the Fourth International Conference on AIDS, Stockholm, June 12–16.

Burke, D. S., Brundage, J. F., Herbold, J. R., Berner, W., Gardner, L. I., et al. (1987) Human immunodeficiency virus infections among civilian applicants for United States military service, October 1985 to March 1986. *New England Journal of Medicine* 317:131–136.

Burke, D. S., Brundage, J. F., Goldenbaum, M., Gardner, L. I., Peterson, M., et al. (1990) Human immunodeficiency virus infections in teenagers: Seroprevalence among applicants for U.S. military service. *Journal of the American Medical Association* 263:2074–2077.

Campbell, B. (1984) National Longitudinal Survey of Labor Force Behavior: Technical Report on Interviewing Submitted to the Center for Human Resource Research. National Opinion Research Center, Chicago.

Caruso, B. A., and Haig, J. R. (1987) AIDS on campus: A survey of college health service priorities and policies. *Journal of American College Health* 36:32–36.

Catania, J. A., Kegeles, S. M., and Coates, T. J. (1988) Towards an understanding of risk behavior: The CAPS' AIDS risk reduction model (AARM). Center for AIDS Prevention Studies, University of California at San Francisco, January.

Centers for Disease Control (CDC). (1986) HTLV III/LAV. Antibody prevalence in U.S. military recruit applicants. *Morbidity and Mortality Weekly Report* 35:421–424.

Centers for Disease Control (CDC). (1987) *Sexually Transmitted Disease (STD) Statistics: 1985.* Atlanta, Ga.: Centers for Disease Control.

Centers for Disease Control (CDC). (1988a) HIV-related beliefs, knowledge, and behaviors among high school students. *Morbidity and Mortality Weekly Report* 37:717–721.

Centers for Disease Control (CDC). (1988b) *AIDS Weekly Surveillance Report—United States*. AIDS Program, Center for Infectious Diseases, Centers for Disease Control, Atlanta, Ga., January 18.

Centers for Disease Control (CDC). (1988c) Trends in human immunodeficiency virus infection among civilian applicants for military service—United States, October 1985—March 1988. *Morbidity and Mortality Weekly Report* 37:677–679.

Centers for Disease Control (CDC). (1988d) Guidelines for effective school health education to prevent the spread of AIDS. *Morbidity and Mortality Weekly Report* 37(Suppl. S-2):1–14.

Centers for Disease Control (CDC). (1988e) *Sexually Transmitted Disease Statistics: 1987*. Atlanta, Ga.: Centers for Disease Control.

Centers for Disease Control (CDC). (1989) *HIV/AIDS Surveillance: AIDS Cases Reported Through September 1989*. Atlanta, Ga.: Centers for Disease Control.

Chiasson, R. E., Osmond, D., Moss, A., Feldman, H., and Bernacki, P. (1987) HIV, bleach and needle sharing (letter). *Lancet* 1:1430.

Clayton, R. R., and Ritter, C. (1985) The epidemiology of alcohol and drug abuse among adolescents. In B. Stimmel, ed., *Alcohol and Substance Abuse in Adolescence*. New York: Haworth Press.

Connell, D. B., Turner, R. R., and Mason, E. F. (1985) Summary of findings of school health education evaluation: Health promotion effectiveness, implementation and costs. *Journal of School Health* 55:317–321.

Consumer Reports. (1989) Can you rely on condoms? *Consumer Reports* March:135–142.

Copello, A. G., Sheets, R., Ross, S., and Curvin, M. (1989) Evaluation of a targeted AIDS/HIV education program for secondary school students in a medium-size USA metropolitan area. Presented at the Fifth International Conference on AIDS, Montreal, June 4–9, 1989.

COSSMHO (The National Coalition of Hispanic Health and Human Services Organizations). (1989) AIDS education for youth enters second year. *The COSSMHO AIDS Update* 3:1–2, May–June.

Coyle, S. L., Boruch, R. F., and Turner, C. F., eds. (1990) *Evaluating AIDS Prevention Programs, Expanded Edition*. Washington, D.C.: National Academy Press.

D'Angelo, L., Getson, P., Luban, N., Stallings, E., and Gayle, H. (1989) HIV infection in adolescents: Can we predict who is at risk. Presented at the Fifth International Conference on AIDS, Montreal, June 4–9.

Darrow, W. W. (1989) Condom use and use-effectiveness in high-risk populations. *Sexually Transmitted Diseases* 16:157–160.

D'Augelli, A. R., and Kennedy, S. P. (1989) An evaluation of AIDS prevention brochures for university women and men. *AIDS Education and Prevention* 1:134–140.

Davies, M., and Kandel, D. B. (1981) Parental and peer influence on adolescents' educational plans: Some further evidence. *American Journal of Sociology* 87:363–387.

Davis, J. A., and Smith, T. W. (1989) *General Social Surveys, 1972–1989: Cumulative Codebook*. Chicago: National Opinion Research Center, University of Chicago.

Des Jarlais, D. C., and Friedman, S. R. (1987) HIV infection among intravenous drug users: Epidemiology and risk reduction (editorial review). *AIDS* 1:67–76.

Des Jarlais, D. C., and Friedman, S. R. (1988) Intravenous cocaine, crack, and HIV infection (letter). *Journal of the American Medical Association* 259:1945–1946.

Des Jarlais, D. C., Friedman, S. R., Sotheran, J. L., and Stoneburner, R. (1988) The sharing of drug injection equipment and the AIDS epidemic in New York City: The first decade. In R. J. Battjes, and R. W. Pickens, eds., *Needle Sharing Among Intravenous Drug Abusers: National and International Perspectives.* National Institute for Drug Abuse Research Monograph 80. Washington, D.C.: U.S. Government Printing Office.

Des Jarlais, D. C., Casriel, C., Friedman, S. R., Rosenblum, A., Rodriguez, R., et al. (1989) AIDS education and the transition from non-injecting to injecting drug use. Presented at the Fifth International Conference on AIDS, Montreal, June 4–9.

DiClemente, R. J. (1989) Prevention of human immunodeficiency virus infection among adolescents: The interplay of health education and public policy in the development and implementation of school-based AIDS education programs. *AIDS Education and Prevention* 1:70–78.

DiClemente, R. J., and DuNah, R. (1989) A comparative analysis of risk behaviors among a school-based and juvenile detention facility sample of adolescents in San Francisco. Presented at the Fifth International Conference on AIDS, Montreal, June 4–9.

DiClemente, R. J., Boyer, C. B., and Morales, E. S. (1988) Minorities and AIDS: Knowledge, attitudes and misconceptions among black and Latino adolescents. *American Journal of Public Health* 78:55–57.

DiClemente, R., Forrest, K., and Mickler, S. (1989) Differential effects of AIDS knowledge and perceived susceptibility on the reduction of high-risk sexual behaviors among college adolescents. Presented at the Fifth International Conference on AIDS, Montreal, June 4–9.

DiClemente, R. J., Zorn, J., and Temoshok, L. (1986) Adolescents and AIDS: A survey of knowledge, attitudes and beliefs about AIDS in San Francisco. *American Journal of Public Health* 76:1443–1445.

DiClemente, R. J., Zorn, J., and Temoshok, L. (1987) The association of gender, ethnicity, and length of residence in the Bay area to adolescents' knowledge and attitudes about acquired immune deficiency syndrome. *Journal of Applied Social Psychology* 17:216–230.

Duncan, M. E., Tibaux, G., Pelzer, A., Reimann, K., Pentherer, J. F., et al. (1990) First coitus before menarche and risk of sexually transmitted disease. *Lancet* 335:338–340.

Dusher, R. W., and Mills, C. A. (1963) The adolescent looks at his health and medical care. *American Journal of Public Health* 53:1928–1936.

Elkind, D. (1985) Cognitive development and adolescent disabilities. *Journal of Adolescent Health Care* 6:84–89.

Ellickson, P. L., and Bell, R. M. (1990) Drug prevention in junior high: A multi-site longitudinal test. *Science* 247:1299–1305.

Elliott, D. S., and Morse, B. J. (1989) Delinquency and drug use as risk factors in teenage sexual activity. *Youth and Society* 21:32–60.

Ensminger, M. E. (1987) Adolescent sexual behavior as it relates to other transition behaviors in youth. In S. L. Hofferth and C. D. Hayes, eds., *Risking the Future: Adolescent Sexuality, Pregnancy, and Childbearing.* Vol. 2, *Working Papers and Statistical Appendixes.* Washington, D.C.: National Academy Press.

Ensminger, M. E., and Kane, L. P. (1985) Adolescent drug and alcohol use, delinquency and sexual activity: Patterns of occurrence and risk factors. Presented at the National Institute for Drug Abuse Technical Review on Drug Abuse and Adolescent Sexual Activity, Pregnancy and Parenthood, March.

Ernst, J. A., Bauer, S., Amaral, L., St. Louis, M., and Falco, I. (1989) HIV seroprevalence at the Bronx Lebanon Hospital Center, a CDC sentinel hospital. Presented at the Fifth International Conference on AIDS, Montreal, June 4–9.

Evans, R. I., Henderson, A., Hill, P., and Raines, B. (1979) Smoking in children and adolescents: Psychosocial determinants and prevention strategies. In N. A. Krasnegor, ed., *The Behavioral Aspects of Smoking*. National Institute on Drug Abuse Research Monograph No. 26. Washington, D.C.: U.S. Government Printing Office.

Faltz, B., and Madoover, S. (1987) Substance abuse as a co-factor for AIDS. In *Women and AIDS Clinical Resource Guide*, 2nd ed. San Francisco: San Francisco AIDS Foundation.

Fay, R. E., Turner, C. F., Klassen, A. D., and Gagnon, J. H. (1989) Prevalence and patterns of same-gender sexual contact among men. *Science* 243:338–348.

Feldblum, P. J., and Fortney, J. A. (1988) Condoms, spermicides, and the transmission of human immunodeficiency virus: A review of the literature. *American Journal of Public Health* 78:52–54.

Fisher, J. D. (1988) Possible effects of reference group-based social influence on AIDS-risk behavior and AIDS prevention. *American Psychologist* 43:914–920.

Flavin, D. K., and Frances, R. J. (1987) Risk taking behavior, substance abuse disorders, and the acquired immunodeficiency syndrome. *Advances in Alcohol and Substance Abuse* 6:23–31.

Flay, B. R. (1985) Psychosocial approaches to smoking prevention: A review of findings. *Health Psychology* 4:449–488.

Flora, J. A., and Thoresen, C. E. (1988) Reducing the risk of AIDS in adolescence. *American Psychologist* 43:965–970.

Fox, G. L. (1981) The family's role in adolescent sexual behavior. In T. Ooms, ed., *Teenage Pregnancy in a Family Context*. Philadelphia: Temple University Press.

Freudenberg, N., Lee, J., and Silver, D. (1989) How black and Latino community organizations respond to the AIDS epidemic: A case study in one New York City neighborhood. *AIDS Education and Prevention* 1:12–21.

Friedman, H. L. (1989) The health of adolescents: Beliefs and behavior. *Social Science and Medicine* 29:309–315.

Friedman, I. M., and Litt, I. F. (1987) Adolescents' compliance with therapeutic regimens: Psychological and social aspects and intervention. *Journal of Adolescent Health Care* 8:52–67.

Friedman, S. R., Des Jarlais, D. C., Neaigus, A., Abdul-Quader, A., Sotheran, J. L., et al. (1989) AIDS and the new drug injector. *Nature* 339:333–334.

Fullilove, R. E., Fullilove, M. T., Bowser, B. P., and Gross, S. A. (1989) Crack use and risk for AIDS among black adolescents. Presented at the Fifth International Conference on AIDS, Montreal, June 4–9.

Fullilove, R. E., Fullilove, M. T., Bowser, B. P., Gross, S. A. (1990) Risk of sexually transmitted disease among black adolescent crack users in Oakland and San Francisco, Calif. *Journal of the American Medical Association* 263:851–855.

Furstenberg, F. F., Morgan, S. P., Moore, K. A., and Peterson, J. L. (1987) Race differences in the timing of adolescent intercourse. *American Sociological Review* 52:511–518.

Gayle, H., Manoff, S., and Rogers, M. (1989) Epidemiology of AIDS in adolescents, U.S.A. Presented at the Fifth International Conference on AIDS. Montreal, June 4–9.

Gayle, H., Rogers, M., Manoff, S., and Starcher, E. (1988) Demographic and sexual transmission differences between adolescent and adult AIDS patients, U.S.A. Presented at the Fourth International Conference on AIDS, Stockholm, June 12–16.

Gayle, H., Keeling, R., Garcia-Tunon, M., Kilbourne, B., and Narkunas, J. (1989) HIV seroprevalence on university campuses, U.S.A. Presented at the Fifth International Conference on AIDS, Montreal, June 4–9.

Gellert, G. A., and Durfee, M. J. (1990) HIV infection and child abuse. *New England Journal of Medicine* 321:685.

Gerstein, D. R., Judd, L. L., And Rovner, S. A. (1979) Career dynamics of female heroin addicts. *American Journal of Drug and Alcohol Abuse* 6:1–23.

Gilchrist, L. D., and Schinke, S. P. (1983) Coping with contraception: Cognitive and behavioral methods with adolescents. *Cognitive Therapy and Research* 7:379–388.

Ginzburg, H. M. (1988) Acquired immune deficiency syndrome (AIDS) and drug abuse. In R. P. Galea, B. F. Lewis, and L. A. Baker, eds., *AIDS and IV Drug Abusers: A Current Perspective.* Owings Mills, Md.: National Health Publishing.

Girodo, M., Dotzenroth, S., and Stein, S. (1981) Causal attribution bias in shy males: Implications for self-esteem and self-confidence. *Cognitive Therapy and Research* 5:325–338.

Goedert, J. J., Kessler, C. M., Aledort, L. M., Biggar, R. J., Andes, W. A., et al. (1989) A prospective study of human immunodeficiency virus type 1 infection and the development of AIDS in subjects with hemophilia. *New England Journal of Medicine* 321:1141–1148.

Gold, M., and Petronio, R. J. (1980) Delinquent behavior in adolescence. In J. Adelson, ed., *Handbook of Adolescent Psychology.* New York: John Wiley and Sons.

Greenblatt, R. M., Catania, J. A., Kegeles, S. M., Schachter, Y., Miller, J., and Coates, T. J. (1989) Predictors of condom use and STDs in a group of sexually active adolescent women. Presented at the Fifth International Conference on AIDS, Montreal, June 4–9.

Haignere, C., Rotheram-Borus, M., Bradley, J., Koopman, C., and Harden, N. (1989) Stressful life events and social supports as mediators of safe behaviors among runaway and gay youths. Presented at the Fifth International Conference on AIDS, Montreal, June 4–9.

Hamburg, B. A., Kraemer, H. C., and Jahnke, W. (1975) A hierarchy of drug use in adolescence: Behavioral and attitudinal correlates of substantial drug use. *American Journal of Psychiatry* 132:1155–1163.

Hamburg, D. (1986) Preparing for life: The critical transition of adolescence. In *The 1986 Annual Report of the Carnegie Corporation of New York.* New York: The Carnegie Corporation.

Hardy, A. M. (1989) AIDS knowledge and attitudes for April–June 1989: Provisional data from the National Health Interview Survey. *NCHS Advance Data* 179:1–12.

Hartgers, C., Buning, E. C., van Santen, G. W., Verster, A. D., and Coutinho, R. A. (1989) The impact of the needle exchange programme in Amsterdam on injecting risk behavior. *AIDS* 3:571–577.

Haverkos, H. W., Bukoski, W. J., and Amsel, Z. (1989) The initiation of male homosexual behavior. *Journal of the American Medical Association* 262:501.

Hayes, C. D., ed. (1987) *Risking the Future: Adolescent Sexuality, Pregnancy, and Childbearing.* Vol. 1. Washington, D.C.: National Academy Press.

Hein, K. (1989a) AIDS in adolescence: Exploring the challenge. *Journal of Adolescent Health Care* 10(Number 3 Supplement):10S–35S. Hein, K. (1989b) Commentary on adolescent acquired immunodeficiency syndrome: The next wave of the human immunodeficiency virus epidemic? *Journal of Pediatrics* 114:144–149.

Hein, K., and DiGeronimo, T. F. (1989) *AIDS: Trading Fears for Facts.* Mount Vernon, N.Y.: Consumers Union.

Hein, K., Marks, A., and Cohen, M. (1977) Asymptomatic gonorrhea: Prevalence in a population of urban adolescents. *Journal of Pediatrics* 90:634–635.

Hein, K., Cohen, M. I., Marks, A., Schonberg, S. K., Meyer, M., and McBride, A. (1978) Age at first intercourse among homeless adolescent females. *Journal of Pediatrics* 93:147–148.

Henricks, L. E. (1985) Establishment of accessible and relevant services for adolescents. In D. Shaffer, A. A. Ehrhardt, and L. L. Greenhill, eds., *The Clinical Guide to Child Psychiatry.* New York: The Free Press.

Hingson, R., and Strunin, L. (1989) Do health belief model beliefs about HIV infection and condoms predict adolescent condom use? Presented at the Fifth International Conference on AIDS, Montreal, June 4–9.

Hingson, R., Strunin, L., and Berlin, B. (1990) Acquired immunodeficiency syndrome transmission: Changes in knowledge and behaviors among teenagers, Massachusetts statewide surveys, 1986 to 1988. *Pediatrics* 85:24–29.

Hingson, R. W., Strunin, L., Berlin, B. M., and Heeren, T. (1990) Beliefs about AIDS, use of alcohol and drugs, and unprotected sex among Massachusetts adolescents. *American Journal of Public Health* 80:295–299.

Hochhauser, M. (1987) Readability of AIDS Educational Materials. Presented at the Annual Meeting of the American Psychological Association, New York, August 30.

Hofferth, S. L. (1987) Factors affecting initiation of sexual intercourse. In S. L. Hofferth, and C. D. Hayes, eds., *Risking the Future.* Vol. 2, *Working Papers and Statistical Appendixes.* Washington, D.C.: National Academy Press.

Hofferth, S. L., Kahn, J. R., and Baldwin, W. (1987) Premarital sexual activity among U.S. teenage women over the past three decades. *Family Planning Perspectives* 19:46–53.

Horan, J. J., and Williams, J. M. (1982) Longitudinal study of assertion training as a drug abuse prevention strategy. *American Educational Research Journal* 19:341–351.

Horton, J., Alexander, L., and Brundage, J. (1989) HIV prevalence among military women: An examination of military applicant, active duty and reserve testing data. Presented at the Fifth International Conference on AIDS, Montreal, June 4–9.

Howard, J., Taylor, J. A., Ganikos, M. L., Holder, H. D., Godwin, D. F., and Taylor, E. D. (1988) An overview of prevention research: Issues, answers, and new agendas. *Public Health Reports* 103:674–683.

Hudson, R. A., Petty, B. A., Freeman, A. C., Haley, C. E., and Krepcho, M. A. (1989) Adolescent runaways' behavioral risk factors, knowledge about AIDS and attitudes about condom usage. Presented at the Fifth International Conference on AIDS, Montreal, June 4–9.

Hummel, R., Rodriguez, G., Brandon, D., and Wells, D. (1989) Outreach model for HIV positive adolescents and adolescents currently at high risk for HIV infection. Presented at the Fifth International Conference on AIDS, Montreal, June 4–9.

Inazu, J. K., and Fox, G. L. (1980) Maternal influence on the sexual behavior of teenage daughters. *Journal of Family Issues* 1:81–102.

Institute of Medicine (IOM). (1988) *Homelessness, Health, and Human Needs.* Washington, D.C.: National Academy Press.

Institute of Medicine/National Academy of Sciences (IOM/NAS). (1986) *Confronting AIDS: New Directions in Public Health, Health Care, and Research.* Washington, D.C.: National Academy Press.

Institute of Medicine/National Academy of Sciences (IOM/NAS). (1988) *Confronting AIDS: Update 1988.* Washington, D.C.: National Academy Press.

Jackson, J., and Neshin, S. (1986) New Jersey community health project: Impact of using ex-addict education to disseminate information on AIDS to intravenous drug users. Presented at the Second International Conference on AIDS, Paris, June 25–26.

Jackson, J., and Rotkiewicz, L. (1987) A coupon program: AIDS education and drug treatment. Presented at the Third International Conference on AIDS, Washington, D.C., June 1–5.

Jaffe, L. R., Seehaus, M., Wagner, C., and Leadbeater, B. J. (1988) Anal intercourse and knowledge of acquired immunodeficiency syndrome among minority-group female adolescents. *Journal of Pediatrics* 112:1005–1007.

Jessor, R., Chase, J. A., and Donovan, J. E. (1980) Psychosocial correlates of marijuana use and problem drinking in a national sample of adolescents.*American Journal of Public Health* 70:604–613.

Jessor, R., Costa, F., Jessor, S. L., and Donovan, J. E. (1983) Time of first intercourse: A prospective study. *Journal of Personality and Social Psychology* 44:608–626.

Jessor, S. L., and Jessor R. (1975) Transition from virginity to nonvirginity: A social-psychological study over time. *Developmental Psychology* 11:473–484.

Job, R. F. S. (1988) Effective and ineffective use of fear in health promotion campaigns. *American Journal of Public Health* 78:163–167.

Johnston, L. D., Bachman, J. G., and O'Malley, P. M. (1984) *Monitoring the Future: Questionnaire Responses from the Nation's High School Seniors, 1983.* Ann Arbor, Mich.: Institute for Social Research.

Johnston, L. D., Bachman, J. G., and O'Malley, P. M. (1989) *Results of the 1988 National High School Senior Survey* (press release). University of Michigan, Ann Arbor, Mich., February 28.

Johnston, L. D., O'Malley, P. M., and Bachman, J. G. (1988) *Illicit Drug Use, Smoking, and Drinking by America's High School Students, College Students, and Young Adults 1975–1987.* Rockville, Md.: National Institute on Drug Abuse.

Jones, E. F., Forrest, J., Goldman, N., Henshaw, S. K., Lincoln, R., et al. (1985) Teenage pregnancy in developed countries: Determinants and policy implications. *Family Planning Perspectives* 17:53–63.

Kahn, J. R., Kalsbeck, W. D., and Hofferth, S. L. (1988) National estimates of teenage sexual activity: Evaluating the comparability of three national surveys. *Demography* 25:189–204.

Kahn, J. R., Rindfuss, R. R., and Guilkey, D. K. (in press) Adolescent contraceptive method choices. *Demography.*

Kandel, D. B. (1975) Stages in adolescent involvement in drug use. *Science* 190:912–914.

Kandel, D. B. (1978) Similarity in real-life adolescent friendship pairs. *Journal of Personality and Social Psychology* 36:306–312.

Kandel, D. B. (1980) Drug and drinking behavior among youth. In J. Coleman, A. Inkeles, and N. Smelser, eds., *Annual Review of Sociology* 6:235–285.

Kandel, D. B. (1984) Marijuana users in young adulthood. *Archives of General Psychiatry* 41:200–209.

Kandel, D. B. (1985) On processes of peer influences in adolescent drug use: A developmental perspective. In B. Stimmel, ed., *Alcohol and Substance Abuse in Adolescence.* New York: Haworth Press.

Kandel, D. B., and Davies, M. (In press) Cocaine use in a national sample of U.S. youth (NLSY): Epidemiology, predictors and ethnic patterns. In C. Schade and S. Scholer, eds., *The Epidemiology of Cocaine Use and Abuse,* National Institute on Drug Abuse Research Monograph. Rockville, Md.: National Institute on Drug Abuse.

Kandel, D. B., and Logan, J. A. (1984) Patterns of drug use from adolescence to young adulthood: I. Periods of risk for initiation, continued use, and discontinuation. *American Journal of Public Health* 74:660–666.

Kandel, D. B., Kessler, R. C., and Margulies, R. Z. (1978) Antecedents of adolescent initiation into stages of drug use: A developmental analysis. *Journal of Youth and Adolescence* 7:13–40.

Kandel, D. B., Murphy, D., and Karus, D. (1985) Cocaine use in young adulthood: Patterns of use and psychosocial correlates. In N. J. Kozel, and E. H. Adams, eds., *Cocaine Use in America: Epidemiologic and Clinical Perspectives.* National Institute on Drug Abuse Research Monograph 61. Rockville, Md.: National Institute on Drug Abuse.

Keating, D. P. (1980) Thinking processes in adolescence. In J. Adelson, ed., *Handbook of Adolescent Psychology.* New York: John Wiley and Sons.

Kegeles, S., Greenblatt, R., Catania, J., Cardenas, C., Gottlieb, J., and Coates, T. (1989) AIDS risk behavior among sexually active Hispanic and Caucasian adolescent females. Presented at the Fifth International Conference on AIDS, Montreal, June 4–9.

Kegeles, S. M., Adler, N. E., and Irwin, Jr., C. E. (1988) Sexually active adolescents and condoms: Changes over one year in knowledge, attitudes and use. *American Journal of Public Health* 78:460–461.

Kelley, P. W., Miller, R. N., Pomerantz, R., Wann, F., Brundage, J. F., and Buck, D. S. (1990) Human immunodeficiency virus seropositivity among members of the active duty U.S. Army 1985–1989. *American Journal of Public Health* 80:405–410.

Kilbourne, B. W., Buehler, J. W., and Rogers, M. F. (1990) AIDS as a cause of death in children, adolescents, and young adults. *American Journal of Public Health* 80:499–500.

Kilbourne, B. W., Rogers, M. F., and Bush, T. J. (1989) The relative importance of AIDS as a cause of death in pediatric and young adult populations in the U.S. 1980–1987. Presented at the Fifth International Conference on AIDS, Montreal, June 4–9.

Kiselica, M. S. (1988) Helping an aggressive adolescent through the "Before, during and after program." *The School Counselor* 35:299–306.

Kleinman, P. H., Goldsmith, D. S., Friedman, S. R., Mauge, C. E., Hopkins, W., and Des Jarlais, D. C. (In press.) Knowledge about and behaviors affecting the spread of AIDS. *International Journal of the Addictions.*

Kolbe, L., Jones, J., Nelson, G., Daily, L., Duncan, C., et al. (1988) School health education to prevent the spread of AIDS: Overview of a national program. *Hygie* 7:10–13.

Kreipe, R. E., and Strauss, J. (1989) Adolescent medical disorders, behavior, and development. In G. R. Adams, R. Montemayor, and T. P. Gullotta, eds., *The Biology of Adolescent Behavior and Development.* Newbury Park, Calif.: Sage Publications.

Lamke, L. K., Lujan, B. M., and Showalter, J. M. (1988) The case for modifying adolescents' cognitive self-statements. *Adolescence* 92:967–974.

Lashley, K. S., and Watson, J. B. (1922) *A Psychological Study of Motion Pictures in Relation to Venereal Disease Campaigns.* Washington, D.C.: U.S. Interdepartmental Social Hygiene Board.

Lawrence, F. C., Tasker, G. E., Daly, C. T., Orhiel, A. L., and Wozniak, P. H. (1986) Adolescent's time spent viewing television. *Adolescence* 21:431–436.

Lemp, G. F., Payne, S. F., Neal, D., Temelso, T., and Rutherford, G. W. (1990) Survival trends for patients with AIDS. *Journal of the American Medical Association* 263:402–406.

Lesnick, H., and Pace, B. (1990) Knowledge of AIDS risk factors in South Bronx minority college students. *Journal of Acquired Immune Deficiency Syndromes* 3:173–176.

Lewis, C. E., and Lewis, M. A. (1984) Peer pressure and risk-taking behaviors in children. *American Journal of Public Health* 74:580–584.

Longini, Jr., I. M., Clark, W. S., Horsburgh, C. R., Lemp, G. F., Byers, R. H., et al. (1989) Statistical analysis of the stages of HIV infection using a Markov model. Presented at the Fifth International Conference on AIDS, Montreal, June 4–9.

Lui, K., Darrow, W. W., and Rutherford, G. W. (1988) A model-based estimate of the mean incubation period for AIDS in homosexual men. *Science* 240:1333–1335.

Mantell, J. E., and Schinke, S. P. (In press) The crisis of AIDS for adolescents: The need for preventive risk-reduction interventions. In A. R. Roberts, ed., *Crisis Intervention Handbook.* New York: Springer.

Marks, A., Malizio, J., Hoch, J., Brody, R., and Fisher, M. (1983) Assessment of health needs and willingness to utilize health care resources of adolescents in a suburban population. *Journal of Pediatrics* 102:456–460.

Marlatt, G. A. (1982) Relapse prevention: A self-control program for the treatment of addictive behaviors. In R. B. Stuart, ed., *Adherence, Compliance and Generalization in Behavioral Medicine.* New York: Brunner/Mazel.

Martin, A. D., and Hetrick, E. S. (1987) Designing an AIDS risk reduction program for gay teenagers: Problems and proposed solutions. In D. G. Ostrow, ed., *Biobehavioral Control of AIDS*. New York: Irvington Publishers, Inc.

Mason, J. O., Noble, G. R., Lindsey, B. K., Kolbe, L. J., Van Ness, P., et al. (1988) Current CDC efforts to prevent and control human immunodeficiency virus infection and AIDS in the United States through information and education. *Public Health Reports* 103:255–260.

Mata, A. G., and Jorquez, J. S. (1988) Mexican-American intravenous drug users' and needle-sharing practices: Implications for AIDS prevention. In R. J. Battjes, and R. W. Pickens, eds., *Needle Sharing Among Intravenous Drug Abusers: National and International Perspectives*. National Institute on Drug Abuse Research Monograph 80. Washington, D.C.: U.S. Government Printing Office.

Mays, V. M., and Cochran, S. D. (1987) Acquired immunodeficiency syndrome and black Americans: Special psychosocial issues. *Public Health Reports* 102:224–231.

McCaul, K. D., and Glasgow, R. E. (1985) Preventing adolescent smoking: What have we learned about treatment construct validity? *Health Psychology* 4:361–387.

McKusick, L., Coates, T. J., and Babcock, K. (1988) Knowledge and attitudes about AIDS and sexual behavior in California high school students. Presented at the Fourth International Conference on AIDS, Stockholm, June 12–16.

Mensch, B. S., and Kandel, D. B. (1988a) Dropping out of high school and drug involvement. *Sociology of Education* 61:95–113.

Mensch, B. S., and Kandel, D. B. (1988b) Underreporting of substance use in a national longitudinal youth cohort: Individual and interviewer effects. *Public Opinion Quarterly* 52:100–124.

Meyer-Bahlburg, H. F. L. (1980) Sexuality in early adolescence. In B. B. Wolman, and J. Money, eds., *Handbook of Human Sexuality*. Englewood Cliffs, N.J.: Prentice-Hall.

Miller, P. Y., and Simon, W. (1974) Adolescent sexual behavior: Context and change. *Social Problems* 22:58–76.

Mitchell, F., and Brindis, C. (1987) Adolescent pregnancy: The responsibilities of policy makers. *Health Services Research* 22:399–437.

Moore, D., and Schultz, N. (1983) Loneliness at adolescence: Correlates, attributions, and coping. *Journal of Youth and Adolescence* 12:187–196.

Moore, K. A., Nord, C. W., and Peterson, J. L. (1989) Nonvoluntary sexual activity among adolescents. *Family Planning Perspectives* 21:110–114.

Moore, K. A., Wenk, D., Hofferth, S. L., and Hayes, C. D., eds. (1987) Statistical appendix: Trends in adolescent sexual and fertility behavior. In S. L. Hofferth, and C. D. Hayes, eds., *Risking the Future*. Vol. 2, Working Papers and Statistical Appendixes. Washington, D.C.: National Academy Press.

Morris, R., Huscroft, S., Roseman, J., Re, O., Baker, C. J., and Iwakoshi, K. A. (1989) Demographic and high-risk behavior study of incarcerated adolescents. Presented at the Fifth International Conference on AIDS, Montreal, June 4–9.

Morisky, D. E., DeMuth, N. M., Field-Fass, M., Green, L. W., and Levine, D. M. (1985) Evaluation of family health education to build social support for long-term control of high blood pressure. *Health Education Quarterly* 12:35–50.

Mosher, W. D., and Bachrach, C. A. (1987) First premarital contraceptive use: United States, 1960–82. *Studies in Family Planning* 18:83–95.

Mott, F. L., and Haurin, R. J. (1988) Linkages between sexual activity and alcohol and drug use among American adolescents. *Family Planning Perspectives* 20:128–136.

Murray, D. M., and Perry, C. L. (1985) The prevention of adolescent drug abuse: Implications of etiological, developmental, behavioral, and environmental models. In C. L. Jones, and R. J. Battjes, eds., *Etiology of Drug Abuse: Implications for Prevention.* National Institute on Drug Abuse Research Monograph 56. Rockville, Md.: U.S. Department of Health and Human Services.

Nahmias, A., Corey, L., Lee, F., Clumeck, N., Cannon, R., and Holmberg, S. (1989) Genital herpes as a possible risk factor for HIV transmission. Presented at the Fifth International Conference on AIDS, Montreal, June 4–9.

National Institute on Drug Abuse (NIDA). (1988) *National Household Survey on Drug Abuse: Main Findings 1985.* Rockville, Md.: National Institute on Drug Abuse.

Newcomb, M. D., and Bentler, P. M. (1988) *Consequences of Adolescent Drug Use: Impact on the Lives of Young Adults.* Newbury Park, Calif.: Sage.

Newcomb, M. D., and Bentler, P. M. (1989) Substance use and abuse among children and teenagers. *American Psychologist* 44:242–248.

Newcomer S. F., and Udry, J. R. (1983) Adolescent sexual behavior and popularity. *Adolescence* 18:515–522.

Newmeyer, J. A. (1988) Why bleach? Development of a strategy to combat HIV contagion among San Francisco intravenous drug users. In R. J. Battjes, and R. W. Pickens, eds., *Needle Sharing Among Intravenous Drug Abusers: National and International Perspectives.* NIDA Research Monograph 80. Washington, D.C.: U.S. Government Printing Office.

New York State Department of Health. (1989) *AIDS in New York State through 1988.* Albany, N.Y.: New York State Department of Health.

Novello, A. C. (1988) *Secretary's Work Group on Pediatric HIV Infection and Disease.* Washington, D.C.: Department of Health and Human Services.

Novick, L. F., Berns, D., Stricof, R., Stevens, R., Pass, K., and Wethers, J. (1989a) HIV seroprevalence in newborns in New York State. *Journal of the American Medical Association* 261:1745–1750.

Novick, L. F., Glebatis, D., Stricof, R., and Berns, D. (1989b) HIV infection in adolescent childbearing women. Presented at the Fifth International Conference on AIDS, Montreal, June 1–4.

O'Donnell, J. A. (1985) Interpreting progression from one drug to another. In L. N. Robins, ed., *Studying Drug Abuse.* New Brunswick, N.J.: Rutgers University Press.

O'Donnell, J. A., and Clayton, R. R. (1982) The stepping-stone hypothesis: Marijuana, heroin, and causality. *Chemical Dependencies* 4:229–241.

Office of Technology Assessment (OTA). (1988) *How Effective is AIDS Education?* Washington, D.C.: Office of Technology Assessment.

Osgood, D. W., Johnston, L. D., O'Malley, P. M., and Bachman, J. G. (1988) The generality of deviance in late adolescence and early adulthood. *American Sociological Review* 53:81–93.

Paget, K. D. (1988) Adolescent pregnancy: Implications for prevention strategies in educational settings. *School Psychology Review* 17:570–580.

Parcel, G. S., Nader, P. R., and Meyer, M. P. (1977) Adolescent health concerns, problems and patterns of obligation in a triethnic urban population. *Pediatrics* 66:157–164.

Pearl, D., Bouthilet, L., and Lazar, J., eds. (1982) *Television and Behavior: Ten Years of Scientific Progress and Implications for the Eighties.* Vol. 1: *Summary Reports.* Rockville, Md.: U.S. Department of Health and Human Services.

Pentz, M. A., Cormack, C., Flay, B., Hansen, W. B., and Johnson, C. A. (1986) Balancing program and research integrity in community drug abuse prevention: Project STAR approach. *Journal of School Health* 56:389–393.

Pentz, M.A., Dwyer, J. H., MacKinnon, D. P., Flay, B. R., Hansen, W. B., et al. (1989a) A multicommunity trial for primary prevention of adolescent drug abuse. *Journal of the American Medical Association* 261:3259–3266.

Pentz, M. A., MacKinnon, D. P., Flay, B. R., Hansen, W. B., Johnson, C. A., and Dwyer, J. H. (1989b) Primary prevention of chronic diseases in adolescence: Effects of the Midwestern prevention project on tobacco use. *American Journal of Epidemiology* 130:713–724.

Perlman, J. A., Kelaghan, J., Wolf, P. H., Baldwin, W., Coulson, A., and Novello, A. (1990) HIV risk difference between condom users and nonusers among U.S. heterosexual women. *Journal of Acquired Immune Deficiency Syndromes* 3:155–165.

Perry, C. L., Klepp, K. I., and Schultz, J. M. (1988) Primary prevention of cardiovascular disease: Community-wide strategies for use. *Journal of Consulting and Clinical Psychology* 56:358–364.

Peterson, M. R., Mumm, A. H., Mathis, R., Kelley, P. W., White S. L., et al. (1988) Prevalence of HIV antibody in U.S. active-duty military personnel, April 1988. *Morbidity and Mortality Weekly Report* 37:461–463.

Polich, J. M., Ellickson, P. L., Reuter, P., and Kahan, J. P. (1984) *Strategies For Controlling Adolescent Drug Use.* Santa Monica, Calif.: The Rand Corporation.

Polit, D. F., and Kahn, J. R. (1986) Early subsequent pregnancy among economically disadvantaged teenage mothers. *American Journal of Public Health* 76:167–171.

Pratt, W. F., Mosher, W. D., Bachrach, C. A., and Horn, M. C. (1984) Understanding U.S. fertility: Findings from the National Survey of Family Growth, Cycle III. *Population Bulletin* 39:3–41.

Price, J. H., Desmond, S., and Kukulka, G. (1985) High school students' perceptions and misperceptions of AIDS. *Journal of School Health* 55:107–109.

Quinn, J. (1988) Natural allies: Youth organizations as partners in AIDS education. In M. Quackenbush, M. Nelson, and K. Clark, eds., *The AIDS Challenge: Prevention Education for Young People.* Santa Cruz, Calif.: Network Publications.

Quinn, T. C., Glasser, D., Cannon, R. O., Matuszak, D. L., Dunning, R. W., et al. (1988) Human immunodeficiency virus infection among patients attending clinics for sexually transmitted diseases. *New England Journal of Medicine* 318:197–203.

Radius, S. M., Dielman, T. E., Becker, M. H., Rosenstock, I., and Horvath, W. J. (1980) Health beliefs of the school-aged child and their relationship to risk-taking behaviors. *International Journal of Health Education* 23:3–11.

Remafedi, G. (1988) Preventing the sexual transmission of AIDS during adolescence. *Journal of Adolescent Health Care* 9:139–143.

Reuben, N., Hein, K., Drucker, E., Bauman, L., and Lauby, J. (1988) Relationship of high-risk behaviors to AIDS knowledge in adolescent high school students. Presented at the Annual Research Meeting of the Society for Adolescent Medicine, New York City, March.

Rizvi, M. H. (1983) An empirical investigation of some item nonresponse adjustment procedures. In W. G. Madow, H. Nisselson, and I. Olkin, eds., *Incomplete Data in Sample Surveys,* Vol. 1, *Report and Case Studies* (Report of the National Research Council Panel on Incomplete Data). New York: Academic Press.

Roberts, E. S., Kline, D., and Gagnon, J. (1981) *Family Life and Sexual Learning of Children.* Vol. 1. Cambridge, Mass.: Population Education, Inc.

Robins, L. N., and Wish, E. (1977) Childhood deviance as a developmental process: A study of 223 urban black men from birth to 18. *Social Forces* 56:448–473.

Rolf, J., Nanda, J., Thompson, L., Mamon, J., Chandra, A., et al. (1989) Issues in AIDS prevention among juvenile offenders. In J. O. Woodruff, D. Doherty, and J. G. Athey, eds., *Troubled Adolescents and HIV Infection.* Washington, D.C.: Child and Adolescent Service System Program (CASSP), Georgetown University Child Development Center.

Rolf, J., Nanda, J., Baldwin, J., Chandra, A., and Thompson, L. (In press) Substance abuse and HIV/AIDS risk among delinquents: A prevention challenge. *International Journal of Addictions,* Silver Anniversary Issue on Prevention (Special Issue No. 3).

Rosenbaum, E., and Kandel, D. B. (In press) Early onset of adolescent sexual behavior and drug involvement. *Journal of Marriage and the Family.*

Rosenberg, M. (1965) *Society and the Adolescent Self Image.* Princeton, N.J.: Princeton University Press.

Rotheram-Borus, M. J., Selfridge, C., Koopman, C., Haignere, C., Meyer-Bahlburg, H., and Ehrhardt, A. (1989) The relationship of knowledge and attitudes toward AIDS to safe sex practices among runaway and gay adolescents. Presented at the Fifth International Conference on AIDS, Montreal, June 4–9.

Rothman, J., and David, T. (1985) Status offenders in Los Angeles County: Focus on runaway and homeless youth. Los Angeles: School of Social Welfare, University of California at Los Angeles.

Santrock, J. W. (1981) *Adolescence: An Introduction.* Dubuque, Iowa: William C. Brown.

Schinke, S. P. (1984) Preventing teenage pregnancy. In M. Hersen, R. M. Eisler, and P. M. Miller, eds., *Progress in Behavior Modification.* San Francisco: Academic Press.

Severson, H. H. (1984) Adolescent social drug use: School prevention program. *School Psychology Review* 13:150–161.

Shaffer, D., and Caton, D. (1984) Runaway and homeless youth in New York City: A report to the Ittleson Foundation. New York: The Ittleson Foundation.

Sharp, E., Cowan, D., Goldenbaum, M., Brundage, J., and McNeil, J. (1989) Epidemiology of HIV infection among young adults in the U.S.: Regional variations and trends. Presented at the Fifth International Conference on AIDS, Montreal, June 4–9.

Siegel, D., Lazarus, N., Durbin, M., Krasnovsky, F., Chesney, M., and Kakimoto, D. (1989) AIDS prevention in junior high school students in an AIDS epicenter: Results of a baseline survey. Presented at the Fifth International Conference on AIDS, Montreal, June 4–9.

Single, E., Kandel, D. B., and Johnson, B. D. (1975) The reliability and validity of drug use responses in a large-scale longitudinal survey. *Journal of Drug Issues* 5:426–443.

Smith, E. A., and Udry, J. R. (1985) Coital and non-coital sexual behaviors of white and black adolescents. *American Journal of Public Health* 75:1200–1203.

Sobol, J. (1987) Health concerns of young adolescents. *Adolescence* 22:739–750.

Sonenstein, F. L., Pleck, J. H., and Ku, L. C. (1989a) At risk of AIDS: Behaviors, knowledge and attitudes among a national sample of adolescent males. Presented at the Annual Meeting of the Population Association of America, Baltimore, Md., March 31.

Sonenstein, F. L., Pleck, J. H., and Ku, L. C. (1989b) Sexual activity, condom use and AIDS awareness among adolescent males. *Family Planning Perspectives* 21:152–158.

Sorenson, R. C. (1973) *Adolescent Sexuality in Contemporary America.* New York: World Publishing Co.

Spencer, B. D. (1989) On the accuracy of current estimates of the numbers of intravenous drug users. In C. F. Turner, H. G. Miller, and L. E. Moses, eds., *AIDS, Sexual Behavior, and Intravenous Drug Use.* Washington, D.C.: National Academy Press.

St. Louis, M. E., Hayman, C. R., Miller, C., Anderson, J. E., Peterson, L. R., and Dondero, T. J. (1989) HIV infection in disadvantaged adolescents in the U.S.: Findings from the Job Corps screening program. Presented at the Fifth International Conference on AIDS, Montreal, June 4–9.

Stall, R., McKusick, L., Wiley, J., Coates, T. J., and Ostrow, D. G. (1986) Alcohol and drug use during sexual activity and compliance with safe sex guidelines for AIDS: The AIDS Behavioral Research Project. *Health Education Quarterly* 13:359–371.

Stark, E. (1986) Young, innocent, and pregnant. *Psychology Today* 20:28–30,32–35.

Sternleib, J. J., and Muncan, L. (1972) A survey of health problems, practices and needs of youth. *Pediatrics* 49:177–186.

Stimson, G. V. (1988) *Injecting Equipment Exchange Schemes: Final Report.* London: Monitoring Research Group, Sociology Department, Goldsmith's College.

Stimson, G. V. (1989) Syringe exchange programmes for injecting drug users. *AIDS* 5:253–261.

Strecher, V. J., DeVellis, B. M., Becker, M. H., and Rosenstock, I. M. (1986) The role of self-efficacy in achieving health behavior change. *Health Education Quarterly* 13:73–91.

Strunin, L., and Hingson, R. (1987) Acquired immunodeficiency syndrome and adolescents: Knowledge, beliefs, attitudes and behavior. *Pediatrics* 79:825–828.

Sutton, S. R. (1982) Fear-arousing communications: A critical examination of theory and research. In J. R. Eiser, ed., *Social Psychology and Behavioral Medicine.* New York: John Wiley and Sons.

Telzak, E. E., Chiasson, M. A., Stoneburner, R. L., Rivera, J., Jaffee, H. W., and Schultz, S. (1989) A prospective cohort study of HIV-1 seroconversion in patients with genital ulcer disease in New York City. Presented at the Fifth International Conference on AIDS, Montreal, June 4–9.

Temoshok, L., Moulton, J. M., Elmer, R. M., Sweet, D. M., Baxter, M., and Shalwitz, J. (1989) Youth in detention at high risk for HIV: Knowledge, attitudes and behaviors regarding condom use. Presented at the Fifth International Conference on AIDS, Montreal, June 4–9.

Tolsma, D. D. (1988) Activities of the Centers for Disease Control in AIDS education. *Journal of School Health* 58:133–136.

Trussell, J. (1988) Teenage pregnancy in the United States. *Family Planning Perspectives* 20:262–272.

Turner, C. F., Miller, H. G., and Barker, L. (1989) AIDS research and the behavioral and social sciences. In R. Kulstad, ed., *AIDS, 1988.* Washington, D.C.: American Association for the Advancement of Science.

Turner, C. F., Miller, H. G., and Moses, L. E., eds. (1989) *AIDS, Sexual Behavior, and Intravenous Drug Use.* Washington, D.C.: National Academy Press.

Udry, J. R., and Billy, J. O. G. (1987) Initiation of coitus in early adolescence. *American Sociological Review* 52:841–855.

U.S. Bureau of the Census. (1985) *Statistical Abstract of the United States: 1985.* 105th ed. Washington, D.C.: U.S. Government Printing Office.

U.S. Bureau of the Census. (1987) *Statistical Abstract of the United States: 1988.* 108th ed. Washington, D.C.: U.S. Government Printing Office.

Valdiserri, R. O. (1989) *Preventing AIDS: The Design of Effective Programs.* New Brunswick, N.J.: Rutgers University Press.

van den Hoek, J. A. R., Coutinho, R. A., van Haastrecht, H. J. A., van Zadelhoff, A. W., and Goudsmit, J. (1988) Prevalence and risk factors of HIV infection among drug users and drug-using prostitutes in Amsterdam. *AIDS* 2:55–60.

van den Hoek, J. A. R., van Haastrecht, H. J. A., and Coutinho, R. A. (1990) Risk reduction among intravenous drug users in Amsterdam under the influence of AIDS. *American Journal of Public Health* 79:1355–1357.

Vermund, S. H., Hein, K., Gayle, H. D., Cary, J. M., Thomas, P. A., and Drucker, E. (1989) Acquired immunodeficiency syndrome among adolescents. *American Journal of Diseases in Children* 143:1220–1225.

Vernon, M. E. L., Green, J. A., and Frothingham, T. E. (1983) Teenage pregnancy: A prospective study of self-esteem and other sociodemographic factors. *Pediatrics* 72:632–635.

Vincent, M. L., Clearie, A. F., and Schluchter, M. D. (1987) Reducing adolescent pregnancy through school and community-based education. *Journal of the American Medical Association* 257:3382–3386.

Vlahov, D., Anthony, J. C., Celentano, D. D., Solomon, L., Choudhury, N., and Mandell, W. (1989) Trends of risk reduction among initiates into intravenous drug use 1982–1987. Presented at the Fifth International Conference on AIDS, Montreal, June 4–9.

Voelker, R. (1989) No uniform policy among states on HIV/AIDS education. *American Medical News* September 15:3.

Walker, D. K., Cross, A. W., Heyman, P. W., Ruch-Ross, H., Benson, P., and Tuthill, J. W. G. (1982) Comparisons between inner-city and private school adolescents' perception of health problems. *Journal of Adolescent Health Care* 3:82–90.

Watters, J. K., (1987) Preventing human immunodeficiency virus contagion among intravenous drug users: The impact of street-based education on risk behavior. Presented at the Third International Conference on AIDS, Washington, D.C., June 1–5.

Wetzel, J. R. (1987) *American Youth: A Statistical Snapshot.* Washington, D.C.: The William T. Grant Foundation.

Wiebel, W. W. (1988) Combining ethnographic and epidemiologic methods in targeted AIDS interventions: The Chicago model. In R. J. Battjes, and R. W. Pickens, eds., *Needle Sharing Among Intravenous Drug Abusers: National and International Perspectives.* National Institute on Drug Abuse Research Monograph 80. Washington, D.C.: U.S. Government Printing Office.

Wigersma, L., and Oud, R. (1987) Safety and acceptability of condoms for use by homosexual men as a prophylactic against transmission of HIV during anogenital sexual intercourse. *British Medical Journal* 295:94.

Yamaguchi, K., and Kandel, D. B. (1984a) Patterns of drug use from adolescence to young adulthood: II. Sequences of progression. *American Journal of Public Health* 74:668–672.

Yamaguchi, K., and Kandel, D. B. (1984b) Patterns of drug use from adolescence to young adulthood: III. Predictors of progression. *American Journal of Public Health* 74:673–681.

Yates, G., MacKenzie, R., Pennbridge, J., and Cohen, E. (1988) A risk profile comparison of runaway and non-runaway youth. *American Journal of Public Health* 78:820–821.

Zabin, L. S., and Clark, S. D. (1983) Institutional factors affecting teenagers' choice and reasons for delay in attending a family planning clinic. *Family Planning Perspectives* 15:25–29.

Zabin, L. S., Kantner, J. F., and Zelnik, M. (1979) The risk of adolescent pregnancy in the first months of intercourse. *Family Planning Perspectives* 11:215–222.

Zabin, L. S., Hardy, J. B., Smith, E. A., and Hirsch, M. B. (1986) Substance use and its relation to sexual activity among inner-city adolescents. *Journal of Adolescent Health Care* 7:320–331.

Zelnik, M. (1983) Sexual activity among adolescents: Perspective of a decade. In E. R. McAnarney, ed., *Premature Adolescent Pregnancy and Parenthood.* New York: Grune and Stratton.

Zelnik, M., and Kantner, J. F. (1977) Sexual and contraceptive experience of young unmarried women in the United States, 1976 and 1971. *Family Planning Perspectives* 9:55–71.

Zelnik, M., and Kantner, J. (1979) Reasons for nonuse of contraception by sexually active women aged 15–19. *Family Planning Perspectives* 11:289–296.

Zelnik, M., and Kantner, J. (1980) Sexual activity, contraceptive use and pregnancy among metropolitan-area teenagers: 1971–1979. *Family Planning Perspectives* 12:230–237.

Zelnik, M., and Shah, F. K. (1983) First intercourse among young Americans. *Family Planning Perspectives* 15:64–70.

Zelnik, M., Kantner, J. F., and Ford, K. (1981) *Sex and Pregnancy in Adolescence.* Beverly Hills, Calif.: Sage Publications.

Zenilman, J. (1988) Sexually transmitted diseases in homosexual adolescents. *Journal of Adolescent Health Care* 9:129–138.

Zewdie, D., Abdurahman, M., Ayhunie, S., Adal, G., Tadesse, M., and Yemane, B. T. (1989) High prevalence of HIV-1 antibodies in STD patients with genital ulcers. Presented at the Fifth International Conference on AIDS, Montreal, June 4–9.

Ziffer, J., Ziffer, A., Bywater, M., and Bywater, L. (1989) Knowledge of HIV transmissions and adolescent sexual behavior. Presented at the Fifth International Conference on AIDS, Montreal, June 4–9.

4

Interventions for Female Prostitutes

In the beginning stages of the AIDS epidemic, many people feared that female prostitutes would become widely infected and spread the AIDS virus to their male clients.[1] At present, this fear appears to be unfounded, at least in the United States. The evidence instead suggests that prostitutes' risk of transmission is more closely associated with drug use than with multiple sexual clients. The evidence also indicates that the risk of transmission through sexual contact is greater in the personal relationships of female prostitutes than in their paying ones.[2] Data to support these inferences are sparse, however, because research on prostitution is limited. For this reason, and because the future dynamics of the epidemic are still unclear, there is a continuing need to monitor any future role that prostitution may play in transmitting HIV.

---

[1] The term *prostitute* is used to denote the diverse group of women who exchange sexual acts for money, goods, or services as a means (or partial means) of their livelihood or survival. Other terms—such as sex workers, sex industry workers, and commercial sex workers—have also been used to describe this population in an effort to avoid the judgments that are often associated with the term prostitute. The committee appreciates this distinction but has chosen to use the terms interchangeably. None of the terms are intended to convey any judgment about individuals who work in this area.

Because so little is known about male prostitutes, the committee has restricted its focus to females, although male prostitutes are also at risk of acquiring and spreading HIV infection. One study of 152 male prostitutes recruited from the streets of Atlanta, Georgia, found that 27 percent were infected. Compared with seronegative respondents, male prostitutes who were HIV positive had spent more years as prostitutes, were more likely to self-identify as homosexual, and had had more encounters involving receptive anal intercourse in the month prior to the interview (Elifson et al., 1989).

[2] The rate of HIV infection appears to be highest among prostitutes who report IV drug use (CDC, 1987). A recent study of the prevalence of related viruses (HTLV-I/II) among female prostitutes also found rates to be highest among women who had injected drugs (Khabbaz et al., 1990). In addition, a recent study of prostitutes who did not use drugs found a significant relationship between infection and the number of personal (i.e., nonpaying) heterosexual partners (Darrow et al., 1988).

As is the case for other individuals believed to be at-risk for HIV infection, the design of effective intervention strategies should be informed by an understanding of the risk-associated behaviors of the prostitute and her partners, as well as the conditions under which the behaviors occur. Unfortunately, information about women who work as prostitutes is scant, and knowledge of their clients is sketchier still.[3] The stigmatized and generally illegal nature of prostitution has meant that studies necessarily have had to rely on small nonprobability samples or on ethnographic research, neither of which yields results that can be generalized to the female sex worker population as a whole. Moreover, such studies cannot provide an accurate estimate of the number of women who work as prostitutes. Instead, estimates of the total population are constructed from informed "guesstimates" of knowledgeable observers or from arrest and imprisonment records that capture the subsets of female sex workers who are most likely to come into contact with the criminal justice system–that is, the poor, the inexperienced, minorities, drug users, and women who work the streets (Turner, Miller, and Moses, 1989). Little is known about the occupational histories of prostitutes, but anecdotal evidence suggests that this is a dynamic population. Thus, despite predictions of "once bad, always bad," women tend to move into and out of prostitution; there are few data about these patterns, however, or about the relative amounts of time women spend as sex workers and about when and why former prostitutes return to this work (Goldstein, 1979; Delacoste and Alexander, 1987; Potterat et al., in press).

In the following section, the committee reviews the literature on prostitution as it relates to the AIDS epidemic in the United States. In presenting this overview, the committee wishes to emphasize that our understanding of this population is far from complete and our knowledge of the widely varied contexts in which its members work is limited. Caution must thus be exercised in deriving generalizations from the findings presented below. Although all prostitutes share the common characteristic of exchanging sexual acts for some kind of payment, there is in fact great diversity in all aspects of the social organization of prostitution and its relations to the larger society in which it is embedded.

THE EPIDEMIOLOGY OF AIDS AND
HIV INFECTION AMONG PROSTITUTES

There are no accurate estimates of the prevalence of HIV infection among female prostitutes in the United States. Serologic surveys capture only

---

[3]For examples of research that reflect the perspective of prostitutes, see Jaget (1980), Perkins and Bennett (1985), and Delacoste and Alexander (1987).

those women who volunteer for testing, those who seek care in public clinics for sexually transmitted diseases (STDs), those involved in drug treatment programs, or those in contact with the criminal justice system. Nonetheless, these data shed some light on the distribution of the disease within the population. An important source of information about HIV infection rates among prostitutes is CDC's ongoing multicenter study of 1,396 women, which relies on nonprobability samples of participants from diverse populations around the country. Samples at eight sites were constructed from volunteers who had engaged in prostitution at least once since 1978. The women were recruited from brothels, detention centers, methadone clinics, STD clinics, and networks of "street walkers" and "call girls." Data from this coordinated study (Table 4-1) indicate that the rates of HIV infection among female prostitutes vary greatly from site to site, ranging from zero to 47.5 percent (Darrow et al., in press.)[4]

Yet despite apparently high seroprevalence rates in some areas, HIV infection is not necessarily an occupational hazard for female prostitutes in the United States. Rather, two other factors are indicated: prostitutes are more likely to become infected as a result of unprotected intercourse in the context of a personal relationship than unprotected intercourse with paying clients, and prostitutes who are IV drug users are more likely to acquire HIV infection from contaminated drug injection equipment than from work-related sexual behavior. The risk prostitutes pose to their male clients appears to be minimal, although data regarding these men are extremely limited, in part owing to the criminalization of prostitution and the reluctance of clients to be identified. Nevertheless, the available data on all of these transmission risks argue for continued attention to the differential risk of infection for prostitutes related to IV drug use and differential risk associated with particular contexts of sexual activity.

Risks Related to Drug Use and Sexual Transmission

Data from the CDC multicenter study show that rates of HIV infection are much higher among female sex workers who report a history of IV drug use than among those for whom no evidence of drug use is found (19.9 percent versus 4.8 percent). As shown in Table 4-1, HIV seroprevalence rates vary by locale but are higher in most sites for IV drug users. In addition, in a separate analysis of respondents in this study who did not report IV drug use and had no physical signs of injection, HIV infection was associated with large numbers of personal (i.e., nonpaying) sexual partners (Darrow et al., 1988). Variations in infection rates by locale may

---

[4]These data correct Table 2.8 of Turner, Miller, and Moses (1989:143), which includes the results of 60 serologic retests that were originally reported to the editors as individual respondents.

TABLE 4-1 HIV Seroprevalence in 1986–1987 Among Women Who Reported Engaging in Prostitution (at least once) since January 1978

Site	No. HIV+/No. Tested (%)			Data Collection Source
	Evidence of IV Drug Use	No Evidence of IV Drug Use	All Women	
Southern Nevada	0/10 (0.0)	0/27 (0.0)	0/37 (0.0)	Brothels, brothel applicants
Atlanta	1/65 (1.5)	0/58 (0.0)	1/123 (0.8)	Street and call girl outreach; tabloid advertisement
Colorado Springs	2/52 (3.8)	0/46 (0.0)	2/98 (2.0)	STD, methadone, and HIV screening clinics
Los Angeles	6/163 (3.7)	6/137 (4.4)	12/300 (4.0)	Detention center
San Francisco	10/101 (9.9)	0/111 (0.0)	10/212 (4.7)	Street outreach
Miami	46/173 (26.6)	20/267 (7.5)	66/440 (15.0)	Detention center
South New Jersey	6/14 (42.9)	0/14 (0.0)	6/28 (21.4)	Street outreach
North New Jersey	67/115 (58.3)	8/43 (18.6)	75/158 (47.5)	Methadone and STD clinics; street outreach
Total	138/693 (19.9)	34/703 (4.8)	172/1396 (12.3)	

SOURCE: Darrow et al. (in press).

reflect different injection patterns or different seroprevalence rates in the heterosexual or IV drug-using populations, or they may be an artifact of the disparate sampling schemes used at the several sites. Follow-up studies are now being conducted in Atlanta, Colorado Springs, and San Francisco; these efforts will include prostitutes and their sexual and needle-sharing partners (Darrow et al., 1989).[5]

Although these studies show that the risk for female sex workers is primarily associated with injecting drugs, the proportion of sex workers who inject drugs is not known with any certainty. One estimate, based on a nonprobability sample of 75 arrested sex workers in New York, found that one-third had injected drugs in the past two years; half had injected drugs at least once in their lives (Des Jarlais et al., 1987). However, data collected from CDC's multicenter study indicate greater uncertainty in these estimates: between 27 and 73 percent of prostitutes recruited from settings as diverse as legal brothels and STD clinics were found to have injected drugs at some time (Darrow et al., 1989).

IV drug use may not be evenly distributed throughout the population of female sex workers. Indeed, ethnographic and survey data indicate that needle use is more common among prostitutes who work on the street and among minorities than it is among other sex workers (Goldstein, 1979; Khabbaz et al., 1990).[6] Lower rates of IV drug use among women who work primarily for escort services or brothels would be consistent with the lower rates of HIV infection reported in this group (Fischl et

---

[5]That the source of infection was contaminated injection equipment rather than multiple professional customers is given further credence by the results of Wolfe and colleagues (1989). Their study of 220 female intravenous drug users recruited from methadone maintenance programs and detoxification treatment facilities in San Francisco found that seropositivity was not in fact associated with "paid sex." Moreover, Khabbaz and colleagues' (1990) analyses of data on the prevalence of HTLV-I/II infection from the CDC multicenter study of female prostitutes found statistically significant positive associations between seropositivity for these viruses and the use of shooting galleries, needle-sharing, duration of injecting career, and frequency of drug use. Infection was not associated with number of sexual partners.

[6]In a survey of 1,305 female prostitutes from the CDC multicenter study, 600 reported that they had injected illicit drugs at some time in their lives or had physical signs (needle marks) of IV drug use (Khabbaz et al., 1990). Slightly more than half (318, or 53 percent) were nonwhite (217 blacks, 73 white Hispanics, 13 black Hispanics, 10 American Indians, and 5 Asians). Other analyses of these data find that 84 percent of IV drug-using women reported street prostitution compared with a significantly smaller proportion (74.3 percent) of women with no history or signs of injection (W. W. Darrow, chief of the Social and Behavioral Studies Section, Center for Infectious Diseases, CDC, personal communication, October 6, 1989). In another study of 60 women who reported drug use, Goldstein (1979) found that 43 also reported prostitution. The vast majority (96 percent) of the 25 streetwalkers interviewed in this study reported regular heroin use. In contrast, none of the 18 prostitutes who worked in massage parlors, as call girls, or as madams reported regular use of heroin, although 22 percent had used the drug at least once. Of the 25 streetwalkers interviewed, 64 percent were black, and 20 percent were Hispanic.

al., 1987; Seidlin et al., 1988).[7] In fact, the causal connection, if any, between prostitution and drug use (or vice versa) is unknown. Given the evidence, however, that HIV infection among female prostitutes has occurred mainly among those who use IV drugs and that prostitutes thus appear to be at increased risk for HIV infection primarily through drug use rather than through sexual practices, **the committee recommends that the National Institute on Drug Abuse and the Centers for Disease Control continue to support and strengthen current efforts to understand and intervene in the relationship between drug use and prostitution.**[8] In its first report, the committee recommended that steps be taken to close the vast gaps in knowledge regarding the relationship between sexual behavior and drug use (Turner, Miller, and Moses, 1989). In the case of drug use and prostitution, the committee found that such steps should include better understanding of the following: variations in drug use across different subpopulations of prostitutes, the effect of drug use on risk-associated behaviors, the relationship between drug use and prostitution and the conditions and antecedents surrounding their initiation, and interventions that might protect prostitutes from the threat of HIV infection and other dangers associated with drug use.

In addition to HIV transmission associated with injection practices, risks related to the evolving drug scene—in particular, the threat now presented by noninjected drugs, such as crack—have increased. As discussed in Chapter 1, the use of crack may foster increased demand for sexual services, which can be supplied by women exchanging sex for the drug itself or for money to buy it. Some of the risk associated with prostitutes' nonpaying sexual partners may be related to the use of crack or other drugs. For example, crack use in New York has been associated with sexual transmission of HIV (Chiasson et al., 1989).[9] In addition,

---

[7] A serologic survey of 90 streetwalking female prostitutes recruited from a depressed inner-city area of south Florida and 25 women who worked for an escort service in a middle-class urban area of that state found that 41 percent of the streetwalkers were infected but none of the women from the escort service were seropositive (Fischl et al., 1987). These results are consistent with findings from the CDC multicenter study, in which brothel workers and applicants constituted the group with the lowest rates of IV drug use and the lowest rates of HIV infection (Darrow et al., in press).

[8] CDC supports ongoing studies of female prostitutes in several cities (see Table 4-1) that are investigating the sexual and social networks of prostitutes as well as strategies for outreach, treatment, and social mobilization of female sex workers. NIDA funds outreach and education programs for a diverse population of women, including prostitutes.

[9] In a study of HIV infection among patients seeking treatment at an STD clinic, Chiasson and coworkers (1989) found that, among twelve infected men who reported no same-gender sexual contact, no IV drug use, and no sexual contact with a person known to be infected with HIV, three had a history of sexual contact with known crack users, one was a crack user himself, and eight reported contacts with prostitutes. Furthermore, of the six seropositive women identified in this study who also reported no

Shedlin (1987) reports that female prostitutes recruited primarily through drug treatment programs in New York City and Bridgeport, Connecticut, identified "crack addiction" as one of the primary reasons for engaging in unprotected intercourse, particularly among younger women who worked on the streets. Friedman and coworkers' (1988) ethnographic research on "crack houses" (buildings in which crack is sold and used) also confirmed the link between crack use and unprotected intercourse and, occasionally, street prostitution. Many of the acts of unprotected intercourse reported by Friedman and colleagues occurred between male IV drug users and female crack users,[10] thus increasing the risk of spread of the virus.

Clearly, the risks associated with crack are related to unprotected intercourse rather than to a specific characteristic of the drug or the route of administration. The context of the sexual encounter is thus an important factor in differential rates of HIV transmission. Also of importance to the level of HIV transmission risk shared by female prostitutes and their clients is the specific set of sexual activities the client purchases. These factors are discussed in the sections that follow.

Context-Related Risks

The context of the sex-for-money exchange involves a variety of elements, from setting and time limitations to cultural preferences and the nature of the relationship between the partners. Most sexual encounters with female prostitutes are brief. For street prostitutes, the time from striking the bargain—which activities for what price—to their return to the street may be only a dozen minutes or so. More extended periods of time and a wider variety of sexual techniques are generally more expensive and primarily characteristic of outcall or other off-street practitioners. Within time-limited contexts, oral sex is frequently preferred by both clients and prostitutes (see, e.g., Shedlin, 1987). Neither partner need remove his or her clothing, and the act is usually over quickly, thus reducing vulnerability for both. It may also reduce transmission risks among female prostitutes and their male clients.

On the other hand, clients' sexual technique preferences vary substantially by class and culture. Although street prostitutes in New York report that oral sex is the activity of preference (Des Jarlais et al., 1987),

---

history of IV drug use or sexual contact with an infected individual, four were prostitutes who used crack.

[10] In this study, ex-addict street outreach workers were used to identify informants among residents of buildings that served as crack houses. They reported that male addicts found female crack users to be an inexpensive and readily available source of sexual gratification.

women who work as prostitutes among newly immigrant Latino populations report that vaginal intercourse is preferred by their clients (Magana and Carrier, in press). In these cases, transmission risks may be higher, particularly if there is a history of STDs or current infection. In addition, some men may choose anal intercourse, which carries an even greater risk of viral transmission, particularly if condoms are not used. The frequency of anal sex in this population is not known.[11] Not all female prostitutes offer this service; others may charge premium rates for anal sex, which may reduce demand. It is clear, however, that the distribution of sexual techniques offered by women and desired by clients in any community could affect rates of viral transmission. The need for safer sex practices and the ability to modify dangerous practices are affected by the degree to which these practices are ingrained in the local culture, as well as by the strength of an individual client's desires.

The use of condoms for protection against HIV and other STDs appears to vary with the nature of the relationship between the sexual partners. Several studies of condom use among female prostitutes report that unprotected intercourse is more likely to occur in the context of a personal relationship than in a paid transaction. In an earlier (1987) report of the ongoing CDC multicenter study, more than 80 percent of the women surveyed reported at least occasional use of condoms, but that use was much more likely to occur with clients (78 percent) than with husbands or boyfriends (16 percent). In a sample of approximately 500 prostitutes living in the San Francisco area (who were recruited by other prostitutes hired to do outreach and through sex-related media), J. B. Cohen and coworkers (1989) found that 90 percent reported at least one instance of condom use with paying customers. In fact, 38 percent said they always used condoms with clients, compared with only 14 percent who sometimes used condoms with husbands or boyfriends. Studies of prostitutes in Europe have also found less reported use of condoms in the context of personal relationships than in professional ones (Day, Ward, and Harris, 1988; Hooykaas et al., 1989).[12] In fact, it is among sex

---

[11] There are, however, some preliminary data on this practice from the CDC multicenter study. More than one-third (36.3 percent) of the women in the study reported at least one episode of anal intercourse (W. W. Darrow, chief of the Social and Behavioral Studies Section, Center for Infectious Diseases, CDC, personal communication, October 6, 1989).

[12] In a study of 91 prostitutes recruited from an STD clinic in London, Day, Ward, and Harris (1988) reported that more than half (59 percent) of the women reported consistent condom use with paying customers. Of the 71 women who reported vaginal intercourse with their boyfriends, 6 percent said they used condoms consistently with these partners. The differential pattern of condom use did not change over the course of the 17-month study; however, the percentage indicating condom use increased for both groups.

workers with large numbers of nonpaying sexual partners that the risk of sexual transmission of HIV infection has been found to be highest (Darrow et al., 1988).

The lower frequency of condom use in personal relationships may have something to do with the distinction both female prostitutes and their husbands or boyfriends make between intimate sexual acts and paid sex (J. B. Cohen, 1989). Shedlin (1987), for example, noted that the prostitutes in her study differentiated between what they did with clients and intimate acts reserved for their personal partners, such as kissing. In another study (Darrow et al., in press), female prostitutes reported that their personal sexual partners saw themselves as having a low risk of infection because they believed the women consistently used condoms with clients. As a result, many prostitutes reported difficulties in persuading their private partners to use condoms.

Client-Related Risks

The extent of the risk of HIV infection for paying customers of prostitutes is not known with certainty, but the number of cases ascribed to contact with female sex workers has not been large, and the few existing studies of prostitutes' clients have found relatively low rates of HIV infection. However, data on clients come from a limited group of studies that have relied on small, nonprobability samples, and their results must be interpreted with caution. Wallace, Mann, and Beatrice (1988) recruited paying customers of prostitutes through advertisements in a New York City weekly newspaper, television and radio news stories about the study, ads placed at union headquarters, and hotline referrals. Interviews and blood specimens were obtained from 340 men with a history of sexual contact with female prostitutes and no other risk factors for infection. Six of the men were found to be infected. Upon reinterview, however, three later admitted other risk behavior, leaving three (0.9 percent) seropositive men whose only alleged risk factor was unprotected sexual contact with a prostitute. These three infected men reported a mean of 575 lifetime contacts with prostitutes (compared to an overall average of 94 contacts for study participants). As noted earlier, although the risk of infection for female sex workers is not clearly related to the number of clients, this study provides some evidence, albeit limited, that for clients a large number of prostitute contacts may be associated with a greater risk of acquiring HIV.

In another study, Chiasson and colleagues (1988) recruited 671 men from a New York City STD clinic and found that 138 men reported no risk factors for AIDS except vaginal intercourse with prostitutes. Of the 138 men, 2 (1.4 percent) were found to be infected. Among 222 respondents who reported no risk factors at all, 3 men (1.4 percent) were found to be seropositive. The following year, the same investigators (Chiasson et al., 1989) collected data from 955 men recruited from another New York STD clinic situated in an area in which the cumulative HIV incidence rate was high and drug use, including the use of crack, was common. Of the 571 men with no identifiable risk factors, 262 reported contacts with prostitutes, and 15 (5.7 percent) of the 262 men were antibody positive. (In addition, five seropositive men reported sexual contact with known crack users.) Neither study reported the average number of prostitute contacts for the infected men. Nevertheless, the higher infection rate in the second study suggests the need for continued monitoring of the population of men who report sexual contact with prostitutes.

Finally, in a CDC follow-up study of 1,138 AIDS cases originally diagnosed in adult males with no reported risk factors, investigators were able to identify a risk factor in all but 281 of the cases. Of these 281 remaining cases with no identifiable risk factor, 178 were reinterviewed. Ninety-six of these men responded to the question on prostitute contact, and 33 reported contact with female sex workers. These 33 men account for only 0.08 percent of the 41,770 adult cases of AIDS diagnosed at the time of the study (Castro et al., 1989), thus suggesting a limited transmission threat posed by female prostitutes.

Although these data affirm the possibility that female prostitutes can transmit infection, questions regarding the accuracy of risk reporting may cast doubt on any conclusion regarding the extent of such transmission. A problem relevant to reporting prostitute contact is response bias attributable to deliberate misreports of behavior to project an image of "social desirability." Castro and colleagues (1989), for example, suggest that men who engage in risk-associated behaviors other than contact with female sex workers may nevertheless report prostitute contact to prevent further investigation of other risk factors the respondent may consider more sensitive or stigmatizing (e.g., same-gender sexual contacts). (Chapter 6 provides a more detailed discussion of the difficulties in validating self-reported data on sexual practices.) Although the number of men who have become infected through contact with female prostitutes is not known, it appears to be small when compared with the number of men who report other risk behaviors.

In its first report, the committee recognized both the need for and the difficulties involved in collecting high-quality data on the clients of female prostitutes. At that time, a number of possible approaches were suggested: studies using household samples in which men are asked about contact with prostitutes; specialized samples of men who might not be reached through household samples but who nonetheless are or have been associated with prostitutes; special studies of men who are particularly likely to use the services of prostitutes; and studies of men from cultures in which the patronage of prostitutes is considered part of the normative repertoire of sexual behavior. The committee reaffirms its support for these suggestions. In addition, because so little is known about the role of prostitutes' clients in the spread of HIV infection, **the committee recommends that the Public Health Service undertake a series of feasibility studies to determine the best ways to gather appropriate information about prostitutes' clients and their role in the spread of HIV to the larger population.**

The segment of the female prostitute population that does not inject drugs appears to pose only a limited threat to clients at this time, and sexual contact with clients appears to be less of a threat to prostitutes than either drug use or personal sexual relationships. However, as other populations have demonstrated, the problem of HIV infection is not static. The risks may, indeed, be limited, but changes seen over the course of the first decade of the epidemic argue for continued vigilance. Given the factors that are known to distinguish the risk profile of many prostitutes (unprotected sexual contacts and IV drug use), **the committee recommends that the Centers for Disease Control continue to monitor the effects of the AIDS epidemic in this population. Activities should include a continuing, systematic effort to track the incidence and prevalence of both HIV infection and sexually transmitted diseases in this group.** To reach both prostitutes and their clients, knowledge of the varying patterns of prostitution and prostitute patronage is critical. The available data on such patterns are presented in the following section.

PATTERNS OF PROSTITUTION

Stereotypical depictions of prostitution tend to present two ends of a spectrum: the pathos associated with streetwalkers and the sophisticated elegance of call girls. The reality is that women who engage in prostitution have a wide range of lifestyles, work in many different milieus, and have varying feelings about their work, ranging from degradation and despair to pride (James, 1977; B. Cohen, 1980; Carmen and Moody, 1985; Perkins and Bennett, 1985; Delacoste and Alexander, 1987; Shedlin, 1987). These differing patterns have important implications for intervention efforts. The place of work, services offered, number of clients served, local prevalence of infection, and availability and use of protective measures are all factors that affect the risk of HIV infection for female prostitutes, and they should be taken into account in the design and delivery of AIDS prevention programs for this population. Several different lifestyles of female prostitutes and their implications for outreach and intervention strategies are described below.

Street Prostitution

The most familiar form of prostitution, and the one that draws the most attention, is street prostitution (James, 1977; Alexander, 1987). Carmen and Moody (1985) report that in this country the preponderance of recreational sex involves random, unplanned activity. Thus, it makes sense that prostitutes congregate around locations where travel may be delayed, tourists are at loose ends, or men find themselves free of work-related obligations, affording them time to spend with sex workers. In the urban setting, street prostitution often occurs in "stroll districts" in which potential clients can be found: streets near hotels (whether downtown or near airports), fast-food restaurants, train stations, and bus stations frequented by tourists and other transients (James, 1977; B. Cohen, 1980; Carmen and Moody, 1985). Rural variations include truck-stop prostitution; female sex workers solicit clients in the parking lots of restaurants where long-haul truckers congregate or make contact with them through CB radios (Luxenberg and Klein, 1984). Other women, traveling in groups of two or three, may work a circuit that might include conventions, migrant labor camps, lumber camps, job training camps, or work camps (James, 1977). Perhaps less obvious to the general public is prostitution that occurs in bars, a pattern in which women solicit clients and leave to have sex in another location, perhaps a hotel room. Women who work the streets are more likely than other groups of prostitutes to have pimps, although an unknown proportion of street prostitutes work independently (James, 1977; Alexander, 1987).[13]

Patterns of street prostitution may be similar across cities of the same size and culture, but they may be dissimilar across regions of the country and across cities of unequal size. The visibility of street prostitution is particularly affected by aggressive law enforcement efforts, which generally focus on women who are openly soliciting business (James, 1977).[14] Indeed, highly proactive police work and long sentences can drive street prostitutes (and massage parlors) out of a specific city or neighborhood, at least temporarily. Few jurisdictions of any size,

---

[13] The female prostitute who works alone—either through circumstances beyond her control or more often by choice—is referred to as an "outlaw" (Carmen and Moody, 1985).

[14] Such differential enforcement often results in an overrepresentation of street prostitutes in statistics generated by the criminal justice system.

however, will expend the level of effort necessary to reduce prostitution substantially. More often, police will engage in management efforts to "keep it within bounds" through periodic sweeps and crusades that increase the work-related expenses of female sex workers (e.g., time off the job, bail and other legal fees) and sometimes inconvenience clients but rarely change the form or prevalence of the activity.

The perception that intermittent police intervention (e.g., harassment, searches, arrests, detention) decreases the prevalence of prostitution is in part a function of removing women from the street to jails. But this is merely a temporary absence, part of what James (1977) calls the "revolving door" of street/jail/street. For women who are not detained, police intervention may result in migration to other areas. The migratory pattern of street work is well recognized by researchers who have studied prostitutes and is referred to as "horizontal mobility" or the "scatter syndrome" (Carmen and Moody, 1985:194). In fact, Carmen and Moody (1985) suggest that short-term police crackdowns have more impact on migratory patterns of female prostitutes than on the practice of prostitution per se. For women who are detained, Alexander (1987) postulates that the usual activities of the police may reinforce reliance on pimps who can arrange for bail or attend to child care needs while the women are in custody, but that such activities are unlikely to be effective in reducing the prevalence of prostitution.

One consequence of migration is the problem it poses for AIDS outreach workers who wish to contact these women or, once reached, to maintain contact with them. There are also other repercussions associated with scatter and mobility. Without repeated contact with the targeted group, intervention staff may find it difficult to develop the credibility and trust needed to convey information and provide services, especially to a population that is suspicious of authority figures. Moreover, women who have migrated to new areas may find themselves more vulnerable and therefore more amenable to enticements offered by pimps. Not only may mobility impair efforts to find and retain street prostitutes in prevention programs but the interpolation of pimps as mediators with the outside world may also undermine the ability of street outreach workers to identify and establish contact with prostitutes.

IV drug use is thought to be more common among street prostitutes than among other sex workers, and streetwalkers are also more likely to be poor and minority women (James, 1977; Goldstein, 1979). Some prostitutes report resorting to drug use as a result of their work; others report starting a career in prostitution to support a drug habit (Goldstein,

1979).[15] (The role of crack in fostering prostitution is addressed later in this chapter.) As noted earlier, the relationship between prostitution and drug use is unclear, but the potential for HIV transmission has been established in situations in which both factors are present. Therefore, directing AIDS intervention efforts toward prostitutes who inject drugs makes eminent good sense.

Bar prostitution coexists with street prostitution but is less likely to result in arrest because police generally have to spend more resources to identify and entrap prostitutes who work in bars (so-called B girls). An observant bartender familiar with local vice squad personnel can either assist or foil police efforts (James, 1977). Some women who work in bars are afforded protection or at least a warning of ongoing police activity by the bartender, but these women must pay for this service by "pushing" drinks. (Whether bar prostitutes are independent or controlled by pimps, they often give large tips to the bartender or owner of the establishment.) At the same time, bar prostitutes are not entirely safe from police intervention. Because bartenders or owners are accountable to the police and other agencies that regulate alcohol sales, they sometimes find it useful to turn prostitutes over to the police intermittently. The usually clandestine activity of bar prostitutes hampers outreach efforts to prevent AIDS in this population.

Brothels

Prostitutes who work in brothels constitute another subgroup of the female sex worker population, and this subset of women can be further subdivided into workers at legal or illegal houses of prostitution. In the United States, brothels are legal places of business only in certain parts of Nevada and are separated from the rest of the town, often with fences (James, 1977; Carmen and Moody, 1985). The movements of women who work in Nevada's legal brothels are severely restricted (Carmen and Moody, 1985; Alexander, 1987). Because prostitutes are required to register with the sheriff (a process that includes fingerprinting), these restrictions are generally enforceable (James, 1977; Alexander, 1987). Registered prostitutes are not allowed to enter or solicit customers in a gambling casino or bar (although other women may be "working" there), be in the company of a man on the street or in a restaurant, or reside in the same community in which they work. They are required to live in the brothel during a three-week work shift; after their shift, they are off

---

[15]In Goldstein's (1979) research, 58 percent of the streetwalkers participating in the study started using heroin once they became prostitutes; 24 percent had used heroin regularly before their entry into prostitution.

duty for a week or more during which time they are expected to leave town.

Prostitutes in Nevada's legal brothels undergo mandatory weekly testing for gonorrhea and monthly testing for syphilis and HIV infection (Alexander, 1987; Rowe and Ryan, 1987), and each woman is required to pay for her own tests, which cost approximately $150 per month. There is little evidence of HIV infection among prostitutes working in legalized brothels (CDC, 1987; Rowe and Ryan, 1987). Moreover, the percentage of legal brothel workers and applicants reporting a history of IV drug use (27 percent) was lower than among any other group of sex workers who participated in the CDC multicenter study (Darrow et al., in press).

Life in illegal brothels may be quite different. Rules of behavior, residence, and personal care are generally more flexible and are set by the local establishment. Typically, a brothel is managed by a "madam," but it may be run by an owner of either sex (James, 1977; Alexander, 1987). Female prostitutes who work in such brothels (on eight-hour shifts) generally live elsewhere (James, 1977). The extent of IV drug use in these establishments is unclear, although it has been reported that sex workers with a reputation for heavy drug use are excluded from employment in some brothels because of the problems associated with drug dependence (Goldstein, 1979).

Compared with drives against street prostitution, the suppression of off-street sex work, such as brothel employment, requires even greater efforts on the part of the law enforcement system, and few jurisdictions are willing to commit the resources necessary to eliminate this type of prostitution. For one thing, brothels are not always easy to identify, although they usually come to the notice of the police if they are of any size. The visibility of illegal brothels and their accessibility to the general public often depend on levels of local tolerance. Historically, "red-light districts" in the United States have housed many illegal yet tolerated brothels. At present, brothels appear to be less open to the general public, but they continue to be known to many individuals (cabdrivers, bartenders, others who may refer business to them). Nevertheless, for the purposes of AIDS prevention, most such organizations are difficult to identify and contact.

Massage Parlors

Other prostitutes work in massage parlors, spas, encounter studios, and other businesses with euphemistic names for essentially the same services. These businesses are generally identifiable from the street (Alexander, 1987). Not all massage parlors offer sexual services, but in those that do, it is customary for the masseuses to make arrangements with the customer regarding the services to be delivered and for the owner to feign ignorance of this illicit activity (James, 1977). The owners and managers of these businesses, who legally are considered pimps and panderers, may be resistant to onsite AIDS prevention programs for workers or clients, in part out of fear that such activities may be a prelude to or a "setup" for arrest.

In several U.S. cities, including San Francisco, massage parlors and their employees are required to obtain work licenses from the police department (Alexander, 1987), establishing a de facto form of legalized prostitution in this one setting. Paradoxically, however, women with a history of arrests for prostitution are denied licenses, and licenses are revoked after an arrest for prostitution.

Outcall Prostitution

Another segment of the prostitute population works on an "outcall" basis. The traditional call girl works independently, with a "book" of steady clients who are contacted by phone. Instead of recruiting clients from the street or meeting them in brothels or other centralized locations, the call girl sets up her own referral system (James, 1977; Alexander, 1987). A call girl may develop a list of phone numbers of potential clients in a variety of ways, including the purchase of names from other call girls (James, 1977). When business is slow, income can often be generated by telephoning known customers and extending invitations. Usually, call girls are more affluent and have better working conditions than most prostitutes (Gagnon and Simon, 1973; James, 1977; B. Cohen, 1980; Shedlin, 1987). Prices for services may vary, but the generally higher socioeconomic status of their clients provides call girls with a higher price per transaction than is received by most prostitutes. In addition, because of their lower public visibility, call girls generally have fewer problems with the police than do streetwalkers.

Over the last two decades, "escort services," originally an outcall feature of massage parlors, have begun to develop as businesses in their own right. The owner of an escort service that employs female sex workers meets the legal definition of a pimp. Unlike pimps who may have sexual or personal relationships with street prostitutes, however, the relationship between the owner of an escort service and a call girl is usually restricted to business. In general, there is little or no personal contact between sex workers and agents.

There are certain legal benefits to this new system of services. Managers of escort agencies can deny knowledge of sexual transactions between clients and employees, claiming that the only service advertised and offered is companionship. Moreover, because the fee is understood to include sexual services, the outcall worker does not have to discuss price, which makes it difficult for law enforcement personnel to collect evidence of solicitation (Perkins and Bennett, 1985). Many cities license escort services through the police department, again barring anyone with a history of prostitution-related arrests from obtaining a license.

The implications for AIDS prevention of this pattern of prostitution are still unclear. For example, the extent of drug use in these establishments is not known, but at least one ethnographic study has reported that many of the "better" agencies forbid drug use (Shedlin, 1987). What is clear is that prostitutes who work on an outcall basis (either through an escort service or on their own) are among the least visible and most independent of all prostitute subgroups.[16] This independence may exacerbate existing problems in gaining access to this subgroup to provide AIDS education.

Crack and Prostitution

In the past, women often engaged in sex with men for a "taste" of heroin or cocaine, or they might work as prostitutes to make money to purchase their own supply. In a number of urban settings a new form of sexual barter has arisen in connection with the widespread use of crack. Crack-related prostitution displays some similarities with past practices involving drug-sex interaction, but certain features of crack suggest that the use of this drug may evoke a qualitatively different situation. For example, crack provides only short-term effects (addicts often require 10 to 20 "hits" per day); there is evidence of increased sexual arousal among men who smoke crack (unlike heroin, which tends to dampen sexual excitement); and because the drug is so inexpensive (a vial may cost less than $5, a "toke" as little as 50 cents), very young people—including girls in their early teens—can afford it. Some of these young women engage in sex with men either directly for the drug or for money with which to purchase it. Men who wish to have sex with these young women (either when they themselves have taken crack or when they have not) can purchase these sexual services quite inexpensively. Some of the women become so-called "crack whores," spending a great deal of time in crack houses and engaging in sex with customers. Because

---

[16]Most male escorts, also known as call boys, work independently, although there are some organized male escort services (Pittman, 1971; Gagnon and Simon, 1973; Perkins and Bennett, 1985).

money may not change hands or is immediately used for drugs rather than subsistence, the women exchanging sex for drugs may not consider themselves to be prostitutes and, indeed, may not view their actions as work.

Researchers in this area report ethnographic evidence that crack has begun to change street prostitution. Outreach workers in Harlem, for example, have found that very young teenage girls engage in sexual intercourse with IV drug users to receive crack (Friedman et al., 1988). In a study of 82 teenage female crack users from the San Francisco area, 24 (29 percent) reported exchanging sexual favors for drugs or money (Fullilove et al., 1990). In some areas, older, more experienced women are leaving the streets because of their fear of AIDS and the violence associated with crack; younger women addicted to this drug are taking their place (Shedlin, 1987).[17]

In the case of crack, the risk of HIV infection is related to the exchange of sex for drugs and the disinhibition associated with crack use that fosters frequent unprotected sex (Friedman et al., 1988; Abramowitz et al., 1989; Worth et al., 1989). Because crack is highly addictive and provides only a short-term "high," supporting a crack habit may require a large number of sexual partners or sexual acts, thus amplifying the risk for HIV infection (Weissman, 1988). Because a woman may have multiple partners during the course of one time period at a crack house, one would predict a significant level of HIV risk associated with the activity if there is infection among local crack users or their sexual partners. The committee has already commented in Chapter 1 on research relating crack use to HIV and other STDs (Chiasson et al., 1989; J. B. Cohen et al., 1989; Fullilove et al., 1989). It reiterates here its counsel on the need to monitor the spread of infection among crack users.

INTERVENTION PROGRAMS

The picture of prostitution that emerges from these limited data is not an integrated one. Rather, it is a composite of very different women, some working independently, others with procurers; soliciting on the streets or working in organized sites; earning subsistence wages or lucrative incomes; living with drug dependence or living drug free. Some women, such as those who exchange sex for crack, do not view their activities as work at all and do not see themselves as part of the sex industry. Many, perhaps most, have other identities in addition to their sex work

---

[17] Once on the street, these young women may also be at increased risk of initiating heroin use (Friedman et al., 1988).

roles. This diversity needs to be considered in designing intervention strategies for reducing HIV risk because it has important consequences for selecting access routes to the various subpopulations and for tailoring the content of interventions. In addition, at least two essential themes have been noted by those who have worked with female prostitutes: for a message to be heard, the source must be trustworthy and nonjudgmental, and the content must reflect sex workers' interests.

Access

At first glance, it might seem sensible to launch AIDS intervention activities from existing institutional bases (such as law enforcement agencies, STD clinics, or other public health programs) because these locations are typical points of contact with some sex workers. However, prostitutes' experiences with these institutions in many instances have not led to relationships of trust. As a result, intervention efforts made by or through these agencies may be severely handicapped in terms of earning participant trust and gaining acceptance of the AIDS prevention messages being delivered (Stephens et al., 1989).

The theory of adoption and diffusion of innovation predicts that trusted and respected leaders in any community are important resources to be mobilized in the design and implementation stages of activities to introduce a new product or procedure (Rogers, 1962; Becker, 1970; Rogers and Adhikarya, 1980). For this reason, involving prostitutes and ex-prostitutes directly in the design and implementation of AIDS prevention programs may instill trust and facilitate access to the population and the recruitment of participants; it may also help to ensure that the implemented programs reflect the needs of prostitutes and the diversity of contexts in which they work. Peer-led programs involve the target audience as part of the solution to the problem rather than as merely the object of their efforts. Several existing AIDS programs for female prostitutes in this country and abroad have used women from the sex industry as part of their outreach and educational efforts (Locking, 1988; Sanchez, 1988; J. B. Cohen et al., 1989; Kinnell and Griffiths, 1989; Monny-Lobe et al., 1989b; Nichols et al., 1989; Rosario et al., 1989; Stephens et al., 1989). The knowledge that these women bring to a project regarding the local population has often been important in encouraging recruitment, maintaining participation, and ensuring follow-up.

Understanding how the business of prostitution is organized is important for designing methods to gain access to the different groups of female sex workers. Prostitutes who work independently (e.g., call girls) are often difficult to contact because they are less visible and accessible than other sex workers. In addition, they may be the most isolated of all sex workers and the least integrated into information networks. Researchers have located independent sex workers through ads in daily newspapers, classified telephone directories, sex-related newspapers, and other media.[18] Ethnographic research may also be used to identify and utilize existing networks of independent sex workers to reach this subpopulation. For example, Shedlin's (1987) model for delivering AIDS prevention education to prostitutes grew out of her work with a group of female street prostitutes who had initially been recruited to receive other social services. (For descriptions of additional programs, see also B. Cohen [1980] and Carmen and Moody [1985].) Finally, current and former street prostitutes may be able to deliver health messages effectively by contacting women who are currently in the industry.

Workers in organized sites, such as brothels, massage parlors, escort services, and the like, are less visible than street workers but may be more accessible for prevention efforts (especially those delivered by former sex workers), even though the illegal nature of prostitution may make managers reluctant to allow educators access to workers. Individuals who have established intervention programs for prostitutes at organized sites offer the following advice for the design and execution of AIDS prevention projects. First, problems can arise if project staff become overly identified with the owners of organized prostitution sites. The prevention efforts offered by these projects should be presented as a resource for sex workers, acting, for example, as an advocacy group to support prostitutes' rights to safe working conditions. Second, in areas where prostitution is illegal, management personnel of organized sites must be convinced of the trustworthiness of AIDS outreach workers and the benefits to be gained from safer sex practices. (Without the cooperation of the management, it will be extremely difficult to identify and contact women working in these establishments.)[19] Finally, managers of organized sites may discourage prostitutes from using condoms because

---

[18] In Holland (Paalman and deVries, 1988), outreach efforts for both female prostitutes and their clients also provide condom-promoting messages in pornographic magazines, on radio stations, and through posters. For additional information on methods of reaching the population of female prostitutes, see J. B. Cohen and colleagues (1988b).

[19] In such cases it may be possible to design health education projects that involve currently employed women as agents of education and training. One such program in the Dominican Republic uses a train-the-trainers strategy wherein working prostitutes are elected by their peers as representatives of the local sex workers' community to participate in a Ministry of Public Health project, the National Struggle Against AIDS. These representatives are trained to provide safer sex information, education, and motivation to their fellow workers (Rosario et al., 1989).

they fear losing business and consequently income. The implementation of AIDS prevention efforts may be particularly difficult if some sites in a community promote the use of condoms and others do not. Because some clients are not willing to use condoms, such a two-tiered system may draw business away from prostitutes who insist on protected sex and contribute to conditions under which HIV and other STDs can spread. Alternatively, with the appropriate introduction, condom use may provide a positive selling point for such businesses, as both prostitutes and clients become more aware of AIDS. The Australian experiment discussed in the next section has tried to implement a universal condom policy in a manner that enhances the attractiveness of a brothel.

Types of Interventions

Ideally, any intervention program for female prostitutes should serve its targeted population in a nonjudgmental fashion, forming partnerships that will help each individual understand her level of risk, make appropriate behavioral changes, and facilitate the development of required skills to sustain those changes over time. In the case of sex workers, it may be particularly important to state the spirit and goals of the program in clear, unambiguous language. Because prostitutes have often been stigmatized by society and labeled as deviant by some research activities, AIDS education and research programs targeting this population need to stress that their goal is to help prostitutes protect themselves from HIV infection. Conversely, if female sex workers perceive the primary purpose of interventions to be the protection of clients, it may be difficult to gain their trust and cooperation.

Because the major risk factor associated with infection among prostitutes appears to be IV drug use, AIDS prevention should highlight drug treatment and safer injection projects, as well as the prevention of IV drug use. As noted earlier, such efforts would surely benefit from a better understanding of the connection between IV drug use and prostitution. It is also vital to provide instructions regarding safer needle use for women who continue to inject drugs. Both referral to treatment and education about safer injection practices can be delivered through street outreach projects. For example, outreach programs to distribute bleach to drug users in New York and San Francisco have incorporated street counseling and drug treatment referral (Des Jarlais, 1987). These program components are being delivered in outreach projects directed toward prostitutes, using mechanisms as innovative as a prostitute collective, which was organized by the New York City ADAPT (Association for Drug Abuse Prevention and Treatment) project for participation in a series of weekly meetings to discuss drug and sex risk reduction techniques (Friedman et al., 1989).

The second increased risk factor for female sex workers is multiple unprotected sex acts. Many of the safer sex education programs designed for the broader population of women at risk may also be appropriate for women who work in the sex industry. In their personal lives, prostitutes enact the same intimate roles (e.g., spouses, lovers) as women in the larger female population. In addition, however, they face unique problems in changing high-risk sexual practices because sex occurs not only in a personal context but also with clients. Intervention programs for prostitutes must take into account the number and diversity of risk behaviors in which sex workers engage and the contexts in which these behaviors are enacted.

Many existing street outreach programs are designed to protect street prostitutes from HIV infection by providing them with information about safer sex and IV drug use practices. An example of such a program is the ongoing California Prostitutes Education Project (CAL-PEP). This program employs former female street prostitutes who walk through stroll districts, introducing themselves and the program as they encounter sex workers. The outreach workers provide information about how AIDS is transmitted and how to prevent infection (both injection based and sexually transmitted). They distribute small bottles of bleach and instructions on how to clean injection equipment, as well as safer-sex kits (small plastic bags containing five different kinds of condoms and safer-sex guidelines) (Alexander, 1988). CAL-PEP also holds monthly workshops for street workers. Training sessions include a number of components: a discussion of how HIV is transmitted and how to prevent infection; a demonstration of how to clean injection equipment; a demonstration of how to use condoms (including instructions on using condoms for oral sex as well as for vaginal and anal intercourse, avoiding breakage, and using a lubricating spermicide for additional protection); and a practice session for newly learned skills and roles, with special emphasis on encouraging the cooperation of both paying clients and nonpaying partners in the use of safer-sex practices. The project has also established support groups to provide a comfortable opportunity for prostitutes to continue to discuss their concerns about AIDS, obstacles to behavioral change, and strategies for facilitating change. Support group sessions have been held in a van, in hotel rooms, and in places where prostitutes congregate.

Similar peer-led intervention workshops have also been conducted for organized workers in brothels, massage parlors, sex clubs, erotic dancing theaters, and other locations that employ sex workers.[20] As noted earlier, many of these projects use current and former prostitutes familiar with a particular work location to win over management and gain access to sex workers.[21] For example, in a program developed by the Australian Prostitutes Collective, outreach teams contacted the managers of brothels to make arrangements for bringing safer-sex and IV drug use training sessions onto the premises (Overs and Hunter, 1989). This program also developed a Safe House Endorsement policy: houses that enacted and enforced mandatory condom policies and maintained good working conditions received a certificate of endorsement from the project. Project planners hoped to encourage the patronage of only those houses that had received endorsements.

Another type of intervention—voluntary anonymous counseling and HIV antibody testing of prostitutes in the context of a supportive environment —has been advocated and implemented in several communities. However, the lack of solid evaluation data on the vast majority of programs precludes drawing firm conclusions about the effectiveness of these efforts in changing behavior.[22] Where mandatory HIV antibody testing has also been implemented (e.g., for convictions of prostitution or as a prerequisite to drug treatment), prostitutes have expressed resentment (Shedlin, 1987). Jurisdictions that encourage voluntary testing while mandating HIV tests for women convicted of prostitution may compromise the usefulness of voluntary testing. At the least, such a policy sends out mixed messages to sex workers, raising serious doubts about the benefits these women may gain from testing and how information on test results is to be used (Decker, 1987; J.B. Cohen, Alexander, and Wofsy, 1988; Rosenberg and Weiner, 1988).

Some intervention programs advocate eliminating prostitution but

---

[20] In Holland, outreach programs for female prostitutes have distributed brochures on protective measures to prevent HIV and other STDs, towels bearing the slogan "Nice and Safe, Use a Condom," and calling cards with this message in eight languages to facilitate communication with clients (Paalman and deVries, 1988). In addition, clients of prostitutes have been organized to serve as distributors of condoms to other prospective clients.

[21] Peer-led programs from several other countries have reported promising results in behavioral change among prostitutes (Ngugi et al., 1988; Monny-Lobe et al., 1989a,b; Plummer et al., 1989). In some studies, self-reports of behavioral change have been supported by decreased rates of HIV seroconversion and of other STDs (Ngugi et al., 1988).

[22] In a prospective study of 240 sexually active women from the San Francisco area, J. B. Cohen and coworkers (1988a) found substantial risk reduction at 6- to 12-month follow-ups after HIV antibody testing. However, 11 percent of the women tested continued to report IV drug use, 24 percent reported anal sex, and 32 percent reported more than 10 sexual partners. For additional information on designs for the evaluation of both counseling and testing projects and community-based outreach, see Coyle, Boruch, and Turner (1990).

neglect important economic realities. Prostitution provides better economic incentives and more flexible work schedules than many other jobs available to women who are likely to have few alternative employment opportunities. If intervention programs do not include vocational training components, they may well be unsuccessful because they do not address the limited occupational skills and survival needs of this population (Decker, 1987). Making the transition to lower-paying legitimate jobs can be difficult for many female sex workers, but the process may be eased with the help of former prostitutes who can provide role models as well as support and counseling (Alexander, 1987; J. B. Cohen, Alexander, and Wofsy, 1988).

Finally, AIDS prevention programs related to prostitution must look at both the supply of and demand for these services. Client demand for unprotected sex can make it difficult for prostitutes to adopt safer-sex technologies (Rosenberg and Weiner, 1988). Thus, safer-sex intervention efforts that focus exclusively on sex workers and fail to include their clients neglect an important aspect of AIDS prevention and may prove unsuccessful. Although the current risk of HIV infection associated with unprotected sex with a female sex worker is small, it will remain so only if both clients and prostitutes adopt safer sexual practices on a wider scale and more consistent basis. Given that there is both a supply of and demand for prostitution and little likelihood that the AIDS epidemic will eliminate either, messages designed to protect the health of all participants should tell men to use condoms if they have sex with prostitutes.

IMPEDIMENTS TO MORE EFFECTIVE INTERVENTIONS

The barriers that have impeded AIDS prevention efforts among prostitutes fall into several categories. In some cases the obstacles to prevention within this population are similar to those hindering interventions among other groups. For example, because the major HIV risk factor in the sex worker population is IV drug use, providing treatment for drug use and information about safer injection practices is of paramount importance. A major barrier to such interventions is the inability of current treatment programs to respond to demand (IOM/NAS, 1988; Turner, Miller, and Moses, 1989). Long waiting lists for admission are common, program retention rates are low, and support services, such as job training, are deficient. The lack of drug-use treatment facilities is of particular concern because the risk of transmission among IV drug users is clear and efforts to prevent this type of transmission have lagged far behind what is needed. Prostitutes who are drug users may have a difficult time securing needed services because there are fewer drug treatment openings for women than for men, especially for women with children.

The illegality and marginality of prostitution constitute another series of barriers to deploying interventions and adopting new behaviors (Decker, 1987; J. B. Cohen, Alexander, and Wofsy, 1988). In particular, the illegal nature of prostitution often forces female sex workers and their agents (pimps, madams, massage parlor and outcall service operators) to conceal their practices, thereby limiting educators' access to these groups and restricting support group and outreach activities. Laws against prostitution have other ramifications for intervention as well, which are discussed in the sections below.

Laws Against Prostitution

It is a crime to solicit or engage in an act of prostitution in all 50 states and the District of Columbia; the only legal exception is brothel prostitution, which is a local option in rural Nevada counties with populations of fewer than 250,000 inhabitants (Decker, 1987; Rowe and Ryan, 1987). Prostitution is defined as a lewd act in exchange for money or other consideration. Violation of these laws is generally a misdemeanor, except in states that have passed AIDS-related legislation increasing the charge to a felony for an individual arrested after testing positive for HIV infection (see, for example, Shaw, 1988). In addition, all states have laws against living off the earnings of a prostitute (pimping), encouraging anyone to work as a prostitute (pandering or procuring), or running a house of prostitution. Various statutes also deal with the abuse of minors in prostitution.

Federal law is applied when a person crosses state lines to work as a prostitute or sends money earned by prostitution in one state to another state. In addition, U.S. immigration laws bar anyone who has ever worked as a prostitute, either legally or illegally, from entering the country. Such laws can also be used to deport aliens who work as prostitutes after entering the United States, even if the work is legal (Alexander, 1987).

Enforcement rates of laws against prostitution appear to vary by state and region as well as over time.[23] A recent AIDS-related concern that has arisen in connection with law enforcement is the use of condoms as probative or indirect evidence of a crime. There is anecdotal evidence that law enforcement officials in some locales seize condoms as evidence of intent to commit or solicit prostitution. In some jurisdictions the practice

---

[23] In most cities, there appear to be periods of intense enforcement, followed by periods of relative inactivity (Alexander, 1987), as indicated by the fluctuating statistics on arrests related to prostitution. There are many possible explanations for such variability include shifts in the overall economic and political climate of the country and perhaps even the fear of AIDS. Alternatively, changes in criminal justice statistics may reflect differences in the way data are collected and tabulated.

has been abolished; as the San Francisco Police Department has stated, "[t]he police value of these materials as indirect evidence of prostitution . . . is exceeded by their AIDS prevention value" (Department Special Order 87-13).[24] Where it continues, the practice of using condoms as evidence of a crime dampens AIDS interventions that seek to persuade prostitutes and others in the sex industry to make condoms available to clients.

Although many prostitution laws were originally enacted to protect women from exploitation, such laws can also have the effect of cultivating secrecy among prostitutes and a wariness of outsiders that impedes outreach efforts to promote health education and risk reduction. Research has shown that in jurisdictions in which prostitution is illegal and the law is enforced, it does not go out of existence but instead goes underground in a way that increases the difficulties of outreach to female sex workers for public health purposes (B. Cohen, 1980; Carmen and Moody, 1985; Alexander, 1987). If police confiscate condoms as evidence of intent to solicit prostitution or if possession of condoms is listed on an arrest record, prostitutes receive a message that is inconsistent with what is being asked of them by public health authorities. Prostitutes may thus be discouraged from carrying condoms on their person, making it even more likely that they will engage in unprotected sex.

AIDS-Related Legislation

In an attempt to control the spread of HIV, some states have proposed or passed special AIDS legislation that targets persons working as prostitutes (Rowe and Ryan, 1987). One type of statute restricts the activities of infected individuals, and another calls for mandatory HIV testing of prostitutes. Not much is currently known about the enforcement of these laws, but both types of legislation have consequences for the implementation of AIDS prevention programs.

Restriction of Infected Individuals

In some locales, local health officers can "restrict" (either through quarantine or isolation) individuals who have a communicable disease that is thought to endanger the public health. In Colorado, for example, the

---

[24] In response to public health concerns, for example, the San Francisco Police Department issued an order on April 10, 1987, that reads in part "this [Police] Department and the District Attorney's Office have examined the current practice of routine confiscation of condoms and bleach containers for evidence during prostitution and drug-related arrests. Effective immediately, . . . [they] shall not be seized as evidence, unless . . . [as] evidence of a crime other than prostitution . . . ." (Department Special Order 87-13).

statute is rather stringent and singles out HIV as an isolable condition. If a person is reasonably believed to be infected with HIV, a representative of Colorado's public health office can issue a cease-and-desist order for specified dangerous conduct (in this case, prostitution); violation can result in a criminal penalty (Gostin and Ziegler, 1987).

The impact of such laws on HIV transmission and on the ability to provide intervention and other services is not known. However, legal provisions for isolation are unlikely to address fundamental problems of HIV transmission, according to a report by the Institute of Medicine (IOM/NAS, 1988). Indeed, the threat of such restrictive action may cause at-risk individuals, including prostitutes, to avoid HIV testing and other help-seeking measures in order to escape identification by the authorities.

Mandatory HIV Testing

A few states have passed legislation or have bills pending that would require anyone convicted or arrested for prostitution to be tested for HIV infection (Gostin and Ziegler, 1987; Rowe and Ryan, 1987). For example, Florida requires women convicted of prostitution to undergo screening for a variety of STDs, including HIV; women who are found to be infected must submit to treatment and counseling as a condition for release (Gostin and Ziegler, 1987). In addition, some states have imposed penalties on HIV-infected persons who are convicted of exposing other individuals to the virus. Prostitutes obviously will be affected by these laws, even when they are not specific targets of the legislation (Gostin and Ziegler, 1987).

It is unclear whether mandatory testing laws are effective in reducing the rate of transmission of HIV infection. Certainly, other attempts to legislate the control of STDs have not met with great success.[25] Without safeguards in place to protect individuals who are found to be infected, female prostitutes may view compulsory HIV testing as harmful, which in turn may nullify any anticipated benefits. Moreover, such laws may divert resources from educational efforts that could be more effective in reducing the epidemic's spread.

Even in locales in which prostitution is legal, the benefits of mandatory HIV testing are not entirely clear. Policies that enforce regular medical examinations of prostitutes may also foster risk taking by engendering a false sense of security (i.e., that one is not at risk) that in reality

---

[25] In an effort to stem venereal disease, Congress passed the May Act in 1941, making "vice activities" near military installations a federal offense; during World War II, the May Act served as a prod to local communities to suppress prostitution. Yet despite the ensuing incarceration of several thousand prostitutes, military physicians found no decline in the "venereal problem" (Brandt, 1988).

cannot be ensured by weekly or monthly checkups to detect syphilis, gonorrhea, HIV infection, or other STDs (J. B. Cohen, Alexander, and Wofsy, 1988). For example, once mandatory HIV testing was instituted in Bavaria, West Germany, clients began to refuse to use condoms because they felt that testing had eliminated the risk of AIDS (Pheterson, 1989). Of course, this perception of eliminated risk does not take into account the possibility that the client could infect the prostitute. Very few countries have begun intervention efforts to educate customers about their responsibility for condom use.

Other Effects of Marginality

Groups such as prostitutes and drug users who live and work on the margins of society often experience subtle consequences of this marginality that may affect any attempts to facilitate behavioral change. The nature of sex work as a marginal profession, for example, creates barriers for some prostitutes that may impede their implementation of safer-sex behaviors. In legitimate workplaces, employees are protected by law from many hazardous conditions; they are able to organize to promote occupational safety and guaranteed fair wages. These patterns and practices are not necessarily available to prostitutes, even though safeguards, such as the technology currently advocated to reduce sexually transmitted HIV infection (latex condoms and spermicides with nonoxinol-9) have been available for decades to prevent other STDs.

At the same time, female prostitutes report problems persuading their partners, both paying and nonpaying, to use condoms (J. B. Cohen, 1987; Shedlin, 1987; Day, Ward, and Harris, 1988; Rosenberg and Weiner, 1988; Monny-Lobe et al., 1989c; Wilson et al., 1989; Darrow et al., in press). A prostitute's precarious financial position may make her vulnerable to customers who offer a higher price for sex without a condom. Moreover, prostitutes are at least as vulnerable as other women in their personal relationships. In contrast to professional relationships, the way in which personal sexual relationships are defined by sex workers and their partners often precludes condom use or other protective measures (J. B. Cohen, 1989).

Finally, the marginality of their profession and prostitutes' need to earn a living may engender a quite practical apprehension about AIDS education. It has been reported that streetwalkers are sometimes reluctant to accept materials labeled as "AIDS" information because the materials might be seen by others who might infer that any prostitute reading such material has already been infected. It thus becomes a wise business decision to refuse risk reduction literature (Shedlin, 1987).

Although female prostitutes do not appear to play an important role in transmitting HIV, a significant proportion of sex workers in some locales are infected with the virus, mainly from IV drug use practices and, to a lesser extent, from sexual contact with infected husbands and boyfriends. For this reason, it is important to extend to sex workers the services and education they need to prevent acquisition of the disease. Options for future HIV prevention efforts are presented below.

FUTURE NEEDS AND OPTIONS FOR HIV PREVENTION

Female prostitutes as drug users mandate a specific set of HIV prevention strategies, the most prominent of which include access to drug treatment centers and, for women who continue injecting, instructions on cleaning injection equipment. These interventions were discussed at length in Chapter 3 of the committee's first report (Turner, Miller, and Moses, 1989). In addition, prostitutes in their capacity as prostitutes have unique needs. The illegality and marginality of the sex industry raise a number of stubborn issues that resist resolution, but some of these issues can be affected by changes that would further the implementation of HIV interventions.

First, nationwide agreement is needed among enforcement and criminal justice personnel that the possession of condoms will not be used as evidence of intent to commit or solicit prostitution or, in the case of brothel owners and managers, as evidence of intent to commit the more serious offenses of pimping, pandering, or procuring. Such an agreement is consistent with recommended public health practices and has already been adopted by a handful of U.S. cities. Moreover, the policy of mandatory HIV testing for arrested or convicted prostitutes is not warranted at this time. Prostitutes' risk of HIV transmission is more closely associated with drug use than with sexual activity and appears to be greater in personal relationships than in paying ones. Mandatory testing programs that focus on female prostitutes as professional sex workers are thus mistargeted and reflect an injudicious use of resources, given that most serologic studies of prostitutes who do not inject drugs find few who are infected. In addition, one-sided testing policies that do not include the clients of prostitutes are not sound public health practice. The committee finds, therefore, that mandatory testing of prostitutes is unlikely to address the real sources of increased risk, which are tied to private, intimate relationships and clandestine use of illicit substances. Recently, the Institute of Medicine's Committee for the Oversight of AIDS Activities rejected the policy of mandatory testing and warned that tying antibody status to criminal activity might also discourage voluntary testing, counseling, and medical referral (IOM/NAS, 1988). The committee concurs with that position and urges the rejection of such policies.

Second, the connection between HIV infection and prostitution needs to be better understood. The known facts about this diverse population are few. There is currently some sense of the prevalence of HIV infection among female prostitutes, although studies to date have relied on small, geographically discrete groups that may or may not be representative of the larger population. Although some information is available on how and why women enter prostitution, little is known about how and why they leave this work (see, for example, Potterat and colleagues [1985]). Most existing studies are based on discrete groups of prostitutes and are outdated. In addition, support is needed for studies of men who are clients of prostitutes. For the purposes of understanding both HIV transmission and the design and implementation of intervention programs, data are needed on the work contexts of prostitutes, their personal social networks, their occupational histories, and their clients.

The committee believes such research efforts will benefit from input by women who have actually worked as prostitutes. Especially important are investigations of individuals who report behaviors recently found to be associated with HIV transmission, such as the young women who are exchanging sex for drugs but do not define themselves as being "in the business"—and so do not protect themselves against any STDs, including HIV infection. The relationship between crack use and sexual transmission of HIV is just beginning to be understood; a fuller understanding requires careful study of the subpopulation of women and men who exchange sex for crack to shed light on emerging patterns and risks. It is likely, however, that IV drug use will continue to be the major route of infection for prostitutes in the industrialized countries.

Finally, there is little information about the effectiveness of recently begun intervention efforts for this population, and the committee urges that this situation be corrected. Longitudinal studies of planned variations accompanied by rigorous evaluation are just as necessary and desirable for this population as for others at risk for HIV infection. Strategies for evaluating the risk reduction projects of community-based organizations have been laid out in Coyle, Boruch, and Turner (1990) and could prove to be useful in this arena as well. Without some evaluation of the effects of a project, be they positive or negative, planners lose the opportunity to understand what best facilitates change and where resources are best expended.

REFERENCES

Abramowitz, A., Guydish, J., Woods, W., and Clark, W. (1989) Increasing crack use among drug users in an AIDS epicenter: San Francisco. Presented at the Fifth International Conference on AIDS, Montreal, June 4–9.

Alexander, P. (1987) Prostitution: A difficult issue for feminists. In F. Delacoste, and P. Alexander, *Sex Work: Writings by Women in the Sex Industry.* San Francisco: Cleis Press.

Alexander, P. (1988) *Prostitutes Prevent AIDS: A Manual for Health Educators.* San Francisco: California Prostitutes Education Project.

Altman, R., Grant, C. M., Brandon, D., Shahied, S., Rappaport, E., and Costa, S. (1989) Statewide HIV-1 serologic survey of newborns with resultant changes in screening and delivery system policy. Presented at the Fifth International AIDS Conference, Montreal, June 4–9.

Becker, M. H. (1970) Sociometric location and innovativeness: Reformulation and extension of the diffusion model. *American Sociological Review* 35:267–282.

Benjamin, H., and Masters, R. E. L. (1964) *Prostitution and Morality.* New York: Julian.

Brandt, A. M. (1988) AIDS in historical perspective. In C. Pierce, and D. VanDeVeer, eds., *AIDS: Ethics and Public Policy.* Belmont, Calif.: Wadsworth Publishing Co.

Carmen, A., and Moody, H. (1985) *Working Women: The Subterranean World of Street Prostitution.* New York: Harper and Row.

Castro, K. G., Lifson, A. R., White, C. R., Bush, T. S., Chamberland, M. E., et al. (1989) Investigations of AIDS patients with no previously identified risk factors. *Journal of the American Medical Association* 259:1338–1342.

Centers for Disease Control (CDC). (1987) Antibody to human immunodeficiency virus in female prostitutes. *Morbidity and Mortality Weekly Report* 36:157–161.

Centers for Disease Control (CDC). (1989) HIV/AIDS surveillance: AIDS cases reported through July 1989. Centers for Disease Control, Atlanta, Ga.

Chiasson, M. A., Stoneburner, R. L., Lifson, A. R., Hildebrandt, D., and Jaffe, H. W. (1988) No association between HIV-1 seropositivity and prostitute contact in New York City. Presented at the Fourth International Conference on AIDS, Stockholm, June 12–16.

Chiasson, M. A., Stoneburner, R. L., Telzak, E., Hildebrandt, D., Schultz, S., and Jaffe, H. (1989) Risk factors for HIV-1 infection in STD clinic patients: Evidence for crack-related heterosexual transmission. Photocopied materials distributed at the Fifth International Conference on AIDS, Montreal, June 4–9.

Cohen, B. (1980) *Deviant Street Networks: Prostitution in New York City.* Lexington, Mass.: Lexington Books.

Cohen, J. B. (1989) Condom promotion among prostitutes. In *Condoms in the Prevention of Sexually Transmitted Diseases.* Research Triangle Park, N.C.: American Social Health Association. Monograph.

Cohen, J. B., Alexander, P., and Wofsy, C. (1988) Prostitutes and AIDS: Public policy issues. *AIDS and Public Policy* 3:16–22.

Cohen, J. B., Poole, L. B., Dorfman, L. E., Lyons, C. A., Kelly, T. J., and Wofsy, C. B. (1988a) Changes in risk behavior for HIV infection and transmission in a prospective study of 240 sexually active women in San Francisco. Presented at the Fourth International Conference on AIDS, Stockholm, June 12–16.

Cohen, J. B., Poole, L. E. Lyons, C. A., Lockett, G. J., Alexander, P., and Wofsy, C. B. (1988b) Sexual behavior and HIV infection risk among 354 sex industry women in a participant based research and prevention program. Presented at the Fourth International Conference on AIDS, Stockholm, June 12–16.

Cohen, J. B., Lyons, C. A., Lockett, G. J., McConnell, P. A., Sanchez, L. R., and Wofsy, C. B. (1989) Emerging patterns of drug use, sexual behavior, HIV infection and STDs in high-risk San Francisco areas from 1986–1989. Presented at the Fifth International Conference on AIDS, Montreal, June 4–9.

Coyle, S. L., Boruch, R. F., and Turner, C. F., eds. (1990) *Evaluating AIDS Prevention Programs, Expanded Edition.* Washington, D.C.: National Academy Press.

Darrow, W. W. (1984) Prostitution and sexually transmitted diseases. In K. K. Holmes, P. Mardh, P. F. Sparling, and P. F. Wiesner, eds. *Sexually Transmitted Diseases.* New York: McGraw-Hill.

Darrow, W. W., Bigler, W., Deppe, D., French, J., Gill, P., et al. (1988) HIV antibody in 640 U.S. prostitutes with no evidence of intravenous (IV) drug abuse. Presented at the Fourth International Conference on AIDS, Stockholm, June 12–16.

Darrow, W. W., Cohen, J. B., Wofsy, C., French, J., Gill, P., et al. (1989) Human immunodeficiency virus infection in female prostitutes. In Guy de Thé, ed., *AIDS: 89–90.* Paris: McGraw-Hill.

Darrow, W. W., Deppe, D. A., Schable, C. A., Hadler, S. C., Larsen, S. A., et al. (In press) Prostitution, intravenous drug use, and HIV-1 infection in the United States. In M. A. Plant, ed., *AIDS, Drugs and Prostitution.* London: Routledge.

Day, S., Ward, H., and Harris, J. R. W. (1988) Prostitute women and public health. *British Medical Journal* 297:1585.

Decker, J. F. (1987) Prostitution as a public health issue. In H. L. Dalton, S. Burris, and the Yale AIDS Law Project, eds., *AIDS and the Law.* New Haven: Yale University Press.

Delacoste, F., and Alexander, P., eds. (1987) *Sex Work: Writings by Women in the Sex Industry.* San Francisco: Cleis Press.

Des Jarlais, D. C. (1987) Research on HIV infection among intravenous drug users: State of the art and state of the epidemic. Presented at the Third International AIDS Conference, Washington, D.C., June 1–5.

Des Jarlais, D. C., Wish, E., Friedman, S. R., Stoneburner, R. L., Yankovitz, F., et al. (1987) Intravenous drug users and the heterosexual transmission of the acquired immunodeficiency syndrome. *New York State Journal of Medicine* 87:283–286.

Elifson, K. W., Boles, J., Sweat, M., Darrow, W. W., Elsea, W., and Green, R. M. (1989) Seroprevalence of human immunodeficiency virus among male prostitutes. *New England Journal of Medicine* 321:832–833.

Eric, K., Drucker, E., Worth, D., Chabon, B., Pivnick, A., and Cochrane, K. (1989) The women's center: A model peer support program for high-risk IV drug and crack-using women in the Bronx. Presented at the Fifth International Conference on AIDS, Montreal, June 4–9.

Fischl, M. A., Dickinson, G. M, Flanagan, S., and Fletcher, M. A. (1987) Human immunodeficiency virus (HIV) among female prostitutes in south Florida. Presented at the Third International Conference on AIDS, Washington, D.C., June 1–5.

Friedman, S. R., Dozier, C., Sterk, C., Williams, T., Sotheran, J. L., and Des Jarlais, D. C. (1988) Crack use puts women at risk for heterosexual transmission of HIV from intravenous drug users. Presented at the Fourth International Conference on AIDS, Stockholm, June 12–16.

Friedman, S. R., Serrano, Y., Torres, L., Sufian, M., Nelson, P., et al. (1989) Organizing intravenous drug users against AIDS. Presented at the Fifth International Conference on AIDS, Montreal, June 4–9.

Froschl, M., and Braun-Falco, O. (1988) Women and AIDS. In H. Jager, ed., *AIDS and AIDS Risk Patient Care*. New York: John Wiley and Sons.

Fullilove, R. E., Fullilove, M. T., Bowser, B. P., and Gross, S. A. (1989) Crack use and risk for AIDS among black adolescents. Presented at the Fifth International Conference on AIDS, Montreal, June 4–9.

Fullilove, R. E., Fullilove, M. T., Bowser, B. P., and Gross, S. A. (1990) Risk of sexually transmitted disease among black adolescent crack users in Oakland and San Francisco, Calif. *Journal of the American Medical Association* 263:851–855.

Gagnon, J. H., and Simon, W. (1973) *Sexual Conduct: The Social Sources of Human Sexuality*. Chicago: Aldine Publishing Co.

Goldstein, P. J. (1979) *Prostitution and Drugs*. Lexington, Mass.: Lexington Books.

Gostin, L., and Ziegler, A. (1987) A review of AIDS-related legislative and regulatory policy in the United States. *Law, Medicine and Health Care* 15:5–16.

Hooykaas, C., van der Pligt, J., van Doornum, G. J. J., van der Linden, M. M. D., and Coutinho, R. A. (1989) Heterosexuals at risk for HIV: Differences between private and commercial partners in sexual behavior and condom use. *AIDS* 3:525–532.

Horton, J., Alexander, L. and Brundage, J. (1989) HIV prevalence among military women: An examination of military applicant, active duty, and reserve testing data. Presented at the Fifth International AIDS Conference, Montreal, June 4–9.

Institute of Medicine/National Academy of Sciences (IOM/NAS) (1988) *Confronting AIDS: Update 1988*. Committee for the Oversight of AIDS Activities. Washington, D.C.: National Academy Press.

Jaget, C., ed. (1980) *Prostitutes—Our Life*. Bristol, U.K.: Falling Wall Press.

James, J. (1977) Prostitutes and prostitution. In E. Sagarin and F. Montanino, eds., *Deviants: Voluntary Actors in a Hostile World*. Morristown, N.J.: General Learning Press.

Khabbaz, R. F., Darrow, W. W., Hartley, T. M., Witte, J., Cohen, J. B., et al. (1990) Seroprevalence and risk factors for HTLV-I/II infection among female prostitutes in the United States. *Journal of the American Medical Association* 263:60–64.

Kinnell, H., and Griffiths, R. K. G. (1989) Measuring and reducing risks of HIV transmission amongst female prostitutes in Birmingham, England. Presented at the Fifth International Conference on AIDS, Montreal, June 4–9.

Kloser, P., Bais, P., Lynch. A., Lombardo, J., and Kapila, R. (1989) Women with AIDS: A continuing study 1988. Presented at the Fifth International Conference on AIDS, Montreal, June 4–9.

Laws, J., and Schwartz, P. (1977) *Sexual Scripts: The Social Construction of Female Sexuality*. Hinsdale, Ill.: The Dryden Press.

Locking, K. C. (1988) Prostitutes as AIDS educators. Presented at the Fourth International Conference on AIDS, Stockholm, June 12–16.

Luxenberg, J., and Klein, L. (1984) CB radio prostitution: Technology and the displacement of deviance. *Journal of Offender Counseling, Services, and Rehabilitation* 9:71–87.

Magana, R., and Carrier, J. (In press) Mexican and Mexican American male sexual behavior and the spread of AIDS in California. *Social Sciences and Medicine.*

Monny-Lobe, M., Nichols, D., Zekeng, L., Salla, R., and Kaptue, L. (1989a) HIV infection and prostitution in Yaounde-Cameroon. Presented at the Fifth International Conference on AIDS, Montreal, June 4–9.

Monny-Lobe, M., Nichols, D., Zekeng, L., Salla, R., and Kaptue, L. (1989b) Prostitutes as health educators for their peers in Yaounde: Changes in knowledge, attitudes and practices. Presented at the Fifth International Conference on AIDS, Montreal, June 4–9.

Monny-Lobe, M., Nichols, D., Zekeng, L., Salla, R., and Kaptue, L. (1989c) The use of condoms by prostitutes in Yaounde-Cameroon. Presented at the Fifth International Conference on AIDS, Montreal, June 4–9.

Ngugi, E. N., Simonsen, J. N., Bosire, M., Ronald, A. R., Plummer, F. A., et al. (1988) Prevention of transmission of human immunodeficiency virus in Africa: Effectiveness of condom promotion and health education among prostitutes. *Lancet* 2:887–890.

Nichols, D. J., Monny-Lobe, M., Koumare, B., Neequaye, A., DeBuysscher, R., et al. (1989) Impact of pilot interventions to reduce the spread of HIV infection among high risk women in Africa. Presented at the Fifth International Conference on AIDS, Montreal, June 4–9.

Overs, C., and Hunter, A. (1989) AIDS prevention in the legalized sex industry. Presented at the Fifth International Conference on AIDS, Montreal, June 4–9.

Paalman, M. E. M., and de Vries, K. J. M. (1988) Condom promotion in The Netherlands: Prostitution. Presented at the Fourth International Conference on AIDS, Stockholm, June 12–16.

Padian, N., Carlson, J., Browning, R., Nelson, L., Grimes, J., and Marquis, L. (1989) Human immunodeficiency virus (HIV) infection among prostitutes in Nevada. Presented at the Fifth International Conference on AIDS, Montreal, June 4–9.

Perkins, R., and Bennett, G. (1985) *Being a Prostitute: Prostitute Women and Prostitute Men.* Boston, Mass.: Allen and Unwin, Inc.

Pheterson, G. (1989) *Vindication of the Rights of Whores.* Seattle: Seal Press.

Pittman, D. J. (1971) The male house of prostitution. *Trans-Action* 8:21–27.

Plummer, F. A., Scarth, J., Ngugi, E. N., Waiyaki, P., Ndinya-Achola, J. O., et al. (1989) Effectiveness of condom promotion in a Nairobi community of prostitutes. Presented at the Fifth International Conference on AIDS, Montreal, June 4–9.

Potterat, J. J., Phillips, L., Rothenberg, R. B., and Darrow, W. W. (1985) On becoming a prostitute: An exploratory case-comparison study. *Journal of Sex Research* 21:329–335.

Potterat, J. J., Woodhouse, D. E., Muth, J. B., and Muth, S. Q. (In press) Estimating the prevalence and career longevity of prostitute women. *Journal of Sex Research.*

Rogers, E. M. (1962) *Diffusion of Innovations.* New York: Free Press.

Rogers, E. M., and Adhikarya, R. (1980) Diffusion of innovations: An up-to-date review and commentary. In D. Nimmo, ed., *Communication Yearbook 3.* New Brunswick, N.J.: Transaction Books.

Rosario, S., Guerrero, E., DeMoya, E. A., Volquez, C., and Alcantara, R. (1989) The agglutinating approach to joint STD/AIDS prevention and control in female sex workers in the Dominican Republic. Presented at the Fifth International Conference on AIDS, Montreal, June 4–9.

Rosenberg, M. J., and Weiner, J. M. (1988) Prostitutes and AIDS: A health department priority? *American Journal of Public Health* 78:418–423.

Rowe, M., and Ryan, C. (1987) *AIDS: A Public Health Challenge: State Issues, Policies and Programs.* Volume 1: Assessing the Problem. Washington, D.C.: Intergovernmental Health Policy Project.

Sanchez, L. (1988) You have to know street talk. In I. Rieder and P. Ruppelt, eds., *AIDS: The Women.* San Francisco: Cleis Press.

Seidlin, M., Krasinski, K., Bebenroth, D., Itri, V., Paolino, A.M., and Valentine, F. (1988) Prevalence of HIV infection in New York call girls. *Journal of Acquired Immune Deficiency Syndromes* 1:150–154.

Shaw, N. S. (1988) Preventing AIDS among women: The role of community organizing. *Socialist Review* 18:76–92.

Shedlin, M. G. (1987) If you wanna kiss, go home to your wife: Sexual meanings for the prostitute and implications for AIDS prevention activities. Presented at the Annual Meeting of the American Anthropological Association, Chicago, Ill., November 18–22.

Silbert, M. H., Pines, A. M., and Lynch, T. (1982) Substance abuse and prostitution. *Journal of Psychoactive Drugs* 14:193–197.

Stephens, P. C., Hayes, B. J., Adams, R., and Gross, M. (1989) Women working as prostitutes: Participatory/consensus-based planning for provision of mobile prevention, risk reduction and seroprevalence activities. Presented at the Fifth International Conference on AIDS, Montreal, June 4–9.

Stevens, R., Wethers, J., Berns, D., and Pass, K. (1989) Human immunodeficiency (HIV) and human T-lymphotropic (HTLV-I/II) viruses in childbearing women: Tests of 24,569 consecutive newborns. Presented at the Fifth International Conference on AIDS, Montreal, June 4–9.

Turner, C. F., Miller, H. G., and Moses, L. E., eds. (1989) *AIDS, Sexual Behavior, and Intravenous Drug Use.* Report of the National Research Council Committee on AIDS Research and the Behavioral, Social, and Statistical Sciences. Washington, D.C.: National Academy Press.

Wallace, J. I., Mann, J., and Beatrice, S. (1988) HIV-1 exposure among clients of prostitutes. Presented at the Fourth International Conference on AIDS, Stockholm, June 12–16.

Weissman, G. (1988) Community outreach and prevention: A national demonstration project. Presented at the 116th Annual Meeting of the American Public Health Association, Boston, November 16.

Wilson, D., Sibanda, B., Mboyi, L., Msimanga, S., and Dube, G. (1989) Health education among commercial sex workers in Zimbabwe, Africa. Presented at the Fifth International Conference on AIDS, Montreal, June 4–9.

Withum, D. G., LaLota, M., Holtzman, D., Buff, E. E., Chan, M. S., et al. (1989) Prevalence of HIV antibodies in childbearing women in Florida. Presented at the Fifth International Conference on AIDS, Montreal, June 4–9.

Wofsy, C. W., Cohen, J. B., Hauer, L. B., Padian, N. S., Michaelis, B. A., et al. (1986) Isolation of AIDS-associated retrovirus from genital secretions of women with antibodies to the virus. *Lancet* 1:527–529.

Wolfe, H., Keffelew, A., Bacchetti, P., Meakin, R., Brodie, B., and Moss, A. R. (1989) HIV infection in female intravenous drug users in San Francisco. Presented at the Fifth International Conference on AIDS, Montreal, June 4–9.

Worth, D., Drucker, E., Eric, K., Chabon, B., Pivnick, A., and Cochrane, K. (1989) An ethnographic study of high risk sexual behavior in 96 women using IV heroin, cocaine, and crack in the South Bronx. Presented at the Fifth International Conference on AIDS, Montreal, June 4–9.

5

AIDS and the Blood Supply

The advent of AIDS and HIV infection has raised new concerns about the safety of the blood supply in the United States. Although safety has been a concern since the beginning of the era of transfusion medicine and is not unique to the AIDS epidemic, the stresses that AIDS places on the blood supply pose serious challenges to those charged with protecting that supply. These challenges will require not only the continuing efforts of the blood banking system, which is responsible for protecting the supply, but the intervention of both the biomedical and the social/behavioral research communities to devise strategies that address three major areas of concern: (1) maintaining an adequate supply of safe blood; (2) ensuring the safety of that supply; and (3) encouraging appropriate use of blood and blood components.

Infectious diseases are of paramount interest to those responsible for protecting the blood supply, but maintaining an adequate supply of safe blood has become increasingly important as the donors who provide that supply receive more scrutiny. Only a small fraction of the people who may be eligible attempt to give blood, and those who do are required to meet increasingly stringent criteria designed to protect blood recipients.[1] If eligibility criteria become even more stringent and the donor pool is not enlarged, the supply will inevitably contract. The demand for blood in this country is substantial but not without some flexibility, as noted in the discussion of the appropriate use of blood at the end of this chapter. Each year, more than 4 million patients receive approximately 20 million

---

[1] In 1986 only a small minority of the age-eligible donors—8.6 percent—donated (Linden, Gregorio, and Kalish, 1988); repeat donors constituted an even smaller proportion.

transfusions of blood or blood components (red blood cells, platelets, leukocytes, or plasma) prepared from about 12.5 million units[2] of blood. Of the 20 million units used, a significant number may be transfused unnecessarily.[3] In the era of AIDS, the question of the inappropriate use of blood has come under renewed examination as the balance between supply and demand becomes increasingly precarious.

Although maintaining an adequate supply of blood is crucial to the delivery of health care, a great deal of concern has also been expressed about the safety of the blood that is being donated. Technological advances provide increasingly expanded capacities to detect evidence of infectious pathogens in the blood itself, but in the case of AIDS the time lag between acquisition of HIV infection and the production of antibodies highlights the limitations of technology to solve all of the problems AIDS brings to blood. Thus, technological solutions must be augmented by behavioral strategies that focus on donor characteristics— who the donors are and whether they engage in behaviors that may have put them at risk for acquiring HIV infection—and emphasize approaches that identify, recruit, and retain only those donors who are least likely to be infected. After 1975, the blood collection system in the United States ceased outright payments, except in a few cases, for the donation of whole blood.[4] Studies of viral hepatitis demonstrated that the rate of this infection was greater in recipients of blood from paid donors than in recipients of blood from volunteers (Walsh et al., 1970; Alter, Holland, and Purcell, 1975; Seeff et al., 1975; Alter, 1987). An all-volunteer system was established to prevent the intrusion of undesirable factors (e.g., financial remuneration) into motivations to donate blood. Yet the question of safety does not stand alone. Indeed, shortages, which have been apparent in some areas of the country for some time, reemerge as a continuing problem that now warrants additional attention. Thus, the issues of adequate supply and safety are integrally connected.

In this chapter, the committee looks at how blood is collected, how the balance between supply and demand can be maintained through intervention strategies targeting the donors that supply the blood and the physicians that prescribe its use, and behavioral mechanisms to protect

---

[2] A unit, which is the standard donation per individual, is generally 450 milliliters, and each unit is, on the average, converted to 1.54 component units (Cumming et al., 1989).

[3] Christine Parker, National Heart, Lung, and Blood Institute, personal communication, February 15, 1990.

[4] Donors with rare blood types may be paid to provide a regular supply of this scarce resource, and a few blood collection organizations (e.g., The Mayo Clinic) provide payment for at least a portion of their regular donors, though this practice is being phased out.

the safety of the blood supply. Because of the connection between an adequate and a safe blood supply, the committee has grouped its recommendations concerning these issues after its review of related substantive material.

BRIEF HISTORY AND OVERVIEW OF THE PROBLEM

Early in the epidemic, suspicions arose that AIDS could be transmitted by transfusion (CDC, 1982; Curran et al., 1984). In the spring of 1983, cases of AIDS diagnosed among hemophiliacs were thought to be related to clotting factor concentrates made from contaminated blood (Evatt et al., 1983). Although the etiologic or causative agent of AIDS had not been identified in the early 1980s and no specific diagnostic tests were available, reports of cases among transfusion recipients and hemophiliacs prompted blood banks to institute a variety of procedures to reduce the risk of AIDS associated with blood transfusions. Such procedures included efforts to exclude donors who were members of groups at high risk for the disease, studies of the use of tests that measured factors considered to be surrogate markers of AIDS (e.g., antibody to hepatitis B core antigen, T-lymphocyte ratios), the increased use of autologous donation (providing one's own blood for personal use), and the reduction of unnecessary transfusions of blood and blood components (Nichols, 1986).

After the etiologic agent, HIV, was identified and blood tests for antibody to the virus became available in March 1985, blood collection organizations added this serologic test to their screening procedures (CDC, 1985; Ward et al., 1986). Yet despite the high sensitivity of HIV antibody tests, they do not detect all infected donors (CDC, 1986; Ward et al., 1988b). A variable length of time elapses between acquisition of the virus and development of a detectable antibody response. Generally, this period is no more than a few months, but in one study virus was isolated from blood samples of 27 men who did not yet exhibit antibodies for periods of as long as three years after the initial positive virus culture (Imagawa et al., 1989). During this so-called "window" period, the blood collected from an infected donor may test negative and thus go undetected by the serologic screening mechanisms employed in most blood banks.[5]

The current incidence of HIV infection from antibody-negative blood in the United States is not known. Estimates vary from a rate of approximately one infection for every 40,000-50,000 units transfused (N. D.

---

[5] Although evidence of infection can be demonstrated among antibody-negative individuals during the window period, the precise risk associated with transmission during this period is not known.

Cohen et al., 1989) to one in every 153,000 units transfused (Cumming et al., 1989).[6] Estimates of the prevalence of detectable HIV infection in donors have ranged from 1.3 to 5 per 10,000 (Ward et al., 1988a; Hughes et al., 1989). These rates, however, are not constant across all donor groups, geographic areas, or time. For example, seroprevalence rates are higher among black and Hispanic donors and among younger males (Ward et al., 1988a; Hughes et al., 1989). It also appears that repeat donors, especially females, are less likely to be infected than are first-time donors (Cumming et al., 1989; Leitman et al., 1989). The proportion of HIV antibody-positive donations has also decreased over time. This decrease is due both to notification and exclusion of donors found to be positive for antibody to HIV and to success in donor self-exclusion measures, donor prescreening, community education efforts, availability of HIV antibody tests in alternative sites for donors who have been using blood collection systems for this service, and a reduction in the incidence of new HIV infections in some populations (Ward et al., 1988a; Hughes et al., 1989).[7] Nevertheless, the risk of HIV transmission through transfusion remains (Kleinman and Secord, 1988; N. D. Cohen et al., 1989).

Although HIV antibody tests cannot eliminate all possibility of transfusion-associated HIV infection, they have vastly improved the safety of the blood supply. Additional methods to detect infected units, such as those based on recombinant-DNA technology, synthetic peptides, and gene-amplification techniques, are being explored to increase the sensitivity of serologic testing (Menitove, 1989). Other safeguards involving improved donor screening and recruitment are also being evaluated and implemented, as described below.

THE BLOOD COLLECTION SYSTEM IN THE UNITED STATES

In the United States there are two separate systems that collect blood for various products: (1) a commercial system that pays donors for plasma[8]

---

[6]Cumming and colleagues (1989) report a range of one infection in 88,000 units transfused to one in 300,000. Earlier in the epidemic, Kleinman and Secord (1988) estimated that the risk of infection from blood that tested negative for HIV antibody was between one in 51,000 units to one in 102,000 units. The lower rates of infection associated with antibody-negative donations that have been derived from more recently collected data may reflect diminishing numbers of HIV-positive donors and a changing donor pool that may include more tested donors (Menitove, 1989).

[7]It should be noted that before testing was available, self-exclusionary and prescreening measures resulted in significant deferral rates among gay men (Wykoff and Halsey, 1986).

[8]Plasma is the fluid component of blood that transports water, nutrients, minerals, oxygen, and hormones to all cells of the body. It also contains important proteins and other substances vital to the clotting capacity of blood and to maintaining the integrity of the circulation. Plasma collected from

used by industry to manufacture albumin, antihemophilic factor, gamma globulin, and various protein derivatives; and (2) a voluntary system for whole blood that uses no monetary incentives to motivate donations. This latter system provides whole blood and blood components such as platelets, red blood cells, cryoprecipitate, and plasma for blood transfusion services. Plasma that is not used for transfusion is provided to pharmaceutical companies for the manufacture of blood products. This report deals only with the voluntary system for whole blood collection.

The volunteer donor system expects healthy individuals to donate blood to meet the needs of their community; those who need blood then receive it at the cost of collection plus processing. Occasionally, individuals make directed donations, donating blood specifically for use by friends or relatives. Before the AIDS epidemic, enough volunteers gave blood to maintain an adequate supply for most parts of the country although only 5 or 6 percent of the adult population donated blood in any given year. Today, however, there is not enough blood available locally in several U.S. communities, and in such cases blood must be acquired from individuals in other locales.

The Organization of Blood Collection

There are three major blood collection organizations operating at the community level: the American Red Cross, the American Association of Blood Banks (AABB), and the Council of Community Blood Centers (CCBC). The American Red Cross currently collects about half of the blood used in the United States (Kalish, Cable, and Roberts, 1986). The AABB and the members of the CCBC and independent hospital blood banks collect the remainder. In the United States, approximately 80 percent of donated blood is collected at mobile sites through blood drives that recruit donors from organizations such as high schools, universities, businesses, and corporations of varying size, as well as the offices of local governments and other public-sector organizations. Equipment to collect blood is brought to the donors, either through a bloodmobile van or in temporary facilities set up at the donors' organization. Blood is also collected at fixed sites (e.g., buildings that house the necessary equipment and staff on a permanent basis). Individuals who come to donate on their own initiative may prefer fixed sites, although few studies link different subpopulations of donors to donation sites. Thus, it is not clear that fixed sites and mobile operations are dealing with the same donor populations.

---

paid donors in the commercial system is treated with detergents or heat to kill infectious pathogens, including viruses (Horowitz, 1987). Thus, the danger of acquiring HIV infection from these products is greatly reduced.

Once the blood has been collected and tested for a variety of infectious agents (including HIV), those units that pass all safety requirements are distributed to blood banks and organizations that transfuse blood and blood products, such as hospitals and dialysis centers. The shelf life of blood and blood components ranges from 72 hours to 42 days, depending on the specific component. However, frozen products can generally withstand longer periods of storage than fresh ones, although some components (e.g., platelets) cannot be frozen.

Exclusionary Procedures

Donor deferral measures have two goals: (1) to protect the donor from potential harm and (2) to ensure the safety of the recipient. People are deferred from donation, either temporarily or permanently, for a number of reasons, including fever, anemia, a history of exposure to malaria, recent infection, signs of symptoms of HIV infection, or a history of risk-associated behavior. Blood banks have established procedures to assist potential donors in their assessment of whether they may have been exposed to HIV and to discourage those at risk from donating.[9] Each donor is given information about the donation process and about infections transmitted by blood, especially HIV, and asked to read it carefully. Those who have signs or symptoms of AIDS or who have engaged in behaviors that put them at risk are asked not to donate (self-defer) and are informed that they may leave the donation site with no explanation required. Potential donors who choose to continue the donation process provide a confidential health history, which is given to or reviewed by a member of the blood collection staff. (Donors are asked a number of health-related questions, including questions about possible exposure to HIV and symptoms consistent with HIV-related illnesses.) Following the health history, donors are asked to attest that they have read and understood the information about risk factors for AIDS.

Because some potential donors feel pressure to donate blood (especially during blood drives) and others may not have been truthful in responding to questions posed during the health history, all donors are offered yet another opportunity to exclude their unit from the blood supply even if they complete the donation process. The donor is asked to choose one of two options for handling the unit of blood indicating either that (1) the blood *may* be used for transfusion or (2) the blood should *not* be transfused. Donors select the option in private or using a code so

---

[9]Minimum donor guidelines for exclusionary criteria have been established by federal regulatory law, but additional restrictions can be imposed by blood collection organizations (Linden, Gregorio, and Kalish, 1988).

that others in the blood collection facility will not learn of the choice. This step is referred to as confidential unit exclusion, or the CUE. Some centers also use a callback system that permits donors after leaving the site to notify the blood bank that they may be at risk. Regardless of subsequent laboratory test results, all units identified by the donors for exclusion from transfusion are removed from the blood distribution pool. This step allows a donor to go through the entire donation process in the presence of friends and associates without revealing potentially sensitive information and without compromising the safety of the blood supply.

Exclusionary Procedures: The Organizational Perspective

Although donors who may be at risk of acquiring HIV infection are discouraged from donating and are given an opportunity to have their blood discarded through self-exclusion mechanisms, these approaches are by no means fully effective. The majority of donors who are found to be HIV antibody positive do not self-exclude. Thus, continuing efforts are needed to improve approaches for discouraging HIV-infected individuals from giving blood and to educate potential donors more effectively to improve self-exclusion. In this section, the committee looks at how the organization of blood collection might affect donor deferral and proposes structural changes that may improve this process. In a later section of the chapter, the committee reviews the impact of exclusionary measures on donor behavior.

Generally, AIDS-related information is only provided to prospective donors when they arrive to give blood. It may also be productive to contact individuals before they come to donate and provide specific information about behaviors that exclude donors. This practice would allow prospective donors time to reflect on their risk status and to make decisions regarding donation in private and under conditions of lower social pressure. In setting the tone for such information, blood collection organizations should stress both the factors that motivate donors to give (which are described below) and the altruistic reasons for not donating if at risk. It should be made clear that appropriate self-deferral is a community-spirited act.

There are other informational issues that blood collection organizations must consider. In addition to providing AIDS-related information, community blood centers may wish at this time of increasing fear and decreasing supply to increase their efforts to educate the public regarding blood donation in general. Such efforts should tap a broader range of individuals and organizations and make more effective use of coordination. The media can also play an important role in providing messages about the need for blood, the need for specific individuals to give, the safety and ease of giving, the collective responsibility for the quality and quantity of the blood supply, and the problems associated with alternative collection systems (such as directed and paid donation).

One approach to improving self-deferral, albeit a controversial one, has been the use of direct questions concerning intimate personal behavior. In August 1989, the American Association of Blood Banks took the tradition-breaking position that donors should be asked specific questions regarding risky behaviors during the health history. Although the presumption had been that donors would not be likely to answer such questions honestly, recent studies suggest that direct questioning may be more effective than previously thought in identifying high-risk donors. Silvergleid, LeParc, and Schmidt (1989) found that 90 percent of donors approved of direct questioning[10] and that direct (as opposed to indirect) questioning resulted in a fivefold increase in deferrals for participation in high-risk activities. Although the Food and Drug Administration (FDA), one of the federal institutions responsible for regulating the blood collection system in this country, has provided recommendations concerning the provision of educational materials to donors, to date no guidelines have been developed concerning direct questioning of potential donors during the health history.

The use of explicit questions during the donation process can create problems related to loss of privacy and confidentiality if one donor can overhear the questions asked and answers given by another. This problem would be most severe in small bloodmobiles or in an instance in which a donor knows others who are giving blood at the same time. Thus, if interviewing is to be effective in eliciting truthful responses to direct questions on sensitive matters, the physical settings in which interviews take place must take privacy into account. One possible solution might be computer-conducted health history interviews, which afford privacy even when space is limited. Computer questioning may also eliminate embarrassment on the part of both interviewer and interviewee when sensitive topics are covered and might lead to greater honesty in reporting risk behaviors. However, the capacity of donors to understand written material and to use computers must be kept in mind when developing such an interview format.

Changes in the "processing" of donors raise staffing issues for blood collection organizations. Increased scrutiny of potential donors involves a more detailed history and currently relies on a face-to-face interview

---

[10] Only 1 percent of donors found the questions to be embarrassing, and only 1 percent said they would stop donating blood because of explicit questioning (Silvergleid, LeParc, and Schmidt, 1989).

concerning behaviors that may be stigmatizing or even illegal. Experience from survey research involving personal interviews shows that adequate interviewer training improves the quality of the data that are collected (Hyman et al., 1975; Fowler, 1989; Fowler and Mangione, 1990; Campbell et al., n.d.). Studies of sexual behavior have revealed that even experienced interviewers require special training to gather valid data on sensitive topics (Reinisch, Sanders, and Ziemba-Davis, 1988). Blood collection staff who are not professionally trained in discussing sensitive personal issues may feel uncomfortable and therefore may not be very effective in this area. Specific training may help these staff overcome this barrier or identify those who should not be entrusted with this task.

Processing donors raises the difficult issue of managing donors who must be deferred. Donors who are temporarily or permanently deferred require careful attention from staff. Donors who are permanently deferred must be made to understand that they should not give blood again. However, donors who are temporarily deferred may be eligible to donate in the future and, in the interest of securing an adequate supply of blood, these donors should be effectively encouraged to return at an appropriate time. Because little is known about the factors associated with successful management of permanent or temporary deferral of donors, this topic could benefit from additional research.

Although organizational issues may be important in fine-tuning donor screening to maintain a safe blood supply, other issues must also be addressed. If blood banks are to reconsider how they recruit and retain sufficient numbers of safe donors, several questions need to be answered. What motivates people to donate? What are the barriers to donation? What characterizes safe donors? The next section discusses available data on donor demographics and behavior and explores areas in which additional information is needed.

MAINTAINING AN ADEQUATE SUPPLY OF SAFE BLOOD

Given the increasing restrictions on donors, it is reasonable to question whether the number of donors will be sufficient to maintain a supply of blood that is adequate to meet current and future demands. The American Red Cross estimates that, of 14.8 million donors who presented at blood collection sites between 1986 and 1987, 1.3 million were deferred. Of 13.2 million units collected, 0.7 million were rejected at the time of testing (Cumming, Schorr, and Wallace, 1987). The impact of exclusionary policies on the adequacy and safety of the blood supply remains an important area of study, although existing data indicate increasingly lower rates of HIV antibody-positive donations over time. These data also show significant decreases in the number of high-risk donors, especially males.[11] As more donors are deferred and as more donations are rejected, the issue of supply shortages will inevitably arise.

Periodic shortages are already occurring, and some regions must obtain blood from other areas.[12] In deciding whether or not to obtain blood from other areas during periods of shortage, administrators of blood collection organizations may balance the cost of more intensive recruitment efforts against the cost of getting blood from another organization. In areas with persistent shortages, management may favor purchasing blood from other areas, as recruitment efforts are very costly and may not result in a supply that will be adequate to meet the demand.

Although the precise number of people whose medical or behavioral history excludes them from the pool of potential donors is uncertain, recent research suggests that more than half of the men and women in the United States should be eligible to give blood (Gregorio and Linden, 1988; Linden, Gregorio, and Kalish, 1988).[13] Thus, factors other than

---

[11] In a New York area study that compared the donor population of 1982 to that of 1983, Pindyck and coworkers (1985) found that male participation in New York City decreased by 6.1 percent; the decrease was particularly striking among 21- to 36-year-old males. Medical screening resulted in rejection of 2 percent of all individuals presenting as donors at the Greater New York Blood Program and the confidential unit of exclusion (CUE) procedure eliminated another 1.4 percent. However, there was an overall increase in blood collections of 1.1 percent, largely due to increases in the participation of women and men from other areas (Pindyck et al., 1985). A review of 818,629 donations collected in three major blood centers in the United States between March 1985 and July 1986 found that 450, or 0.05 percent, were HIV antibody positive (Ward et al., 1988a). Between May 1988 and September 1989, 756 HIV antibody-positive donations (0.029 percent) were found among 2.65 million donations at 19 different blood centers (Council of Community Blood Centers, 1989).

[12] Anecdotal information indicates that the Irwin Memorial Blood Bank in San Francisco is encountering the worst shortage of donors in its 50-year history. (See David Perlman, "Major Blood Bank Facing Worst-Ever Shortage of Donors," *San Francisco Chronicle,* February 1, 1989.) For example, normal inventory would include 350 units of type O-positive blood, but on January 31, 1989, only 9 units were available; 60 units were flown in from Milwaukee. However, the cause of this shortage is less than clear; blood bank officials indicated that flu viruses were in part to blame (see George Raine, "Bay Area Supplies of Blood at Crisis," *San Francisco Examiner,* February 1, 1989).

[13] The eligible donor population was estimated by subtracting from the number of 17- to 75-year-olds identified in the 1980 census the number of individuals meeting American Red Cross exclusion criteria for (1) low hematocrit levels, (2) inadequate body weight, (3) recent pregnancy, (4) heart disease, (5) diabetes requiring insulin, (6) high blood pressure, (7) male homosexual activity since 1977, (8) intravenous drug use, (9) sexual contact with a member of a high-risk group, (10) transfusion within the previous six months, (11) history of cancer, and (12) other factors, including a history of hepatitis, medications, and certain types of foreign travel. (See Linden, Gregorio, and Kalish [1988] for criteria definition, data sources, and estimates of individuals meeting exclusionary criteria as well as estimated overlap across criteria.) The authors estimate that 57 percent of women and 70 percent of men are eligible to donate blood. Screening for hepatitis C (non-A, non-B) virus would further reduce these numbers but only slightly.

eligibility, including willingness to give blood, play an important role in maintaining an adequate blood supply. The current challenge lies in utilizing available information on the characteristics of individuals who donated in the past and on factors that motivate people to participate to devise effective strategies for safe donor recruitment.

Who Donates Blood?

In the United States most blood is given by donors who have given blood before (American Red Cross Mid-America Regional Blood Services, 1980; Piliavin and Callero, in press). Epidemiological studies find that repeat blood donors—especially repeat female donors—have the lowest rates of infections transmitted through transfusion (Dondero et al., 1987; Cumming et al., 1989). Consequently, both supply and safety issues highlight the importance of retaining safe donors once they have been identified.

Prior to the AIDS epidemic most blood donors were men (Oswalt, 1977); depending on when and where the data were collected, men constituted between 49 and 91 percent of the donor population (Boe, 1976; American Red Cross Mid-America Regional Blood Services, 1980; American Red Cross Blood Services, Los Angeles-Orange Counties Region, 1981; Lightman, 1981). In a recent survey, 8 percent of men and 5 percent of women in the general population claimed to have given blood in the past year (Dawson, 1989). Among first-time donors, however, females predominate (Mell, 1979; Callero, 1983). Because the majority of AIDS cases have been diagnosed among men, blood drives have looked to women as potential sources of safer blood. Unfortunately, fewer women than men are repeat donors, and gender discrepancies therefore become more apparent with subsequent donations (Mell, 1979; American Red Cross Mid-America Regional Blood Services, 1980; Callero, 1983; American Red Cross Greater Buffalo Chapter, 1985). Less than a third of blood donors who have given one gallon or more are women (Mell, 1979; Piliavin and Callero, in press).

A factor that may be related to the loss of women from the donor pool is low hemoglobin levels and depletion of iron stores, which can lead to temporary deferral. Unfortunately, even temporary discouragement from donation may have permanent effects. One remedy to this problem is routine provision of iron supplements to permit such women to remain regular donors (Gordeuk et al., 1987). In an experiment using "VIP" donors—a special group whose members volunteer to donate at least four times a year—administering iron supplements to menstruating female donors prevented depletion of iron stores and retained these donors in the donor pool (Gordeuk et al., 1987).

Most donors are between 20 and 40 years of age (Wallace and Pegels, 1974; Bettinghaus and Milkovich, 1975; Leibrecht et al., 1976; Moss, 1976; Lightman, 1981). As individuals reach age 50, they become increasingly less likely to donate blood; individuals in their 60s make up only 2 to 3 percent of the donor population (Brewer, Rappaport, and Waterfield, 1974; Pindyck et al., 1987; Dawson, 1989). There are also racial differences between donor and nondonor groups. Surveys find higher rates of blood donation among whites than among minorities. Data from the National Health Interview Survey indicate that 32 percent of blacks interviewed said that they had donated blood at least once compared with 41 percent of whites. Only 4 percent of blacks versus 7 percent of whites reported donating in the past 12 months (Dawson, 1989).

After collections from paid donors ceased in 1975 for the most part, the socioeconomic status of donors increased as individuals who donated blood to augment their income dropped out of the donor pool (Grindon et al., 1976; Surgenor and Cerveny, 1978). A recent study conducted for the Blood Center of Southeastern Wisconsin found that frequent donors had incomes that were approximately 30 percent higher than nondonors, and frequent donors reported higher educational levels than occasional donors or nondonors (Blood Center of Southeastern Wisconsin, 1986). Recent data from the National Health Interview Survey showed that interviewees with higher levels of educational achievement were more likely than those with lower levels of education to report ever donating blood; individuals with more education were also more likely to report donation in the past 12 months (Dawson, 1989).[14] In a separate study of six Red Cross regions (Piliavin and Callero, in press), individuals with some college education, college graduates, and people with some postgraduate education were overrepresented in the donor samples, whereas men and women with less than a high school education and female high school graduates were underrepresented. Moreover, workers in the managerial, professional, and technical categories are more heavily represented among donors than in the general population. Overall, blue-collar and clerical workers are underrepresented in the donor population.

As in the past, current recruitment efforts are looking to major

---

[14]Of individuals with more than 12 years of education, 50 percent reported donating blood at least once; among respondents with less than 12 years of education, 29 percent reported donating. In the group with higher levels of education, 10 percent reported donating in the past 12 months versus 2 percent in the lower educational group (Dawson, 1989).

untapped or underrepresented sources of donors to augment the blood supply. It is likely that additional attention and research will be needed to encourage participation by individuals from these groups. However, in addition to recruiting new donors, blood collection organizations are also trying to get current donors to give blood more often. Indeed, tapping the current donor population more frequently may be less expensive, more efficient, and, in some areas, safer than recruiting new donors. Recruitment strategies for untapped or underutilized groups and repeat donors are discussed in more detail in a later section of this chapter on maintaining the safety of the blood supply.

What Motivates Donors to Give Blood?

Why do some people give blood and others refuse to give? Answers to this question are critical to the development of more effective strategies to recruit and retain donors. Data from donor surveys and theories of the behavioral and social sciences provide some sense of productive areas for exploration but unfortunately give no definitive answers.

The AIDS epidemic raises further questions about motivation and the effect of incentives on the safety of the blood supply. The earlier threat to safety produced by the use of paid donors was eliminated by the move to an all-volunteer system. Yet there are other strategies and approaches (e.g., those that employ social pressure to motivate donation) still used in blood drives to generate sufficient numbers of donors that must now be reevaluated in the light of HIV infection.

Extrinsic and Intrinsic Rewards and Incentives

When asked why they donate blood, most donors report an altruistic reason for their actions (Oborne, Bradley, and Lloyd-Griffiths, 1978; Staallekker, Stammeijer, and Dudok de Wit, 1980; Piliavin, Evans, and Callero, 1984). In some studies, donors report that giving blood provides emotional gratification, making them feel heroic and heightening their sense of self-esteem (Szymanski et al., 1978; Burnett, 1982). Although feeling special or altruistic may be a motivational factor, it may not be sufficient to induce actual donation. Attempts to determine the social-psychological dimensions of altruistic motivations, however, find few variables that discriminate donors from nondonors (Condie, Warner, and Gillman, 1976). Complex acts such as blood donation are more likely to be motivated by multiple factors.

Other research, for example, finds that donation is increased by incentives like the "mini" medical exam, blood typing, or cholesterol testing (where available) (Condie, Warner, and Gilman, 1976; Murray,

1988; Rzasa and Gilcher, 1988).[15] Organizations that use incentives, competitions, and raffles to recruit donors obtain significantly higher rates of donation than do organizations that do not use these techniques (Jason, Jackson, and Obradovic, 1986). However, the relative importance of various incentives in motivating donation is not clear. One study of nondonors found that a monetary reward would not be sufficient to motivate this sample to become donors (Drake, 1978). From his literature review, Oswalt (1977) concluded that, "only some people report donating for a reward, such as money, or time off from work; for most donors, reward does not appear to be a major motivational factor."

Qualified support for the effectiveness of incentives was found by Ferrari and colleagues (1985b), who investigated the impact on donation of coupons redeemable for free or reduced-price merchandise and the possibility of winning a raffle. These incentives proved more effective than appeals to altruistic feelings but only among first-time donors. In fact, there is some evidence that rewards may actually decrease donations by regular donors. Piliavin and Callero (in press) found that feelings of moral obligation at first donation, coupled with a lack of external incentives, predicted repeat donation in a prospective longitudinal study of college donors. In an earlier study of older donors, Upton (1974) found that a combination of high levels of altruistic motivation and low levels of extrinsic reward was more effective in producing donors. Finally, although an altruistic communication before donation enhanced the likelihood of future donation for repeat donors, this effect was not seen among first-time donors in a study by Paulhus, Shaffer, and Downing (1977).

Perceived Community Needs and Community Support

Donors interviewed in several studies reported that a perceived need within the community prompted their blood donations (Grace, 1957; M. A. Cohen and Pierskalla, 1975; Leibrecht et al., 1976; Oswalt, 1977; Mell, 1979). Indeed, an appeal to individual perceptions of community need was an approach used in New Mexico in the successful conversion from a paid to a volunteer donor system (Surgenor and Cerveny, 1978). The message in the appeal noted that many lives could be saved by an adequate supply of blood and that each person's contribution was needed.

Community norms that are congruent with donating may encourage

---

[15] Offering "mini" medical examination as an incentive does not appear to satisfy all donors, however. Staallekker, Stammeijer, and Dudok de Wit (1980) reported that a number of individuals who had discontinued donating complained that the mini exam was not enough of an incentive to maintain their interest in the program.

individuals who are undecided about blood donation. Foss (1983) found that, at two universities known to donate substantially different amounts of blood, the one that produced more units of blood had more individuals who perceived a greater degree of community support for donation. A similar relationship between the perceived strength of support for blood donation and the success of blood drives was found by Piliavin and Libby (1986) across 17 small Wisconsin communities. Thus, the literature appears to suggest that people are most willing to respond to appeals stressing the need for blood if they perceive both the existence of the need and the existence of community support for blood donation.

As the committee noted in its first report (C. F. Turner, Miller, and Moses, 1989), communities can be defined by various criteria: shared behavioral patterns (e.g., basketball players), a common geographic area or organization (e.g., a town or a school), or a common racial, ethnic, or sexual identity (e.g., lesbian women). Thus, "community" support for donation may come from any of these levels. For example, the Irwin Memorial Blood Bank in San Francisco appealed to the lesbian community to help meet the community's blood needs while protecting the safety of the blood supply. Since the summer of 1985, the blood bank has conducted 17 successful blood drives whose main recruitment target was lesbians, a group at low risk for HIV infection.[16]

On the individual level, a personal experience with the need for blood, either through family or friends, may be associated with donation (Drake, Finkelstein, and Sopolsky, 1982; Piliavin and Callero, in press). Indeed, some blood banks have developed recruitment strategies directed toward members of families who are familiar with the use of blood and blood components. Newman and colleagues (1988) found that blood drives targeting families and friends of patients who had recently received large quantities of blood were more productive than drives that targeted first-time donors from the general population.

Social Pressure

Pressure to conform to the expectations of others may be a factor motivating blood donation (Condie, Warner, and Gillman, 1976; Drake, Finkelstein, and Sopolsky, 1982). The belief that social pressure increases donations certainly underlies the recruitment strategy of blood bank "drives" at various organizations or businesses. Social pressure is also obviously applied in personal face-to-face solicitation, a recruitment technique that is reported to be highly effective (Swain and Balscovich,

---

[16]Teresa Kelly, Irwin Memorial Blood Bank, San Francisco, personal communication, August 29, 1989.

1977; McBarnette et al., 1978; Jason et al., 1984). A variation on this approach is a personal telephone call to remind the prospective donor the night before a pledged donation; Ferrari and colleagues (1985a) found this method to be quite effective in helping donors keep their appointments. Personal contact may also help in converting nondonors to donors. Drake and his colleagues (Drake, 1978; Drake, Finkelstein, and Sopolsky, 1982) found in their studies that almost one-fifth of eligible nondonors reported that they did not give blood because no one had asked them to give.[17] These authors also contend that most eligible ex-donors do not consciously decide not to continue to donate but rather have not been recontacted. A similar important finding comes from a study by Condie (1979). Respondents in that study who claimed never to have been asked did not consider mass media appeals to donate as "having been asked."

Despite the advantages intense social pressure appears to offer in recruiting adequate numbers of donors, this strategy also has a number of drawbacks, especially in the context of AIDS. For example, to keep from revealing their risk status to friends or colleagues, some at-risk donors who cannot think of a socially acceptable excuse may give blood when pressured in a social setting. In one survey of 304 seropositive donors, almost one-third (29 percent) reported that they had been pressured to donate by colleagues at their work site, and 36 percent reported pressure from blood center personnel (Doll et al., 1989). Other studies of seropositive donors found that between 15 and 29 percent felt pressure to donate (Williams et al., 1987; Leitman et al., 1989).[18] Not all such donors will understand the CUE option for excluding their donation from use in transfusions. In fact, most seropositive donors do not exclude their blood through CUE, including those who subsequently admit to traditional risk behaviors. Presumably, the same problem applies to the specific donors CUE is designed to eliminate, those who are in the "window" period in which they do not yet have antibodies but are infected. Because blood testing procedures will not eliminate such units of blood from the donor pool, it is hoped that CUE will do so. Although imperfect, CUE may help decrease the risk associated with blood and blood components as donors who do elect to exclude their blood from the transfusion pool through the CUE option have been found to be much more likely to be infected

---

[17] Respondents were asked to rate the importance of six reasons for nondonation. Nondonors gave their highest ratings to "nobody asked me personally."

[18] There are some problems in interpreting these data because no comparison groups were included. Thus, it is not known what proportion of safe donors give blood because they feel pressured to do so or what proportion of donors would have given without pressure.

with HIV than donors who do not defer through CUE (Nusbacher et al., 1986; Gaynor et al., 1989b).

The AIDS epidemic requires a reexamination of recruitment strategies that emphasize social pressure and the use of incentives. Strategies that appeal to more intrinsic motivations may hold greater promise, especially when trying to solicit first-time donors and those whose blood is safe. The use of strong social pressure, on the other hand, may increase the likelihood that high-risk donors will fail to self-exclude. The competing forces of asking prospective donors to self-defer while simultaneously pressuring individuals to participate in blood drives work against each other. Both professional blood bank recruitment personnel and volunteer mobile drive coordinators should be educated regarding the implications of various recruitment strategies. Given the autonomy of local blood collection organizations in setting recruitment policies and procedures, it may be helpful to establish and disseminate guidelines for recruitment strategies that are consistent with current needs for a safe blood supply.

Factors That Inhibit Donation

Oswalt (1977) claimed that medical ineligibility, fear (of needles, the sight of blood, weakness, finger or ear pricking), reactions, apathy, and inconvenience were all factors that prevented people from donating blood. More recent data (AABB, 1984) indicate that ill health, ineligibility, inconvenience, and age prevented a substantial portion of those interviewed from donating blood, but the list of factors now included the unfounded fear of contracting AIDS from the donation process.[19]

Medical Ineligibility

A number of studies cite medical problems as one of the reasons listed most often for nondonation (Leibrecht et al., 1976; Gibson, 1980; Boe and Ponder, 1981). Oswalt (1977) notes, however, that it is not clear whether these reports reflect actual medical conditions or beliefs, excuses, or rationalizations for not donating. Disseminating comprehensible information about criteria for donor eligibility may aid in dispelling incorrect preconceptions and correcting invalid assumptions. In turn, such measures may

---

[19]In 1984, telephone interviews were conducted with 758 individuals from San Diego, Chicago, Miami, and the Baltimore-Washington area (AABB, 1984). Of the 69 individuals who had decreased or stopped giving blood, 11.6 percent believed they were too old, 21.7 percent feared exposure to AIDS, 29.0 percent reported ill health or ineligibility, 15.9 percent had no time to donate, and 1.4 percent reported that they had not been asked to donate. Of the 544 participants who did not donate regularly, 7.7 percent reported ill health, 30.5 percent feared needles, 25.7 percent believed they were ineligible, 4 percent feared AIDS, 5.5 percent found donation to be inconvenient, and 11.8 percent reported that they had never been asked to donate.

ultimately increase the donor pool (Farrales, Stevenson, and Bayer, 1977; Simon, Hunt, and Garry, 1984).

Fear

The association of fear (of the needle, of pain, of the sight of blood, or of weakness and dizziness) with the avoidance of donation has been well documented in the literature (Leibrecht et al., 1976; Boe, 1977; Oborne, Bradley, and Lloyd-Griffiths, 1978; Wingard, 1979; Boe and Ponder, 1981). Yet, in general, only a minority of nondonors report fear as their reason for nondonation, but at least in one instance fully 61 percent of "hard core" nondonors in "intense collection environments" gave fear as a reason when asked an open-ended question (Drake, Finkelstein, and Sopolsky, 1982; AABB, 1984). Fear is reported as well by individuals who give blood. In in-depth interviews with first-time donors, 30 percent claimed that they had considered the pain involved as a drawback to donation, and 32 percent had worried about possible weakness, fainting, or nausea (Piliavin and Callero, in press).

Physiological indicators of anxiety have been used to substantiate self-reported levels of fear. In several studies, both self-reported fear and high heart rates as measures of anxiety were found more often before donation than during the collection process (Kaloupek, White, and Wong, 1984; Kaloupek, Scott, and Khatami, 1985; Kaloupek and Stoupakis, 1985). Anxiety by all measures is highest among first-time donors but decreases with donation experience (Kaloupek, White, and Wong, 1984; Piliavin and Callero, in press). Moreover, "regular" donors have been found to report less physical discomfort and fear than "irregular" donors (Edwards and Zeichner, 1985). If decreased anxiety reflects the knowledge and experience acquired from the donation process itself, anxiety in anticipation of the unknown might be allayed by prior reassurance regarding donation and by information about the actual donation process.

The groundless fear of contracting AIDS from donating blood became a problem with the association of disease with contaminated needles and receiving blood transfusions. In November 1985 and again in April 1988, the AABB carried out a national survey of attitudes about blood donation and transfusion (Hamilton, Frederick, and Schneiders, 1988). In 1985, 34 percent of those polled believed that it was at least somewhat likely that they could get AIDS from donating blood. In 1988, approximately one in four Americans still held this erroneous belief. Among individuals who actually donate, this misconception apparently does not exist. The incorrect perception of risk associated with donating blood is thus more likely to affect new donors than repeat donors.[20] Blood banks and other organizations that provide AIDS education for the general public need to continue and improve efforts to correct the misperception that donation poses a risk of becoming infected with HIV.

Reactions to Donation

The incidence of syncope (fainting), which reportedly occurs in only a minority of donors, has been found to be related to prior donation experience, age, predonation anxiety, and several different styles of emotional coping (Kaloupek, Scott, and Khatami, 1985). Donors experiencing such untoward reactions said that they were less likely to donate again (Kaloupek, Scott, and Khatami, 1985). Among first-time high school and college donors, between 8.8 and 11.7 percent experienced either mild or moderate reactions to donating blood (Piliavin and Callero, in press) whereas repeat donors were significantly less likely to report syncope, pain, or anxiety during donation. The predonation moods of reacting donors tended to be more negative than those of nonreacting donors. In addition, much greater numbers of those who had reactions reported that "I am the kind of person who should not give blood," as well as decreased intentions to return, than were found among people who had not experienced reactions. Indeed, rates of return donation were significantly lower among those who had experienced reactions.

Deferral

Being deferred from donation, either temporarily or permanently, is distressing for many individuals. Yet deferral is becoming more and more common as the list of behaviors associated with HIV transmission is expanded and tests for other blood-borne pathogens are introduced. Some individuals are free to donate when the condition that prompted temporary deferral has been remedied.[21] However, temporarily deferred donors are more likely than nondeferred donors to perceive that they should not give blood and are therefore less likely to return. Studies have shown that temporarily deferred donors consistently show a lower rate of intending to return than do nondeferred donors, although this effect is stronger among early-career donors than among repeat donors (Evans, 1981; Piliavin, 1987).

---

[20]It is not known, however, if incorrectly perceived donation risk is associated with a history of any of the behaviors that transmit HIV infection.

[21]Individuals are deferred temporarily for a variety of reasons, including fever, anemia, body weight of less than 110 pounds, or pregnancy.

As strategies to protect the blood supply result in more individuals who are permanently deferred, permanent losses to the donor pool could have more serious consequences. Because adequate supplies of blood are an important component of health care delivery, potential losses due to temporary and permanent deferral warrant further investigation. A more quantitative estimate of the impact of temporary deferral on the adequacy of the blood supply would require additional information, including measurement of actual return rates as opposed to presently available measures of the intention to return. Permanent deferral raises additional data needs, including quantitative measures of loss to the donor pool and the blood supply as a result of exclusionary procedures.

Inconvenience

The lack of a convenient donation opportunity is seen as a major reason for not donating blood (Caruso, 1978; Drake, 1978; Talafuse, 1978; Staallekker, Stammeijer, and Dudok de Wit, 1980; American Red Cross Blood Services, Los Angeles-Orange Counties Region, 1981; Drake, Finkelstein, and Sopolsky, 1982). Donors and nondonors alike have cited the length of time it takes to donate blood as a constraint to donation (Oswalt and Zack, 1976; Paulhus, Shaffer, and Downing, 1977; Mell, 1979; Callero and Piliavin, 1983; Piliavin and Callero, in press). Unfortunately, there are no studies that examine the association between actual time spent at the donation site and the perception of time spent. However, inconveniences other than time also appear to affect donation. Perceived delays, inconvenient blood collection hours, and locations that are not readily accessible are factors that inhibit repeat donations (American Red Cross Blood Services, Los Angeles-Orange Counties Region, 1981). Blood collection organizations have addressed the issue of convenience in part by collecting blood at mobile sites. The limited space available in these small facilities, such as bloodmobile vans, however, creates special problems related to privacy, especially when donors are questioned regarding behaviors that may be sensitive or illegal.

If the screening process becomes more involved as efforts increase to eliminate donors who are at risk of AIDS, it may take longer to complete intake interviews, further increasing the level of inconvenience. As yet, optimal conditions for collecting all relevant data to screen donors while minimizing inconvenience have not been established. The use of separate "tracks" for first-time donors and repeat donors may alleviate some problems of convenience for regular donors. A separate and faster track for those who are familiar with the information, interview, and donation process may be more convenient for repeat donors and for staff who should spend more time with first-time donors. However, the design of faster track processing would need to ensure that significant changes in risk-associated behavior or other eligibility criteria would not be missed in repeat donors assigned to fast-track processing.

The ideal donor experience is one involving personal attention, professional treatment, and a clear exchange of information in a setting that expresses concern for the donor and his or her privacy. The quality of the donation experience, from registration through the health history, venipuncture, and donation, is critical in leading individuals to commit themselves to continued giving. The need of blood collection organizations to proceed in an efficient manner for economic reasons must be weighed against the need to inform donors adequately about HIV infection and the importance of deferral for those who may be at risk.

Behavioral Theory and Its Application to Donor Recruitment

Research on blood donation has been largely empirical; theoretical work in this area has been more limited. Applying relevant theories of the social and behavioral sciences to the problem of donor recruitment may help in developing new strategies appropriate to the concerns of the post-AIDS era. This section discusses several such theories and their applicability to donor recruitment strategies including the operation of personal norms and a factor called the attribution of responsibility to the self, the use of role models, the theory of reasoned action, and attribution theory.

Internal Versus External Antecedents to Action

Any action including blood donation is preceded by a series of events both internal and external to the individual. Such events include internal states, such as a belief or attitude, or external forces, such as peer pressure or community norms.[22] Psychologists and sociologists have a long-standing interest in these antecedents of behavior and have proposed a variety of theories to predict the conditions under which specific behaviors will occur.

Attribution theory (Heider, 1958; Kelley, 1967) looks at how people make causal judgments about their behavior, how they decide whether to "attribute" an action of theirs to internal or external sources. Indeed, psychologists have found that people often make inferences about their

---

[22] Norms are shared expectations that guide behaviors, such as table manners or sexual behaviors; they may be seen as the "shoulds and oughts" for individual behavior. They are the standards to which a society or group expects its members to adhere.

attitudes and the kind of person they are by reviewing their external behavior rather than their internal cognitions or affect. But internal factors play other important roles in motivating behavior. People prefer to see themselves as inner directed and helpful. According to attribution theory, people who appear to be directed by internal forces are seen as more powerful and are accorded more status; a strong person who performs an altruistic or helpful act without coercion of any kind is seen as a better person than another individual who performs the same act but is perceived as weaker and externally controlled. Other things being equal, people who perceive that they have taken action without external coercion or reward are likely to attribute to themselves a predisposition toward that action. In turn, once such an attribution has been made—once they decide that "I am the kind of person who does such things"—they are more likely to act in ways consistent with that attribution in the future.

Several studies have shown that people see themselves as acting less altruistically if they provide help after being offered money as an incentive, if they act under reciprocity pressures (that is, if the person they helped had previously helped them), or if expectations to help have been made obvious (Batson et al., 1978; Thomas and Batson, 1981; Thomas, Batson, and Coke, 1981). A review of research on donor motivation by Batson and colleagues concludes: "These studies suggest that, over time, the use of extrinsic pressure to elicit help from morally mature adults can backfire" (Batson et al., 1987:595).

Two strategies based on attribution theory have been applied to efforts to improve donor recruitment: the "foot-in-the-door" and the "door-in-the-face" approaches. The foot-in-the-door technique involves an initial small request (e.g., to put up a recruitment poster), followed by a larger critical request (e.g., to give blood). Theoretically, after individuals comply with the initial request, they define themselves as "helping people" and will continue to comply in order to maintain that self-perception. The door-in-the-face technique involves an initial request that is so large (e.g., commitment to a long-term donor program) that the individual will surely refuse. This initial contact is then followed by a lesser, more manageable request (e.g., one blood donation). Theoretically, refusing the first request makes one uncertain of one's helpfulness whereas agreeing to the lesser restores one's initial self-appraisal.

Studies that have applied these concepts to blood donation have had varying results. Cialdini and Ascani (1976), in face-to-face interviews with prospective donors, found that the door-in-the-face technique obtained greater verbal compliance than either the foot-in-the-door approach or to a single request. It did not, however, result in more donations. The foot-in-the-door procedure was generally found to be ineffective in this study. Later research (Foss and Dempsey, 1979) varied the delay between the small and large requests of the foot-in-the-door method, as well as the strength of the initial small requests. In all cases, the effect of the foot-in-the-door approach was insignificant.

In a more recent study, Hayes and coworkers (1984) contacted active donors, inactive donors, and nondonors by telephone. Their initial small request was to place the individual's name on a "list of potential donors to be called and asked to donate blood in the event of a shortage." Agreement to this request varied by donor group: 85 percent of active donors agreed to be included on the list and 33 percent of those on the list actually donated; 71 percent of inactive former donors signed up and 33 percent donated; but only 40 percent of nondonors complied with the initial request and only 11 percent gave blood. However, for all groups in this study, the foot-in-the-door approach was more effective than a single request for an actual donation and was significantly more effective in producing actual donations than the door-in-the-face approach.[23]

Thus, studies that have applied attribution theory to donor recruitment strategies have produced inconsistent results. Overall, they provide some evidence that the foot-in-the door approach has merit, especially when the initial request is a meaningful one. It is probably not the self-attribution "I am a helpful person" that is critical here but the more specific, internalized self-definition of "I am a blood donor" (Callero, 1983; Piliavin and Callero, in press).

Other theories are also concerned with the internal versus external stimuli for action, including the role of social norms in motivating behavior. People learn about their community's norms or standards for behavior in a variety of ways; for example, children are socialized to community standards at home, in school, and by their peers. After this socialization process is complete, however, some of the community norms become internalized; that is, they are incorporated into the individual's personal set of attitudes and beliefs and become internal standards of behavior. Again, studies of blood donors have found that internal factors are more potent motivators than external forces; that is, internal, personal norms are more powerful predictors of blood donation than external community norms (Piliavin and Libby, 1986).

---

[23] Of the 286 participants who were asked if they would put their name on a donor's list (the so-called foot-in-the-door approach), 189 (66 percent) signed up for future donation and 55 (or 29 percent of the list) actually gave blood. The door-in-the-face approach was attempted with 316 subjects, 299 (or 95 percent) of whom agreed to sign up for a long-term donor program. However, only 10 individuals who signed up actually gave blood.

Schwartz (1970) found that individuals who joined a bone marrow donor pool scored significantly higher than nondonors on scales that assessed the degree to which people ascribed their actions to an internal factor called attribution of responsibility to the self. This personality characteristic is thought to predict the willingness of individuals to engage in a variety of altruistic acts. Blood donors were more likely to score higher rather than lower on scales for attribution of responsibility to the self (Zuckerman, Siegelbaum, and Williams, 1977).[24]

This internal sense of responsibility to others may be linked to the economic concept of free ridership. Free ridership is the tendency of some people to let others pay the costs of public goods and services that are available to all (e.g., public radio and television). Because the blood supply is a public resource, it may be useful to consider the implications of the concept of free ridership when trying to understand why some individuals choose not to donate blood. In one study that attempted to discern differences between donor and nondonor populations, nondonors were found to be more likely to display characteristics consistent with free ridership (Condie, Warner, and Gillman, 1976). Thus, donation may be associated with a belief that one should contribute to public resources that one might reasonably expect to use in the future.

Intention and Action

The theory of reasoned action provides insight into how individuals make decisions to take action (Fishbein and Ajzen, 1975). In general, it is assumed that information will change beliefs and attitudes, which will ultimately result in a specific behavior. The theory of reasoned action finds that the intention to act is the immediate determinant of behavior but that four factors precede the establishment of an intention: (1) the person's attitude toward the behavior (e.g., that donating blood is good), (2) the person's beliefs about the behavior (e.g., that donation is the responsibility of every eligible individual), (3) the person's perception of what others will think of the behavior (e.g., donors are seen as helpful and inner directed), and (4) the value the person places on the approval of others. This theory would predict that a person who values the approval of peers, who believes that they support donating blood and that blood donation is a good thing to do, is more likely to give blood than a person who does not share these beliefs.

Empirical work in blood donation confirms the theoretical postulate

---

[24] A study of blood donors found that 34 percent of individuals with high attribution scores gave blood when solicited, as compared with 10 percent of individuals with low scores (Zuckerman, Siegelbaum, and Williams, 1977).

that intention is the antecedent to action (Schwartz and Tessler, 1972; Pomazal and Jaccard, 1976). However, the relationship between the perception that others expect one to donate blood and either an intention to donate or actual donation is far from clear (Bagozzi, 1981a,b, 1986). Methodological complications posed by very heterogeneous samples may cloud such a relationship if it in fact exists. Indeed, Charng, Piliavin and Callero (1988) found that the perception that others expected donation to occur had some effect on the donation behavior of early-career donors; it had less effect on the behavior of more experienced repeat donors.[25]

One way to reinforce an intention and impel the resulting donation of blood is to persuade a perspective donor to schedule an appointment, a practice that makes it more likely that blood will actually be given. A study of intentions conducted by Walz and Coe (1984) compared the influence on donation rates of three different strategies: (1) prospective donors were informed that a bloodmobile would be in their area; (2) prospective donors were informed about the bloodmobile and were sent a checklist of dates to which they could commit themselves; and (3) prospective donors were not given any information other than mass media messages about the blood drive. Individuals who were sent the checklist of dates and asked to commit to a scheduled appointment were more likely to give blood than individuals in either of the other two groups. Similarly, studies using planned variations of phone call reminders to prospective donors have found that strategies leading to a specific commitment to donate produce more donors than mere reminders of a blood drive (Lipsitz et al., in press). One blood center applied these findings over a three-year period during which all donors were asked to schedule a specific appointment to donate. The researchers claimed that the "show" rate of donors more than tripled over that period (Walz and Coe, 1984).

Following temporary deferral, reports indicate that future donations are most likely if specific appointments are made. In one study (Walz, McMullen, and Simpson, 1985), potential donors were contacted two days after they were deferred and asked if they would be willing to try to give again. Those who were willing were scheduled or called again near the time when they would be eligible. For those deferred for upper respiratory infections, the return rate was 67.5 percent, and the deferral rate at the second intake was only 2.6 percent. For donors with a low

---

[25]The evidence provided by Charng and colleagues is correlational (i.e., it demonstrates a relationship between two variables but does not elaborate on the nature of the relationship). Thus, one cannot rule out the possibility that behavior influences perception.

hematocrit, the return rate was 59.6 percent, and the deferral rate at the second intake was only 8.2 percent.

Strategies to establish intentions to donate may also be helpful in developing repeat donors. A recent study of 180 first-time donors who had responded to an emergency appeal compared the effectiveness of two follow-up strategies intended to encourage repeat donation. All donors received a personalized thank-you letter. Half also received a postcard reminder about scheduling another donation, followed by a telephone call to set up an appointment. In the test group, 33 percent returned within 4.5 months; in the control group (no postcard or telephone call), only 11 percent of donors returned (Freiburger and George, 1988).

Role Models

Many learned behaviors reflect the observed and interpreted actions of others. In attempting to learn by example, people may look to and mimic individuals they perceive to be powerful or successful or individuals who provide a believable example of a desired demeanor that is possible to imitate. Such individuals serve as role models and can effectively influence the behavior of others.

The family provides role models that are critical in the primary socialization of children. The family can influence behavior in three important ways to encourage donation: it can develop values that are consistent with helping others and positive involvement in the community; it can provide information; and it can offer role models. Family role models may be the most powerful of all of these influences on children's behavior. One would expect that children who observed their parents donating blood would themselves be likely to do the same in the future, and some data support such an expectation. Almost 60 percent of a sample of 237 first-time college donors said that someone in their families gave blood; of that 60 percent, nearly half stated that their family members gave regularly (Piliavin and Callero, in press).[26] These figures are striking when one considers that only between 6 and 8 percent of people who would be eligible in the general population give blood each year.

As part of a more general strategy to use regular donors as recruiters, blood drives have looked to family members with a history of blood donation to serve as role models, introducing children and teenagers to the blood donation process and recruiting those who are eligible to donate. Bringing children to the donation center may help to demystify blood donation and link it to everyday life. Educational programs provided

---

[26] However, there was no comparison of donors reporting a family history of donation to donors whose family members do not give blood.

through school-based courses in health and human sexuality can reinforce messages provided by the family and supply additional information on the function of blood, the use of blood and blood components, and even the connection between lifestyle and deferral criteria. Parents who are regular donors might use their teenager's seventeenth birthday to introduce him or her to blood donation.

Role models for donation need not rely exclusively on the family. The experimental design of one study (Rushton and Campbell, 1977) paired an older woman confederate[27] with female students ostensibly to go together to an office where the student was to receive payment for participating in the study. On the way, they were recruited for a blood donation. In some of the cases the confederate was asked first and agreed to give blood, serving as a positive role model; in other cases the student was approached first. When students were asked first, only 25 percent agreed to donate, but none actually appeared for the appointment, even after receiving four reminder cards. Of the students exposed to the role model provided by the confederate, 67 percent agreed, and 33 percent actually donated.

The notion of using committed, regular donors as role models and to recruit new donors is a recently implemented strategy that perhaps deserves more attention in future efforts. For example, the "Adopt A Donor" program (Cox, 1987) relies on committed donors to motivate donors who have given once but have not returned. This activity uses repeat donors as role models for other donors and capitalizes on their willingness to extend their volunteer contribution.

Linking Organizational and Theoretical Issues in Donor Recruitment Strategies

Several years ago, Piliavin, Evans, and Callero (1984) proposed a four-step model to enhance donor commitment: (1) identify and neutralize the negative aspects of donation, (2) develop internalized motives for donation and integrate them into the self-concept, (3) develop a behavioral intention to continue giving blood, and (4) develop an actual habit of donation. Piliavin and coworkers suggested that donors move through stages that roughly parallel these processes. Negative perceptions associated with donation tend to decay over time and with repeat donations, as shown in a study in which individuals who became regular donors were interviewed at two different times: at their first donation and approximately 18 months later (Piliavin, Evans, and Callero, 1984). On both

---

[27]In psychological experiments, a confederate is a member of the experimental team who interacts with subjects in a prescribed fashion but does not reveal his or her role to the subject.

occasions, donors were asked to identify the negative aspects they had considered over the course of their donor history. At their first donation, 30 percent said they remembered thinking about pain; 12 percent thought of inconvenience; 32 percent considered the possibility of weakness, fainting, or nausea; and 11 percent thought of possible deferral, mistakes by the staff, or fear of the unknown. In the later interview, most of the donors could not remember considering any drawbacks at their most recent donation.

A study that explored factors related to decisions to donate a second, third, and fourth time found interesting differences (Callero and Piliavin, 1983). All participants were asked to evaluate retrospectively their motivations for donating blood, and the pain, anxiety, and inconvenience associated with the experience. Individuals who reported an external stimulus for the first donation (e.g., participating because of a blood drive) were nevertheless likely to make a second donation; whether they made a third donation, however, depended on internal factors (e.g., a belief that donation is important or a positive self-definition as a blood donor). Pain and anxiety associated with the first donation experience had a negative correlation with the return for a second donation but were not related to later donations. Finally, recall of a short waiting time was related to the decision to donate a second and third time but was more strongly associated with the third donation. These findings are consistent with the model suggested above: first, the donor must deal with the negative aspects of donation such as pain and anxiety; later, internal motivations begin to contribute to an increasing commitment to blood donation.

Change in attitudes and perceptions quite often result from the donation experience. Studies that follow donors prospectively have found that later donation experiences are less stressful than first donations. It appears that motivations for donation also change over the course of a donor's "career." Lightman (1981) found that external motivations (e.g., the company of a friend, persuasion or encouragement by others, the existence of a blood drive or emergency) became less important over time. However, internal motives (e.g., a general desire to help others, a sense of duty, support for the work of the Red Cross) were rated as more important motivators with subsequent donations.[28] The author concluded that, "[w]ith the repeated performance of a voluntary act over time, the sense of personal, moral obligation assumed increasing importance as a

---

[28] It is not possible to infer a causal relationship, however. Indeed, it is not possible to rule out alternative explanations, e.g., that upon subsequent donation, more repeat donors reported such motivations or that donors "susceptible" to such motivations go on to become repeat donors.

motivator; a supportive and favorable context in general became much less vital" (Lightman, 1981:64). A recent prospective longitudinal study of college students supports this conclusion (Piliavin and Callero, in press).

Theories such as those discussed above can serve as the basis for developing new strategies of donor recruitment and can augment existing social marketing approaches that have been used to divide the potential donor population into homogeneous segments and to target recruitment efforts to specific segments (Kotler and Roberto, 1989). In addition, new target groups, as defined by various demographic characteristics (discussed below), may present further opportunities for specialized recruiting efforts to safely augment the donor population and the blood supply.

PROTECTING THE BLOOD SUPPLY FROM HIV INFECTION

Protecting the blood supply from HIV infection rests on recruiting individuals who do not engage in behaviors that transmit the virus, excluding those who are at even minimal risk, and testing donations to detect antibody to HIV. Because of the close interconnection between the safety of the blood supply and its adequacy, however, recruitment, exclusionary, and testing procedures must be implemented with great care. Attempts to ensure the adequacy of the blood supply by using social pressure to increase donations or by seeking donations from social and ethnic groups currently underrepresented in the donor population may raise concerns about safety if high-risk behavior is not adequately considered. Efforts to enhance the safety of the supply by excluding individuals who report high-risk behaviors or by providing HIV antibody testing at blood centers raise other issues. Such efforts must deal with complex issues related to the perception of risk, the types of mechanisms used to encourage self-deferral, and the inappropriate use of blood centers for HIV antibody testing. The changing nature of the epidemic—its extension to broader age groups and to women—further complicates efforts to balance the demands of safety and supply.

The delicate balance between safety and adequacy of supply is illustrated by the response of recruitment strategies to a problem posed by donor demographics. Minority group members are underrepresented among donors, resulting in an excess of certain blood types (e.g., Group A, which is more common among white donors) and a shortage of others (e.g., Group B, which is more common among blacks). Yet intensified recruitment strategies that attempt to redress the problem by focusing on minorities would have to take into account the fact that minorities in some areas are more heavily affected by the AIDS epidemic than are whites. Recruiting "safe" donors thus becomes a challenge that parallels that of obtaining sufficient supplies of blood across all blood groups. With these considerations in mind, in the following section the committee looks at donor recruitment issues as they pertain to the safety of the blood supply.

Recruiting "Safe" Donors

Designing effective strategies to recruit healthy donors requires an understanding of the differences between donors found to be infected with a blood-borne disease (in particular, HIV) and those whose blood is "safe." Surveys of HIV infection among blood donors find more infection among men than among women, more infection among younger donors than among older ones, and more infection among minorities than among whites. Overall, this pattern is consistent with the trends seen in serologic surveys of the general population. However, individuals with no identifiable risk factors comprise a significant portion of blood donors who are found to be infected (Cleary et al., 1988; Ward et al., 1988a; Petersen et al., 1989).[29] In contrast to the pattern in reported AIDS cases, very few HIV-infected blood donors are intravenous drug users. In at least one study, a new trend is reported: the proportion of HIV-infected blood donors exposed through heterosexual contact has increased over time as the proportion of cases ascribed to homosexual contact has declined (Leitman et al., 1989). The same kind of shift has also been reported in New York City, where between 1985/1986 and 1988 there has been a clear shift in risk factors among HIV-infected blood donors away from homosexual contact and toward heterosexual contact, especially sexual contact with intravenous drug users (Gaynor et al., 1989a).

Unfounded assumptions and changing risk patterns thus complicate the effort to devise donor recruitment strategies that will ensure both a safe and adequate blood supply. The practice of directed donation, for example, raises safety as well as supply issues even though recipients and their families perceive this form of donation as safer than donation by unknown volunteers from the general population. Directed donation has been questioned by some blood bankers who believe that implementing it on a wide scale could undermine or disrupt the nation's blood supply. Existing data are insufficient to test this belief, which assumes that many

---

[29]The fact that intravenous drug users are underrepresented in surveys does not indicate that they are entirely absent from the donor population. Surveys of intravenous drug users have found that approximately 25 percent have donated or sold blood in the past ten years; the majority reported selling their blood to commercial plasma collection organizations (Chitwood et al., 1989; Nelson et al., 1989).

regular donors would cease to donate except to meet the specific needs of family and friends. Available data do suggest, however, that directed donation poses safety problems. Directed donors are more likely than the larger donor population to be first-time donors, and first-time donations are more likely to be positive for markers to infectious diseases, such as hepatitis A and B and HIV (Starkey et al., 1989).[30] Many blood bankers, moreover, believe that blood from family and friends who give under pressure may not be as safe as that from volunteers. In fact, the available evidence suggests that there may be no significant difference in the rates of HIV or other viral infections in blood from directed donation and in units from the general donor pool (Fischer et al., 1986; Starkey et al., 1989).[31]

Given the need to enhance donations in general and to increase donations from underrepresented groups (e.g., minorities) in particular, it is critical for blood centers to fine-tune their recruitment strategies and to identify the most promising variations of these strategies. The adequacy of the blood supply in the past has depended on age and gender groups (e.g., 20 to 40 year old men) that parallel those at increased risk for HIV infection. At the same time, relatively safe groups, such as the elderly, have been underrepresented among donors. Yet among all these groups are certainly individuals who could provide safe blood. Some of the strategies that could be used to discriminate between high- and low-risk prospective donors within subpopulations are discussed below.

Racial and Ethnic Minority Groups

Even though minorities are overrepresented in every AIDS risk group[32]

---

[30] Starkey and colleagues (1989) found that first-time directed donations ($N = 5,946$) were 2.8 times more likely to be positive for hepatitis B surface antigen than donations from the total volunteer group ($N = 444,637$).

[31] It should be noted, however, that there are methodological problems that make interpretation of comparisons between volunteer and directed donations complex. In their review of studies of directed and volunteer donors, Strauss and Sacher (1988) found that (1) the comparison groups were often very different in size; (2) it was unclear whether comparison groups were tested concurrently; (3) the methods and results of statistical analyses were often missing; (4) the male-to-female ratio of donors was often absent from reports of studies; (5) the proportion of first-time and repeat donors was not always known; and (6) no study followed transfusion recipients prospectively to note the incidence of transfusion-associated infections.

[32] Rates of hepatitis B, another infectious disease that may be sexually transmitted and is incompatible with blood donation, also exhibit racial differences in population-based samples of the noninstitutionalized civilian population. Data from the second National Health and Nutrition Examination Survey (NHANES II), which collected blood from 14,488 participants between 1976 and 1980, found evidence of hepatitis B infection in 13.7 percent of blacks and 3.2 percent of whites (Centers for Disease Control, 1989). For all age groups, rates of infection were significantly lower for whites than blacks.

and minorities generally bear a disproportionate burden of illness, HIV infection is not arbitrarily or evenly distributed within minority subgroups. Moreover, it is participation in high-risk behaviors and not membership in any particular group that confers a risk of AIDS. Therefore, strategies to recruit blood donors that are directed toward minorities should seek those whose behavior predicts a low risk of HIV infection. Efforts to recruit such low-risk donors may wish to target specific organizations and institutions (i.e., work sites and schools) in communities with large and stable minority populations.

Presumably, the general principles of using local social networks, role models, and convenient donation settings to recruit and retain donors would apply to these special groups as well. Wingard (1979), for example, had considerable success in recruiting blacks for blood donation at work places that employed large numbers of black workers and involved black volunteers in recruitment efforts. Another blood center staged a highly successful blood drive by working with a black fraternity and the Black Caucus on a major Eastern university campus (C. Schroeder, 1987). The center invited a nationally known speaker, who stressed to the black student leaders that one-third of the individuals who require transfusion of rare blood types are black. He also discussed the special needs of patients with sickle-cell anemia, a disease almost exclusively found among blacks. The student leaders then disseminated the information to their groups. The goal set by the organizers of the blood drive was 50 units; the yield was 70, including 18 first-time participants. Donors stated that after this "tailored" experience, they would be much more likely to donate at one of the main campus drives.

A different approach to enhance minority recruitment and to tap segments of the black population presumed to be at lower risk was used for a blood drive scheduled during Black History Month in Florida (Eckert and Neal, 1984). The local blood center offered sickle-cell screening to the community and publicized the opportunity to donate blood in connection with the screening. Black community leaders were involved during the planning stage, and various media strategies were employed to inform people of the event. More than 500 first-time black donors gave blood during the month (a 20 percent increase), and more than 600 individuals were screened for sickle cell, including one male who was found to have the disease. Although these strategies have proven successful, additional work is needed to find the best strategies for targeting those segments of the diverse minority populations at lowest risk for HIV infection.

Age Groups

A somewhat different set of issues applies to strategies for targeting particular age segments of the population of potential blood donors. Because the prevalence of AIDS and HIV is low among the elderly and late middle-aged, these subpopulations are an obvious focus for blood drives. The likelihood of high-risk behavior is also presumed to be low, so that these groups represent relatively "safe" candidates for blood donors. Nonetheless, the elderly and the late middle-aged segments of the population are also underrepresented in the blood donor pool.

Arguments against recruiting those over age 65 have centered on the possibility that they will be taking medication that is inconsistent with donor eligibility guidelines and on the notion that they would be more prone than younger people to adverse reactions associated with donation. These considerations may have made sense decades ago, but in view of the health and vigor displayed by many older people today, they are being reevaluated by many blood collection centers. As a result, recruitment of older people in those states in which it is legally permissible has increased in recent years. Indeed, targeted recruitment programs are already in effect in some areas of the country that have concentrated populations of older individuals. Schmidt (1984) reported on a program in southwest Florida that has actively recruited senior citizens since 1978. In 1981, 2.5 percent of the center's donors were over the age of 65, and by 1984 the figure had increased to 5 percent. Furthermore, this study did not support the notion of increased incidence of adverse reactions among older donors. On the contrary, "senior donors" were less likely than other donors (0.04 percent versus 2 percent) to experience untoward reactions.

A study conducted in New York (Pindyck et al., 1987) supports Schmidt's conclusion that older individuals can be a significant resource for blood collection. In a comparison of approximately 600 donors between the ages of 66 and 78 with a group 52 to 65 years old, no differences were found in reaction rates following donation, and there was only a small difference (18 versus 9 percent) in onsite deferral rates. As the authors point out, blood donation may also have a positive psychosocial impact on older donors. The psychological rewards that accrue to all regular donors may be particularly valuable to senior donors, whose opportunities to contribute to the community in other ways may be somewhat restricted.

Thus, recruitment efforts may wish to reconsider the current strategies that may overlook both older and younger age groups (e.g., drives conducted at work sites). However, successfully reaching more diverse age groups may require additional information on motivational and eligibility factors.

Genders

Of all the demographic factors related to donation, the issues posed by gender may be the most important. Women, especially women who are repeat donors, have in the past been considered to be relatively safe in terms of the risk of HIV infection (Cumming et al., 1989). Indeed, Cumming and colleagues recommend that "every effort should be made to recruit and retain female donors" (1989:945). Now, however, the changing risk profile of women as the epidemic enters its second decade (see Chapters 1 and 2) raises new concerns about efforts to step up recruitment of women as donors. Moreover, many women are unaware of being at risk because their exposure to the virus is indirect (i.e., their risk is related to the behaviors of their sexual partners which may be clandestine and may include bisexuality or occasional drug injection), thus posing significant and increasing problems for self-deferral mechanisms. In one large study, for example, the proportion of infected women who were unable to identify a risk factor for HIV infection was equal to that reporting heterosexual contact with an at-risk man (Ward et al., 1988a).[33] For such women, who do not perceive that they are at risk, voluntary self-deferral is not possible (Cleary et al., 1988).

Even if the safety concerns related to the changing risk status of women and the adequacy of self-deferral mechanisms could be resolved, the problem of recruiting women for regular, repeated donations remains. Currently, more than 50 percent of first-time donors are female, but women constitute less than 30 percent of the committed long-term cadre of donors. Considering the potential importance of women to the donor pool, research on the causes of the attrition could be crucial to blood donor recruitment. A variety of informational and structural barriers may inhibit women from donating blood, including the need for child care at the donation site and education regarding when to return to donate after pregnancy and nursing. Additional research to pinpoint such barriers to regular donation and identify their solutions should be part of any overall strategy to correct the underrepresentation of women. One reason women withdraw from the pool of donors is deferral for low hemoglobin levels. As suggested earlier, this problem can be addressed for many women by

---

[33] Of the 818,629 participants, less than half (42 percent) were females; 54 women were found to be seropositive. Of the 34 infected women who were interviewed, 15 reported heterosexual contact as their risk factor, and 15 cited no identifiable risk (Ward et al., 1988a.)

providing iron supplements. Exactly what proportions of female donors are lost as a result of other factors is not currently known.

In addition to the above focus on recruiting underrepresented groups, issues related to not recruiting or deferring individuals who are at higher risk for HIV infection remain a problem. This problem relates especially to men, because most at-risk individuals in the United States are men. Men who have sex with other men but do not consider themselves to be homosexual present a particularly difficult problem. Men who self-identify as homosexual are more likely to self-defer than men who are bisexual. Delivering comprehensible messages to male donors who report sexual contact with both men and women is thus a high priority task. The following section deals with issues related to excluding at-risk donors.

Exclusionary Procedures: The Donor Perspective

It is clear that HIV antibody testing detects the majority of but not all individuals who are infected with the virus. Self-deferral mechanisms are intended to eliminate infected donors who are not identified through antibody testing. Self-deferral has apparently achieved some of its desired end of protecting the blood supply. Even in the early years of the epidemic, many at-risk individuals were aware of the need to self-exclude and acted accordingly (Pindyck et al., 1985). In March 1983, blood collection organizations introduced the request for self-deferral of homosexual or bisexual men with multiple partners, a practice that resulted in halving the rate of blood donation by an at-risk group of 187 donors who were studied retrospectively (Wykoff and Halsey, 1986). Perkins, Samson, and Busch (1988) also found sizable decreases (from 100 in 1982 to 45 in 1983) in the number of blood donations provided by individuals later diagnosed as having AIDS after introduction of an information sheet requesting male donors with multiple male sex partners to defer themselves from donating. In September 1985, the Red Cross introduced new, more restrictive wording ("If you are a male who has had sex with another male at any time since 1977, you must not give blood or plasma") in the informational materials given to all donors. Following the introduction of this statement, a statistically significant reduction in the percentage of confirmed HIV antibody-positive donors was observed in selected regions of the country.[34] Reductions in seropositive donations

---

[34] In one study from the American Red Cross Blood Services, Connecticut Region, the rate of Western blot-positive donors dropped from 0.034 percent identified in the nine weeks preceding the addition of this wording to 0.0084 percent in the following nine weeks (Kalish, Cable, and Roberts, 1986). In a second study (Perkins et al., 1987), decreases were also reported in the proportion of HIV-positive donors over time (from 0.0272 percent in the period June 28, 1984, to September 4, 1984, to 0.0033

were also observed following the introduction of a self-exclusion call-back system described earlier (Perkins, Samson, and Busch, 1988). In addition to the effects of self-deferral of high-risk individuals (Pindyck et al., 1985; Kalish, Cable, and Roberts, 1986; Wykoff and Halsey, 1986; Hughes et al., 1989; Leitman et al., 1989), some of the change is the product of elimination of donations from individuals who had already been tested by a blood collection organization and the request that donors found to be positive not return to donate again (Ward et al., 1988a; Cumming et al., 1989).

Despite indications of success, however, concerns remain regarding the effectiveness of self-exclusionary procedures. There are important questions related to the perception of risk and nondeferral among high-risk donors that remain to be answered. A significant number of donors infected with HIV did not self-exclude because they did not believe they were at risk. These donors cite the following reasons for this belief: they had changed their behavior, they had not engaged in risky behaviors recently, they did not feel sick or have HIV-related symptoms, they had only limited numbers of sexual partners (one to three), they had been in a monogamous relationship, they lived a healthy lifestyle, or they did not find their behavior congruent with their personal interpretation of "promiscuous" activity (Williams et al., 1987; Doll et al., 1989; Leitman et al., 1989). Donors who cannot identify a risk factor, of course, do not perceive a risk (Williams et al., 1987; Doll et al., 1989; Gaynor et al., 1989b; Leitman et al., 1989). Williams[35] interviewed 158 HIV antibody-positive donors from three American Red Cross blood service regions in 1985 and 1986; 17 percent of male donors and 56.5 percent of female donors had no identifiable risk factor. Fewer than half (44 percent) indicated that they knew or suspected that they were in a high-risk category for AIDS at the time of their donation.

In a survey of more than 800,000 donors from three urban areas in the United States (Ward et al., 1988a), more than half of infected men who reported same-gender sexual contact also reported intercourse with women. An anonymous questionnaire administered to 867 homosexual and bisexual men in Boston between October and November 1984 found that 7 percent reported donating blood in the year immediately preceding the survey (Seage et al., 1988). The men who had donated most recently were younger, less likely to know someone with AIDS, and less likely

---

percent for the second half of 1986). These figures include a drop from 0.0108 to 0.0065 percent after the introduction (in 1985) of the wording.

[35] Alan E. Williams, American Red Cross, Jerome H. Holland Laboratory, personal communication, April 30, 1990.

to have received information about not donating from gay-oriented publications than the men who had not donated recently. The most recent donors were also less likely to be open about their risk status and less likely to perceive themselves to be at risk for HIV infection. This lack of perception of risk among male donors found to be infected (as well as among females who may not know about risk behaviors of their sexual partners) has been reported in several studies and has obvious implications for self-exclusion strategies (Williams et al., 1987; Doll et al., 1989; Leitman et al., 1989).[36]

The changing face of the epidemic makes it essential that donor screening techniques continue to be monitored for effectiveness. One recently adopted change in the health history interview is to focus on risk behavior rather than on populations at risk. This change reflects the realization that many people who engage in risky behavior do not identify themselves as members of a population at risk. For example, some men who engage in same-gender sex nevertheless do not identify themselves as homosexual (Doll et al., 1989). The extension of the epidemic to individuals who have been considered "safe" donors (e.g., women) further emphasizes the need to screen potential donors by risk behavior rather than risk groups.

Both donors and blood collection personnel complain about the complexity of the AIDS risk information materials provided to donors. Misunderstanding information or instructions used in self-deferral was apparent in a small study that considered how well donors understood the informational materials. When 31 seropositive donors were interviewed regarding their understanding of the "What You Should Know About Giving Blood" pamphlet used by the Red Cross (Chambers et al., 1986), 90 percent said they had read the pamphlet. However, more than half of those who were members of a high-risk group indicated that they did not understand the self-deferral requirement, which is based on HIV-associated risk behaviors. Other studies confirm donors' difficulties in comprehending predonation information brochures. A survey of 304 seropositive donors found evidence of misperceptions and misunderstanding of deferral information in a small but worrisome subset: 16 percent did not understand that their blood would be tested for HIV antibody, and only 5 percent elected to exclude their blood through the CUE option (Doll et al., 1989). These findings point to particular problems for individuals with low educational levels (Cleary et al., 1988).

---

[36] A study of 113 seropositive blood donors in New York found that those who perceived themselves to be at risk were more likely to self-exclude than donors who did not perceive a risk (Gaynor et al., 1989b).

Almost half (47 percent) of seropositive donors in another study reported by Williams assumed that the screening tests used by blood collection organizations could detect all contaminated donations and would ensure that their blood, if infected, would not be used for transfusion.[37] Williams suggests that the pamphlet on self-exclusion provided by the American Red Cross may present comprehension problems, especially for Hispanic donors. Other researchers have posited that higher rates of infection among minority donors may reflect a disproportionate level of misunderstanding as well as a disproportionate background prevalence of infection in these subpopulations (Ward et al., 1988a).

Studies that identify the most effective materials to communicate the criteria, mechanisms, and reasons for self-deferral are clearly needed. The Food and Drug Administration is currently sponsoring a research project to develop and test such materials.[38] There is also a need to determine the efficacy of other modes of communication, such as posters listing the risk behaviors displayed in waiting areas, or the use of audiocassettes (especially for donors whose first language is not English) or videotaped presentations.

Studies designed to examine specifically the effectiveness of confidential unit exclusion (CUE) indicate that donors who exclude their donation through the CUE option are more likely to be HIV antibody-positive than are donors who indicate that their blood should be safe for transfusion (Nusbacher et al., 1986; Gaynor et al., 1989b). However, CUE is not completely effective. Cleary and colleagues (1988) found that, among the HIV antibody-positive donors in their study, most indicated that their blood could be used for transfusion. Subsequently, most of the men in the study reported risk behavior even though they did not self-exclude. Among HIV-seropositive women who participated in the study, 92 percent directed their blood for transfusions, and more than half had no identified risk factor. Other studies report variation in self-exclusion rates by risk factors, with homosexually active males being the most likely to remove their donation from the transfusion pool (Gaynor et al., 1989b). Variations in the CUE process itself may also affect its success in appropriately excluding donations. Loicano and coworkers (1988) found that seropositive donors were more likely to self-exclude when either a confidential ballot or a bar code was used than when the

---

[37] Alan E. Williams, American Red Cross, Jerome H. Holland Laboratory, personal communication, April 30, 1990.

[38] Donna Mayo, American Institutes for Research, personal communication, May 4, 1989.

CUE process involved a callback procedure.[39] CUE procedures are often difficult for donors to understand, and one study indicated that fewer than 5 percent of donors understood the purpose of the CUE (Leitman et al., 1989). The most effective CUE mechanisms need to be identified if this process is to add significantly to the safety of the blood supply.

The Inappropriate Use of
Blood Collection Agencies for HIV Testing

From the beginning of HIV antibody testing, blood centers have been concerned that some people will give blood in order to be tested rather than using alternative testing sites. In fact, Leitman and coworkers (1989) and Williams and colleagues (1987) found that approximately one-quarter of seropositive donors had donated in order to undergo HIV antibody testing. Blood donation centers were preferred because of the stigma associated with these other test sites. In a study by Doll and coworkers (1989), fewer seropositive donors (6 percent) reported using blood collection organizations for HIV testing, but 17 percent were unable to identify another testing site. Because there will probably continue to be some individuals at risk for HIV infection who donate blood as a way of being tested, every effort should be made to reach these donors and refer them to alternative testing sites or to ensure that they use CUE if they elect to donate blood. A survey in Wisconsin found lower rates of infection among donors in communities that provided readily accessible testing and counseling at alternative sites (Snyder and Vergeront, 1988).[40] Referral networks to alternative testing sites that are consistent with the needs of the donor may also decrease the inappropriate use of blood collection organizations for testing.

RESEARCH TO IMPROVE THE EXISTING SYSTEM

This section summarizes the committee's recommendations for a research agenda in this area and identifies both general and specific issues for further attention. However, the recommendations that follow are not intended to be an exhaustive enumeration of suitable research topics. Rather, the general categories of research provide a point of departure

---

[39] The self-excluding donors using either the bar code or ballot were more likely than the total sample (1.15 percent versus 0.033 percent) to be Western blot positive.

[40] It should be noted, however, that Wisconsin has very low rates of HIV infection. Of the 197,751 units of blood donated between April 1, 1985 and December 31, 1987 in communities with alternative testing programs, 4 were found to have antibodies to HIV. Of the 182,720 units donated during this period in communities without alternative counseling and testing sites, 9 were found to be antibody positive (Snyder and Vergeront, 1988).

for what the committee hopes will become a continuing effort to identify areas and problems to which the social and behavioral sciences can make a meaningful contribution and to be a dialogue that cuts across the various disciplines that can bring expertise (empirical and theoretical) to bear on the behavioral mechanisms for maintaining an adequate supply of safe blood for this country.

Although much previous research on donor behavior points to potentially useful strategies to improve donor recruitment as well as donor screening, additional research is needed that is specific to the context of AIDS and that reflects the evolving nature of the epidemic. The next iteration of research on intervention strategies is likely to require on the one hand more tightly controlled methodologies and on the other hand more far-reaching, imaginative approaches to help donors who are at risk to self-defer and to encourage those who are not at risk to donate regularly. Moreover, effective strategies for recruiting and retaining safe donors from different subgroups of the donor population need to be established. Previous efforts have used the theories and methods of marketing; recruitment drives have surveyed community structures for potential groups of donors and sites for blood collection, segmented populations, and targeted drives to specific subgroups. Now, in the light of the AIDS epidemic, there is a need to assess whether the theories and tools of marketing and other relevant business-related areas can be applied to the development of recruitment programs that take into account current needs and HIV transmission. The need to evaluate new programs will continue.

The specific research efforts proposed here would take either a correlational or experimental approach. Correlational studies would be appropriate to explore questions for which control over the independent variable of interest is not possible. Questions that might be investigated by correlational methods include the following: How do donors decide to designate their units "not for transfusion" on the CUE form? How can misunderstandings regarding the procedure be corrected? Why do some donors with identifiable risk factors continue to donate? How many donors without risk factors incorrectly indicate that their blood should not be used for transfusion, and why do they do so?

Areas that would be amenable to experimental research include new recruitment techniques, alternative formats (computer-assisted, audiotaped or videotaped) for presentations of risk information and health screening, and various educational programs in schools designed to increase general knowledge about risk factors and the importance of donation to the community. Exploration of recruitment techniques could evaluate the impact on donation of various incentives and motivational factors, different recruiters, and different structural formats for the donation process itself. Impacts should be assessed considering both first-time and repeat donors.

Several methodological issues must be considered in assessing currently available data on donor behavior and in designing future research. One of the methodological limitations of existing studies that makes their interpretation so difficult is the absence of control groups. For example, studies on the use of CUE have largely relied on samples of seropositive donors. Much less is known about how seronegative donors have approached this self-exclusionary mechanism, and yet it is a small subset of this population—the infected seronegative donor who is in the "window" between acquisition of infection and the development of an immunologic response—for which the CUE was designed. Changing current sampling strategies could improve our understanding of these protective procedures, but additional work is needed. For example, the failure to separate first-time and repeat donors has made it difficult to assess the relative risk of directed versus volunteer donations.

At the heart of intervening to protect the blood supply is the problem of understanding risk perceptions. If we cannot help donors to appreciate behaviors that may have put them at risk in the past, we will have compromised our ability to prevent further transmission. Recent studies of donors who are labeled as homosexual but report sexual contact with both men and women highlight the need to separate bisexual men from gay men in data analyses. Our capacity to elicit accurate data is limited and will require significant resources and sustained attention (see Chapter 6 of this report).

Refining intervention tools calls for improvement in the measurement of motivational factors associated with donation. Vague conceptualizations of factors such as social pressure, internal incentives, and the like, have precluded the development of sound understanding of the impact of these factors on appropriate and inappropriate donation.

Protecting the blood supply requires accurate, up-to-date information. Unfortunately, much of the available research on blood donation processes and donors was published prior to the AIDS epidemic and is therefore of questionable relevance to the current situation. In addition, much early work was carried out by local blood collection organizations, largely to guide their own efforts; their findings, when reported, were brief. Important details, such as research design, sampling, and response rates, are often missing. Even when the details of design and analysis are available, the quality of the work varies greatly, and generalizations are difficult to make. Behavioral research expertise has not been strongly represented in surveys of donor populations. As additional behavioral research is called for, the need for such expertise increases. Progress in solving current donor-related problems depends on a cadre of experienced researchers. In addition, training in how to conduct surveys of donor populations is needed. Most studies have looked at donors and nondonors at one point in time; such cross-sectional efforts are not suited to understanding motivations for donation, repeat donation, and exclusion. Thus, the committee finds there is a need for additional, well-designed research that takes current conditions into account. These studies are needed to improve our understanding of the factors that influence both the quantity and quality of blood donations.

At present, considerable pressure is being placed on recruitment, screening, and collection personnel for the efficient "production" of units of blood. This pressure reflects both the need to maintain an adequate supply of blood and the need to keep blood collection costs to a minimum. Added to this pressure is the countervailing emphasis on blood safety with its focus on screening and deferring at-risk donors. Reconciling these seemingly contradictory objectives will require continuing efforts and innovative strategies. Methods to develop a total "community responsibility" system that uses no pressure tactics, rewards, or incentives could contribute to blood safety and a greater probability of intrinsically motivated donation, which, as noted earlier, holds considerable promise for continued donorship.

To increase the blood supply, **the committee recommends that:**

- **blood collection organizations prepare and deliver (in cooperation with the mass media) clear and accurate information concerning both the need for donation and the absence of health risks from donation;**
- **the National Heart, Lung, and Blood Institute support research on the design, systematic testing, and implementation of new methods for attracting healthy first-time donors, retaining and encouraging repeat donations, and enlisting the aid of repeat donors in donor recruitment;**
- **blood collection organizations undertake to make the actual donation process as comfortable, friendly, and efficient as possible through changes in scheduling procedures, physical accommodations, donor processing, and staff training;**

- blood collection agencies, **Public Health Service agencies, and community leaders employ innovative recruitment approaches among populations such as minority and certain age groups that traditionally have not been represented in the donor pool;** and

- **physicians and blood banks encourage autologous donation** (i.e., predeposit of an individual's own blood) in cases in which surgery is anticipated (see later section on the appropriate use of blood).

To improve the safety of the blood supply, **the committee recommends that:**[41]

- blood collection agencies strive for clearer communication of the exclusion criteria to potential and actual donors;

- blood collection agencies work to increase donation by those who can safely give and abstention by those who are at even minimal risk through recruitment approaches that stress altruistic appeals rather than the use of competitions, incentives, and social pressure; and

- the National Heart, Lung, and Blood Institute continue its support for research to investigate why some donors with identifiable risk factors continue to donate while others without risk factors inappropriately exclude themselves.

REDUCING THE RISK OF HIV INFECTION THROUGH APPROPRIATE USE OF TRANSFUSED BLOOD AND BLOOD COMPONENTS

In addition to focusing on the donor to reduce the risk of HIV infection from transfused blood, strategies to reduce HIV infection can also focus on decreasing the patients' exposure to blood and blood components that have been collected from other individuals.[42] Reducing the exposure of potential transfusion recipients to donated blood can be accomplished in

---

[41] The committee's recommendations are consistent with the World Health Organization's guidelines for the recruitment of safer donors (1.1, 1.2, 1.3) provided in the 1989 "Consensus Statement on Accelerated Strategies to Reduce the Risk of Transmission of HIV by Blood Transfusion" (World Health Organization, 1989).

[42] The risk of HIV infection is estimated to increase linearly with the volume of blood transfused; that is, the less blood transfused, the lower the risk of HIV infection (Cumming et al., 1989).

several ways, depending on the circumstances that prompt transfusion. In principle, these approaches involve more appropriate use of blood products by decreasing the unnecessary use of blood and blood components, increasing autologous donations, reducing the need for transfusion, and inactivating viruses that may be present in blood products. Educating physicians and their patients and modifying behavior are necessary to achieve these goals. This section presents background information on practices and trends in blood utilization, potential points for reducing transfusion exposure (with an emphasis on changing the behavior of prescribing physicians and patients who may be recipients), and the committee's recommendations for further research.

Trends in Blood Utilization

In recent years, blood centers have encouraged a shift from the transfusion of whole blood to transfusion of the specific component needed. This trend is considered sound medical practice and had the added benefit that a single donation could be used to treat as many as four different patients, thus relieving some of the strain on the blood supply. Currently, only 10 to 20 percent of transfusions are given as whole blood; the other 80 to 90 percent of donations are split into two or more blood components (red blood cells, platelets, leukocytes, or fresh-frozen plasma). The benefit of the trend away from transfusion of whole blood has been that patients receive the specific component they need and are not exposed to other components unnecessarily. A drawback of this practice, however, is that two to four patients may be exposed to blood components from one donation.

The various blood components are used for different purposes. Packed red blood cells are generally used for chronic blood loss and anemias or in combination with saline or a colloid supplement for acute intraoperative or traumatic blood loss. Platelets are used for a variety of acute and chronic platelet deficiency conditions, including iatrogenic thrombocytopenias associated with cancer chemotherapy or with massive intraoperative blood loss, especially during cardiovascular surgery. To achieve adequate therapeutic levels, platelets derived from regular blood donations from several donors are pooled, thus multiplying the risk of exposure. An alternative to pooling donations from several donors is the collection of larger quantities of platelets from a single donor through plateletapheresis, which selectively removes only platelets. Leukocytes are mainly used to treat severe infections in patients with leukopenias associated with chemotherapy. Leukocytes may also be derived from regularly donated blood or from single donors through leukopheresis.

Fresh-frozen plasma is used in a number of ways, some of which may not be medically indicated. The most appropriate use of fresh-frozen plasma is to correct certain clotting factor deficiencies when the factor is not present in other blood products. Yet fresh-frozen plasma is often given simply to expand blood volume when other, sterile volume expanders could be used instead. It is also common for fresh-frozen plasma to be given with a transfusion of red blood cells to reconstitute whole blood. The only possible benefit of such a practice might be an enrichment of clotting factors. However, the practice is often used when there is no therapeutic justification. Moreover, the benefits of such concomitant transfusion have not been established (Snyder, Gottschall, and Menitove, 1986). This practice also increases the risk of infection by exposing the recipient to two donors instead of one.

There is evidence that blood transfusion utilization in the United States has been affected by concern over the risk of HIV transmission. Prior to the AIDS epidemic, national surveys revealed that transfusions of blood and blood components doubled between 1971 and 1980 (National Heart, Lung, and Blood Institute, 1972; Surgenor and Schnitzer, 1985). A shift in this trend was observed between 1980 and 1985 (inclusive) in four sets of U.S. hospitals that together accounted for 4.8 percent of red blood cell transfusions in the United States in 1980 (Surgenor et al., 1988). Total red blood cell transfusion rates (total red blood cell transfusions per 1,000 hospital admissions) increased between 1980 and 1982 but remained nearly constant between 1982 and 1985. Plasma transfusion followed a similar pattern. In contrast, total platelet transfusion rates continued to increase by a total of 76 percent over the six-year period. Thus, the AIDS epidemic may have been a moderating factor in the use of red cells and plasma, but any impact on platelet transfusion rates is not apparent. An increasing demand for platelets during the period, however, may have obscured any moderating effect.

Under certain conditions, patients can predeposit their own blood for transfusion during elective surgery. Such transfusion is referred to as "autologous," in contrast to transfusion of blood from other donors ("homologous"). Before 1985, autologous blood transfusions were rarely used, and many blood centers in the United States did not have procedures for handling predeposited blood. From the perspective of the HIV epidemic, the infrequent use of autologous transfusion is regrettable.

Autologous blood transfusion would have been especially beneficial between 1978 and 1985 when the prevalence of HIV in the blood supply was greatest but before a specific test was available to screen donor blood. Surveys conducted between 1980 and 1985 show an increase in autologous blood transfusions (Surgenor et al., 1988). However, even after recognition of the dangers HIV presents to transfusion recipients, autologous blood transfusions were underutilized. Among 18 university hospitals surveyed in 1986, only 0.9 percent of total transfused red cell units were autologous, when as much as 10 percent of such transfusions could have been made using autologous donations (Toy et al., 1987). Since then, the percentage of autologous units transfused at these same hospitals has increased (to 1.3 percent in 1987 and 2.6 percent in 1988), but the rate showed insignificant change in 1989 (Toy, 1989). Thus, predeposited blood is now used in only one-quarter of the surgeries in which it could be used. Because transfusion with autologous blood is the safest form of transfusion, its infrequent use warrants further attention, as do methods to reduce inappropriate use of transfusions of blood and blood components.

Reducing Transfusion Exposure

Decreasing Unnecessary Use of Blood Products

In 1985 the Office of Technology Assessment (1985) reported to Congress that both the suppliers and users of blood agreed that blood was often overused or used inappropriately. The report indicated, however, that suppliers and users differed in their assessment of the extent to which blood was misused and in their suggestions for promoting more appropriate use. At present, there are no absolute standards or criteria regarding the appropriate use of blood and blood components. In the absence of such standards, it is difficult to determine with certainty whether transfusions are given appropriately. National data on transfusion practices, whether appropriate or inappropriate, do not exist. Nevertheless, a number of studies on a more limited scale have audited transfusion practices and support the contention that some transfusions of red cells, platelets, and plasma are, indeed, inappropriate and could be reduced.

For example, it has been common practice to postpone surgery or give preoperative blood transfusions to patients who have a hemoglobin level of less than 10 grams per deciliter (gm/Dl) or a hematocrit of less than 34 percent. Using these criteria, Stehling and Esposito (1987) found that 19 percent of all red cell intraoperative transfusions were not indicated. In addition, data from studies of Jehovah's Witnesses (Carson et al., 1988) who refuse transfusion because of religious convictions revealed no excess morbidity or mortality among patients who underwent surgery with hemoglobin levels of as low as 8 gm/Dl. In another study, Tartter and Barron (1985) found that 25 percent of red cell units given to elective colorectal cancer surgery patients were unnecessary because either the preoperative hematocrit exceeded 36 percent or the postoperative hematocrit exceeded 33 percent prior to transfusion. Excessive intraoperative transfusion or giving red cell units in pairs accounted for 90 percent of the unnecessary transfusions. It should be noted, however, that because the amount of bleeding during surgery is difficult to estimate, some transfusions that are retrospectively considered to be excessive may have seemed unavoidable at the time. Such considerations contribute to the difficulties in assessing how much transfusion is inappropriate and how to improve the situation.

There is evidence that platelet transfusions are used inappropriately in some cases. To assess the appropriateness of platelet transfusions, Simpson (1987) screened all platelet requests made to a blood bank. Of 984 requests, 226 (23 percent) were deemed inappropriate; an additional 305 requests (31 percent) needed modification. The most common inappropriate requests were for patients with platelet counts greater than 20,000 per microliter with no evidence of bleeding (70 requests), multiple platelet transfusions with no platelet count taken between transfusions (56 requests), and cardiopulmonary bypass patients without evidence of hemostatic dysfunction (63 requests). McCullough and colleagues (1988) reviewed platelet transfusions in their institution that were given prophylactically to prevent bleeding. Of 165 prophylactic transfusion episodes, 46 (22 percent) had pretransfusion platelet counts greater than 20,000 per microliter and no special factors that would justify the need for platelets (e.g., fever, coagulopathy, antiplatelet drug therapy). Such platelet transfusions could probably have been avoided.

With the increase in component production in recent years, the use of fresh-frozen plasma has risen dramatically. The indications for its use, however, are often not apparent (Office of Medical Applications of Research, NIH, 1985). Fresh-frozen plasma may be used prophylactically in cases that involve massive transfusion such as cardiopulmonary bypass operations. The rationale for its use under these circumstances is to replace clotting factors that may be depleted because of extreme blood loss. Although this use may be reasonable for patients who lose more than one to two times their blood volume, fresh-frozen plasma is also used for blood volume expansion when albumin or another sterile solution could be used just as effectively (Snyder, Gottschall, and Menitove, 1986). In addition, the practice of reconstituting packed red blood cells with fresh-frozen plasma is common (Snyder, Gottschall, and Menitove, 1986). The advantage of such concomitant transfusion has not been established, and, indeed, this practice may increase the risk of infection by exposing the recipient to two donors. Blumberg and colleagues (1986), however, have found suspect the assumption that this practice is of benefit to the patient. A consensus development conference, sponsored jointly by NIH's Office of Medical Applications of Research and the National Heart, Lung, and Blood Institute (1985) has stated that use of fresh-frozen plasma as a volume expander or to reconstitute red blood cells has no demonstrated benefit to the patient and unnecessarily exposes the recipient to additional donors.

The extent to which fresh-frozen plasma is misused is unknown but is expected to be high. In one retrospective audit of transfusion practices in a hospital in Minnesota, 17 percent of fresh-frozen plasma transfusions were questionable, and an additional 11 percent were found not to be indicated (Coffin, Matz, and Rich, 1989). Another study conducted at the Puget Sound Blood Center in which all orders for fresh-frozen plasma have been audited by the blood bank for years showed that 20 percent of the fresh-frozen plasma requests in 1988 were considered not to be indicated (Price, 1989).

Increasing Autologous Donation

Autologous blood is the safest source of blood for transfusion because there is no possibility of transfusion reactions (as a result of blood group incompatibility) or of acquiring an infectious agent. The use of autologous blood reduces or may even eliminate the need for homologous blood from other donors. However, despite the benefits associated with the use of autologus blood, it has not been universally adopted. Barriers to increased use of autologous donation include insufficient knowledge about the procedure among surgeons (Strauss et al., 1988), a failure to incorporate the procedure into standard preoperative routines, and unnecessarily rigid eligibility criteria adopted by many blood collection organizations (Anderson and Tomasulo, 1988). Patient ineligibility to donate also limits autologous blood use to some extent. In a study of 180 candidates for autologous donation (Kruskall et al., 1986), 47.8 percent were deferred at least once, and 25.5 percent of attempts to use only autologous blood were abandoned because of deferral. Of those who were able to predeposit, 36.9 percent used only autologous components, and almost two-thirds used no homologous blood.

Several successful interventions have increased the use of autologous donation by focusing on physician education and improving the system so that predeposited blood can be gathered, stored, and delivered when needed (Kruskall et al., 1986). For example, at the Beth Israel Hospital in Boston, blood bank personnel now review the surgical schedule, and, if the scheduled surgery is two or more weeks away, they initiate the process of autologous donations (Kruskall et al., 1986). In other successful programs, surgeons instruct their office staff to incorporate autologous donation into routine preoperative procedures. When possible, surgery is scheduled four weeks later to allow time for donation. Despite these successes, predepositing blood is still underutilized, pointing to the need for better application of mechanisms known to promote autologous donation as well as research to develop more effective ways of increasing autologous transfusion rates.

For planned surgical procedures that are expected to result in sufficient blood loss to require transfusion, autologous transfusion strategies should be considered. The options for autologous transfusion are several: preoperative autologous blood donation, perioperative blood salvage, and acute normovolemic hemodilution (National Blood Resource Education Program, 1990). Each of these strategies can be used alone or in combination to reduce or eliminate the need for homologous blood.

Preoperative Autologous Blood Donation. A candidate for preoperative donation is a patient who has two or more weeks before a scheduled surgery, who is healthy, and who has a hemoglobin level of 11 gm/Dl (hematocrit of 33 percent) or higher. Patients undergoing orthopedic surgical procedures, for example, such as elective total hip replacement or scoliosis repair, are often ideal candidates for autologous donation. For patients who need more immediate surgery, the benefit of decreased exposure to homologous blood should be weighed against the risk of delaying surgery for the time needed for preoperative donation. Even elderly and pediatric patients can successfully predeposit blood. Autologous donations should not be routinely encouraged for pregnant women because transfusion is rarely needed during a normal delivery. Women with placenta previa,[43] however, are highly likely to need a transfusion and can be encouraged to predeposit blood (Herbert, Owen, and Collins, 1988; McVay et al., 1989).

Despite the benefits of autologous donation, there are practical considerations that must be addressed if its use is to be maximized. The relatively short shelf life of red blood cells (approximately one month) limits the time available between donation and use of blood unless they are frozen and stored. The optimal donation period begins four to six weeks before surgery. Because most patients are able to donate once a week, three or more units can usually be collected before surgery, especially if the patient also takes a therapeutic dose of oral iron. Although

---

[43] Placenta previa, a form of placental development, often produces hemorrhage in the last trimester of pregnancy, particularly during the eighth month.

many blood centers maintain autologous donor programs for long-term storage of frozen red blood cells, for practical reasons these programs are usually limited to patients with very rare blood types. Autologous donor programs for frozen red blood cells for the general population have thus far usually failed because of logistic and cost considerations (Meryman, 1989).

Perioperative Blood Salvage. This form of autologous donation involves the collection and reinfusion of the patient's own blood during or after surgery (Hartz, Smith, and Green, 1988). It is especially beneficial in cases in which preoperative donation is impossible or inadequate and during procedures in which large amounts of blood are lost but can be salvaged. It is not appropriate for procedures with little blood loss or for patients with infection or malignant tumors (American Medical Association, Council on Scientific Affairs, 1986). The amount of blood recovered in this manner is small, usually not exceeding one or two units. Thus, although salvage may provide some benefit, its potential is not nearly as great as that of predonation.

Acute Normovolemic Hemodilution. By this procedure, a portion of the patient's blood is removed before surgery and is replaced with nonblood solutions. The result is hemodilution and a decrease in the viscosity of blood and changes in several other physiologic parameters during surgery (American Medical Association, Council on Scientific Affairs, 1986). At the end of surgery, the blood collected from the patient before surgery is reinfused. Because the blood lost during surgery is relatively dilute, the amount of red cells lost in a given volume is minimized. However, the safe lower limit of the hemodilution of hematocrit is unknown, and this uncertainty has limited the use of this procedure.

Decreasing Patient Need for Blood Products

Another strategy for reducing exposure to homologous blood involves shortening the patient's bleeding time or enhancing the patient's own red blood cell production. Desmopressin acetate has been shown to reduce blood loss in patients undergoing complex cardiac surgery (Salzman et al., 1986), and the hormone erythropoietin can substantially increase red blood cell production in certain patients with chronic anemia. Recent reports, for example, indicate that many chronic renal failure patients on hemodialysis who are transfusion dependent can maintain adequate hemoglobin/hematocrit levels with erythropoietin treatment alone (Eschbach et al., 1989; Zanjani and Ascensao, 1989). The use of erythropoietin in chronic renal failure can reduce red blood cell transfusion requirements overall by as much as 2 to 3 percent. Other potential uses of erythropoietin have not been fully explored, but one use might be to increase preoperative red blood cell levels in anemic patients. Additional uses of this kind could theoretically reduce nationwide red blood cell transfusion requirements by as much as 5 to 10 percent. The cost of the hormone, however, may limit its applicability for this purpose.

Inactivating Viruses

Only two strategies could completely eliminate all risk of infection through blood transfusions: removing or inactivating viruses from blood and blood components, and using blood substitutes. Using blood substitutes would have the additional benefit of alleviating shortages in the blood supply. Unfortunately, neither an effective inactivation method for all blood products nor an effective blood substitute is on the immediate horizon. Viruses present in clotting factor concentrates can now be inactivated either by heat or by solvent detergent treatment (Horowitz, 1987), but viral inactivation is not yet viable for whole blood, fresh-frozen plasma, or such cellular components as packed red blood cells, platelets, and leukocytes (Horowitz, 1987). Therefore, efforts to reduce the risk of transfusion-transmitted HIV infection must continue to rely on donor screening and on modifying physician practices and patient behavior.

Modifying Physician Behavior

Few studies have been done to date on modifying physician practices regarding transfusion. Nonetheless, the literature on modifying physician behavior in other areas of medical practice suggests that modifying physician transfusion practices will probably also require more sophisticated interventions than simply providing printed materials or continuing education lectures (Soumerai et al., 1987). Reliance on such approaches reflects a commonly held belief that changes in a physician's behavior and attitudes will follow changes in knowledge, but the availability of printed information may not lead to new knowledge or in turn to changes in behavior. Several studies indicate that the provision of classroom tutorials and written educational materials, primary educational tools in physician training, has little impact on some physician behavior (Inui, Yourtee, and Williamson, 1976; Avorn and Soumerai, 1983; Schaffner et al., 1983; Maiman et al., 1988). Moreover, there may be dissociation between knowledge and behavior. In studies of physician prescribing practices, innovative printed materials led to changes in a physician's knowledge and attitudes but were not accompanied by changes in behavior (Soumerai and Avorn, 1984). These studies do not negate the role of print-based educational materials as an integral component of more effective strategies, but they do show that print information alone cannot be relied on to produce change (Soumerai and Avorn, 1984).

Giving physicians feedback about their behavior, often in conjunction or comparison with accepted guidelines, has been used to induce behavioral change. This approach assumes that feedback pertaining to the physicians' own cases will motivate them to modify their behavior to adhere more closely to recommended practices. Studies of the effect of feedback on physician behavior, however, have had mixed results (Avorn and Soumerai, 1982; S. A. Schroeder et al., 1984). This inconsistency may reflect the manner and context in which feedback is given in various studies. The length of time between the behavior and the feedback or the extent to which feedback is individualized may influence its potential impact. Soumerai, McLaughlin, and Avorn (1989) noted that feedback programs are more often administrative rather than educational in that they focus on criticism and correction of errors rather than on modifying beliefs about appropriate medical practice and changing behaviors. In one successful intervention to improve physician performance of colorectal cancer screening, physicians given feedback regarding their individual performance did better than those who did not receive feedback (Winick-off et al., 1984).[44] It has been suggested that the effectiveness of feedback might be enhanced if opinion leaders in the medical community and the physicians to be monitored all participate in program design (Tierney, Hui, and McDonald, 1986).

Hospital audits of blood usage, such as those required by the Joint Council of the Administration of Healthcare Organizations (JCAHO) could provide valuable information for feedback to physicians as part of transfusion intervention programs (Coffin, Matz, and Rich, 1989). These audits have provided the impetus for studies of the impact of prospective or daily review systems on transfusion practices in a number of hospitals. Prospective review involves an audit prior to transfusion, thus offering an opportunity to provide immediate feedback to the physician, coupled with education at the point of requesting blood and intervention if requests are not appropriate. Prospective audits in conjunction with transfusion

---

[44] An educational program to improve physician performance in colorectal cancer screening was implemented in a department of internal medicine and evaluated. The program included: 1) an educational meeting for the department's physicians at which a standard of care for colorectal cancer screening was conveyed (the standard included a digital examination and stool test for occult blood to be obtained at all initial or periodic check-ups of patients over age 40); 2) a follow-up meeting at which the rate of adherence to the standard by the physicians as a group was presented; and 3) for a subset of the physicians, an experiment in which physicians were given monthly individual feedback, comparing their performance to that of their peers. The results showed that the physicians receiving individualized feedback significantly improved in adherence when compared with those who were not given feedback; behavior changes persisted at 6 and 12 months after intervention.

education led to a 50 percent reduction of fresh-frozen plasma use in one study (R. R. Solomon, Clifford, and Gutman, 1988) and reductions in platelet use of 14 percent (McCullough et al., 1988) and 56 percent (Simpson, 1987) in two others. Daily review systems involve retrospective review of transfusion, which may also affect transfusion practices. In one study, daily audit reviews reduced inappropriate red cell transfusions from 37 to 10 percent (Giovanetti et al., 1988). Similar audits decreased fresh-frozen plasma use by 77 percent (Shanberge, 1987).

Personalized, face-to-face educational interventions appear to give the best results in modifying physician behavior. In studies involving physician prescription practices, personal intervention resulted in significantly improved decisions when compared with education limited to print materials (Avorn and Soumerai, 1983; Schaffner et al., 1983). Face-to-face interventions also increased the effectiveness of physicians' efforts to educate their patients on adherence to medication (Maiman et al., 1988). There is some evidence that direct intervention with physicians results in greater behavioral change than can be achieved by training faculty who in turn pass training messages on to physicians under their supervision (Kramer, Ber, and Moore, 1987).[45]

Once behavior has changed, it is important to reinforce the new practices physicians adopt. Some researchers have observed that changes in physician behavior diminish after training programs are removed (Patterson, Fried, and Nagle, 1989). Reminders, such as checklists affixed to patient charts, appear to increase physician compliance (McDonald et al., 1984). Such reminders are more effective if they are provided close to the time at which the physician will engage in the targeted behavior. For example, in a study by Tierney, Hui, and McDonald (1986), reminders attached to patient charts were more effective in stimulating behavioral change than general reminders of recommended practices given at monthly intervals. With regard to transfusion practices, checklists for preparing patients for elective surgery could prompt physicians

---

[45] Medical students and physicians (who also would later be used to tutor a group of medical students) participated in an interpersonal skills workshop on supporting behaviors in the medical interview. The workshop consisted of ten 90-minute meetings held twice a week for five weeks. The workshops taught openness, flexibility, and empathy among group members. "The assumption behind these objectives was that developing these reactions in the group members toward each other would allow the students to transfer the use of these skills toward patients." (p. 906). The topics covered in the meetings were: patient admission, diagnosis of a life-threatening disease, death and dying teamwork, uncertainty, and chronic disease. Time was spent role-playing and in group discussion. The results showed that both medical students and physicians who participated in the workshop showed a significant reduction in rejecting behaviors (i.e., ignoring emotions, not listening, or evading eye contact during patient interviews). However, a group of students who were taught by physicians who had been through the workshop did not show a reduction in rejecting behaviors.

to consider autologous donation and also provide a summary of donation guidelines. Similarly, request forms for transfusion could prompt physicians to consider the appropriateness of their request by including standard criteria for transfusion (Avorn et al., 1988).

Modifying Patient Behavior

Patients—potential recipients of blood products—have not been included in research on transfusion practices, and that absence has produced gaps in information that need to be filled. Undoubtedly, patient concerns regarding transfusion-transmitted HIV have contributed to the changes seen in blood use (Surgenor et al., 1988). Pressure from patients, however, depends on the individual patient's knowledge of the issues. Thus, patients could be educated regarding the risks and benefits of transfusion so as to play a more active part in decisions regarding transfusion practices. For example, they could be made aware of the potential risks associated with directed donation. Most important, patients could be more effectively taught about the advantages of autologous donation so that they might be more willing to endure its "costs"—the slight discomfort of blood donation, the time and travel that may be required to donate, the postponement of surgery when medically appropriate, and the necessity of taking oral iron as prescribed.

The committee recommends that agencies of the Public Health Service sponsor the development, systematic testing, and implementation of transfusion-related intervention and education programs to facilitate change in physicians' attitudes and behaviors with regard to:

- **encouraging healthy patients to donate blood;**
- **encouraging autologous donation where medically appropriate;**
- **eliminating the unnecessary use of blood and blood components; and**
- **employing appropriate procedures (e.g., perioperative blood salvage, use of erythropoietin) that reduce the need for transfusion.[46]**

Directions for Future Research

Determining the appropriateness of blood and blood component use requires that standards or criteria be established against which to measure

---

[46]The committee's recommendations are consistent with the World Health Organization's (1989) consensus statements (3.1, 3.2, 3.3) concerning the use of fewer transfusions.

current practices. To develop such standards requires more accurate data on the extent of such use (to discern trends or patterns), together with standardized information on the medical history of the candidates for blood transfusion that make up this data base. Currently, trends in transfusion practices are derived from surveys of individual hospitals in discrete geographic locations that collected data (Surgenor et al., 1988). To detect patterns across locations (which later may be used to target education programs) requires careful consideration of how the hospitals are selected and the types of data that are being collected. It would be helpful to know, for example, whether transfusion practices vary across different types of health care facilities (e.g., university-affiliated hospitals, public institutions). Similarly, data are needed on patterns of use for the different health problems for which transfusions may be ordered. (At least one ongoing national study examining blood use in first-time coronary artery bypass surgery suggests wide variation in transfusion practices for this cardiovascular procedure [Goodnough et al., 1988].) Data that indicate changes in usage over time will also be needed to monitor blood use and the effectiveness of education programs. Data on autologous donation (Toy et al., 1987) have provided an impetus for educational efforts, such as the National Blood Resource Education Program.

To achieve a more solid basis for the formulation of guidelines on appropriate blood use, **the committee recommends that the Public Health Service sponsor research to monitor trends in transfusion practices nationally to permit evaluation of the appropriateness of blood and blood component utilization and to identify targets for change. It further recommends that the PHS develop and evaluate effective strategies for informing patients about the risks and benefits of transfusion.** The burden of developing widely accepted standards of blood and blood component use largely rests with those individuals who are responsible for the supply and distribution of blood. Yet, the consumers of that blood (i.e., the patients) also require education regarding the conditions under which transfusion is necessary and the current need to balance concerns about safety and appropriate use.

* * * * * * * * * *

The enigma of silent, undetected HIV infection thus poses a particularly serious challenge for the biomedical and social/behavioral research communities in relation to the nation's blood supply. The progress achieved to date has come from the concerted efforts of a variety of scientists, who continue to confront the problem of securing an adequate supply of safe blood. Future research may not achieve the quantum leap in risk reduction provided by the introduction of the HIV antibody test in 1985, but incremental improvement is clearly possible, given a long-term commitment to such systematic acquisition of valid and reliable information. Carefully planned and coordinated research programs that can assess and strengthen donor education, screening, and deferral mechanisms, improve testing technologies, modify donor recruitment strategies, and facilitate change in the behaviors that lead to unnecessary use of blood will further reduce the margin of risk.

REFERENCES

Ahlering, R. F. (1979) Recruitment of Blood Donors: A Field Test of Fishbein's Behavioral Intention Model. *Dissertation Abstracts International* 4095–B.

Alter, H. J. (1987) You'll wonder where the yellow went: A 15-year retrospective of post-transfusion hepatitis. In S. B. Moore, ed., *Transfusion-Transmitted Viral Diseases.* Arlington, Va.: American Association of Blood Banks.

Alter, H. J., Holland, P. V., and Purcell, R. H. (1975) The emerging pattern of post-transfusion hepatitis. *American Journal of the Medical Sciences* 270:329–334.

American Association of Blood Banks (AABB). (1984) Telephone Survey on AIDS Conducted by the Dominion Research Corporation. American Association of Blood Banks, Arlington, Va.

American Medical Association, Council on Scientific Affairs. (1986) Council report: Autologous blood transfusions. *Journal of the American Medical Association* 256:2378–2380.

American Red Cross Blood Services, Los Angeles-Orange Counties Region. (1981) The donor experience in the Los Angeles-Orange counties Red Cross blood services. Report prepared by the UCLA Management Field Study Team, Los Angeles, Calif.

American Red Cross Greater Buffalo Chapter. (1985) Blood donor report. Report prepared by Tower Market Research, Buffalo, N. Y.

American Red Cross Mid-America Regional Blood Services. (1980) Red Cross blood donor inquiry. American Red Cross, Chicago, Ill.

Anderson, B. V., and Tomasulo, P. A. (1988) Current autologous transfusion practices. *Transfusion* 28:394–396.

Avorn, J., and Soumerai, S. B. (1982) Use of computer-based Medicaid drug data to analyze and correct inappropriate medication use. *Journal of Medical Systems* 6:377–386.

Avorn, J., and Soumerai, S. B. (1983) Improving drug-therapy decisions through educational outreach: A randomized controlled trial of academically based "detailing." *New England Journal of Medicine* 308:1457–1463.

Avorn, J., Soumerai, S. B., Taylor, W., Wessels, M. R., Janousek, J., and Weiner, M. (1988) Reduction of incorrect antibiotic dosing through a structured educational order form. *Archives of Internal Medicine* 148:1720–1724.

Bagozzi, R. P. (1981a) An examination of the validity of two models of attitude. *Multivariate Behavioral Research* 16:323–359.

Bagozzi, R. P. (1981b) Attitudes, intentions, and behaviour: A test of some key hypotheses. *Journal of Personality and Social Psychology* 41:607–627.

Bagozzi, R. P. (1986) Attitude formation under the theory of reasoned action and a purposeful behaviour reformulation. *British Journal of Social Psychology* 25:95–107.

Baker, J. (1981) Blood component therapy and transfusion reactions. In R. E. Condon, and L. M. Nyhus, eds., *Manual of Surgical Therapeutics.* Boston: Little Brown.

Banks, P. (1989) Blood, tests, and fears: Is a "zero-risk" blood supply possible? *Journal of NIH Research* 1:27–28.

Batson, C. D., Coke, J. S., Jasnoski, M. L., and Hanson, M. (1978) Buying kindness: Effect of an extrinsic incentive for helping on perceived altruism. *Personality and Social Psychology Bulletin* 4:86–91.

Batson, C. D., Fultz, J., Schoenrade, P. A., and Paduano, A. (1987) Critical self-reflection and self-perceived altruism: When self-reward fails. *Journal of Personality and Social Psychology* 53:594–602.

Becker, H. S. (1963) *Outsiders: Studies in the Sociology of Deviance.* New York: The Free Press.

Bettinghaus, E. P., and Milkovich, M. B. (1975) Donors and non-donors: Communication and information. *Transfusion* 15:165–169.

Blood Center of Southeastern Wisconsin. (1986) A lifestyle profile of blood donors. Report prepared by Needham Harper Worldwide, Chicago, Ill.

Blumberg, N., and Heal, J. M. (1989) Transfusion and host defenses against cancer recurrence and infection. *Transfusion* 29:236–245.

Blumberg, N., Laczin, J., McMican, A., Heal, J., Arvan, D. (1986) A critical survey of fresh-frozen plasma use. *Transfusion* 26:511–513.

Boe, G. P. (1976) A survey of the attitudes and motivations of college students regarding blood donations. *Journal of American Medical Technologists* 38:166–169.

Boe, G. P. (1977) A descriptive characterization and comparison of blood donors and non-donors in a community blood program. *Dissertation Abstracts International* 3789–B.

Boe, G. P., and Ponder, L. D. (1981) Blood donors and non-donors: A review of the research. *American Journal of Medical Technology* 47:248–253.

Brecher, M. E., Moore, S. B., and Taswell, H. F. (1988) Minimal-exposure transfusion: A new approach to homologous blood transfusion. *Mayo Clinic Proceedings* 63:903–905.

Brewer, T., Rappaport, F., and Waterfield, J. (1974) Special holiday blood donor campaign. American Red Cross, Washington, D.C.

Briggs, N. C., Piliavin, J. A., Lorentzen, D., and Becker, G. A. (1986) On willingness to be a bone marrow donor. *Transfusion* 26:324–330.

Burnett, J. J. (1982) Examining the profiles of the donor and nondonor through a multiple discriminant approach. *Transfusion* 22:138–142.

Callero, P. L. (1983) Role-identity commitment and regular blood donation. *Dissertation Abstracts International* 44:1582.

Callero, P. L., and Piliavin, J. A. (1983) Developing a commitment to blood donation: The impact of one's first experience. *Journal of Applied Social Psychology* 13:1–16.

Campbell, B., Phillips, P., Zahavi, R., Williams, E., and Murphy, S. (1989) Establishing the comfort zone: Developing interviewer competence and confidence in a survey on a sensitive topic. In F. J. Fowler, Jr., ed., *Conference Proceedings: Health Survey Research Methods*. DHHS Publ. No. PHS 89–3447.

Carson, J. L., Poses, R. M., Spence, R. K., and Bonavita, G. (1988) Severity of anemia and operative mortality and morbidity. *Lancet* 2:727–729.

Caruso, M. J. (1978) Blood donation attitudes and behavior. Technical Report No. 139. Operations Research Center, Massachusetts Institute of Technology.

Casati, S., Passerini, P., Campise, M. R., Graziani, G., Cesana, B., et al. (1987) Benefits and risks of protracted treatment with human recombinant erythropoeitin in patients having haemodialysis. *British Medical Journal* 295:1017–1020.

Centers for Disease Control (CDC). (1982) Possible transfusion-associated acquired immune deficiency syndrome (AIDS)—California. *Morbidity and Mortality Weekly Report* 31:652–654.

Centers for Disease Control (CDC). (1985) Provisional Public Health Service interagency recommendations for screening donated blood and plasma for antibody to the virus causing the acquired immunodeficiency syndrome. *Morbidity and Mortality Weekly Report* 34:1–5.

Centers for Disease Control (CDC). (1986) Human T-lymphotropic virus type III/lymph-adenopathy-associated virus antibody prevalence in U.S. military recruit applicants. *Morbidity and Mortality Weekly Report* 35:421–424.

Centers for Disease Control (CDC). (1989) Racial differences in rates of hepatitis B virsus infection—United States, 1976–1980. *Morbidity and Mortality Weekly Report* 38:818–821.

Chambers, L. A., Volpp, J. L., Page, P. L., and Popovsky, M. A. (1986) Failure of self-deferral of high-risk anti-HTLV-III positive volunteer blood donors. *Transfusion* 26:591(A28).

Charng, H. W., Piliavin, J. A., and Callero, P. L. (1988) Role identity and reasoned action in the prediction of repeated behavior. *Social Psychology Quarterly* 51:303–317.

Chitwood, D. D., Comerford, M., McCoy, C. B., and Trapido, E. J. (1989) Blood sale and donation behavior of IVDUs. Presented at the Fifth International Conference on AIDS, Montreal, June 4–9.

Cialdini, R. B., and Ascani, K. (1976) Test of a concession procedure for inducing verbal, behavioral, and further compliance with a request to give blood. *Journal of Applied Psychology* 61:295–300.

Cleary, P. D., Singer, E., Rogers, T. F., Avorn, A., Van Devanter, N., et al. (1988) Sociodemographic and behavioral characteristics of HIV antibody-positive blood donors. *American Journal of Public Health* 78:953–957.

Coffin, C., Matz, K., and Rich, E. (1989) Algorithms for evaluating the appropriateness of blood transfusion. *Transfusion* 29:298–303.

Cohen, M. A., and Pierskalla, W. P. (1975) Management policies for a regional blood bank. *Transfusion* 15:58–67.

Cohen, N. D., Munoz, A., Reitz, B. A., Ness, P. K., Frazier, O. H., et al. (1989) Transmission of retroviruses by transfusion of screened blood in patients undergoing cardiac surgery. *New England Journal of Medicine* 320:1172–1176.

Condie, S. J. (1979) When altruism fails: The logic of collective action and blood donor behavior. In D. J. Oborne, M. M. Gruneberg, and J. R. Miser, eds., *Research in Psychology and Medicine.* Vol. 2. *Social Aspects: Attitudes, Communication, Care and Training.* New York: Academic Press.

Condie, S. J., Warner, W. K., and Gillman, D. C. (1976) Getting blood from collective turnips: Volunteer donation in mass blood drives. *Journal of Applied Psychology* 61:290–294.

Cordell, R. R., Yalon, V. A., Cigahn-Haskell, C., McDonough, B. P., Perkins, H. A., et al. (1986) Experience with 11,916 designated donors. *Transfusion* 26:484–486.

Council of Community Blood Centers (CCBC). (1989) CDC study looks at why HIV-seropositive individuals donate blood. *CCBC Newsletter* November 10:1.

Cox, J. (1987) Adopt a donor, an innovative recruitment concept. *Transfusion* 27:569(A68).

Crowley, J. P., Guadagnoli, E., Pezzullo, J., Fuller, J., and Yankee, R. (1988) Changes in hospital component therapy in response to reduced availability of whole blood. *Transfusion* 28:4–7.

Cumming, P. D., Schorr, J. B., and Wallace, E. L. (1987) *Annual Blood Facts United States Totals—1986–1987.* Washington, D.C.: American Red Cross National Headquarters.

Cumming, P. D., Wallace, E. L., Schorr, J. B., and Dodd, R. Y. (1989) Exposure of patients to human immunodeficiency virus through the transfusion of blood components that test antibody-negative. *New England Journal of Medicine* 321:941–946.

Curran, J. W., Lawrence, D. N., Jaffe, H., Kaplan, J. E., Zyla, L. D., et al. (1984) Acquired immunodeficiency syndrome (AIDS) associated with transfusions. *New England Journal of Medicine* 310:69–75.

Dawson, D. A. (1989) AIDS knowledge and attitudes for January-March, 1989: Provisional data from the National Health Interview Survey. In *Advance Data from Vital and Health Statistics* 176:1–12. Hyattsville, Md.: National Center for Health Statistics.

Dodd, R. Y., and Barker, L. F. (1989) Early markers of HIV-1 infection in plasma donors. *Journal of the American Medical Association* 262:92–93.

Dodd, R. Y., and Barker, L. F., eds. (1985) *Infection, Immunity and Blood Transfusion.* New York: Alan R. Liss.

Doll, L. S., Peterson, L., Ward, J., White, C., Bush, T., et al. (1989) Behavioral determinants of blood donations among HIV-seropositive persons: A multi-center study. Presented at the Fifth International Conference on AIDS, Montreal. June 4–9.

Dondero, T. J., and the HIV Data Analysis Team. (1987) Human immunodeficiency virus infection in the United States: A review of current knowledge. *Morbidity and Mortality Weekly Report* 36(S–6):1–48.

Drake, A. W. (1978) Public Attitudes and Decision Processes with Regard to Blood Donation: Final Report and Executive Summary. National Center for Health Services Research, Hyattsville, Md.

Drake, A. W., Finkelstein, S. N., and Sopolsky, H. M. (1982) *The American Blood Supply.* Cambridge, Mass.: Massachusetts Institute of Technology.

Eckert, N., and Neal, D. (1984) Sickle cell screening—a public relations and donor recruitment success story. *Transfusion* 24:445(A37).

Edwards, P. W., and Zeichner, A. (1985) Blood donor development: Effects of personality, motivational and situational variables. *Personality and Individual Differences* 6:743–751.

Eschbach, J. W., Egrie, J. C., Downing, M. R., Browne, J. K., and Adamson, J. W. (1987) Correction of the anemia of end-stage renal disease with recombinant human erythropoietin: Results of a combined Phase I and II clinical trial. *New England Journal of Medicine* 316:73–78.

Eschbach, J. W., Kelly, M. R., Haley, N. R., Abels, R. I., and Adamson, J. W. (1989) Treatment of the anemia of progressive renal failure with recombinant human erythropoietin. *New England Journal of Medicine* 321:158–163.

Evans, D. E. (1981) Development of intrinsic motivation for voluntary blood donation among first-time donors. *Dissertation Abstracts International* 42:3777.

Evatt, B. L., Francis, D. P., McLane, M. F., Lee, T. H., Cabradilla, C., et al. (1983) Antibodies to human T-cell leukemia virus-associated membrane antigens in hemophiliacs: Evidence for infection before 1980. *Lancet* 2:698–700.

Farrales, F. B., Stevenson, A. R., and Bayer, W. L. (1977) Causes of disqualification in a volunteer blood donor population. *Transfusion* 17:598–601.

Ferrari, J. R., Barone, R. C., Jason, L. A., and Rose, T. (1985a) Effects of a personal phone call prompt on blood donor commitment. *Journal of Community Psychology* 13:295–298.

Ferrari, J. R., Barone, R. C., Jason, L. A., and Rose, T. (1985b) The use of incentives to increase blood donations. *Journal of Social Psychology* 125:791–793.

Fischer, A., Pura, L., Smith, L., and Goldfinger, D. (1986) Safety and effectiveness of directed blood donation in a large teaching hospital. *Transfusion* 26:600(A61).

Fishbein, M., and Ajzen, I. (1975) *Belief, Attitude, Intention and Behavior: An Introduction to Theory and Research.* Reading, Mass.: Addison and Wesley.

Fisher, J. D. (1988) Possible effects of reference group-based social influence on AIDS-risk behavior and AIDS prevention. *American Psychologist* 43:914–920.

Foss, R. D. (1983) Community norms and blood donation. *Journal of Applied Social Psychology* 13:281–290.

Foss, R. D., and Dempsey, C. B. (1979) Blood donation and the foot-in-the-door technique: A limiting case. *Journal of Personality and Social Psychology* 37:580–590.

Fowler, F. J., Jr. (1989) Evaluating special training and debriefing procedures for pretest interviews. In C. Cannell, L. Oksenberg, G. Kalton, K. Bischoping, and F. J. Fowler, eds., *New Techniques for Pretesting Survey Questions.* (mimeo). Final Report to the National Center for Health Services Research and Health Care Technology Assessment. Survey Research Center, University of Michigan and Center for Survey Research, University of Massachusetts.

Fowler, F. J., and Mangione, T. W. (1990) *Standardized Survey Interviewing.* Newbury Park, Calif.: Sage.

Freiburger, C. A., and George, W. R. (1988) It's as easy as 1, 2, 3: 1st-time donors will come back. *Transfusion* 28:(Suppl. 6):55S(A55).

Gaynor, S., Kessler, D., Berge, P., Andrews, S., and Del Valle, C. (1989a) Risk factors for HIV among New York blood donors in 1988. Presented at the Fifth International Conference on AIDS, Montreal, June 4–9.

Gaynor, S., Kessler, D., Andrews, S., and Del Valle, C. (1989b) Self-exclusion by HIV antibody positive blood donors. Presented at the Fifth International Conference on AIDS, Montreal, June 4–9.

Gibson, T. (1980) Notes on East Anglian blood donors. *Transfusion* 20:716–719.

Giovanetti, A. M., Parravicini, A., Baroni, L., Riccardi, D., Pizzi, M. N., et al. (1988) Quality assessment of transfusion practice in elective surgery. *Transfusion* 28:166–169.

Goldfinger, D. (1989) Directed blood donations: Pro. *Transfusion* 29:70–74.

Goodnough, L. T., Kruskall, M., Stehling, L., Johnson, M., Kennedy, M., et al. (1988) A multicenter audit of transfusion practice in coronary artery bypass (CABG) surgery. *Blood* 72:277a.

Gordeuk, V. R., Brittenham, G. M., Bravo, J. A., Hughes, M. A., and Keating, L. J. (1987) Carbonyl iron for short-term supplementation in female blood donors. *Transfusion* 27:80–85.

Grace, H. A. (1957) Blood donor recruitment: A case study in the psychology of communication. *Journal of Social Psychology* 46:269–276.

Greenwalt, T. J., and Jamieson, G. A., eds. (1975) *Transmissible Disease and Blood Transfusion.* New York: Grune and Stratton.

Gregorio, D. L., and Linden, J. V. (1988) Screening prospective blood donors for AIDS risk factors: Will sufficient donors be found? *American Journal of Public Health* 78:1468–1471.

Grindon, A. J., Winn, L. C., Kastal, P., and Eska, P. (1976) Conversion of professional donors to volunteer donors. *Transfusion* 16:190.

Haigh, J. D. (1987) A plan to educate elementary school children, recruit their parents and maintain an adequate blood supply. *Transfusion* 27:570(A69).

Hamilton, Frederick, and Schneiders. (1988) Recent trend survey research findings. Memorandum to the American Association of Blood Banks, June 15. Hamilton, Frederick, and Schneiders, Washington, D.C.

Handler, S. (1983) Does continuing medical education affect medical care: A study of improved transfusion practices. *Minnesota Medicine,* March:167–180.

Hartz, R. S., Smith, J. A., and Green, D. (1988) Autotransfusion after cardiac operation: Assessment of hemostatic factors. *Journal of Thoracic Cardiovascular Surgery* 96:178–182.

Hayes, T. J., Dwyer, F. R., Greenwalt, T. J., and Coe, N. A. (1984) A comparison of two behavioral influence techniques for improving blood donor recruitment. *Transfusion* 24:399–403.

Heider, F. (1958) *The Psychology of Interpersonal Relations.* New York: Wiley.

Herbert, W. N. P., Owen, H. G., and Collins, M. L. (1988) Autologous blood storage in obstetrics. *Obstetrics & Gynecology* 72:166–170.

Hochschild, A. R. (1983) *The Managed Heart: Commercialization of Human Feeling.* Berkeley, Calif.: University of California Press.

Hocking, B., O'Collins, M., Pulsford, R. L., Woodfield, D. J., Arnold, P., et al. (1974) Blood donor motivation in Papua New Guinea. *Medical Journal of Australia* 2:670–674.

Horowitz, B. (1987) Inactivation of viruses in blood derivatives. In S. B. Moore, ed., *Transfusion-Transmitted Viral Diseases.* Arlington, Va.: American Association of Blood Banks.

Hughes, M. J., Winter, S. L., Perkins, C. I., Kizer, K. W., Capell, F. J., and Trachtenberg, A. I. (1989) Prevalence of HIV antibody among blood donors in California. *New England Journal of Medicine* 321:974–975.

Hyman, H. H., Cobb, W. J., Feldman, J. J., Hart, C. W., and Stember, C. H. (1975) *Interviewing in Social Research.* Chicago, Ill.: The University of Chicago Press.

Imagawa, D. T., Lee, M. H., Wolinsky, S. M., Sano, K., Morales, F., et al. (1989) Human immunodeficiency virus Type 1 infection in homosexual men who remain seronegative for prolonged periods. *New England Journal of Medicine* 320:1458–1462.

Inui, T. S., Yourtee, E. L., and Williamson, J. W. (1976) Improved outcomes in hypertension after physician tutorials: A controlled trial. *Annals of Internal Medicine* 84:646–651.

Jason, L. A., Jackson, K., and Obradovic, J. L. (1986) Behavioral approaches in increasing blood donations. *Evaluation and the Health Professions* 9:439–448.

Jason, L. A., Rose, T., Ferrari, J. R., and Barone, R. (1984) Personal versus impersonal methods for recruiting blood donations. *Journal of Social Psychology* 123:139–140.

Kalish, R. I., Cable, R. G., and Roberts, S. C. (1986) Voluntary deferral of blood donations and HTLV-III antibody positivity. *New England Journal of Medicine* 314:1115–1116.

Kaloupek, D. G., and Stoupakis, T. (1985) Coping with a stressful medical procedure: Further investigation with volunteer blood donors. *Journal of Behavioral Medicine* 8:131–148.

Kaloupek, D. G., Scott, J. R., and Khatami, V. (1985) Assessment of coping strategies associated with syncope in blood donors. *Journal of Psychosomatic Research* 29:207–214.

Kaloupek, D. G., White, H., and Wong, M. (1984) Multiple assessment of coping strategies used by volunteer blood donors: Implications for preparatory training. *Journal of Behavioral Medicine* 7:35–60.

Kelley, H. H. (1967) Attribution theory in social psychology. In D. Levine, ed., *Nebraska Symposium on Motivation.* Lincoln, Neb.: University of Nebraska Press.

Kleinman, S., and Secord, K. (1988) Risk of human immunodeficiency virus (HIV) transmission by anti-HIV negative blood: Estimates using the lookback methodology. *Transfusion* 28:499–501.

Kotler, P., and Roberto, E. L. (1989) *Social Marketing: Strategies for Changing Public Behavior.* New York: The Free Press.

Kramer, D., Ber, R., and Moore, M. (1987) Impact of workshop on students' and physicians' rejecting behaviors in patient interviews. *Journal of Medical Education* 62:904–909.

Kruskall, M. S., Glazer, E. E., Leonard, S. S., Willson, S. C., Pacini, D. G., et al. (1986) Utilization and effectiveness of a hospital autologous preoperative blood donor program. *Transfusion* 26:335–340.

LaQue, C., Bailey, G., Odell, T., Heal, J., and Nusbacher, J. (1982) Hemapheresis donors as volunteer recruiters. *Transfusion* 22:446(A43).

Leibrecht, B. C., Hogan, J. M., Luz, G. A., and Tobias, K. I. (1976) Donor and non-donor motivations. *Transfusion* 16:182–189.

Leitman, S. F., Klein, H. G., Melpolder, J. J., Read, E. J., Esteban, J. I., et al. (1989) Clinical implications of positive tests for antibodies to human immunodeficiency virus Type 1 in asymptomatic blood donors. *New England Journal of Medicine* 321:917–924.

Levine, E. A., Gould, S. A., Rosen, A. L., Sehgal, L. R., Egrie, J. C., et al. (1989) Perioperative recombinant human erythropoietin. *Surgery* 106:432–438.

Lightman, E. S. (1981) Continuity in social policy behaviours: The case of voluntary blood donorship. *Journal of Social Policy* 10:53–79.

Lima, V. M., and D'Amorim, M. A. (1985) Application of Fishbein and Ajzen's theory of persuasion to the recruitment of voluntary and periodic blood donors. *Arquivos Brasileiros de Psicologia* 37:110–119.

Linden, J. V., Gregorio, D. I., and Kalish, R. I. (1988) An estimate of blood donor eligibility in the general population. *Vox Sang* 54:96–100.

Lipsitz, A., Kallmeyer, K., Ferguson, M., and Abas, A. (1989) Counting on blood donors: Increasing the impact of reminder calls. *Journal of Applied Social Psychology* 19:1057–1067.

Loicano, B., Carter, G., Leitman, S. F., and Klein, H. G. (1988) Efficacy of various methods of confidential unit exclusion in identifying potentially infectious blood products. *Transfusion* 28(Suppl. 6):54S(A51).

London, P. (1970) The rescuers: Motivational hypotheses about Christians who saved Jews from the Nazis. In J. Macaulay and L. Berkowitz, eds., *Altruism and Helping Behavior.* New York: Academic Press.

Maiman, L. A., Becker, M. H., Liptak, G. S., Nazarian, L. F., and Rounds, K. A. (1988) Improving pediatricians' compliance-enhancing practices. *American Journal of Diseases of Children* 142:773–779.

Marrow, A. J. (1969) *The Practical Theorist.* New York: Basic Books, Inc.

McBarnette, L., Rosner, F., Blake, M. V., and Kahn, A. E. (1978) The rejected blood donor: Comparison between a voluntary and municipal hospital. *Transfusion* 18:69–72.

McCall, G. J., and Simmons, J. L. (1978) *Identities and Interactions.* Rev. ed. New York: The Free Press.

McCullough, J., Steeper, T. A., Connelly, D. P., Jackson, B., Huntington, S., and Scott, E. P. (1988) Platelet utilization in a university hospital. *Journal of the American Medical Association* 259:2414–2418.

McDonald, C. J., Hui, S. L., Smith, D. M., Tierney, W. M., Cohen, S. J., et al. (1984) Reminders to physicians from an introspective computer medical record. *Annals of Internal Medicine* 100:130–138.

McVay, P. A., Hoag, R. W., Hoag, M. S., and Toy, T. (1989) Safety and use of autologous blood donation during the third trimester of pregnancy. *American Journal of Obstetrics and Gynecology* 160:1479–1488.

Mell, G. W. (1979) Research findings of Red Cross blood donor profile. American Red Cross, Muskegon-Oceana Chapter.

Menitove, J. E. (1989) The decreasing risk of transfusion-associated AIDS. *New England Journal of Medicine* 321:966–968.

Meryman, H. T. (1989) Frozen red cells. *Transfusion Medicine Reviews* 3:121–127.

Moore, S. B., ed. (1987) *Transfusion-Transmitted Viral Diseases.* Arlington, Va.: American Association of Blood Banks.

Moss, A. J. (1976) Blood donor characteristics and types of blood donations. In *Vital and Health Statistics.* DNEW 76–1533. Series 10, No. 106:1–19. Rockville, Md: National Center for Health Statistics.

Murray, C. (1988) Evaluation of on-site cholesterol testing as a donor recruitment tool. *Transfusion* 28(Suppl. 6):56S(A59).

National Blood Resource Education Program. (1989) *Transfusion Alert: Use of Autologous Blood.* NIH Publication No. 89–3038. Bethesda, Md.: National Heart, Lung, and Blood Institute.

National Blood Resource Education Program. (1990) The use of autologous blood: The national blood resource education program expert panel. *Journal of the American Medical Association* 263:414–417.

National Heart, Lung, and Blood Institute (NHLBI). (1972) Summary report: National Heart, Lung and Blood Institute's resource studies. U.S. Department of Health, Education, and Welfare Publication No. (NIH) 73–416. Bethesda, Md.: U.S. Department of Health, Education, and Welfare.

National Heart, Lung, and Blood Institute (NHLBI). (1988) AIDS and blood resources. Presented at the meeting of the Committee on AIDS Research, National Academy of Sciences. Washington, D.C., December 22.

Nelson, K. E., Vlahov, D., Margolick, J., and Bernal, M. (1989) Blood and plasma donations among a cohort of IV drug users. Presented at the Fifth International Conference on AIDS, Montreal, June 4–9.

Newman, B. H., Burak, F. Q., McKay-Peters, E. H., and Pothiawala, M. A. (1988) Patient-related blood drives. *Transfusion* 28:142–144.

Nichols, E. K. (1986) *Mobilizing Against AIDS: An Unfinished Story of a Virus.* Cambridge, Mass.: Harvard University Press.

Nusbacher, J., Chiavetta, J., Naiman, R., Buchner, B., Scalia, V., and Herst, R. (1986) Evaluation of a confidential method of excluding blood donors exposed to human immunodeficiency virus. *Transfusion* 26:539–541.

Oborne, D. J., Bradley, S., and Lloyd-Griffiths, M. (1978) The anatomy of a volunteer blood donation system. *Transfusion* 18:458–465.

Office of Medical Applications of Research (OMAR), National Institutes of Health. (1985) Consensus Conference: Fresh-frozen plasma indications and risks. *Journal of the American Medical Association* 253:551–553.

Office of Medical Applications of Research (OMAR), National Institutes of Health. (1987) Consensus Conference: Platelet transfusion therapy. *Journal of the American Medical Association* 257:1777–1780.

Office of Medical Applications of Research (OMAR), National Institutes of Health. (1989) Perioperative red cell transfusion: National Institutes of Health Consensus Development Conference. *Transfusion Medicine Reviews* 3:63–68.

Office of Technology Assessment (OTA). (1985) *Blood Policy and Technology.* Washington, D.C.: Office of Technology Assessment.

Oswalt, R. M. (1977) A review of blood donor motivation and recruitment. *Transfusion* 17:123–135.

Oswalt, R. M., and Zack, L. A. (1976) The motivation and recruitment of pheresis donors. Presented at the 29th Annual Meeting of the American Association of Blood Banks, San Francisco, October 30–November 5.

Page, P. L. (1989) Controversies in transfusion medicine: Directed blood donations: Con. *Transfusion* 29:65–70.

Patterson, J., Fried, R. A., and Nagle, J. P. (1989) Impact of a comprehensive health promotion curriculum on physician behavior and attitudes. *American Journal of Preventive Medicine* 5:44–49.

Paulhus, D. L., Shaffer, D. R., and Downing, L. L. (1977) Effects of making blood donor motives salient upon donor retention: A field experiment. *Personality and Social Psychology Bulletin* 3:99–102.

Perkins, H. A., Samson, S., and Busch, M. P. (1988) How well has self-exclusion worked? *Transfusion* 28:601–602.

Perkins, H. A., Cordell, R., Bueno, C., Shiota, J., Hitchcock, B., et al. (1987) The progressive decrease in the proportion of blood donors with antibody to the human immunodeficiency virus (HIV). *Transfusion* 27:502–503.

Petersen, L., and the HIV Blood Donor Study Group. (1989) Surveillance for unusual modes of HIV transmission in the USA: A 5-year multicenter study of blood donors. Presented at the Fifth International Conference on AIDS, Montreal, June 4–9.

Piliavin, J. A. (1987) Temporary deferral and donor return. *Transfusion* 27:199–200.

Piliavin, J. A., and Callero, P. L. (In press) *Giving the Gift of Life to Unnamed Strangers: The American Community Responsibility Blood Donor.* Baltimore, Md.: Johns Hopkins University Press.

Piliavin, J. A., and Libby, D. (1986) Personal norms, perceived social norms, and blood donation. *Humboldt Journal of Social Relations* 13:159–194.

Piliavin, J. A., Callero, P. L., and Evans, D. E. (1982) Addiction to altruism? Opponent-process theory and habitual blood donation. *Journal of Personality and Social Psychology* 43:1200–1213.

Piliavin, J. A., Evans, D. E., and Callero, P. L. (1984) Learning to "give to unnamed strangers:" The process of commitment to regular blood donation. In E. Staub, D. Bar-Tal, J. Karylowski, and J. Reykowski, eds., *Development and Maintenance of Prosocial Behavior: International Perspectives on Positive Morality.* New York: Plenum.

Pindyck, J., Waldman, A., Zang, E., Oleszko, W., Lowry, M., and Bianco, C. (1985) Measures to decrease the risk of acquired immunodeficiency syndrome transmission by blood transfusion. *Transfusion* 25:3–9.

Pindyck, J., Avorn, J., Kuriyan, M., Reed, M., Ibgal, M. J., et al. (1987) Blood donation by the elderly. *Journal of the American Medical Association* 257:1186–1188.

Pomazal, R. J., and Jaccard, J. J. (1976) An informational approach to altruistic behavior. *Journal of Personality and Social Psychology* 33:317–326.

Price, T. H. (1989) Prospective audits: An approach for improving transfusion practice. In S. R. Kurtz, S. H. Summers, and M. S. Kruskall, eds., *Improving Transfusion Practice: The Role of Quality Assurance.* Arlington, Va.: American Association of Blood Banks.

Reinisch, J. M., Sanders, S. A., and Ziemba-Davis, M. (1988) The study of sexual behavior in relation to the transmission of human immunodeficiency virus. *American Psychologist* 43:921–927.

Rosenhan, D. (1970) The natural socialization of altruistic autonomy. In J. Macaulay and L. Berkowitz, eds., *Altruism and Helping Behavior.* New York: Academic Press.

Rushton, J. P., and Campbell, A. C. (1977) Modeling, vicarious reinforcement and extraversion on blood donating in adults: Immediate and long-term effects. *European Journal of Social Psychology* 7:297–306.

Ryan, T. (1987) Junior high school student blood drive—A community education program for non blood donors. *Transfusion* 27:571(A75).

Rzasa, M., and Gilcher, R. (1988) Cholesterol testing: Incentive or health benefit? *Transfusion* 28(Suppl. 6):56S(A60).

Salzman, E. W., Weinstein, M. J., Weintraub, R. M., Ware, J. A., Thurer, R. L., et al. (1986) Treatment with desmopressin acetate to reduce blood loss after cardiac surgery: A double-blind randomized trial. *New England Journal of Medicine* 314:1402–1406.

Schaffner, W., Ray, W. A., Federspiel, C. F., and Miller, W. O. (1983) Improving antibiotic prescribing in the office practice: A controlled trial of three educational methods. *Journal of the American Medical Association* 250:1728–1732.

Schmidt, P. J. (1984) Senior donors. *Transfusion* 24:445(A38).

Schroeder, C. (1987) Recruiting blacks as blood donors. *Transfusion* 27:570(A70).

Schroeder, S. A., Myers, L. P., McPhee, S. J., Showstack, J. A., Simborg, D. W., et al. (1984) The failure of physician education as a cost containment strategy: Report of a prospective controlled trial at a university hospital. *Journal of the American Medical Association* 252:225–230.

Schwartz, S. H. (1970) Elicitation of moral obligation and self-sacrificing behavior: An experimental study of volunteering to be a bone marrow donor. *Journal of Personality and Social Psychology* 15:283–293.

Schwartz, S. H. (1973) Normative explanations of helping behavior: A critique, proposal and empirical test. *Journal of Experimental Social Psychology* 9:349–364.

Schwartz, S. H., and Tessler, R. C. (1972) A test of a model for reducing measured attitude-behavior discrepancies. *Journal of Personality and Social Psychology* 24:225–236.

Seage, G. R., Barry, A., Landers, S., Silvia, A. M., Lamb, G. A., et al. (1988) Patterns of blood donations among individuals at risk for AIDS. *American Journal of Public Health* 78:576–577.

Seeff, L. B., Wright, E. C., Zimmerman, H. J., and McCollum, R. W. (1975) VA cooperative study of post-transfusion hepatitis, 1969–1974: Incidence and characteristics of hepatitis and responsible risk factors. *American Journal of the Medical Sciences* 270:355–362.

Shanberge, J. N. (1987) Reduction of fresh-frozen plasma use through a daily survey and education program. *Transfusion* 27:226–227.

Shilts, R. (1988) *And the Band Played On: Politics, People, and the AIDS Epidemic.* 2nd ed. New York: Viking Penguin, Inc.

Silvergleid, A. J., Leparc, G. F., and Schmidt, P. J. (1989) Impact of explicit questions about high-risk activities on donor attitudes and donor deferral patterns: Results in two community blood centers. *Transfusion* 29:362–364.

Simon, T. L., Hunt, W. C., and Garry, P. J. (1984) Iron supplementation for menstruating female blood donors. *Transfusion* 24:469–472.

Simpson, M. B. (1987) Prospective-concurrent audits and medical consultation for platelet transfusions. *Transfusion* 27:192–195.

Skettino, S., Sorenson, D., and Perkins, H. A. (1988) A medical history question used to help identify donors in risk groups for AIDS. *Transfusion* 28(Suppl. 6):54S(A49).

Snyder, A. J., and Vergeront, J. M. (1988) Safeguarding the blood supply by providing opportunities for anonymous HIV testing. *New England Journal of Medicine* 319:374–375.

Snyder, A. J., Gottschall, J. L., and Menitove, J. E. (1986) Why is fresh-frozen plasma transfused? *Transfusion* 26:107–112.

Solomon, R. L. (1980) The opponent-process theory of acquired motivation: The costs of pleasure and the benefits of pain. *American Psychologist* 35:691–712.

Solomon, R. R., Clifford, J. S., and Gutman, S. I. (1988) The use of laboratory intervention to stem the flow of fresh frozen plasma. *American Journal of Clinical Pathology* 89:518–521.

Soumerai, S. B. (1988) Factors influencing prescribing. *Australian Journal of Hospital Pharmacy* 18(Suppl.):9–16.

Soumerai, S. B., and Avorn, J. (1984) Efficacy and cost-containment in hospital pharmacotherapy: State of the art and future directions. *Milbank Memorial Fund Quarterly* 62:447–474.

Soumerai, S. B., McLaughlin, T. J., and Avorn, J. (1989) Improving drug prescribing in primary care: A critical analysis of the experimental literature. *Milbank Quarterly* 67:268–317.

Soumerai, S. B., Avorn, J., Gortmaker, S., and Hawley, S. (1987) Effect of government and commercial warnings on reducing prescription misuse: The case of propoxyphene. *American Journal of Public Health* 77:1518–1523.

Staallekker, L. A., Stammeijer, R. N., and Dudok de Wit, C. (1980) A Dutch blood bank and its donors. *Transfusion* 20:66–70.

Starkey, J. M., MacPherson, J. L., Bolgiano, D. C., Simon, E. R., Zuck, T. F., and Sayers, M. H. (1989) Markers for transfusion-transmitted disease in different groups of blood donors. *Journal of the American Medical Association* 262:3452–3454.

Stehling, L. C., and Esposito, B. (1987) Appropriate intraoperative blood utilization. *Transfusion* 27:545(AS152).

Strauss, R. G., and Sacher, R. A. (1988) Directed donations for pediatric patients. *Transfusion Medicine Reviews* 2:58–64.

Strauss, R. G., Ferguson, K., Black, D., Stone, G., Stehling, L. C., et al. (1988) Surgeon knowledge and attitude of preoperative autologous donation. Presented at the 41st Annual Meeting of the American Association of Blood Banks, Kansas City, Mo., October 8–13.

Stryker, S. (1980) *Symbolic Interactionism: A Social Structural Version.* Menlo Park, Calif.: Benjamin/Cummings.

Surgenor, D. M. (1987) The patients' blood is the safest blood. *New England Journal of Medicine* 316:542–544.

Surgenor, D. M., and Cerveny, J. F. (1978) A study of the conversion from paid to altruistic blood donors in New Mexico. *Transfusion* 18:54–63.

Surgenor, D. M., and Schnitzer, S. S. (1985) The nation's blood resource: A summary report. National Institutes of Health Publication No. 85–2028. Bethesda, Md.: U.S. Department of Health and Human Services.

Surgenor, D. M., Wallace, E. L., Hale, S. G., and Gilpatrick, M. W. (1988) Changing patterns of blood transfusions in four sets of United States hospitals, 1980–1985. *Transfusion* 28:513–518.

Swain, H. L., and Balscovich, J. J. (1977) Effects of solicitor variables on obtaining pledges to donate blood. *Public Health Reports* 92:383–385.

Szymanski, L. S., Cushna, B., Jackson, B. C. H., and Syzmanski, I. O. (1978) Motivation of plateletpheresis donors. *Transfusion* 18:64–68.

Tabor, E., ed. (1982) *Infectious Complications of Blood Transfusion.* New York: Academic Press.

Talafuse, D. W. (1978) Blood donor attitudes and decisions: An exploratory analysis. Technical Report No. 137. Operations Research Center, Massachusetts Institute of Technology.

Tartter, P. I., and Barron, D. M. (1985) Unnecessary blood transfusions in elective colorectal cancer surgery. *Transfusion* 25:113–115.

Therkelsen, D. J., Korent, H. M., Haugen, J. D., Undis, J. M., Jensen, J., et al. (1988) Factors influencing aggregate level of blood donation. *Transfusion* 28(Suppl. 6):43S(A6).

Thomas, G. C., and Batson, C. D. (1981) Effect of helping under normative pressure on self-perceived altruism. *Social Psychology Quarterly* 44:127–131.

Thomas, G. C., Batson, C. D., and Coke, J. S. (1981) Do good Samaritans discourage helpfulness? Self-perceived altruism after exposure to highly helpful others. *Journal of Personality and Social Psychology* 40:194–200.

Tierney, W. M., Hui, S. L., and McDonald, C. J. (1986) Delayed feedback of physician performance versus immediate reminders to perform preventive care: Effects on physician compliance. *Medical Care* 24:659–666.

Titmuss, R. M. (1971) *The Gift Relationship: From Human Blood to Social Policy.* New York: Pantheon.

Toy, P. T. C. Y. (1989) Autologous transfusion. Presented at the Annual Meeting of Transfusion Medicine Academic Awardees, Bethesda, Md., June 1–3.

Toy, P. T. C. Y., Strauss, R. G., Stehling, L. C., Sears, R., Price, T. H., et al. (1987) Predeposited autologous blood for elective surgery: A national multicenter study. *New England Journal of Medicine* 316:517–520.

Turner, C. F., Miller, H. G., and Moses, L. E., eds. (1989) *AIDS, Sexual Behavior, and Intravenous Drug Use.* Washington, D.C.: National Academy Press.

Turner, R. H. (1978) The role and the person. *American Journal of Sociology* 84:1–23.

Upton, W. E., III. (1974) Altruism, attribution and intrinsic motivation in recruitment. In *Selected Readings in Donor Motivation and Recruitment.* Washington, D.C.: American National Red Cross.

Wallace, E. L., and Pegels, C. C. (1974) Analysis and design of a model regional blood management system. In *Selected Readings in Donor Motivation and Recruitment.* Washington, D.C.: American National Red Cross.

Walsh, J. H., Purcell, R. H., Morrow, A. G., Chanock, R. M., and Schmidt, P. J. (1970) Posttransfusion hepatitis after open-heart operations. *Journal of the American Medical Association* 211:261–265.

Walz, E. L., and Coe, N. A. (1984) A three-year evaluation of telephone recruitment with a composite study of scheduled appointments as related to non-scheduled. *Transfusion* 24(Suppl. 5):441(A23).

Walz, E., McMullen, D., and Simpson, L. (1985) The recruitment of donors who have been temporarily deferred for upper respiratory infection or low hematocrit. *Transfusion* 25:485(A10).

Ward, J. W., Grindon, A. J., Feorino, P. M., Schable, C., Parvin, M., and Allen, J. R. (1986) Laboratory and epidemiologic evaluation of an enzyme immunoassay for antibodies to HTLV-III. *Journal of the American Medical Association* 256:357–361.

Ward, J. W., Kleinman, S. H., Douglas, D. K., Grindon, A. J., and Holmberg, S. D. (1988a) Epidemiologic characteristics of blood donors with antibody to human immunodeficiency virus. *Transfusion* 28:298–301.

Ward, J. W., Holmberg, S. D., Allen, J. R., Cohn, D. L., Critchley, S. E., et al. (1988b) Transmission of human immunodeficiency virus (HIV) by blood transfusions screened as negative for HIV antibody. *New England Journal of Medicine* 318:473–478.

Ward, J. W., Bush, T. J., Perkins, H. A., Lieb, L. E., Allen, J. R., et al. (1989) The natural history of transfusion-associated infection with human immunodeficiency virus: Factors influencing the rate of progression to disease. *New England Journal of Medicine* 321:947–952.

Wasman, J., and Goodnough, L. T. (1987) Autologous blood donation for elective surgery: Effect on physician transfusion behavior. *Journal of the American Medical Association* 258:3135–3137.

Weisenthal, D. L., and Emmot, S. (1979) Explorations in the social psychology of blood donation. In D. F. Oborne, M. M. Gruneberg, and J. R. Miser, eds., *Research in Psychology and Medicine,* Vol. 2. New York: Academic Press.

Westphal, R. G., and Toy, P. (1988) Inaccurate transfusion medicine information in clinical manuals. *Transfusion* 28:61S(A77).

Williams, A. E., Kleinman, S., Lamberson, H., Popovsky, M., Williams, K., et al. (1987) Assessment of the demographic and motivational characteristics of HIV-seropositive blood donors. Presented at the Third International Conference on AIDS, Washington, D.C., June 1–5.

Winearls, C. G., Oliver, D. O., Pippard, M. J., Reid, C., Downing, M. R., and Cotes, P. M. (1986) Effect of human erythropoietin derived from recombinant DNA on the anemia of patients maintained by chronic haemodialysis. *Lancet* 2:1175–1178.

Wingard, M. (1979) Recruiting the black blood donor. Presented at the Third Annual Meeting of the American Association of Blood Banks, Las Vegas, November 3–8.

Winickoff, R. N., Coltin, K. L., Morgan, M. M., Buxbaum, R. C., and Barnett, G. O. (1984) Improving physician performance through peer comparison feedback. *Medical Care* 22:527–534.

World Health Organization (WHO). (1989) Global blood safety initiative: Consensus statement on accelerated strategies to reduce the risk of transmission of HIV by blood transfusion (brochure). Geneva: World Health Organization, Global Programme on AIDS, March 20–22.

Wykoff, R. F., and Halsey, N. A. (1986) The effectiveness of voluntary self-exclusion on blood donation practices of individuals at high risk for AIDS. *Journal of the American Medical Association* 256:1292–1293.

Zanjani, E. D., and Ascensao, J. L. (1989) Erythropoietin: A review. *Transfusion* 29:46–57.

Zuckerman, M., Siegelbaum, H., and Williams, R. (1977) Predicting helping behavior: Willingness and ascription of responsibility. *Journal of Applied Social Psychology* 7:295–299.

6

Methodological Issues in AIDS Surveys

Surveys or, more generally, the method of asking questions and recording answers, continue to be one of the most important methods for obtaining essential information about the epidemiology of AIDS and HIV, the behaviors that spread HIV, and the effectiveness of AIDS prevention efforts. Previous chapters included numerous examples of surveys and observations about the methodological difficulties that often attend these measurements.

Because of the central role surveys play in research on AIDS and HIV, this chapter focuses on methodological aspects of this data-gathering method that have important consequences for the usefulness of survey data. The technical material and methodological details in this chapter make it more difficult to read than preceding sections of the committee's report. The committee's aim in presenting this material is to provide researchers conducting AIDS surveys or analyzing data collected in such surveys with a detailed review of the current state of methodological research in this area. Readers who seek only a synopsis of the committee's conclusions and recommendations may wish to consult pages 27–34 of the summary chapter.

Before turning to specifics, it may be useful to consider data gathering in general and the types of problems that may compromise the collection of accurate and informative data. One may usefully distinguish five aspects of survey data collection: (1) the *definition* of the population to be studied and the drawing of a target sample from that population; (2) the *execution* of the sample design, that is, finding the persons in the target sample and enlisting their cooperation in the survey; (3) the *posing of questions* to elicit the desired information; (4) the *answering of those questions* by the respondent; and (5) the *recording of those answers* (and subsequent data processing and analysis).

To examine these elements, let us consider a hypothetical survey (much like the decennial census) that targeted all households in a particular jurisdiction of the state of Texas. Let us suppose further that the information to be obtained concerned automobile ownership (e.g., how many automobiles were owned by each household, the make and year of the autos, etc.). This survey, although not simple to conduct, would nevertheless be considerably less difficult to conduct than a survey seeking to assess behaviors that transmit HIV; in particular,

- the survey involves matters of fact that are both open to direct observation and matters of public record (e.g., make and year of automobiles owned by household);
- the topic is unlikely to be regarded as sensitive or "private" by respondents, although—as in any survey—some respondents may not wish to take the time to respond;
- developing questions about this topic can draw on a widely shared vocabulary (i.e., there is little ambiguity about what constitutes a "car" or "ownership");
- respondents who are not well informed can consult with other household members or check records (e.g., registration certificates);
- checks of survey accuracy can be made at the group level (by comparing the rates of auto ownership found in the survey and in registration records) and at the individual level (by checking individual registrations[1]); and
- census data on income and statewide auto registration data are available to target the survey efficiently toward segments of the population of particular interest (e.g., current or "potential" owners of Belchfire 500s).

Surveys that inquire about sexual behaviors or IV drug use differ in several ways from the foregoing example, and these differences provide a much greater challenge to the survey (or question-and-answer) method. First, many of the logical "target populations" for drug use and sexual behavior surveys cannot be identified reliably from official statistics. There are few reliable data on the distribution across the nation of persons who engage in behaviors that risk HIV transmission.

---

[1] The survey may, however, produce detailed information that cannot be verified from public records—for example, the proportion of Belchfire 500s owned by persons with 16+ years of education.

Furthermore, the behaviors in question occur in private and cannot be verified by direct observation or public records. Many of the behaviors are actively concealed because they are considered illicit (IV drug use is illegal throughout the nation, and many sexual behaviors of interest in preventing HIV transmission are illegal in some states). Thus, the topics these surveys cover are likely to be highly sensitive, which may create difficulties in enlisting the cooperation of persons in a target sample and in obtaining permission from "gatekeepers" (e.g., high school authorities) who control access to particular populations (e.g., high school students).

This chapter considers these problems and reviews the available empirical evidence gathered from surveys of sexual and drug use behaviors. Before beginning this review, however, some cautionary words are in order. The evidence presented here regarding errors in data about sensitive behaviors might lead some readers to unwarranted and wholesale rejection of survey findings on these important topics.[2] Indeed, considering the litany of difficulties presented in this chapter, some readers may ask whether anything at all can be learned from surveys or whether surveys have a useful role to play in research on AIDS and HIV transmission. The following considerations prompt the committee to answer "yes" to these questions.

The most important consideration arises directly from the nature of the disease. HIV infection occurs through the joint operation of the biology of this particular infectious virus and the human behaviors that transmit it. In the absence of vaccines, *all* interventions that seek to retard the spread of HIV infection focus on changing human behaviors to diminish the probability that the virus will be transmitted. Data on these behaviors are needed for a number of important purposes—for example, to understand the factors that motivate and shape the behaviors and to determine whether behaviors that transmit HIV are becoming less frequent in the population.

It might, of course, be argued that merely monitoring changes in the prevalence of HIV would be sufficient to determine whether behavioral change was occurring. Although this argument is true to some extent, there are important deficiencies in any strategy that eschews direct measurement of the behaviors themselves. Reliable data on HIV prevalence and incidence, although of great value for many purposes, are only a final accounting of the number of infected and uninfected persons in the population. From the viewpoint of prevention, such statistics serve best as a catalog of failures. Yet, those who are uninfected are not necessarily

---

[2]The following pages borrow heavily from the discussion of errors in survey measurements in Turner and Martin (1984:Vol. 1, 14–16) and Turner (1989).

successes. For example, the very low rate of HIV infection in states like Wyoming does not necessarily imply that the population has adopted protective behaviors. Instead, the low rate of HIV prevalence could be attributable to an epidemiological happenstance (e.g., isolation—in terms of sexual contacts and injection equipment sharing—from populations with high HIV prevalence.)

Determining whether protective behavioral changes have occurred (in Wyoming or anywhere else) requires asking questions about these risky behaviors. This activity, in turn, raises a host of methodological issues that are germane to survey research of all types plus some questions that are specific to surveys of drug use and sexual behavior. The questions may be quite basic: Are the respondents telling the truth? Do they understand the meaning of the survey questions in the same way the investigator does? Simple or complex, such questions inevitably introduce a degree of uncertainty into the interpretation of all survey data. Grappling with these issues forces an appreciation of the human interactions that produce survey measurements.

Elsewhere it has been argued that fundamental aspects of the survey process

> are quintessentially social psychological in character. They arise from a complex interpersonal exchange, they embody the subjectivities of both interviewer and interviewee, and they present their interpreter with an analytical challenge that requires a multitude of assumptions concerning, among other things, how respondents experience the reality of the interview situation, decode the "meaning" of survey questions, and respond to the social presence of the interviewer and the demand characteristics of the interview. (Turner, 1984:202)

Although this "analytical challenge" may be substantial, researchers are aided in their task by several decades of methodological research (see, for example, Sudman and Bradburn [1974], Bradburn and Sudman [1979], Rossi, Wright, and Anderson [1983], Turner and Martin [1984], and Catania et al. [in press,a,b]). A further reason for not abandoning behavioral measurement is that many of the problems encountered in this arena are not unique. Useful lessons may thus be learned from other disciplines that also confront such challenges.

FALLIBILITY OF MEASUREMENT IN OTHER SCIENCES

Fallibility and error are not confined to behavioral measurements, as evidenced by the decade-long controversy surrounding the population statistics produced by the decennial censuses.[3] Furthermore, just as falli-bility of measurement is not limited to behavioral measurements, neither is it limited to surveys or social statistics. For example, Hunter (1977) and Lide (1981) have noted the variability among measurements of such elementary physical phenomena as the thermal conductivity of copper (Figure 6-1). As Hunter observed, "although each analyst measured a physical quality that did not vary with location or time, it is clear that a remarkable variability attended the measurements" (1977:2). He concluded: "The variation in attempting to evaluate the same physical constant is obvious. This example is not unusual. Similar plots of thermal conductivity as a function of temperature for approximately 400 common metals and materials can be found in a supplement to the *Journal* (Ho, Powell, and Liley, 1974). Nor is the observed variation in the measure-ment of 'thermal conductivity' unique among physical parameters . . ." (p. 2).

Common biological measurements have shown similar fallibility. Examples include data collected by CDC that show substantial variation in the estimates made by different laboratories of the amount of lead in identical samples of blood. For a sample of blood with a putative lead concentration of 41 milligrams per deciliter (mg/Dl), 100 cooperating laboratories produced measurements that ranged from 33 to 55 mg/Dl; this result prompted the reviewer to observe: "Clearly, whatever the true amount of lead in a sample, the variability demonstrated [in these measurements] guarantees numerous false alarms or—perhaps more im-portant when the true level is high—nonalarms" (Hunter, 1980:870).

Another category of fallibility in the physical sciences involves "dis-coveries" that are later shown to be experimental artifacts. For example, between 1963 and 1974 more than 500 journal articles (including some in *Science* and *Nature*) discussed a supposed new substance: anomalous water, or polywater. Although it resembled ordinary water, polywater allegedly had a greater density, a reduced freezing point, and an elevated boiling point, among other anomalous properties. In the end, however, it was discovered that this "new substance" was nothing more than an impure solution of ordinary water (Franks, 1981; Eisenberg, 1981).

Such examples indicate that the problems AIDS researchers confront when they seek to assess sexual and drug-using behavior are not unique in the annals of scientific measurement. As Quinn McNemar observed more than 40 years ago, "[a]ll measurement is befuddled with error.

---

[3] By October 1981, more than 50 lawsuits had been filed challenging the accuracy of the 1980 Cen-sus results and their use in legislative apportionment and fund allocation decisions (Citro and Cohen, 1985:9).

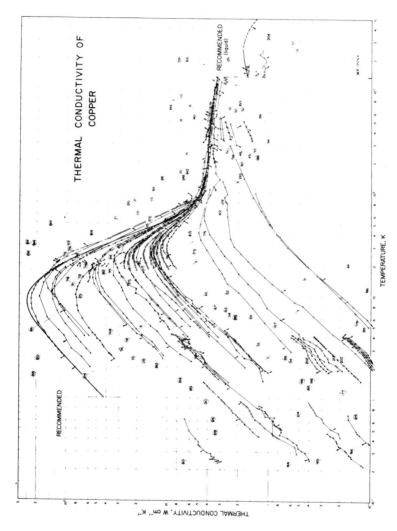

FIGURE 6-1 Display of all reported measurements of the thermal conductivity of copper as a function of temperature (reported by Ho, Powell, and Liley, 1974). NOTE: Each set of connected points corresponds to the data given in a single literature source. The recommended curve is based on an evaluation by Ho, Powell, and Liley (1974). SOURCE: Lide (1981).

About this the scientist can and does do something; he ascertains the possible extent of the error, determines whether it is constant (biasing) or variable, or both, and ever strives to improve his instruments and techniques" (1946:294).

In the following pages the committee reviews what is currently known about the errors that afflict measures of sexual and drug-using behavior and offers some prescriptions for how future measurements might be improved. The first section of the chapter reviews the experience to date in mounting surveys and obtaining responses from the public. The second section considers the reliability and validity of responses obtained in surveys of sexual and drug use behaviors. The final section reviews the use of anthropological research strategies that may provide important complementary information to that obtained in surveys and that may also be crucial in questionnaire development to improve the accuracy and completeness of responses.

RECRUITMENT OF RESPONDENTS IN
SEX AND SEROPREVALENCE SURVEYS

Much of what is now known about the epidemiology of AIDS has come from small-scale, local studies among subgroups thought to be at high risk for infection. Participants in these studies were recruited through various sources and means—from the clientele of local clinics or treatment facilities or the membership rosters of local organizations, through newspaper advertisements and physician referrals, and occasionally from "street sampling." The yield from this research has been remarkably rich. From these studies, researchers have identified the principal mechanisms of HIV infection (i.e., transmission through sexual contact, sharing injection equipment in IV drug use, transfusion of contaminated blood products); verified sexual transmission of HIV from male to male, female to male, and male to female; measured the efficiency of transmission in specific kinds of sexual contacts; and discovered some of the basic features of the long natural history of this devastating disease. As valuable as these studies are, however, the data drawn from them cannot address many other important public health questions that arise because of AIDS, such as: How large is the epidemic? What is the potential for general spread of HIV infection? Can an HIV epidemic be sustained through heterosexual contact alone? To answer questions like these, the knowledge gained from measurements and observations carried out in local studies of special subgroups must be applied in large-scale investigations of populations chosen not because of convenient or ready access but because of their importance in understanding the general course of the epidemic.

This section considers the feasibility of sex and seroprevalence surveys as a means of measuring the distribution of sexual behaviors that risk HIV transmission and the distribution of HIV itself in general populations. Although such surveys may be designed in a variety of ways, all of the studies discussed here employ the same general procedures for participant selection: an unambiguous definition of the population to be studied and a form of sampling from this population that allows the probabilities of selection to be known. The potential advantages of a probability sampling program for selecting survey participants are well known. In principle, probability sampling permits the use of a large body of statistical theory to make inferences from the sample to the larger population and avoids the possible biases inherent in recruitment by other means.

The suggestion to use probability sampling for surveys of sexual behavior was made more than three decades ago in connection with a review of the statistical methods used in Kinsey, Pomeroy, and Martin's *Sexual Behavior in the Human Male* (1948) (Cochran, Mosteller, and Tukey, 1953). The authors of this suggestion were a committee of the Commission on Statistical Standards of the American Statistical Association. At the invitation of Dr. Kinsey and the National Research Council's Committee for Research on Problems of Sex, they were asked to provide counsel on ways to improve the statistical methods used in the Kinsey research. They recommended a step-by-step program of probability sampling, beginning with a small pilot effort. They argued that research of this kind would provide a check on the results obtained with Kinsey's large, nonprobability sample. The committee was aware that problems of cost and potentially high rates of nonparticipation in such surveys would present special challenges. Their comments about the limits of this approach are worth quoting at length because the issues they raised more than 30 years ago in relation to Kinsey's work remain germane in evaluating the potential value of contemporary surveys of sexual behavior.

> In our opinion, no sex study of a broad human population can expect to present incidence data for reported behavior that are known to be correct to within a few percentage points. Even with the best available sampling techniques, there will be a certain percentage of the population who refuse to give histories. If the percentage of refusals is 10 percent or more, then however large the sample, there are no statistical principles which guarantee that the results are correct to within 2 or 3 percent, . . . but any claim that this is true must be based on the undocumented opinion that the behavior of those who refuse to be interviewed is not very different from that of those who are interviewed. These comments, which are not a criticism of [Kinsey, Pomeroy, and Martin's] research, emphasize the difficulty of answering the

question: "How accurate are the results?", which is naturally of great interest to any user of the results of a sex study. (Cochran, Mosteller, and Tukey, 1953:675)

The rationale for using response rates as a "yardstick" to assess the accuracy of survey estimates is twofold: (1) high response rates reduce the influence of selective participation in surveys and hence the potential for bias in the estimates, and (2) for a given target sample size and sample design, the higher the response rate, the larger the actual sample and the smaller the standard error of estimate. In other words, high response rates are better than low rates, provided the procedures used to achieve high response rates do not increase the degree of selectivity or inaccuracy of the responses.

Few contemporary surveys on any topic achieve response rates higher than the 90 percent figure cited in Cochran, Mosteller, and Tukey's review of the Kinsey report; indeed, response rates in most surveys are considerably below that mark. In principle, then, questions about selective participation (i.e., about differences between respondents and nonrespondents) are of concern in judging the accuracy of most survey estimates, not only those that derive from surveys of sexual behavior. Such concerns have generated a substantial literature on the character of nonresponse in surveys and what to do about possibly biased estimation resulting from nonresponse (see, for example, Goyder's 1987 synthesis of nonresponse research and the series of volumes on incomplete data in sample surveys edited by Madow, Nisselson, and Olkin [1983]).

Surveys with response rates that are much lower than 90 percent may still provide useful estimates of population characteristics if it can be established that participation or nonparticipation is unrelated to the characteristic for which an estimate is sought. Furthermore, response rates higher than 90 percent do not guarantee accurate estimation if survey participation is highly selective. Thus, in most cases, the value of the response rate by itself is insufficient justification for claims of accuracy or "representativeness" of survey estimates or for counterclaims that estimates fail in this respect. Such claims should be based on careful study, documentation, and possibly adjustment for bias as a result of refusals and other sources of nonresponse.

In the following review, the committee examines recent efforts to survey sexual behavior and related HIV risk factors that use probability samples from general populations. The review focuses on participation in such surveys and is motivated by the same concerns about nonresponse in probability samples that were expressed in the review of the Kinsey report. It attempts to answer three main questions: (1) What response rates have been achieved in recent surveys of sexual behavior? (2) What survey designs and procedures appear to be associated with higher versus lower levels of participation? and (3) What can be said, at present, about differences between sample persons who participate in sex surveys and sample persons who refuse to participate or do not participate for other reasons? (There is as yet too little information to hazard general statements about differences between participants and nonparticipants in seroprevalence surveys.) Questions about the validity and reliability of survey responses about sexual behavior, which were also noted in reviews of the Kinsey report, will be discussed in the later sections in this chapter.

Scope of the Review

The committee chose 15 surveys for its review, including some that are national in scope and some that target local populations. Most of these studies were initiated after the AIDS epidemic began in response to the need for population-based estimates of sexual behaviors known to be associated with HIV transmission. Both telephone and face-to-face interviewing methods are represented, along with data collection through self-administered questionnaires. There are wide variations among the surveys in the proportion of questions they devote to measuring sexual practices and other risk behaviors. Four surveys were included because of their potential importance for monitoring the prevalence of HIV infection; these surveys attempted to collect a blood specimen for HIV serologic testing from each sample person.

The committee used four criteria for including studies in its review: (1) there was at least a minimal attempt to collect data on personal sexual behavior and, in some cases, other HIV risk factors as well; (2) some form of probability sampling was employed; (3) a response rate of the form (number of survey participants)/(number of sample persons) could be calculated; and (4) enough documentation was available to identify the principal characteristics of the survey design and sampling procedures. Information about the designs, sampling procedures, and participation rates of these surveys appears in Table 6-1.

For the most part, the committee collected information about these surveys from published accounts in books, journal articles, and survey field reports. (The source documents are cited in Table 6-1.) Occasionally, it was necessary to rely on conversations with survey field managers, especially for surveys that had been completed at the time of this writing. In several other cases, documentation is partial because of incomplete reporting or recordkeeping, or both. For these reasons, and because the total number of surveys is small, the committee has not attempted a statistical analysis of participation rates in relation to survey characteristics. Nevertheless, the review does identify differences in response rates in sex surveys that appear to be associated with procedural and design variations. It also reveals several opportunities for learning more about patterns of participation and nonparticipation.

Participation in Sex Surveys

Data Collection Procedures and Response Rates

Each of the surveys listed in Table 6-1 asked respondents to report on certain aspects of their past and present sexual behavior. For the most part, the questions used in recent surveys (i.e., those initiated after the AIDS epidemic began) attempt to measure the occurrence of sexual behaviors associated with HIV infection and transmission and fall into three general categories: sexual orientation (with a focus on homosexuality), selection of sexual partners (number and characteristics of partners, presence of same-sex partnerships), and manner of sexual intercourse (e.g., anal, vaginal, oral). Because of the sensitive and highly personal nature of these questions, virtually all of the surveys made some provision to permit respondents to reveal the details of their sexual behavior without undue embarrassment or fear of disclosure to third parties. Most of the surveys included one or more of the following: special guarantees that responses would be kept confidential; assurance of anonymity—that is, that the person viewing the results would not know the identity of the respondent; privacy during the interview; and placement of the sensitive questions near the end of the interview.

Apart from these similarities, the 15 surveys differ widely with respect to basic methods of data collection and number of questions about sexual behavior. Interviewing was conducted by telephone in four of the surveys (nos. 3, 4, 9, and 10 in Table 6-1), by face-to-face interview in five cases (nos. 7, 8, 12, 13, and 14), and by a combination of face-to-face interview and self-administered questionnaire (SAQ) in six (nos. 1, 2, 5, 6, 11, and 15). Virtually all of the surveys that contained long, detailed inventories of sexual questions were conducted through face-to-face or telephone interviews. When SAQs were used, the length of the self-administered forms varied considerably (some did not exceed 1 or 2 pages whereas others [e.g., survey no. 1] were more than 10 pages long).

The most frequently used data collection procedure was a face-to-face interview followed by a relatively brief SAQ that focused on sexual behavior. In all instances, after the respondent completed the SAQ, it was placed in an envelope (stripped of identifying information except

TABLE 6-1 Methods and Execution of Sampling Designs in Recent Surveys of Sexual Behavior and HIV Seroprevalence

Survey	Dates of Fieldwork	Target Population	Sampling Methods	No. of Completed Interviews	Data Collection Methods — Non-HIV risk items	Data Collection Methods — HIV risk items	Participation Rates	Checks for Nonresponse Bias (in reference document)	Probable Non-Response Bias
				General Population Surveys					
1. Kinsey/ NORC survey	Late in 1970	U.S. residents aged 21+	Multistaged probability sample to block or segment (quotas at person level); interviewed one eligible person per household	3,018	Face-to-face interview in household	SAQ with sealed envelope	None can be calculated; 15% nonresponse on homosexual item among male respondents	Census comparisons; comparisons with 1988 GSS estimates	Probable underrepresentation of "difficult respondents" owing to refusals and lack of callbacks; underrepresentation of older men and black men
2. Danish Institute for Clinical Epidemi-ology	Feb.–June 1987	Danish men aged 16–55	Random sample from Danish population register (list sample)	1,155	Face- to-face interview in household	SAQ and respondent mailback	Interview RR = 78.3%; sex SAQ RR = 54.8%	Compared age distribution of respondents and non-respondents	Possible higher prevalence of HIV risk factors among nonrespondents
3. Los Angeles Times poll	July 1987	U.S. residents aged 18+ living in households with telephones	RDD with oversampling in Los Angeles, New York City, San Francisco, Miami, and Newark	2,095	Telephone interview	Telephone interview	Interview RR = 33%	Census comparisons	Probable underrepresentation of blacks and persons with less than high school diploma
4. Communication Technologies, Inc./ California Dept. of Health Svcs	Oct. to Dec. 1987	California residents aged 18+ living in households with telephones	Two RDD sampling frames; one RSA per household	2,012	Telephone interview	Telephone interview	RR of identified sample not calculable; interview completion rate = 71%	Comparison with state finance department's demographic estimates	Unknown

Survey	Date	Population	Sampling	N	Mode 1	Mode 2	Response rate	Comparison	Bias
5. British National Pilot Survey	Oct. to Nov. 1987	English-speaking residents of Britain aged 16–64	Multistaged probability sample; one RSA per household	785	Face-to-face interview in household	SAQ with sealed envelope	Interview SAQ RR = 47.5%	Comparison with British population projections	Probable underrepresentation of men, persons aged 16–24, and ethnic minorities
6. NORC General Social Survey	Feb. to April 1988	U.S. residents aged 18+	Multistaged probability sample of households; one RSA per household	1,481	Face-to-face interview in household	SAQ with sealed envelope	Interview RR = 77.3%; SAQ RR = 72.6%, item nonresponse = 6%	Comparison with census and current population surveys	Matches census and CPS population estimates
7. National Survey of Family Growth	March to Aug. 1988	U.S. residents, women, aged 15–44	Probability sampling based on HIS enumeration lists	8,450	Face-to-face interview in household	Face-to-face interview in household	Interview RR = 79%; sexual behav. item nonresponse = 4%	Information on non-respondents who were interviewed in HIS	Unknown
8. Sexual Behavior of Young People	1963	Unmarried youth aged 15–19 living in seven London districts	Random sample from lists in NHSAO, supplemented by market research	1,873	Face-to-face interview in local office	Face-to-face interview in local office	RR = 66.2%	None	Unknown
9. Communication Technologies, Inc., San Francisco survey	Aug. to Sept. 1987	Self-identified gay/bisexual men in San Francisco, aged 18+, in households with telephones	Commercial sample of names and telephone numbers; interviewed one eligible person in household	500	Telephone screening for eligibility	Telephone interview	None can be calculated	None	Unknown
10. Seattle pilot study	1985–1986	Selected Seattle area residents, aged 18–45, in households with telephones	Samples from telephone and reverse directories, using RDD	389	Telephone interview	Telephone interview	RR = 55.7%	None	Overrepresentation of persons keeping same telephone number and address over time

Continued

TABLE 6-1 *Continued*

Survey	Dates of Fieldwork	Target Population	Sampling Methods	No. of Completed Interviews	Data Collection Methods		Participation Rates	Checks for Nonresponse Bias (in reference document)	Probable Nonresponse Bias
					Non-HIV risk items	HIV risk items			
11. Contra Costa County survey, Wave II	Nov. 1988 to June 1989	Persons aged 18+ living in Contra Costa County	Multistaged probability sample; one RSA per household	969	Face-to-face interview in household	SAQ with sealed envelope	Interview RR = 65.8%; SAQ RR = 60.9%	Comparison with census data	Unknown
Local Area Seroprevalence Surveys									
12. San Francisco Men's Health Study, Wave I	May 1984 to April 1985	Currently unmarried men, aged 25–54, living in central San Francisco	Multistaged probability sample of households; all eligible persons in household	1,034	Face-to-face interview in clinic	Face-to-face interview in clinic	Interview RR = 56.2%; blood donation rate = 56.2%, clinic venipuncture	Comparison with census data; analysis of RR and variations over census tracts	Probable underrepresentation of younger and older men, black men, and heterosexual men
13. Belle Glade, Florida survey	Feb. to Oct. 1986	Persons aged 18+ living in 12 neighborhoods of Belle Glade	Probability sample of households; all eligible persons in household	877	Face-to-face interview in household	Face-to-face interview in household	73.1% of contacted households participated; individual RR not reported	None	Unknown

Survey	Dates	Population	Sample design	No.	Screening method	Data collection method	Response rate	Analysis	Findings
14. San Francisco Home Health Survey	Aug. 1988 to June 1989	Currently unmarried men and women aged 20–44, living in 16 San Francisco census tracts	Multistaged probability sample of households; interviewed any eligible persons in household	1,780	Face-to-face interview in household	Face-to-face interview in household	Interview RR = 59.4%; blood donation rate = 46.2% (venipuncture in home)	Comparison with census data; analysis of data in nonrespondents who were enumerated in screening interview	Not yet available
15. National Household Seroprevalence Survey pilot study	Jan. 1989	Residents of Allegheny County, Pa.; persons aged 18–54	Multistaged probability sample of households; one RSA per household	263	Face-to-face eligibility screening in household	SAQ in sealed envelope	SAQ RR = 81.2%; blood donation rate = 81.2% (venipuncture or finger stick in home)	Analysis of screening RR by sample segment; analysis of sample person RR by enumeration data and interviewer observations	Lower screening RRs outside Pittsburgh and in areas with more married persons (and fewer black persons); lower sample person response rates among married nonblack persons

NOTES: NORC: National Opinion Research Center; SAQ: self-administered questionnaire; GSS: General Social Survey; RR: response rate; RDD: random digit dialing; RSA: randomly selected adult; CPS: Current Population Survey; HIS: Health Interview Survey; NHSAO: National Health and School Attendance Office.

Reference documents for surveys:: (1) Fay et al. (1989); (2) Schmidt et al. (1989); (3) Turner, Miller, and Barker (1989); (4) Communication Technologies, Inc. (1988); (5) Johnson et al. (1988); (6) Michael et al. (1988), Smith (1988); (7) Pratt (1989); (8) Schofield (1965); (9)Communication Technologies, Inc. (1987); (10) Borgatta, Blumstein, and Schwartz (1987); (11) K. Trocke, Pacific Medical Center, San Francisco, personal communication, July 14 1989; (12) Winkelstein et al. (1987); (13) Castro et al. (1988); (14) Wiley (1989); (15) Research Triangle Institute (1989).

for a serial number, which permitted the questionnaire responses to be linked with interview data), sealed in the presence of the respondent, and collected by the interviewer. In one study (no. 15), the interviewer invited the respondent to accompany him or her to the nearest mailbox from which the questionnaire could be mailed directly to the field office for data entry.

In theory, the SAQ sealed envelope procedure should induce greater cooperation (and perhaps more candid answers) by eliminating the need to verbalize responses to sensitive questions. A potential disadvantage is loss of control over the administration of the questions and recording of responses. Illiteracy or other language problems may prevent the respondent from completing the questionnaire without assistance. In addition, it is easy for a respondent to avoid filling out the questionnaire or to skip questions without refusing directly; on-the-spot checks for item or form nonresponse cannot be conducted without destroying the quasi-anonymous character of the procedure.

Figure 6-2 displays response rates for 13 of the surveys[4] classified by type of data collection: face-to-face interview with SAQ, face-to-face interview only, and telephone interview. The response rates for face-to-face and telephone interviewing were calculated by dividing the number of completed interviews by the total number of sample persons. For surveys that used an SAQ, the response rate is the number of completed SAQs divided by the number of sample persons. In three of the surveys (nos. 4, 10, and 13), the reported response rates should be regarded as upper-bound estimates. Item nonresponse rates were generally low or not reported in the available survey documentation.

As noted earlier, the response rate in a study is conventionally used as one yardstick for measuring the potential accuracy of survey estimates. The response rates in Figure 6-2 span a wide range, from a low of 33 to a high of 81 percent, with most falling between 50 and 80 percent. Several of the surveys reported levels of participation that compared favorably with rates achieved in surveys dealing with less sensitive issues. The majority of them, however, failed to attain response rates that exceed the usual survey standard of 70 to 80 percent. Given such rates, it is difficult to rule out the possibility of substantial bias from selective participation in surveys of sexual behavior. It is therefore crucial to document any claims of representativeness by a careful study of patterns of nonresponse.

No obvious association between response rate and the three methods of data collection was found, although response rates in the telephone

---

[4]Response rates could not be computed for surveys no. 1 and 9.

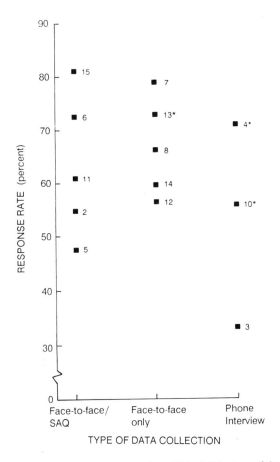

FIGURE 6-2 Response rates in selected surveys (from Table 6-1) by type of data collection used.

surveys appear to be somewhat lower than those in surveys using other procedures. (The reader should note that the response rates reported for surveys no. 4 and 10 are probably overestimates; for details, see the section "Use of Telephone Surveys" below.) Similarly, additional comparisons (not shown in Figure 6-2) indicate that there is no correlation between response rates and the scope of the sampling (local versus national), the size of the sexual behavior component of the interview, or (surprisingly) whether sample persons were asked to donate blood specimens for serologic testing. Although the variation in response rates appears to be largely unrelated to easily documented characteristics of survey sampling and design in this group of surveys, more specific and detailed comparisons yield some plausible explanations for some of the observed differences. These explanations are discussed below.

Survey Configurations Associated with
High Response Rates

Four of the surveys listed in Table 6-1 report response rates higher than 70 percent. The two that are local seroprevalence surveys will be discussed later with other surveys that include a blood component. The focus here is on two large-scale surveys based on national samples of U.S. residents: the 1988 General Social Survey (GSS) and the 1988 National Survey of Family Growth (NSFG).

These two surveys differ in substantive focus, definition of the target population, sampling methodology, and details of survey procedure. Nonetheless, they share certain characteristics that may help to explain why they achieved relatively high rates of participation: they are each part of a series of periodic surveys that have consistently had good response rates; the sexual items consist of a relatively small set of "add-on" questions; the surveys are conducted by the same survey organizations[5] and to some extent by the same supervisory and field staff that have been responsible for previous surveys in the series; and the field procedures include provisions for large numbers of callbacks and special attention to the conversion of refusers.

The 1988 GSS is the fourteenth in a series of annual opinion surveys conducted by the National Opinion Research Center (NORC) under a grant from the National Science Foundation. Since 1977 the GSS sample has been selected using full probability sampling of adults, 18 years and older, living in U.S. households. The GSS interview, which is approximately 90 minutes long, is conducted face to face in the home and is sometimes followed by SAQs dealing with special topics.

In 1988, GSS interviewers gave each respondent a one-page, self-administered questionnaire that included the following questions:

- How many sex partners have you had in the last 12 months?
- Was one of the partners your husband or wife or regular sexual partner?
- If you had other partners, please indicate all categories that apply to them
  - close personal friend;
  - neighbor, coworker, or long-term acquaintance;
  - casual date or pick-up;
  - person you paid or person who paid you for sex;

---

[5]NORC for the General Social Survey and Cycle 1 of the NSFG; Westat for the NSFG cycles 2, 3, 4.

- other (specify).

- Have your sexual partners in the last 12 months been: exclusively male, both male and female, exclusively female?

The marked questionnaire was placed in an envelope, sealed, and collected by the interviewer.

The conduct of fieldwork was similar to that of previous GSS efforts. One hundred thirty interviewers, most of whom had worked on earlier rounds of the survey, were recruited from NORC's interviewer pool and trained in 1988 GSS procedures by supervisory staff. The target response rate for the survey was 77 percent, with a minimum acceptable response rate per sampled area[6] of 65 percent. NORC employed special procedures to minimize nonresponse. Two hundred preselected respondents living in areas in which recruitment difficulties had been encountered in previous rounds of the GSS were offered $10 to complete the interview and SAQ. In addition, NORC assembled a mobile squad of expert interviewers who were assigned to do refusal conversion interviews. In the later stages of fieldwork, field management authorized interviewers to pay respondent fees from $10 to $50 for completion of interviews after an initial refusal. The field staff completed 1,481 interviews during the 10-week period for a total survey response rate of 77.3 percent. Of those who completed the interview portion of the survey, 93.9 percent returned the SAQ, yielding an SAQ response rate of 72.6 percent. The response rate for fully completed SAQs was somewhat lower (66.7 percent), owing to nonresponse on various items.

The 1988 National Survey of Family Growth (Cycle IV of the series that began in 1973) was conducted for the National Center for Health Statistics by Weststat Corporation survey staff from January to August 1988. The target population for this survey consisted of noninstitutionalized civilian women, aged 15 to 44, living in the United States. The target sample for Cycle IV consisted of more than 10,000 eligible and randomly selected women who were listed on household rosters[7] from NCHS's National Health Interview Surveys (NHIS)[8] conducted between October 1985 and April 1987. About 80 percent of the sample persons

---

[6]That is, per primary sampling unit (PSU).

[7]The NHIS attempted to enumerate all persons living in each household included in its target sample. This was possible for 96 percent of the target households. The names entered on the resulting NHIS "household rosters" provided the basis for the NSFG sampling.

[8]The NHIS is an annual survey of approximately 50,000 households conducted by the Bureau of the Census. The response rate for this survey is more than 95 percent.

were located through address correction requests and telephone contacts before the beginning of fieldwork.

After a series of screening questions to verify eligibility, interviewers conducted a one-hour face-to-face home interview that dealt with family planning practices, family size expectations and preferences, sources of family planning services, and aspects of maternal and child health. The interview included several questions about personal sexual behavior (e.g., age at first intercourse, frequency of intercourse, lifetime number of male partners, a series of items on beliefs and attitudes about AIDS, and 19 questions about sexually transmitted diseases.

A field staff of 240 interviewers, the majority of whom had at least one year of prior interviewing experience, completed a total of 8,450 interviews by the end of the data collection phase of the survey. This number of completed interviews yielded a total survey response rate of approximately 79 percent (figured by multiplying the 82.1 percent response rate among NSFG sample persons by a 96 percent enumeration response rate[9] in the NHIS). This rate was achieved after considerable investment by reaching sample persons who were not at home during the initial calls and by converting refusals. The response rate (among NSFG sample persons) after the initial interviewer assignments was approximately 69 percent. It increased to 78 percent after nonrespondents were reassigned and contacted by local interviewers; it increased still further (to 82 percent) in a subsequent follow-up of a random half of the remaining nonrespondents who were assigned to a special core of conversion interviewers. Nonresponse to specific questions about sexual behavior averaged about 4 percent.

Judging by the response rates in these surveys, "piggybacking" a small number of questions about sexual behavior onto established surveys appears to be a feasible strategy for obtaining estimates of the prevalence of certain risk factors for sexual transmission of HIV in general populations. Adding sex-related items to the protocols for the 1988 GSS and NSFG[10] had little effect on the response rates normally obtained in those surveys, although item nonresponse may have been slightly higher for the sexual questions than for the nonsexual material. As noted earlier, relatively high rates of participation are typical of these surveys, and the ingredients for such success are well known to survey practitioners: prior experience with similar surveys, continuity of staff, a high "target

---

[9] The NHIS household rosters were used to sample respondents in the NSFG. Household rosters were missing for approximately 4 percent of the households included in the NHIS target sample.

[10] The NSFG traditionally had some items on sexual behaviors (e.g., age at first intercourse); in 1988 the number of items was increased.

response rate" combined with a field operation that promotes diligent follow-up of nonresponding sample persons, and an ample budget. Under these conditions, response rates for small subsets of sex-related items can be similar to rates achieved in well-conducted surveys that do not inquire about sensitive personal behaviors.

The above remarks, however, do not necessarily apply to surveys with a greater number of questions about sexual behavior or with questions of a more intimate nature than those in the GSS and NSFG. In both of these surveys, questions about sexual behavior constituted a relatively minor part of the interview and were not emphasized in preinterview contacts with potential respondents. Furthermore, neither survey asked about the details of sexual encounters, such as the full range of types of sexual contact. Surveys dominated by sexual questions, especially those that include long Kinsey-like inventories and sexual histories, may encounter more serious problems of nonresponse than are encountered in piggyback surveys. For example, the demands of prior informed consent in true sex surveys will require more complete advance warning about the nature of the questions to be asked, perhaps increasing respondent concerns about embarrassment and disclosure. Whether the relatively high levels of participation that characterized the 1988 GSS and NSFG can be achieved in more extensive piggyback surveys or in true sex surveys remains an open question.

Use of Telephone Surveys

The collection of survey data through telephone interviews has become an increasingly popular alternative to face-to-face interviewing as a result of the generally lower costs of telephone surveys and developments in sampling and interviewing technology (notably, sampling through random-digit dialing [RDD] and computer-assisted telephone interviewing [CATI]). Comparisons between face-to-face and telephone interviewing in the context of national surveys indicate that the overall response rates for telephone surveys are on the order of 5 percent lower than those expected in personal interviews (Groves and Kahn, 1979). Although response rates for the two methodologies tend to converge when unanswered telephone calls are ignored, acceptable standards (e.g., Council of American Survey Research Organizations, 1982) for reporting response rates mandate that a fraction of the numbers not contacted be included in the denominator when calculating response rates for telephone surveys.[11]

---

[11] The ratio of eligible to noneligible contacts found among telephone numbers that *do* answer may be used to deflate the total number included in the denominator. This practice assumes that the proportion of telephone numbers that have no eligible respondents (e.g., business numbers, households without

The generally lower response rates of telephone surveys, along with studies of respondent reactions to the two forms of interviewing, suggest that the rapport and trust between interviewer and respondent attained in face-to-face surveys are harder to achieve in the telephone interview.[12] Thus, it is reasonable to expect somewhat lower rates of participation in telephone surveys that contain explicit sexual content, compared with similar surveys using face-to-face interviewing or a combination of face-to-face interviewing and an SAQ.

Unfortunately, there is only a limited empirical basis for judging the feasibility of conducting interviews about sexual behavior by telephone. Few such surveys have been conducted (four are listed in Table 6-1), and only one of the four reviewed by the committee gives an indication of the utility of telephone interviewing for measuring sexual behavior in general populations. Nevertheless, a brief review of response rates in these surveys is warranted, if only to indicate the character of the attempts thus far.

The two local area telephone surveys (nos. 9 and 10)—one of which was conducted in San Francisco, the other in Seattle—are examples of the use of targeted sampling of phone numbers and telephone interviewing to find and interview persons who may be considered to be at higher than average risk of HIV infection. Yet such surveys are not without their drawbacks. Although probability sampling was ostensibly employed, peculiarities in the definition of the target populations and in the execution of the surveys make generalizations about participation in these surveys hazardous.

The 1987 San Francisco survey (conducted by Communication Technologies, Inc.) was undertaken to determine levels of high-risk sexual behavior among gay and bisexual men living in San Francisco. It was conceived as a baseline survey, the first in a series that would document changes in risk behavior that might be related to educational campaigns directed at gay and bisexual men. The sampling frame, which consisted of male names and linked telephone numbers, was constructed from commercial lists of households that were stratified by census tract.

---

persons meeting screening criteria, etc.) is the same among nonanswers as among those for which responses are obtained.

[12] As part of their comparison of parallel telephone and personal interview surveys, Groves and Kahn (1979:97–99) asked respondents whether they "felt uneasy" discussing various topics that had been included in parallel telephone and personal interview surveys that were conducted in tandem. Survey topics included finances, health, voting, and political attitudes. Groves and Kahn reported finding that larger proportions of respondents interviewed by telephone said they "felt uneasy" about each of these topics. The greatest differences were found for questions on income (17.9 percent "uneasy" in telephone survey versus 15.3 percent in personal interview) and political attitudes (12.1 versus 8.5).

By oversampling telephone numbers from tracts with a large proportion of unmarried males, the researchers composed 24 replicate samples of 500 names and numbers to be released in sequence to interviewers until 500 interviews had been completed with eligible respondents. Eligibility in this case consisted of being male, 18 years of age or older, and self-identifying in the screening interview as a gay or bisexual man.

Interviewers made as many as four attempts to contact a household and, after initial questioning to determine the presence of a male aged 18 or older, attempted to screen for gay or bisexual behavior. Persons who identified themselves as gay or bisexual were asked a series of questions about their sexual behavior. The report of this survey cited a refusal rate of 19.4 percent. It is not clear, however, whether this rate referred to the initial screening for the presence of an adult male or to the subsequent screening for gay or bisexual behavior. Although there is no mention of the number of households that were not contacted or of the eligibility rate per contacted household, the authors hazard the opinion that "[w]ith a sample size of 500, results were projectable to the universe of self-identifying gay and bisexual men in San Francisco within ±4.5% at the 95% level of confidence" (Communication Technologies, Inc., 1987:25).

The 1985–1986 Seattle survey was a pilot study of the use of telephone interviewing to collect data on sexual behavior in subgroups of the general population who were likely to be at risk of acquiring HIV infection. The target population consisted of persons aged 18 to 45 years living in selected localities of Seattle. Based on census data and "local knowledge," the investigators sampled households in census tracts that were considered likely to include large numbers of homosexual and bisexual men and heterosexually active persons. Households were selected from reverse telephone directories[13] so that names and phone numbers could be recorded prior to the telephone contact with the household. This procedure was necessary because the investigators required that an advance letter be sent to all persons to be contacted indicating the kinds of questions to be asked and the voluntary nature of participation. Of the nearly 3,000 advance letters sent, approximately one-third were returned (as undelivered mail, wrong addressees, or business addresses). Contact was made with seventy-two percent of the remaining households; of these, 46 percent contained no eligible respondents, and 16 percent refused to be interviewed prior to the household enumeration. At the end of fieldwork, 389 interviews had been completed. No interviews were attempted with persons who said they had not received the advance

---

[13]Reverse telephone directories are arranged in numerical order by telephone number and give the name and address associated with each listed number.

letter. The response rate was estimated to be 55.7 percent, based on the assumption that about one in three of the nonresponding households contained a person who was eligible to be interviewed.

The two telephone surveys targeted to a broader population include a national and a statewide survey. The national survey, conducted by the *Los Angeles Times* in July 1987 (no. 3 in Table 6-1), included a short series of questions about sexual behavior at the end of a series of opinion questions. The response rate (reported in a secondary analysis of the poll data) was quite low—about 33 percent—no doubt because fieldwork was completed in five days and only three callbacks were permitted. Low response rates are not unusual in short-term commercial surveys; nevertheless, they provide little indication of what can be achieved in more rigorously executed telephone surveys. Surprisingly, the analysis of reports of one aspect of sexual behavior in this survey appear quite consistent with those obtained in another survey that achieved a much higher response rate (see the discussion below).

The 1987 California survey (no. 4 in Table 6-1) was commissioned by the California State Department of Health Services to produce statewide estimates of the distribution of HIV risk factors among adults 18 years of age and older. The investigators generated a sample of telephone numbers by random-digit dialing with deliberate oversampling of prefixes associated with areas containing high proportions of minorities. At first contact, the interviewers attempted to collect information on household composition and to select at random one eligible person to be interviewed. Potential respondents were told in advance about the nature of the questions to be asked. The interviewer then administered a 15-minute series of questions that included screening items pertaining to HIV risk status (e.g., same-gender sexual contact among men, heterosexual contacts with multiple partners or partners in a known HIV risk group, use of recreational drugs). Any respondent who reported one or more of these risk factors was asked additional questions about specific risk behaviors. The interviewers were instructed to make up to 12 attempts to contact each sampled telephone number. Initial refusals were reassigned to other interviewers who made further attempts to complete the interview. At the end of fieldwork, 2,012 persons had been interviewed from a total of 2,834 persons known to be eligible—a completion rate of 71 percent; the 29 percent of incomplete interviews included sample person refusals and interview break-offs. Because noncontacts and enumeration nonresponses were ignored, however, 71 percent must be regarded as a rather generous upper bound on the response rate as conventionally calculated.

The response rates in these few telephone studies appear to be somewhat lower than those obtained in face-to-face interviews of sexual behavior. This conclusion holds true as well for the statewide California survey because the true response rate is undoubtedly lower than the reported completion rate. Experience with sex surveys conducted by telephone is too limited, however, to determine the levels of participation that can be achieved in such surveys and whether the lower response rates in the available cases are a generic feature of telephone surveys or simply the result of early and somewhat idiosyncratic first attempts.

In view of the substantially lower cost of telephone versus face-to-face surveys, as well as the limited scope of current experience, carefully designed experiments should be encouraged to test the feasibility of this methodology for surveys of sexual behavior in general populations. Because noncontacts are a major component of nonresponse in existing surveys, such experiments should include provision for large numbers of callbacks and extended interview periods. Additional increases in response rates may be achieved through research on the best ways to introduce questions about sexual behavior over the phone, improvements in questionnaire design, and more diligent attempts to complete interviews after initial refusals. Another area of possible investigation is to compare—at least at the aggregate and possibly at the individual levels—the results of telephone and personal interview surveys of the same target population.

Participation in Seroprevalence Surveys

If sex surveys are properly executed, they can provide important clues about the potential for sexual transmission of HIV infection in general populations. Survey estimates of the distribution of behaviors associated with HIV transmission, combined with epidemiological findings on the transmission efficiency of HIV in sexual contacts and biological aspects of the natural history of HIV infection, are the raw material for model-based inferences about the future spread of AIDS in known risk groups and in populations not yet considered to be at risk (May and Anderson, 1987; Anderson and May, 1988; May, Anderson, and Blower, 1989; Turner, Miller, and Moses, 1989:Ch. 2). Yet even if the data on sexual behavior in general populations were far more complete than they are at present, the validity of model-based inferences and predictions would be suspect owing to uncertainties about a variety of other forces that govern the epidemic growth of infection. At best, sex surveys of representative samples can indicate degrees of vulnerability to sexual transmission of HIV in individuals and in population subgroups. In this way they can make a significant contribution to prevention and control. Sex surveys cannot, however, substitute for direct assessment of the prevalence of infection.

The most attractive design for direct measurement of the prevalence of infection is the seroprevalence survey.[14] A seroprevalence survey applies well-established principles of probability sampling and survey methodology to the problem of collecting sample blood specimens with the aim of estimating the prevalence of infection in a population. In theory, such surveys could eliminate most of the outstanding uncertainties regarding the size of the AIDS epidemic, the prevalence of infection in major risk groups, and the degree to which HIV has entered populations that are not presently considered to be at significant risk for infection. Yet, the practical difficulties of mounting a seroprevalence survey on a local or national basis are formidable. Not the least of these are the problems of potentially high levels of noncooperation among sample persons and possible correlations between participation and HIV serostatus.

Currently, a national seroprevalence survey is in the planning and development stage under a contract between the National Center for Health Statistics (now a part of CDC) and Research Triangle Institute (RTI). The goal of the first phase of this work, which consists of pilot and pretest surveys, is to select a design that meets several objectives simultaneously: protection of respondent anonymity; attainment of participation rates high enough to justify confidence in prevalence estimates derived from the survey; development of procedures to assess nonresponse bias; and identification of cost-effective fieldwork strategies. Choosing an optimum design requires extensive experimentation with alternative combinations of design characteristics. Among the challenges are determining the best ways: to introduce the study to sample persons and the general public, to maintain anonymity, to collect blood specimens, to ask questions about risk factors, to compensate respondents for the time required for participation, and to minimize fears of disclosure. Survey developers hope that preliminary testing will result in a feasible strategy for a national survey of approximately 50,000 households.

To date, knowledge of what can be accomplished in seroprevalence surveys rests on the results of four local efforts. Only one of these studies, RTI's small-scale pilot seroprevalence survey in Allegheny County, Pennsylvania (which includes the city of Pittsburgh), is part of a program of research to explore alternative designs for a national seroprevalence survey. The other efforts were designed to provide local estimates of the

---

[14]Lengthy discussions of the merits of seroprevalence surveys and of the problems of implementing them on a national scale can be found in Turner and Fay (1987/1989) and De Gruttola and Fineberg (1989).

extent of HIV infection in connection with intensive study of the epidemiological factors associated with transmission. In all four surveys, sample persons were selected from local, residentially defined target populations through multistaged probability sampling procedures.

It will be obvious from the descriptions given below that these surveys occupy vastly different positions in the "design space" of potential options for seroprevalence surveys. The RTI Allegheny County (Pittsburgh) pilot survey (no. 15 in Table 6-1) is one extreme—a one-time anonymous survey in which blood is collected in the home by venipuncture or finger-stick, accompanied by an SAQ about risk factors. In contrast, the two San Francisco seroprevalence surveys (nos. 12 and 14 in Table 6-1) were the first cycles of longitudinal studies that involved periodic collection of blood specimens, extensive personal interviews to obtain risk factor information, and, in one case, routine physical examinations in a clinic setting. Not surprisingly, there is a gradient of response rates in these four studies that corresponds roughly to the intensity and duration of the participation required from each respondent: the response rates for blood samples range from 46 to 81 percent. The highest rates were obtained in the least demanding surveys.

The San Francisco Men's Health Study (no. 12 in Table 6-1) is believed to be the first seroprevalence survey of HIV infection conducted in the United States. The baseline survey, which was designed as the recruitment phase of a longitudinal study, began in the spring of 1984 and continued until April 1985. The target population was defined as currently unmarried men, aged 25 to 54 years, living in the 19 census tracts of central San Francisco that in 1984 had the highest cumulative incidence of AIDS for the city. The investigators anticipated that a majority of the eligible men living in the target area, known locally as the Castro District and considered to be a "gay" area, would have had recent homosexual contact. Within the sample strata (census tracts), the sample was drawn by strict probability sampling at the level of households, and all eligible men within each household (with no advance screening for type of sexual activity or sexual orientation) were invited to participate in the study. Interviewers made the initial contact in a visit to each selected household during which they attempted to complete a household enumeration, to identify persons eligible for participation, and to schedule appointments for a visit to a local clinic—where participants were to be interviewed, given a physical examination, and asked to donate blood and other specimens for laboratory assay. Throughout the 12 months of fieldwork for the baseline survey, there were numerous callbacks for hard-to-reach sample persons, frequent rescheduling of missed clinic appointments, and sustained efforts to convert those who initially refused to participate. At the end of the recruitment phase, 1,034 sample persons had completed their first clinic visit, representing a response rate of 56.2 percent (of approximately 1,839 eligible sample persons, including an estimated 157 eligible men in sample households in which the initial household enumeration could not be completed).

In 1986, CDC conducted a seroprevalence survey in Belle Glade, Florida, as part of an investigation of the causes of an AIDS outbreak in that area (see survey no. 13 in Table 6-1). The target population comprised persons 18 years of age and older and, with parental consent, children aged 2 to 10 years. Households were selected by stratified random sampling from comprehensive lists for 12 locally defined neighborhoods. Approximately 70 percent of the selected households were located in neighborhoods with the largest numbers of reported AIDS cases in the city. After signing a written informed consent document, sample persons were interviewed at home using a standardized questionnaire; they were then asked for a blood sample (obtained by venipuncture) and examined for signs of HIV infection. The report describing this survey indicates that 557 of the selected households were visited while someone was home, and of these households, 73 percent ($N = 407$ households) agreed to participate in the study, yielding a total of 877 persons who completed the full study protocol. The 557 households do not include those in which no contact was made;[15] thus, 73 percent should be considered an upper bound of the household response rate. The study report did not indicate the response rate for individual sample persons.

A second seroprevalence survey of San Francisco neighborhoods was initiated in 1988-1989, this time to monitor HIV infection in areas thought to be likely candidates for transmission through IV drug use or heterosexual contact, or both. The target population was defined as currently unmarried men and women, aged 20 to 44 years, living in three areas (16 census tracts) characterized by high rates of STDs among women, high rates of admission to drug detoxification programs, and AIDS cases among their residents that were not attributable to male homosexual contacts. Full probability sampling was employed at the household level, and all eligible persons within the selected households were invited to participate in the study. The field protocol included an advance letter to each sample household, signed informed consent, a lengthy personal interview in the home covering HIV risk factors in great detail, and collection of blood (venipuncture in the home or at a local

---

[15]Three attempts to contact the household were made at different times of the day (K. G. Castro, Centers for Disease Control, personal communication, May 2, 1990).

clinic) by interviewers who were certified phlebotomists. Participants were paid $20 as compensation for completing the protocol. Repeated callbacks, rescheduling of home visits, and refusal conversion strategies were employed throughout the 10 months of fieldwork. Based on an estimated 2,983 sample persons living in the selected households, the 1,781 sample persons who completed the interview portion of the protocol constituted an interview response rate of 59.7 percent. The response rate for the blood component of the survey was 46.3 percent because blood specimens were not obtained from 401 of the 1,781 persons interviewed (owing to refusal and, in a few cases, the inability to complete the blood draw).

The initial pilot study to test procedures for a national seroprevalence survey was conducted in January 1989 in Allegheny County, Pennsylvania. As is planned for the national study, the target population for this small-scale pilot consisted of the civilian, noninstitutionalized population aged 18 to 54 years old at the time of the survey. A sample of 539 households was selected by area probability sampling methods, and one eligible adult in each household was randomly chosen as the sample person. The fieldwork protocol called for an enumeration interview (which included questions about the age, sex, race, and marital status of each person in the household), selection of the sample person, signed informed consent (which was left with the respondent at the end of the interview to ensure anonymity), collection of a blood specimen (venipuncture or finger-stick by a phlebotomist who accompanied the interviewer), a $50 incentive payment that was promised before the blood draw, and, finally, completion of a brief SAQ (covering demographic characteristics and basic HIV risk factors) that was subsequently placed in a sealed envelope. Videotapes were shown during the contact with the respondent to explain the survey and motivate participation. Earlier, the existence of the survey and its importance had been stressed on all local television news stations. No names were taken at any time during the visit to the household. At the end of fieldwork, 95.1 percent of the 450 occupied households were successfully screened, and 263 (85.4 percent) of 308 enumerated sample persons completed the survey protocol. The response rate thus was (.951 x .854) 81.2 percent.

The Allegheny County pilot study indicates that relatively high response rates can be obtained in seroprevalence surveys that involve public (e.g., TV news) appeals to participate, that make limited demands on participants' time and that offer substantial monetary incentives. The design of the pilot study stands in sharp contrast to the more epidemiologically oriented surveys that employ lengthy personal interviews covering a much wider range of behavioral risk factors, repeated blood draws (as in the San Francisco longitudinal studies), and invitations to learn antibody status through disclosure counseling. In the Allegheny survey, participation was anonymous: no names were recorded, the risk factor information was obtained by the SAQ/sealed envelope procedure, and there was no feedback of HIV antibody test results to respondents. It is not surprising that response rates in the pilot study were substantially higher than those in more demanding epidemiologically oriented surveys.

These comparisons indicate the trade-off that must often be made between maximizing response rates in a streamlined design and intensive epidemiological investigation with lower response rates. The discussions of the design options for a national seroprevalence survey anticipated the necessity of such a trade-off (Turner and Fay, 1987/1989). Thus, the Allegheny experience suggests that the selection of a survey design that limits the demands on respondents—by making participation relatively easy, anonymous, and nonthreatening—may have been a wise choice. Further testing and refinement of this approach on a larger scale will establish whether it constitutes a feasible design for a national survey.

Nonresponse Bias in Sex and Seroprevalence Surveys

Nonresponse bias[16] occurs when participation in a survey is selective with respect to a characteristic whose distribution is to be estimated from survey responses. A high response rate tends to minimize the effects of such selectivity on survey estimates as long as the procedures used to attain it do not in fact increase the correlation between the characteristic of interest and the act of participation. Response rates in most surveys, however, usually are not high enough to justify ignoring problems of selective participation, and there is in fact, a literature that indicates that certain kinds of persons (notably those of low socioeconomic status) are likely to be underrepresented in most samples in ways that may compromise survey estimates (Turner and Martin, 1984:Vol. 1, Fig. 3-1; Goyder, 1987). The committee's review likewise indicates that the response rates achieved in contemporary sex and seroprevalence surveys leave ample opportunity for selective participation to affect the validity of survey estimates of sexual behavior and HIV seroprevalence. (The reader should note that response bias—that is, misleading or inaccurate survey responses—can have similar effects. This issue is addressed later in this

---

[16]Nonresponse bias is the deviation between the distribution of responses obtained from persons who participated in the survey and who responded to the survey question, and the response that would have been obtained if all persons in the target sample had participated in the survey and answered the question.

chapter; this section deals only with biases that result from selective nonresponse.)

There are three kinds of selective participation that have somewhat different effects on estimates of sexual behavior or HIV infection: (1) selective participation with respect to characteristics that are *independent* of sexual behavior and HIV serostatus; (2) selective participation related to attributes (e.g., marital status) that may be correlated with sexual behavior or HIV infection; and (3) selective participation that is directly related to sexual behavior or serostatus. The first kind of selection can be ignored in the construction of estimates of the sort being considered here because (by definition) this type of nonresponse is unrelated to sexual behavior or infection status. Selection of the second kind does result in biased estimates, but the bias might be remedied if, given the selection factors, the (conditional) distribution of sexual behavior (or serostatus) is known to be the same for respondents and nonrespondents and the distribution of the selection factors among nonrespondents can be ascertained. Let us suppose, for example, that participation in a sex survey is correlated with marital status in such a way that single men are underrepresented. If the marital status of male nonrespondents is known (from, for example, a household enumeration interview) and if there were a good basis[17] for the belief that, for any particular marital status, the sexual behaviors of respondents and nonrespondents were similar, sample estimates of the distribution of sexual behavior might be adjusted, using imputation or maximum likelihood procedures, to adjust for this nonresponse bias. Fay and colleagues (1989) provided a rather sophisticated example of this form of adjustment in connection with estimates of the frequency of male same-gender sexual behaviors from the Kinsey/NORC national survey conducted in 1970.

The most troublesome kind of selectivity is participation that depends directly on sexual behavior or serostatus—for example, when the decision to participate is made in relation to fears about reporting socially proscribed sexual practices or the disclosure of a positive antibody result. In this case, simple imputation from observed data will rarely lead to unbiased estimates of prevalence, although in some cases it may be possible to anticipate the direction of bias. Concerns about this form of selection have motivated the development of strategies that make participation in sex and seroprevalence surveys less threatening. Nevertheless, there is likely to be some degree of selection bias attributable to fears about

---

[17] Such a basis might, for example, have been provided by a methodological study that did more intensive follow-up of a subsample of nonrespondents.

disclosing sexual practices (particularly those considered "deviant") or about revealing one's HIV serostatus in the best executed surveys.

Current knowledge about the structure of nonresponse bias in sex and seroprevalence surveys comes from two kinds of comparisons: comparisons of survey estimates with census data and internal analysis of the correlates of different levels of nonresponse. Roughly half of the 15 surveys reviewed here attempted some form of comparison of survey estimates with census data. There is an apparent positive correlation between years of schooling and participation in several of the surveys but few other regularities in the deviations between survey estimates and census figures could be detected. (See Table 6-1 for a summary of the comparisons reported in the source documents.) In any case, a good match between census and sample survey distributions, although encouraging in some respects, does not guarantee that estimates of prevalence rates for sexual behavior or HIV infection are unbiased.

The other major source of information about nonresponse bias comes from analyzing the characteristics associated with nonresponse at different stages of a survey interview. Although such stages vary from study to study, a seroprevalence survey might typically include the following: (1) completing a household enumeration form, which includes basic demographic information about each member of the household; (2) completing the personal interview, which might include an SAQ dealing with sexual behavior and other HIV risk factors; (3) completing every item on the SAQ form; and (4) allowing blood to be drawn for serologic testing. Most of the 15 surveys reviewed here involved some degree of staging of this kind, although not always in this order. In many cases, it is possible to study nonresponse at a given stage in terms of information collected at a previous stage—for example, by comparing (in terms of the responses given by both groups in the personal interview) the characteristics of persons who agreed to give a blood specimen with those who refused.

There were many opportunities for such comparisons in the surveys examined by the committee, but few of those opportunities had been seized. Smith's (1988) study of nonresponse bias in the 1988 GSS is an important exception. Because the GSS consisted of a lengthy personal interview followed by an SAQ covering sexual risk factors, it was possible to examine correlations between the interview responses and two types of nonresponse: nonresponse to the entire SAQ form and nonresponse to specific items. On the basis of this analysis, Smith draws an encouraging conclusion: "In general, the non-response does not appear to be related to differences in sexual behavior. Non-response differentials appear to be absent among those variables most closely related to sexual behavior. Non-response instead is related to general factors such as low education, low political interest, and general uncooperativeness that are not highly related to sexual behavior. As a result, non-response bias to the supplement (i.e., the sex SAQ) appears to be negligible." Smith's conclusion raises an interesting question about the basis for inferring the presence of nonresponse bias. Namely, on what basis can the absence of selection with respect to known or assumed correlates of sexual behavior be taken as evidence of the absence of direct selection (i.e., the third type of selection distinguished above)?

There is clearly a need to encourage further analyses of existing sex and seroprevalence surveys to learn more about the structure of nonresponse. When surveys are organized in a series of stages, which is the case in many instances, analysis can probe more deeply into the potential cause of nonresponse bias than is possible using simple comparisons of survey estimates with external data. Such analyses should provide a firmer basis for estimating population characteristics in the presence of nonresponse, and it would thereby engender increased confidence in the prevalence estimates derived from sex and seroprevalence surveys and surveys of sexual behavior.[18]

NONSAMPLING ISSUES IN AIDS SURVEYS

This section focuses on the survey measurement procedures that yield data for basic and applied studies of the behaviors that transmit HIV. The emphasis here is on nonsampling factors that affect the quality of these data. In this regard, it is important to remember that behind every n–way tabulation, logistic regression, or other analytical model using such data lies a human encounter between two individuals, an interviewer and a respondent. The situational, cognitive, social, and psychological factors that arise within that interpersonal exchange affect the answers that are given and the data that are thereby generated. To understand the sexual and drug-using behaviors that are at issue in survey research on HIV transmission, one must ultimately confront the uncertainties introduced by this question-and-answer process.

Terms and Concepts

In discussing the complex array of factors that can distort survey (and other) measurements, various interrelated terms are used with a reasonably standardized meaning by statisticians and researchers in the behavioral and social sciences. The constellation of sampling and nonsampling

---

[18] A major aim of the NCHS pilot studies for the national HIV seroprevalence survey is the investigation of the nonresponse bias in surveys that seek to estimate HIV prevalence.

factors that influence a particular measurement define the *error structure* of that measurement. Sampling factors can include incompleteness or other errors in the sampling frame used to draw the sample, failure to obtain data from all sampled persons, and so forth. (This type of nonresponse is discussed in the preceding section.) Nonsampling factors that affect measurements include misunderstanding of questions, respondent unwillingness to reveal sensitive information, interviewer mistakes in reading questions, clerical and other errors made during coding and processing of data, and so forth.

Although the factors that affect measurements are diverse, the effects they produce can be divided into two classes: systematic and random. To appreciate this distinction, let us restrict the discussion to phenomena, such as chronological age, for which it seems conceptually simple to sustain the notion of a *true value*.[19] Although any particular measurement procedure might produce inaccurate readings, most people would agree that there does exist a "true" chronological age for all people.

Random errors made in ascertaining age affect the *reproducibility* (widely called "reliability" in this context) of those measurements. Let us imagine, for example, a situation in which interviewers checked one of two boxes: 0-39 years or 40+ years. Assume further that 50 percent of the population were, in fact, 0-39 years old, and 50 percent were 40+. If interviewers accidentally checked the wrong box for 1 in 100 random persons whose true age was less than 40, and there was an equal error rate in coding persons whose true age was 40+, the *aggregate* distribution of ages in the resultant survey data would be identical to the true age distribution for the population. Nevertheless, 1 percent of all individuals in the sample would have been assigned erroneous ages. Random measurement errors of this type produce measurement unreliability, which can be detected in a survey by reinterviewing respondents and asking the relevant questions again. Responses that are inconsistent between the two interviews provide evidence of measurement unreliability.

Systematic errors directly affect the *validity* of a measurement, without altering its reliability. Continuing with the example of chronological age, let us assume that, in some survey, interviewers made neither random nor systematic errors but that 10 percent of respondents who were actually 40+ told the interviewer that they were 39. In this case, there would be

---

[19] In fact, when the argument is pushed far enough, there will always be cases for which the notion of true value becomes difficult to sustain (see Turner and Martin, 1984:97-106). Indeed, even chronological age cannot be known with arbitrarily high levels of precision without careful specification of the precise starting point for life. (The time of birthing, for example, does not readily accommodate specification in milliseconds.)

a systematic error[20] in the aggregate data. The estimates generated from the survey would yield 55 percent who were under 40 and 45 percent who were 40+.[21] This discrepancy between the true distribution and the observed distribution is known as the measurement *bias*. It should be understood that such biases may occur with perfectly reliable measurements. So, for example, the 10 percent of respondents who reported a lower age might well do so again on a reinterview, which would result in perfectly consistent responses in the two interviews: the results would be reproducible, and therefore reliable, but biased nonetheless.

To assess bias in measurements, evidence can often be sought from independent sources. In the case of age, for example, public birth records might be compared with the survey reports to detect bias. (This record check might be performed for a small subsample selected for a validation study rather than for the entire sample.)

Survey Measurement of Sexual Behaviors

Overview

In this section the committee reviews what is currently known about measurement problems that beset surveys of sexual behaviors. Although the survey literature contains much methodological research on nonsampling issues (for reviews, see Bradburn et al., 1979; Rossi, Wright, and Anderson, 1983; Turner and Martin, 1984), there is good reason to suspect that the problems encountered in studying sexual behavior are unique in some respects.[22] There appears to be little that is theoretically unique, however, about the problems of *random* error and the resultant unreliability in survey measurements of sexual behavior, and there is ample evidence in the literature (see below) that respondents do provide reasonably consistent responses to survey questions on sexual behaviors.

When it comes to validation of responses, however, the problems are much more numerous, and they introduce considerable uncertainty into the interpretation of almost all survey data derived from self-reports of sexual behavior and drug use. Moreover, these problems do not appear to be amenable to quick or easy solutions. Indeed, although the committee later notes a number of reasonably secure inferences that can be drawn from available data and offers several recommendations for improvements

---

[20] Systematic error (bias) affects measures of central tendency such as averages and medians, as well as the variability in the distribution of measurements.

[21] This again assumes that the true distribution was 50 percent under age 40 and 50 percent over 40.

[22] For a review see Catania and colleagues (in press,a).

in methodology, researchers and other readers of this chapter will find many more questions than answers in the following pages. In addition, these questions will involve the most fundamental matters, such as the issues raised in a question of the sort:

> Given the observation in a survey that X percent of a (probability) sample reported that they had engaged in unprotected anal intercourse during the previous week, and given the possibility that some respondents may knowingly or unknowingly distort their responses, what can be inferred about the actual proportion of the population that engaged in this practice?

A scrupulous answer to this question might well be that it is uncertain how many persons engaged in this behavior.

There are many approaches that might help reduce (but could not eliminate) this uncertainty. Careful investigations of respondents' understanding of a question, for example, could allow an assessment of biases introduced by subjects who did not comprehend the concepts. (There are anecdotal reports, for example, that researchers occasionally find a few heterosexual respondents who confuse rear-entry vaginal intercourse with anal intercourse.) Experiments with alternative question wordings might also be conducted to evaluate the extent to which the wording of a question influenced the responses given. Similarly, investigators could test alternative questioning procedures that afforded the respondent more privacy (e.g., by using self- or computer-administered questionnaires). Simple, probing questions might be used to gauge the extent of misreporting.[23] In addition, the accuracy of summary responses involving, for example, numbers of partners or rates of sexual contact, could be checked by asking a subsample of respondents to keep diaries.

Although each of these tactics provides valuable ancillary information that would reduce some of the uncertainties, none of them provides a completely satisfactory validation of these measurements. There is, for example, good reason (see Table 6-4 below) to expect that the sensitivity of the topic is more of an obstacle to accurate measurement than the inherent cognitive complexity of the questions (when the time period being recalled is brief) or the unfamiliarity of the terminology. That is to say, questions such as, "Have you had sexual contact to orgasm with another man in the last week?" may be more prone to bias induced by the sensitivity of the topic than by the respondents' inability to understand the question or remember the event.

Furthermore, although there is ample reason and sufficient empirical

---

[23]Newcomer and Udry (1988), for example, had success with the straightforward strategy of asking respondents whether they had given false responses.

evidence to justify experimentation with alternative methods of ensuring respondents' privacy, there is also reason to believe that some respondents may conceal behaviors even in the most private reporting setting and that subsequently they will not admit that they did so. This possibility must be given considerable weight in the face of statutes in many states that classify some sexual behaviors (including oral sex, male-female and male-male anal intercourse) as crimes.[24] Finally, there is the possibility that behaviors in which the respondent engages while under the influence of excessive drugs or alcohol may be poorly recalled, if at all.

Given these considerations, lingering concern about the trustworthiness of such survey estimates is virtually inevitable. Nonetheless, some inferences may be made with relative certainty if one is prepared to make assumptions about the direction of reporting biases.

Inference in the Presence of Bias

It could reasonably be argued that the preponderant source of bias in reports of sexual behaviors or drug use for many (but not all) populations and measurement procedures will be caused by respondents underreporting their behaviors. It might be hypothesized further that this underreporting will follow the norms and taboos of the respondents' society. If this hypothesis were true, one would expect the most extreme underreporting for behaviors that are most disparaged and that carry the most severe penalties for discovery (e.g., adult-child sex, rape, etc.). Similarly, one would expect the least reporting bias for behaviors that are sanctioned or encouraged (e.g., vaginal sex between spouses). (Indeed, in this latter case, one might anticipate an exception to the rule of underreporting. For married couples, it might be reasonable to anticipate some pressure to conceal a low rate or absence of sexual contact between spouses.)

For cases in which underreporting is a reasonable assumption, a safe inference from well-collected survey measurements is that the resultant estimates represent a reasonable lower bound on the true prevalence of the behavior in the population. Such a tack has been explicitly taken in methodological studies of sexual and other sensitive behaviors. For example, investigators who seek to improve the reporting of sexual behaviors such as masturbation (Bradburn et al., 1979) and the reporting of

---

[24]In 1986, the Supreme Court ruled that states could enforce criminal sanctions against consensual homosexual behaviors, even when practiced by adults in the privacy of their own home (*Bowers* v. *Hardwick*, No. 85-140, June 30, 1986). The statute at issue (Georgia Code Annotated at 16-6-2, 1984) held that "(a) A person commits the offense of sodomy when he performs or submits to any sexual act involving the sex organs of one person and the mouth or anus of another . . . ." The argument and opinion in that case implied, however, that although the application of this statute was upheld in the case of male-male sex, it would not be held constitutional if applied to a married male-female couple.

alcohol and drug use (e.g., Waterton and Duffy, 1984) typically assume that the net reporting bias for those behaviors is negative, that is, more persons conceal behaviors in which they have engaged than report behaviors in which they have not engaged. Consequently, these investigators attempt to identify survey procedures (e.g., the use of SAQs) that would increase reporting of these behaviors (in the aggregate). Similarly, a recent attempt to estimate the prevalence of same-gender sex among men in the United States (Fay et al., 1989) argued that the resultant estimates should be treated as lower-bound estimates, on the assumption that the net reporting bias would be negative.

Although this strategy does allow lower bound inferences to be made with relative confidence, it is not an entirely satisfying solution because point estimates (e.g., actual frequencies or means) are, after all, of considerable interest. Indeed, these estimates figure centrally in two of the most important research challenges of the epidemic's second decade: determining whether there are declines over time in the incidence of sexual behaviors that risk transmitting HIV, and assessing the effectiveness of AIDS education and prevention programs by comparing the behaviors of persons who participate in those programs with the behaviors of those who do not. Both of these tasks require comparison of the distribution of behaviors reported by different samples or by the same sample at different points in time to detect differences. Changes in behavior over time or the superior effectiveness of particular interventions in changing behavior could then be inferred. If the only statements about these issues that can be made with certainty must be phrased in terms of lower bounds, these important questions cannot be answered.

Assumption of Constant Bias in Measurements

To answer the questions referred to above, it is neither theoretically necessary to make measurements without bias, nor always required to have accurate assessments of the magnitude and direction of the bias. One can detect change (or intergroup differences) without ever knowing the "true" value, providing it is possible to *assume* that the reporting bias is equivalent at the two points in time (or across the two groups). If the study makes no attempt to validate the self-reports, this assumption is considered to be implicit in studies of time trends or intergroup differences in behavior. This assumption, however, is often problematic.

It is quite possible, for example, that the reporting bias itself will vary over time. Respondents (and the population at large) may become more accustomed to questions about sexual behavior and may be less likely to conceal sensitive behaviors. (For example, condoms, anal intercourse, and other topics that were rarely discussed in the media prior to the AIDS epidemic now appear with greater frequency.) On the other hand, as the result of an educational program or other intervention effort, respondents may become less likely to report unsafe behaviors. Indeed, it might plausibly be argued that the same social and psychological pressures used by intervention programs to encourage behavioral change also make it less likely that respondents will report these same behaviors.[25] Thus, the group receiving an intervention may also have its reporting bias modified in the direction of *less* complete reporting of risky behaviors.)[26]

Approaches to Validation

Measures of sexual behaviors may have much in common with measurements of subjective phenomena (e.g., attitudes, opinions, intentions).[27] Although sexual behavior can, in theory, be observed, there are only a few special circumstances in which the testimony of independent observers could be used to validate respondents' self-reports.[28] Outside these special circumstances, there are no obvious independent measurements that could provide a basis for directly assessing the extent of bias in self-reports of sexual behavior. As discussed below, however, there may be indirect approaches that could be used for such assessments.

---

[25] There is also evidence, however, that in some interventions directed toward IV drug users, increased rapport between clients and program staff over time results in more honest reporting of risky behaviors. D. Worth, Department of Epidemiology and Social Medicine, Montefiore Medical Center, personal communication, June 19, 1989.

[26] Similar arguments apply to efforts to study the "association" between reports of sexual behavior and other variables. Bias in measurements may covary with variables of substantive interest and thus produce spurious correlations. For example, studies of same-gender sexual contact indicate that respondents with college educations report more contacts in childhood and as adults than are reported by those with less than a college education. Although this variation may reflect a true difference between groups with different levels of education, it is also possible that college-educated respondents may be less likely than those with no college education to conceal same-gender sexual behaviors in the context of a survey. To the extent that such differential concealment occurred, a spurious correlation would arise between education and the prevalence of same-gender sexual contacts as a result of the nonequivalent measurement biases in the groups.

[27] In 1984, another NRC panel published a review of concepts and methods for assessing the error structure of survey measurements of subjective phenomena (Turner and Martin, 1984). The report concluded that validation for such measurements might best be sought in demonstrations at an aggregate level that time-series of these measurements were related in a theoretically reasonable fashion to independent time-series that measured objective phenomena to which the subjective phenomena ought to be related. Sufficiently long time-series are not available for most survey measurements of subjective phenomena, but the available data indicate that self-reported attitudes toward the safety of different contraceptives (Beniger, 1984), public perceptions of national "problems" (MacKuen, 1981, 1984), and presidential popularity (MacKuen and Turner, 1984) do show the expected relationships over time.

[28] One such circumstance involves the report of sexual contact by a couple in which each respondent is reporting on the same behavior—for example, the frequency of coitus or the use of a condom; see A.L. Clark and Wallin [1964] and Levinger [1966] for examples.

Validation Using STD Rates. To assess the validity of reports of sexual behavior, the committee's first report recommended consideration of a strategy parallel to that used with subjective measurements. The committee argued:

> It may be possible, for example, to construct a convincing validation by demonstrating that an independent series of measurements of change in the incidence of gonorrhea in a population over time could be predicted from a concurrent time-series monitoring the self-reported incidence of unprotected sexual contacts with new partners in the same population. Although there are many potential pitfalls to executing a successful validation in this way, the committee believes that the feasibility of using such indirect procedures should be given further, careful consideration. (Turner, Miller, and Moses, 1989:150)

The tentativeness of the committee's advice on this validation strategy reflected the practical and theoretical difficulties that attend the use of sexually transmitted disease (STD) statistics for this purpose. The committee noted, for example, that national statistics on STDs may be in need of improvement. It recommended a careful review of these data systems and, if necessary, an increase in resources to improve them (Turner, Miller, and Moses, 1989:167). Furthermore, for any group, the trends in STD rates over time will reflect phenomena such as the changes, if any, in the behaviors of group members that expose them to infection, trends in the rates of STDs among the population from which the group selects its new sexual contacts, and changes in reporting practices. It is thus possible to observe in a particular group a rise in STD rates over time that occurs concurrently with a true decline in the rates of "risky" behaviors. This seemingly paradoxical outcome can result from rising STD rates in the population at large, which mask the protective effect of behavioral change in the smaller subgroup. (That is, although "risky behaviors" are less frequent in number, they are practiced with partners who are more likely to be infected.)[29] Nevertheless, despite the attractiveness of the strategy of conducting validation studies of sexual behavior using STD rates, no assurance currently exists that such a strategy could be made to work.

Psychometric Approaches to Validity. The approaches discussed above follow from measurement traditions in the physical sciences. Yet there is also a robust tradition of measurement in psychology, which has added to the literature both a substantial body of empirical work

---

[29] Numerous other artifacts bedevil this strategy as well. For example, it has been observed that the institution of aggressive STD control programs may inflate the number of cases of STDs that are actually reported. Contact tracing may also serve to bring more STD cases to the attention of public health workers.

and, more important, alternative ways of viewing the error structure of measurements for variables, like intelligence, that are never subject to direct observation. The psychometric literature is vast, and it would be impossible to summarize it here. Excellent texts and reviews are available elsewhere (Gulliksen, 1950; Cronbach and Gleser, 1965; Anastasi, 1976; Wigdor and Garner, 1982). For the purposes of this report, it may suffice to note the approaches to validation offered in this literature. Most important among these are criterion validity, content validity, and construct validity.[30]

- *Criterion validity* for an intelligence test refers to the extent to which a given measurement or test is predictive of the properties it purports to measure. Consider, for example, the Scholastic Aptitude Test, or SAT, which is supposed to measure the test taker's aptitude for college-level course-work. Its criterion validity could be assessed by measuring the correlation between the scores of individuals on the test and some direct indicator of the performance of these individuals in college.[31]

- *Content validity* (sometimes called face validity) is not as-sessed empirically. Rather, it involves a judgment that the questions being asked are appropriate (or inappropriate) to the characteristic being measured. Thus, it might be judged that questions that tested reading comprehension and written composition had high content validity (i.e., were "appropri-ate") for a measure that purported to assess the likelihood an individual would succeed in college. In contrast, a measure of the person's athletic prowess might be judged to have low face validity for success in most college programs.

- *Construct validity* refers to the extent to which a set of measurements relate to one another in a coherent way as specified by some (formal or informal) theory. Unlike crite-rion validity, construct validity cannot be reduced to a single correlation coefficient. Construct validity instead involves a judgment about the extent to which a given measurement fits

---

[30] The discussion in this paragraph draws heavily on that in Turner and Martin (1984:Vol. 1, 120–125).

[31] This example simplifies matters somewhat. The criterion validity could be directly assessed by admitting all students to the same college program and then measuring their performance. In real-ity, practical considerations make such an uncomplicated assessment impossible (e.g., low-scoring students are not admitted to many colleges and universities). These complications require various adjustments and simplifying assumptions.

together with other measurements in a manner that is theoretically meaningful. (In assessing a questionnaire measure of psychological depression, for example, psychologists expect to find a coherent pattern of associations between feelings of helplessness and despair, self-destructive fantasy or behavior, somatic complaints such as sleep disturbances, and negative emotions [Hamilton, 1960; Beck et al., 1961; Himmelweit and Turner, 1982].)

While these three psychometric notions of validity can be helpful in approaching the problems involved in validating survey measures of sexual behaviors, their past use has sometimes been less than optimal. One of the most important failings results from overreliance on correlation coefficients in reporting on the validity of measurements. Although ideal self-report measurements of a phenomenon ought to be perfectly correlated with (error-free) direct observations of the same phenomenon, the presence of a very high or even perfect correlation does not, in itself, guarantee that the survey measurement is not contaminated by significant biases. Consider, for example, hypothetical reporting biases that caused the frequency of anal sex to be underreported by 20, 40, and 60 percent from its "true" incidence in three measurements. Such biases would yield three measurements that differed substantially, but that were, nonetheless, perfectly correlated ($r = 1.0$) with one another. These correlations would occur even though the mean frequency of anal sex observed using these three measuring instruments would be quite different.

If one imagines these different reporting biases to be characteristics of different time periods (or different intervention conditions in an evaluation study), one could conceivably report equivalent "validity coefficients" over time (or experimental conditions), although there were, in fact, substantially different and undetected biases in the measurements.[32] It is unfortunately the case that the current literature contains numerous instances in which researchers report only the bivariate correlations as evidence of validity (or reliability). Indeed, readers will note in the following pages numerous instances in which the committee has had to rely exclusively on such coefficients because the published reports of studies do not provide other needed information.

In this regard, the committee also notes that, when examining the validity and reliability of their measurements, researchers would be well advised to avoid a premature rush to rely on statistical procedures that

---

[32] These differences *could*, of course, be detected by examining the means or the intercept of the regression of one measurement on the other.

assume (multivariate) normality. Many measurements of epidemiological interest have distributions that are not normal. Indeed, there may be strong reasons to focus special concern on biases that disproportionately affect extreme segments of the response distribution. For example, persons with very large numbers of sexual and drug-using partners play a disproportionate role in the spread of HIV. It is for this reason that the committee previously recommended that reports of "averages" or tabular displays that hide the long "tails" of the distributions of these variables be avoided whenever possible (Turner, Miller, and Moses, 1989:Ch. 2). For the same reason, researchers who analyze and report on the error structure of their survey measurements should attend not only to the overall performance of their instruments but also to biases and errors that may disproportionately affect the reports of persons who are in the high-activity end of the response distribution.

EMPIRICAL STUDIES OF SEXUAL BEHAVIORS

Validation

There is only a very limited range of evidence that can be collected to provide independent corroboration of the validity of self-reported sexual behaviors. In the past, three broad types of research evidence have been collected:

- partner reports, in which regular sexual partners respond to the same questions as the study respondent;
- "invalidation evidence," which is derived from longitudinal studies in which it is possible to obtain some measure of reporting accuracy by examining the temporal patterns for impossible temporal sequences (e.g., persons who report having engaged in sexual intercourse when interviewed at age 15 but who report at a later age that they have never had intercourse); and
- clinical evidence of sexual activity that can be used to verify the fact that a particular sexual activity has occurred (the committee is aware of only one study in which this sort of evidence has been gathered).

Partner Reports

Kinsey and his colleagues reported the first empirical study of which the committee is aware in which the self-reports of two sexual partners were compared to explore the reports' accuracy. The Kinsey team used

TABLE 6-2 Findings of Kinsey et al.'s (1948) validation study of sexual behaviors reported by spouses.

COMPARING DATA FROM 231 PAIRS OF SPOUSES

CASES	ITEMS INVOLVED	UNIT OF MEASURE-MENT	IDENT. RSPNS. %	WITH-IN 1 UNIT OF IDENT. %	COEFFIC. OF CORREL.	MEAN OF HUSBAND'S REPORTS	MEAN OF WIFE'S REPORTS	DIFF. OF MEANS: ♂ − ♀
	Vital Statistics				Pears. r			
229	Years married	1 year	88.6	96.1	0.99	6.35 ± 0.42	6.40 ± 0.42	−0.05
214	Pre-marital acquaint.	12 mon.	57.9	86.9	0.88	42.11 ± 2.83	40.88 ± 2.74	+1.23
156	Engagement	4 mon.	57.1	78.2	0.83	12.64 ± 1.03	12.85 ± 1.07	−0.21
226	Age, ♂ at marr.	1 year	68.6	97.3	0.99	27.27 ± 0.37	27.17 ± 0.37	+0.10
228	Age, ♀ at marr.	1 year	61.8	92.5	0.63	24.88 ± 0.32	24.75 ± 0.32	+0.13
231	No. children	1 child	99.6	100.0	0.99	0.90 ± 0.09	0.90 ± 0.09	0.00
185	No. abortions	1 event	90.3	98.4	0.76	0.32 ± 0.06	0.41 ± 0.08	−0.09
227	Lapse, first coitus—marr.	6 mon.	74.4	89.4	0.85	5.09 ± 0.88	4.72 ± 0.86	+0.37
87	Lapse, marr. —first birth	6 mon.	66.7	89.7	0.96	28.05 ± 1.99	28.19 ± 2.01	−0.14
220	Educ. level, ♂	2 years	84.1	99.1	0.97	16.23 ± 0.26	16.16 ± 0.25	+0.07
223	Educ. level, ♀	2 years	79.4	97.8	0.92	14.41 ± 0.21	14.67 ± 0.21	−0.26
219	Occup. class, ♂	1 of 9	91.8	98.6	0.98	5.32 ± 0.14	5.27 ± 0.14	+0.05
	Coital Freq.							
223	Max. freq., marit. coitus	2/wk.	33.2	68.2	0.54	6.72 ± 0.31	6.74 ± 0.31	−0.02
225	Av. freq., early marr.	1/wk.	34.7	73.3	0.50	2.73 ± 0.13	3.00 ± 0.14	−0.27
226	Av. freq., now	1/wk.	56.6	88.1	0.60	1.91 ± 0.11	2.21 ± 0.13	−0.30
218	% with orgasm, ♀	10%	55.0	71.1	0.75	69.82 ± 2.16	66.83 ± 2.26	+2.99
	Techniques in coital foreplay				Tetra-choric r	% Husbands Reporting Yes	% Wives Reporting Yes	
229	Kiss	Yes, No	97		0.92	95.6 ± 1.35	99.1 ± 0.62	−3.5
228	Deep kiss	Yes, No	85		0.72	85.1 ± 2.36	82.0 ± 2.54	+3.1
228	Hand—♀ breast	Yes, No	95		0.78	95.6 ± 1.36	96.5 ± 1.22	−0.9
228	Mouth—♀ breast	Yes, No	89		0.79	90.4 ± 2.04	86.0 ± 2.43	+4.4
229	Hand—♀ genitalia	Yes, No	90		0.61	92.6 ± 1.73	92.2 ± 1.77	+0.4
226	Hand—♂ genitalia	Yes, No	85		0.70	83.6 ± 2.46	85.8 ± 2.32	− .2
220	Mouth—♀ genitalia	Yes, No	82		0.84	35.9 ± 3.23	37.3 ± 3.26	−1.4
226	Mouth—♂ genitalia	Yes, No	85		0.93	33.6 ± 3.14	35.4 ± 3.18	−1.8
	Coital techniq.							
228	Male above	Yes, No	93		0.75	94.3 ± 1.54	93.5 ± 1.63	+0.8
228	Female above	Yes, No	76		0.74	54.8 ± 3.30	49.1 ± 3.31	+5.7
224	On side	Yes, No	76		0.68	39.3 ± 3.26	37.1 ± 3.23	+2.2
221	Sitting	Yes, No	81		0.63	19.0 ± 2.64	17.6 ± 2.56	+1.4
227	Standing	Yes, No	89		0.64	10.1 ± 2.00	7.9 ± 1.79	+2.2
224	Rear entrance	Yes, No	83		0.77	24.6 ± 2.88	17.4 ± 2.53	+7.2
186	Coitus nude	Yes, No	90		0.82	87.1 ± 2.46	89.2 ± 2.28	−2.1
223	Multiple orgasm, ♂	Yes, No	95		0.74	4.9 ± 1.45	4.1 ± 1.33	+0.8

231 pairs of spouses who appear to have been individually interviewed[33] following the normal procedures used in the Kinsey studies (see Gebhard and Johnson, 1979; Turner, Miller, Moses, 1989:80–83). The results obtained from comparing the reports of each spouse regarding coital frequency and technique are summarized in Table 6-2. The table shows— as Kinsey, Pomeroy, and Martin (1948:125) themselves remark—"[a]n amazing agreement between the statements of the husbands and of the wives in each marriage . . . " Given the relatively small sample size, few instances of bias in this study would reach conventional standards of significance. There is, however, a modest trend for females to report less frequently than their male partners the practice of female superior and rear-entry coitus; females also tended to report a higher average frequency of coitus both in their early marriage and at the time of the interview. In assessing the rather high degree of congruence between the reports of spouses in Kinsey's study, one is also well advised to note the interpretive caveat that Kinsey, Pomeroy, and Martin (1948:125) offered, namely, that "allowance must be made for the possibility that there may have been collusion between some of the partners, and a conscious or unconscious agreement to distort the fact[s]."

Following the example set by Kinsey, subsequent sexual behavior researchers have on occasion gathered data from spouses and other partners to gauge the accuracy of self-reported data. With some exceptions, these studies do not cover as comprehensive a range of sexual behaviors as Kinsey explored. They are, nonetheless, perhaps of more relevance for understanding the qualities of the behavioral data that are routinely used in AIDS research. This is so not only because the social norms regarding sexual activity have changed since the 1940s but also because the methodologies employed in recent studies tend to involve standardized interviews or self-administered questionnaires rather than the Kinsey-type interviews that last many hours.

Table 6-3 summarizes the results of selected recent studies that use spousal reports to gauge the accuracy of reporting of sexual behaviors. One of the first things regarding this tabulation that will be noted—and lamented—is the relative dearth of information on response congruence that is typically supplied. Kinsey and colleagues presented the proportions of spousal pairs who were in perfect agreement and who agreed within ±1 unit; in addition, they supplied correlation coefficients and means and standard deviations for reports by husbands and wives. In

---

[33]The description of this research (Kinsey et al., 125–128) does not indicate whether the same interviewer questioned both spouses. The text does indicate, however, that "in many instances there were intervals of two to six years or more between the interviews with the two spouses" (p. 127).

TABLE 6-3 Post-Kinsey Validation Studies of Self-Reported Sexual Behaviors Comparing Reports of Sexual Partners

Study	Sample	Method	Findings
Clark and Wallin (1964)	428 male-female couples (married)[a]	SAQ; frequency of coitus[b]	Correlations of .57 to .61 between husbands' and wives' reports; roughly equal means for husbands and wives
Levinger (1966)	60 male-female couples (married)[c]	Interview question; frequency of coitus (average in relationship)[d]	Mean frequency reported: 7.78 (wives) and 6.96 (husbands); correlation not reported
Seage et al. (1989)	170 male-male couples	Interview	Spearman correlations between number of occurrences reported by two partners: .63 to .76 for oral sex without ejaculation;[e] .63 to .80 for oral sex with ejaculation; .60 to .92 for anal sex without ejaculation; .75 to .79 for anal sex with ejaculation; .73 to .87 for rimming; .48 to .99 for fisting
Jacobson & Moore (1981)	36 male-female couples (married) including 16 "distressed" & 20 non-distressed	Daily checklists of various sexual behaviors[f]	60 percent agreement[g] between spouses in "distressed" couples; 67 percent agreement between spouses in nondistressed couples; (difference was not significant)
Blumstein & Schwartz (1983, 1989)[h]	3,600 male-female couples (married); 650 male-female couples (unmarried); 965 male-male couples; and 770 female-female couples	SAQ	Correlations of .78 to .86 for frequency of intercourse over last year;[i] .66 to .70 for how frequently cunnilingus is part of sex;[j] .71 (heterosexuals) and .38 (gay men) for how frequently fellatio is part of sex;[j] .65 (gay men) for how frequently anal intercourse is part of sex[j]
Coates et al. (1988)	75 male-male couples (one partner with AIDS)	Interview	Correlations between frequency reported by index case and by partner: .82 to .88 for mouth-penis contact;[k] .72 to .75 for ejaculation in partner's mouth;[l] .90 to .91 for insertion of penis in rectum; .85 to .89 for ejaculation in rectum; .57 for insertion of finger in partner's anus;[m] .53 to .71 for tongue-anus contact;[n] .68 to .81 for insertion of object in anus;[o] .49 to .69 for insertion of hand in anus[p]

NOTES: SAQ: Self-Administered Questionnaire.

[a] "White, native born, and when first studied were predominantly residents of Chicago. Only a fifth of the men and a third of the women lacked some college education" (Clark and Wallin, 1964:168).

[b] Question: "About how many times a month have you had sexual relations with your wife [husband] in the past 12 months? (Give the number that tells the average number of times per month.)"

[c] "60 middle class couples, all of whom had children, had been married four to twenty-two years, and who lived in the Greater Cleveland area. The average couple was in its late thirties, had been married 13.6 years, had three children ..."

[d] Question: "Ordinarily, how many times a month do you have sexual relations with your wife [husband]? (Except during periods of pregnancy or physical illness)."

[e] The range reflects correlations reported for three groups: concordant HIV-negative couples (both partners are HIV negative), concordant HIV-positive couples (both partners are HIV positive), and discordant couples (one partner is HIV positive, the other is HIV negative).

[f] Spouse Observation Checklist (SOC): "The SOC, consisting of 409 items, is a comprehensive list of potential events that can occur in a marital relationship" (Jacobsen and Moore, 1981:271). Self-Monitoring Checklist (SMC): The SMC was a parallel checklist of behaviors that required the spouse of the respondent also to track his or her own behaviors. "Sex" behaviors included items such as: "we engaged in sexual intercourse; spouse petted me; spouse caressed me with his mouth."

[g] Results were calculated as the total number of individual behaviors checked by both spouses divided by the number checked by both plus the number checked by one spouse but not the other. Unfortunately, the report of the study does not break down the results by different behaviors. It is reasonable to suspect that there might be more agreement about intercourse than about ambiguous and possibly less memorable events such as "spouse caressed me with his mouth."

[h] Original research reported in Blumstein and Schwartz (1983); reliabilities reported by Blumstein (personal communication, June 21, 1989).

[i] Eight-point scale: (1) daily or almost daily, (2) 3–4 times a week, (3) 1–2 times a week, (4) 2–3 times a month, (5) once a month, (6) once every few months, (7) a few times in last year, (8) never.

[j] Five-point scale: (1) always, (2) usually, (3) sometimes, (4) rarely, (5) never.

[k] Note that two correlations are reported: one for insertion by the index case and one for insertion by the partner. They are not, however, markedly different.

[l] Note that two correlations are reported: one for ejaculation by the index case and one for ejaculation by the partner. They are not, however, markedly different.

[m] Reliabilities were identical for case-partner and partner-case contacts.

[n] .53 is reliability reported for index case having tongue contact with partner's anus; .71 is correlation for partner having tongue contact with index case's anus.

[o] .68 for index case inserting object in partner's anus; .81 for the reverse case.

[p] .49 for index case inserting hand in partner's anus; .69 for the reverse case.

contrast, recent studies typically present only correlation coefficients. As noted previously, these coefficients do not provide some of the information that is most crucial in understanding the error structure of measurements. They do not, for example, allow any statement about bias—for example, for heterosexual couples, the extent to which husbands' reports systematically differ from those provided by wives.

Overall, the results in Table 6-3 together with the Kinsey results suggest that there is substantial but not complete agreement between sexual partners in describing the behaviors in which a couple has engaged. Indeed, in some of the instances reported in Table 6-3, the nature of the questions makes the levels of agreement that were obtained somewhat surprising. Coates and coworkers (1988), for example, requested that the gay men in their study report the total number of sexual encounters they had with a particular partner and the total number of times (or percentage of encounters) during which they engaged in specific sexual behaviors. Given that these men reported a mean of more than 250 encounters with their partners occurring over an average of more than two years, accurate reporting from memory was clearly beyond the ability of most respondents. Nonetheless, the correlational evidence suggests that sexual partners provided quite similar reports of their behaviors.

Similarly, Levinger (1966) asked heterosexual married couples to estimate the mean frequency of intercourse during their marriage. (The couples were married an average of approximately 14 years.) Although one would prefer some report of the joint distribution of spouses' reports, it is impressive nonetheless that the mean monthly frequency of intercourse reported by husbands and wives in this study varied by less than one act per month. Blumstein and Schwartz (1983) report parallel evidence from male-male, male-female, and female-female couples indicating that reports of the frequency of intercourse over the preceding year were quite consistent between partners ($r = .78$ to $.86$), although somewhat lower levels of consistency were found for questions about other sexual behaviors.

Other Validation Techniques

Although partner validation provides the most obvious source of independent information on sexual behavior, it is not the only validation method that has been used.[34] In 1966 J.P. Clark and Tifft reported the use of a polygraph (lie detector) to motivate respondents to correct

---

[34] Occasionally, the literature reports studies that use expert judgments to validate behavioral measurements. For example, Koss and Gidycz (1985) reported the use of a self-administered questionnaire to identify "hidden" rapes (i.e., those not reported to police) in samples of college students (242 female and 144 male). Validity was subsequently assessed by comparing questionnaire responses with the

misreports they may have made in a previously completed questionnaire. By monitoring the changes made by the respondents, Clark and Tifft obtained a measure of the magnitude and direction of reporting biases that may occur in surveys of sexual behavior. Clark and Tifft's subjects were 45 college males who reported on (lifetime) experiences with prostitutes, sexual coercion, homosexual contacts, masturbation, and nonmarital sex. (It should be emphasized that the criterion measure was not the polygraph judgment but rather the subjects' behavior in "correcting" their answers to the questionnaire when confronted with the polygraph.)[35]

Table 6-4 presents selected results from this study. It will be seen that for every measurement a substantial fraction of the sexual behaviors that were finally reported were reported only after the possibility of lie detection was introduced. Thus, although virtually every male (95 percent), when confronted with the polygraph, indicated that he had masturbated, 30 percent of the men in the sample denied masturbating on the initial questionnaire and subsequently changed their response. Similarly, although 22.5 percent of these college men ultimately reported some male-male sexual contact, 15 percent of the men initially denied such contact and subsequently changed their answers.

As these results indicate, the response bias in questionnaire measures can be substantial. Furthermore, the net bias (i.e., the difference between the percentages overreporting and underreporting) is typically weighted in the direction of underreporting. Empirical evidence such as this underlies the common assumption that survey measurements of sexual and drug

---

results of interviews with a "post-master's level psychologist." Twenty-five percent of survey respondents consented to the interview, and the author reported correlations of .73 (female) and .61 (male) when questionnaire data and judgments made by psychologists were aggregated in categories (no victimization, sexual coercion, sexual abuse, and sexual assault). The interpretation of these results is problematic, however, because there is no assurance that the judgments made by the "psychologist" were more accurate than those obtained from the survey questionnaire.

[35] Subjects were given multiple opportunities to change their initial answers. In postsurvey interviews, researchers would ask a respondent for his "utmost cooperation in making his response accurate and [the researchers] strongly alluded to the likelihood of inaccurate responses being given on questionnaires administered in group situations" (J.P. Clark and Tifft, 1966:519). The respondent was then asked to retrieve his questionnaire using the identification number that had been assigned and "to make whatever modifications (in private) that were necessary to bring it to 100 percent accuracy."

Subsequently, subjects were told that the researchers would like them to submit voluntarily to a polygraph examination. (No subjects refused the polygraph.) During the polygraph examination, the researchers reported that "when an indication of deception occurred with one of our respondents, the examiner asked the respondent if he wanted to make a change in his response." The responses supplied by respondents after all "corrections" had been made are taken to be more accurate than those originally supplied in the survey. Although this assumption seems fair, there is, nonetheless, some possibility that respondents may have altered their answers for reasons that would not result in increased accuracy (e.g., to comply with covert social pressure).

TABLE 6-4 Selected Results Reported in Clark and Tifft's Study of Bias in Questionnaire Measurements of "Deviant" Behavior: Percentage of college men ($N = 45$) who: (a) report selected sexual behaviors when confronted with lie detector, (b) deny behavior in questionnaire but report it when confronted with lie detector (underreporting), and (c) report behavior in questionnaire but deny it when confronted with lie detector (overreporting)

Behavior	Percent Reporting Behavior With Lie Detector (a)	Estimate of Bias	
		Under-reporting (b)	Over-reporting (c)
Had sex relations with a person of the same sex	22.5	15.0	5.0
Masturbated	95.0	30.0	5.0
Attempted to force or forced a female to have sexual intercourse with me	15.0	7.5	2.5
Had sex relations with a person of the opposite sex (other than my wife)	55.0	17.5	15.0
Gotten a female other than my wife pregnant	7.5	2.5	2.5
Visited a house of prostitution	17.5	2.5	2.5
Had in my possession pictures, books, or other materials which were obviously obscene and prepared to arouse someone sexually	50.0	12.5	7.5

SOURCE: J.P. Clark and Tifft (1986).

use behaviors may set lower bounds on the actual frequency of these behaviors in the population.

Udry and Morris (1967) used a different strategy to study a behavior that may have been less sensitive to report—that is, intercourse for married women. These investigators collected daily urine specimens for a period of 90 days and tested the specimens for the presence of sperm to validate the women's self-reports of intercourse (which were also obtained daily). Although the absence of sperm does not provide definitive evidence that intercourse had *not* occurred, the presence of sperm can be taken as evidence that intercourse had occurred at some point in the recent past.[36] Fifteen (of 58) women in this study showed

---

[36]There is some uncertainty about how long sperm may be found after intercourse. Udry and Morris adopted the standard that the sighting of three or more intact sperm was consistent with a report of

evidence of sperm in their urine on one or more occasions. For 12 of the women, all 32 reports of the presence of sperm in their daily urines corresponded with *prior* reports of coitus. Among the other 3 women, there were 5 (of 9) instances in which sperm were present but the subject had not reported intercourse during the preceding 48 hours.

Independent evidence validating self-reports is precious. Yet for many studies, obtaining such evidence is impossible (owing to the "private" nature of the behavior) or so difficult as to become infeasible. Consequently, other evidence is required to sustain the claim that a particular data collection method is useful for research.

Replication of Surveys on Samples of the Same Population

In lodging a claim that measurement in a particular domain is "scientific," one may legitimately pose the question: Do independent attempts to measure the same phenomenon produce consistent results? Given the litany of possible contaminants that can corrupt the measurement process, there is substantial interest in knowing whether similar answers about characteristics of the same population can be obtained by different survey organizations using roughly comparable techniques. Because of the dearth of basic research on sexual behavior in particular and the lack of investment in methodological research in general, there is no ample stock of material from which to make such comparisons. There are, however, two examples that demonstrate the important point that survey measurements of sexual behaviors can produce reliable measures of behavior in well-defined populations.

Proportion of Teenagers Who Are Sexually Active

The most thorough demonstration is offered in the literature on teenage sexual activity (an area that fortunately received some investment prior to AIDS to pursue studies to understand patterns of sexual behavior). Kahn, Kalsbeek, and Hofferth (1988) recently published a comparison of rates of teenage sexual activity reported by the 1959-1963 birth cohort in three independent surveys:

- the 1979 national survey of young women undertaken by Zelnik and Kantner (1980) and the Institute for Survey Research of Temple University (KZ79 in Figure 6-3);
- the 1982 National Survey of Family Growth conducted by

---

coitus during the previous 48-hour period. (In making these judgments, the authors centrifuged the urine specimens and analyzed one drop of the sediment for 10 minutes.)

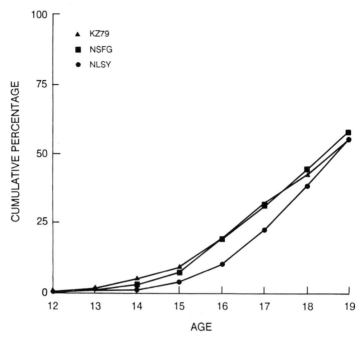

FIGURE 6-3 Estimates derived from three independent surveys of the cumulative percentage of teenagers sexually active, by exact ages. NOTE: Survey estimates have been adjusted to make surveys as comparable as possible by, for example, eliminating population segments that are not included in all three surveys. SOURCE: J. R. Kahn, Kalsbeek, and Hofferth (1988).

Westat for the National Center for Health Statistics (NSFG in Figure 6-3); and

- the 1983 wave of the National Longitudinal Survey of Youth conducted by the National Opinion Research Center (NORC, University of Chicago) for a consortium of federal agencies (NLSY in Figure 6-3).

The comparison undertaken by Kahn, Kalsbeek, and Hofferth involved surveys that had several systematic differences in methodology. The three studies differed, for example, in the precise wording of the question, the age of the respondents at the time they were asked to recall their early sexual experiences, and study design. Adjustments were made (e.g., eliminating population segments that were not included in all surveys) to make the studies as comparable as possible; the adjusted proportions of women reporting sexual activity by each age are shown in Figure 6-3.[37] This plot shows that there is a very close correspondence

---

[37] Respondents in the 1979 survey by Zelnik and Kantner (1980) were asked: When was the first time

between two of the three surveys and that the third survey (the National Longitudinal Survey of Youth) produces estimates that are quite similar for ages 12 to 15 and 18 to 19; however, it provides substantially lower estimates of sexual activity for this cohort of women at ages 16 and 17. Although these observed discrepancies are not trivial and are much larger than would be expected to occur as a result of sampling error alone, one cannot lose sight of the very substantial similarity of the findings obtained by the three surveys. Furthermore, Kahn, Kalsbeek, and Hofferth (1988) go on to demonstrate that the three surveys produce statistically equivalent estimates of the net *association*[38] between sexual activity (i.e., having engaged in intercourse at a given age) and various background variables. The background variables used in this analysis included the exact year of birth, mother's education, whether the respondent was Catholic, and whether the respondent lived with both natural parents at age 14. Of 93 tests for survey-specific differences in the net association between the background variable and sexual activity, in only one case was the estimated discrepancy judged to be different from zero with a p less than 0.05.[39]

The discrepancies observed among young women aged 16 to 17 are large enough to suggest that naive comparisons of results obtained in different surveys can be misleading if the basis for inference is sampling error alone. It has come to be a well-accepted notion in the literature on survey measurements (as it long has been in analytical measurements in other disciplines) that variability in measurements among procedures, investigators, and laboratories cannot be determined by a simple extrapolation of the variances observed in measurements from a single experiment. Rather, different procedures, investigators, and laboratories typically produce measurements that converge on values over repeated measurements that are nevertheless not the grand mean of all measurements. Thus it is not unusual to find that the effects of minor variabilities

---

you had intercourse? That is, in what month and year? How old were you at the time? Respondents in the National Survey of Family Growth were asked: Thinking back after your first menstrual period, when did you have sexual intercourse for the first time—what month and year was that? (If date was not known): How old were you at that time? Was it before your n–th birthday, or after? Respondents in the National Longitudinal Survey were asked: At what age did you first have sexual intercourse? (Source: Kahn, Kalsbeek, and Hofferth, 1988:193, Table 3).

[38]The net association was tested by entering as dummy variables the product of the dichotomous variable reflecting the characteristic of interest (e.g., Catholic or not) and dummy variables for the surveys.

[39]Note that with 100 independent comparisons, one expects random fluctuations to produce five discrepancies of this magnitude when the true discrepancy across all tests is zero (and the significance level is set at .05).

in the particular procedures used by different investigators and research organizations may contaminate individual measurements to some degree. In the case of the three surveys discussed above, however, the overall impact of this effect, although large enough to be statistically detectable, is not so large as to lead to markedly different inferences about the patterns of teenage sexual behavior in this cohort of young women. Indeed, it is somewhat comforting to note that the two cross-sectional surveys (by Zelnik and Kantner and the NSFG) produced very similar results at all ages.

As for the discrepant results of the longitudinal survey, surveys that perform repeated measurements of the same respondent may have many characteristics that can affect typical survey measurements. At a minimum, the design of the longitudinal survey must not only accommodate nonresponse at the initial interview stage but is also subject to attrition of respondents from the sample over time. Furthermore, the experience of repeated interviewing can create a different interview climate which may influence the results that are obtained.[40]

Number of Sexual Partners Reported by Adults

A second example is provided by surveys performed in 1987 by the *Los Angeles Times* and by the 1988 NORC General Social Survey (GSS). Both surveys asked respondents about the total number of sexual partners they had had during the past year.[41] The responses to this question yielded a number of interesting results. Of most interest for methodological purposes was the substantial similarity of results obtained in the two surveys. This similarity is surprising owing to the following:

- The quality of survey execution varied markedly. As noted in Table 6-1 the GSS obtained one of the highest response rates of the surveys reviewed by the committee and the *Los Angeles Times* survey obtained the lowest.

- The surveys differed in the wording of questions, survey content, and mode of administration (phone survey versus self-administered questionnaire in a face-to-face survey).

- The 12-month time period did not cover the same dates. (The time periods were approximately July 1986 to June

---

[40] Careful studies of the responses of persons interviewed in the Bureau of the Census Current Population Survey indicated that employment experience reporting was subject to artifacts resulting from repeated interviewing (Bailar, 1975; Brooks and Bailar, 1978).

[41] The following questions were posed to respondents: About how many sexual partners would you say you have had in the last year? (*Los Angeles Times*); and, How many sex partners have you had in the last 12 months? (NORC).

1987 for the *Los Angeles Times* survey versus March 1987 to February 1988 for the NORC survey.)

Nonetheless, analysis[42] of a five-way crosstabulation of the two surveys by using five age groups, gender (male, female), marital status (married, not married), and number of partners (0, 1, 2, 3+) provided surprising evidence of consistency in the survey findings. (This table is presented in the Appendix.) In this five-way tabulation, once the demographic marginals of the two surveys were made comparable,[43] it was virtually impossible to discriminate statistically among the results obtained in the two surveys with regard to the number of sexual partners in the last year or in the patterns of association found between this variable and marital status, gender, or age.[44]

Replication of Measurements Using Same Respondents

A parallel approach to the replication of entire surveys on new samples from a population is the repeated measurement of a (stable) characteristic of the same respondent, a method that effectively reduces some of the sources of "noise" in comparisons (e.g., differences that arise from variations in the methods of survey measurement). Indeed, for characteristics that are unchangeable during the interval between repeated measurements, such as age of first intercourse (for nonvirgin respondents), a survey measurement that was perfectly reliable might be expected to produce 100

---

[42] See Turner, Miller, and Moses, 1989:104-108.

[43] The four-way demographic marginals (age by marital status by gender by survey) differed owing to divergences in the populations included in telephone versus personal interview surveys and to the substantial differences in the quality of the execution of the sampling plans.

[44] Using a stratified jackknife procedure to fit a hierarchical series of log-linear models to the five-way table (Turner, Miller, and Moses, 1989:104-108), it was found that a model that fit the $\{PAGM\}$ and $\{AGMS\}$ marginals (where P = partners, A = age, M = marital status, G = gender, and S = survey) could be improved slightly by also constraining the model to fit the $\{PS\}$ marginal (jackknifed likelihood-ratio chi-square for comparison of two alternate models: $J^2 = 1.49$, d.f. = 3, p = .051). This improvement is of borderline statistical "significance." An examination of estimates of the $\lambda^{\{PS\}}$ parameters for this "improved" model indicates that the observed intersurvey discrepancy was largely attributable to minor variations between the surveys in the numbers of persons with no sexual partners and with one partner. Estimates of the $\lambda^{\{PS\}}$ parameters (and standard errors) for a log-linear model constrained to fit $\{PAGM\}$ $\{SAGM\}$ $\{PS\}$ marginals were .127 (s.e. =.070) for zero partners; -.123 (.063) for one partner; .035 (.073) for two partners; and -.040 (.072) for the category three or more partners. (Model parameters are [arbitrarily] coded so that positive values indicate an "excess" of NORC cases in the specified category.) With the effects of weighting and the complex sample design in the range of *deff* = 1.6, significant effects were not found for other multivariate parameters involving P and S (e.g., $\{PAS\}$, $\{PGS\}$, $\{PMS\}$, etc.). It should be noted that all model comparisons fit the $\{SAGM\}$ marginals, which allows for intersurvey differences in the demographic composition of the samples drawn by the two surveys.

percent consistency of response between two separate interviews. In reality, however, errors of recall, misunderstanding of questions, miscoding of responses, and a host of other factors may cause two survey measurements made at two different times to be less than perfectly consistent. This lack of consistency is true not only for questions that might be "sensitive" (e.g., those about sexuality), but also for seemingly innocuous inquiries about demographic characteristics.

As a standard component of careful survey practice, it is common for surveyors to recontact a (random) subsample of respondents and to repeat questions that provide crucial measurements. The tabulation of these repeated measurements against the original survey responses provides an index of the reliability of the survey measurements. That is, it provides a way of assessing the consistency of survey response. As noted earlier, consistency alone is no guarantee that the measurements are meaningful or valuable. However, survey measures that have zero (or very low consistency) between repeated measurements are inherently suspect (if the trait being measured is stable over time).

Because repeated measurements can be performed within the context of a single survey, there is opportunity for amassing these measurements, and the published literature (as well as unpublished technical documents) provides greater detail than is available on replicated surveys. Table 6-5 summarizes some of the relevant results, which indicate substantial levels of consistency between answers to questions about sexual behavior obtained at two different points in time.

The observed consistency, however, is not as great as the consistency obtained for some other topics. Saltzman and colleagues (1987), for example, report test-retest reliabilities for two administrations of a questionnaire asking about sexual orientation, sexual behaviors, and change in sexual behaviors. Respondents were 116 gay men participating in an HIV study being conducted at the Fenway Community Health Center in Boston.[45] Compared with the test-retest reliabilities of .94 obtained for questions about smoking behavior and .79 for dietary habits, the reliabilities for reports on sexual behaviors were in the range of .40 to .99. The lowest reliabilities were found for number of nonsteady partners during last six months (.53) and number of partners for insertive anal intercourse without a condom (.61).

Other studies summarized in Table 6-5 found test-retest reliabilities in the range of approximately .5 to .9. The retests in several studies assessed behaviors in a different time period than the first measurements

---

[45] Respondents with AIDS or AIDS-related complex were excluded.

(e.g., this past week). As a result, temporal instability in actual behaviors masquerades as "unreliability" in some of these studies.

Although the reliability analyses reported in Table 6-5 encourage the belief that respondents can report consistently on their sexual behaviors, they do not, in themselves, tell anything directly about the systematic distortions that may occur in reporting. In an enlightening analysis of similar test-retest data, Rodgers, Billy, and Udry (1982) used data from successive waves of a longitudinal survey of adolescents (ages 11 to 16) to deduce evidence of invalidity. In this study, 408 adolescents completed two parallel sexual behavior questionnaires at an interval of 12 months. Rodgers and colleagues reported reliability analyses using items for which different responses at the two points in time are logically impossible. For example, teens who said they had had intercourse one or more times in their life in the first survey should give the same answer in all subsequent surveys. However, 43 percent of adolescents who reported "ever masturbating" in the first survey reported no such experience in the second survey; for intercourse the comparable figure was 19 percent. As a comparison, a similar analysis was conducted for reports of using alcohol; this effort yielded an inconsistency rate of 6 percent. The authors also reported results for an extremely vague question ("Have you ever grown several inches in height very quickly?"), which produced a 34 percent inconsistent response rate.

Across a series of 11 behavior measurements, the authors reported that adolescent respondents were most likely to rescind reports (between times 1 and 2) of touching of sex organs and, to a lesser extent, sexual intercourse. Less intimate behaviors (hand-holding, kissing) were less likely to be rescinded. For masturbation (in wave 1) and sexual intercourse (in waves 1 and 2), reliability was also assessed within each interview by asking questions at the beginning and end of the session. Inconsistent responses within interviews averaged 7.8 percent for intercourse and 8.3 percent for reports of masturbation in the first survey,[46] but there was substantial variation by race and sex. For both intercourse and masturbation, the greatest inconsistency in reporting was observed among black males.[47]

---

[46] Results for the second survey are reported for intercourse alone, for which 4.3 percent of respondents gave inconsistent responses within the interview.

[47] In the first survey, 23.7 percent of black male respondents gave inconsistent responses within the interview to the question on sexual intercourse, and 26 percent gave inconsistent responses to the questions on masturbation. In the second survey, 13 percent of black male respondents gave inconsistent responses to the question on sexual intercourse; no results were reported for masturbation.

Table 6-5 Reliability Studies of Self-Reported Sexual Behaviors

Study	Sample	Method	Findings
Saltzman et al. (1987)	116 asymptomatic gay men, volunteers from community health center in Boston, who were homosexually active in 6 months prior to study	SAQ[h] with retest at 6 weeks (retest ranged from 2 to 18 weeks later): frequency of sexual acts and numbers of partners	Kappa statistic (measure of agreement relative to that expected by chance). For frequency of practice in last 6 months: .52 for insertive oral sex; .45 for receptive oral sex; .53 for insertive anal sex without condom; .50 for insertive anal sex with condom; .56 for receptive anal sex; .47 for kissing. For number of partners in last 6 months: .60 for insertive oral sex; .52 for receptive oral sex; .46 for insertive anal sex without condom; .60 for insertive anal sex with condom; .50 for receptive anal sex; .53 for kissing.
Koss and Gidycz (1985)	386 college students (242 women, 144 men)	SAQ[a] test with QI retest; sexual victimization and aggression	Pearson correlation between SAQ test and QI retest: .73 between women's levels of victimization and .61 between men's levels of aggression
DeLamater (1974)	237 unmarried undergraduates at University of Wisconsin	Interviews varying the order of measures: (1) Current partners—depth of relationship and sexual behaviors; (2) Ideology (sexual attitudes)—personal ideology and peers' ideology	Analysis of variance showed no significant differences among respondents of either sex in measures of current partners' sexual behaviors or in measures of depth of relationship when the item order was varied. Among female respondents only, analysis of variance showed more liberal ideology when personal ideology was measured prior to peers' ideology.
DeLamater and MacCorquodale (1975)	432 single male undergraduates, 429 single female undergraduates, 220 single male nonstudents, and 293 single female nonstudents from Madison, Wisconsin	Three measures were compared: (1) SAQ and QI[b]; (2) location (middle or end of list about sexual experience), and (3) order of measures on current behaviors, partner characteristics, and partner ideology	Analysis of variance showed no significant differences by type of questionnaire administration, location of questions, or order of measures

Reference	Sample	Procedure	Results
Anderson and Broffitt (1988)	57 healthy and 66 women with gynecological disorders	Face-to-face interviews; test with retest at three 4-month intervals using the SES, which assesses the range of current activities	Pearson correlation statistics showed a range in stability in SES responses from .55 to .85 for healthy women and from .62 to .85 for women with gynecological disorders[c]
Catania et al. (1986)	193 college students (66 males, 127 females)	Test with retest at 2 weeks using SAQs[d]; additional retest at second 2-week interval by face-to-face interview using the SSD to study sexual experiences and activities	Pearson correlation of SSD showed high internal consistency (.92); no significant order effects were found within the SAQs
Zuckerman et al. (1976)	221 male and 331 female college students enrolled in personality psychology (control group) or human sexuality courses (experimental group)	Test at beginning and retest at end of 15-week course; SES	For the four sex-course groups, correlations on the 14-item heterosexual experience scale ranged from .80 to .95. The range for the 4-item homosexual experience scale was from .49 to .84. The range for the item on masturbation was from .63 to .90
Allen and Haupt (1966)	56 male and 28 female college students at University of Miami	Test with retest at 3 months; sex inventory of 200 true-false items forming 10 scales of sexual behaviors and attitudes	Intraclass correlation coefficients on the scales ranged from .67 to .89
Marks and Sartorius (1968)	17 psychiatric hospital patients with sex deviations	Test with retest at 24 hours; 260-item questionnaire forming 13 scales on attitudes toward sexual and nonsexual concepts	Pearson correlation coefficients for the 13 sexual scales ranges from .44 to .80, with only 2 scores below .64
LoPiccolo and Steger (1974)	15 heterosexual couples recruited through ads placed on university bulletin boards	Test with retest at 2 weeks; 11-item scale of sexual adjustment and satisfaction	Pearson correlation coefficients for the 11 scales ranged from .53 to .90

continued

TABLE 6-5 *Continued*

Study	Sample	Method	Findings
Harbison et al. (1974)	15 subjects	Test with retest at 3 to 5 months; 140-item sexual interest questionnaire forming 5 subscales and 1 overall scale	Pearson correlation coefficients for the 6 scales ranged from .68 to .92
Derogatis and Melisaratos (1979), Derogatis (1980)	Normal and sexually dysfunctional individuals[e]	Test with retest at 2 weeks; sexual functioning inventory of 258 items forming 10 subtests on sexual behavior and attitudes	Correlations for the subtests ranged from .42 to .96
Coates et al. (1986)	26 gay men in Toronto, recruited through local gay organizations	Face-to-face interviews with retest at least 72 hours after initial interview: volume of sexual partners, percentage frequency of certain sexual activities	Pearson correlation coefficients for the variables regarding number of sexual partners ranged from .71 to .99, with one exception.[f] The range for the percentage frequency of specific sexual activities was from .40 to .99, with most .70 or higher
Catania et al. (in press a)	Sample of sexually active adolescent women	Questions asked at two different points within a SAQ: sexual activity in prior 2 months	The reliability coefficient for frequency of total intercourse (unprotected and protected across partners) was .98, and for frequency of condom use it was .97. Reliability was slightly lower for those with three or more partners versus those with one partner
Catania et al. (in press a)	Sample of heterosexual college undergraduates	SAQ test with retest at 2 weeks: frequency of intercourse for varying retrospective periods	Longer retrospective intervals were associated with lower test-retest reliability (one month = .89, six months = .65, one year = .36)

| Millstein and Irwin (1983) | 108 adolescent female patients recruited from three university hospital clinics | Comparison of: (1) SAQ, (2) computer-assisted SAQ, and (3) face-to-face interview in obtaining sexual histories | Girls assigned to the face-to-face interview reported lower levels of sexual activity than girls assigned to either of the SAQ types. (Roughly 74% of the girls responding to SAQs reported ever having sexual intercourse, compared with 63% of the other girls.) |
| Rolnick et al. (1989) | 268 females at Midwestern University, identified through health service visits for STD treatment or to obtain contraceptives. | Comparison of: (1) face-to-face interview with multiple questions on heterosexual history, (2) mail SAQ with multiple questions, and (3) mail SAQ with only 2 sexual history questions. | Contingency table comparisons showed little difference by method in tendency to give "socially acceptable" responses. |

NOTE: SAQ: self-administered questionnaire; QI: questionnaire interview; SES: sexual experience scale; SSD: sexual self-disclosure scale.

Table includes only studies reporting test-retest analysis of measurements or analysis of measurements made under different conditions (e.g., variations in question order, mode of administration). Studies reporting on scalability or internal consistency of sets of items that were not intended to measure the same behaviors have not been included (e.g., Podell and Perkins, 1957; Brady and Levitt, 1965; Bentler, 1968a,b; Zuckerman, 1973).

[a] SAQ administered in university class. [b] QI was face-to-face and SAQ was given as part of face-to-face interview. [c] The authors expected lower correlations for the women with gynecological disorders than for the healthy group, but the correlations for the two groups were similar. [d] SAQs administered to sample in classroom with alternate seating. [e] Information in Schiavi et al. (1979) suggests that these studies are reporting on 200 normal and slightly fewer than 200 dysfunctional individuals. [f] The exception was a coefficient of .24 for the variable "percentage of male partners since 1978 with whom sexual contact has occurred more than 5 times." [g] Checks on validity of responses (comparing answers with medical histories) showed no differences by methods. [h] Study coordinator reviewed completed SAQ with respondent for missing or inconsistent information.

EMPIRICAL STUDIES OF DRUG-USING BEHAVIORS

Many of the methodological issues investigators face in studying drug use behaviors are identical to those found in studying sexual or other sensitive or illegal behaviors (see, for example, Siegel and Bauman, 1986; Kaplan et al., 1987; Zich and Temoshok, 1987; Kaplan, 1989). Yet some of the difficulties encountered in studying drug use behaviors are unique to this area of inquiry. Some of the most difficult research challenges arise from the fact that patterns of drug availability and injection behaviors may change rapidly. In the last several years, for example, considerable evidence has accumulated that drug-using populations in some communities have changed their needle use practices to avoid HIV infection (Chaisson et al., 1987; Friedman et al., 1987b; Des Jarlais, Friedman, and Stoneburner, 1988; Des Jarlais et al., 1988; Robertson, Skidmore, and Roberts, 1988). These changes have included both decreased needle-sharing and increased use of disinfection regimens for injecting equipment.

As noted in Chapter 1, however, changing patterns of cocaine use complicate this picture. The 1980s saw a dramatic increase in the use of cocaine (Drug Enforcement Administration [DEA], 1988); in a related development, trade in "crack" (smokable) cocaine burgeoned from initial reports in 1981 of its availability in 3 cities, to its availability in 47 states and the District of Columbia during 1987 (DEA, 1988). Similarly, some observers[48] believe that "ice," a synthetic amphetamine that is smoked, may play a major role in drug use in the United States in coming years.

Changes in the illicit drugs in most common use can have important implications for HIV transmission. Studies presented in 1988 and 1989, for example, indicated that the injection of cocaine was associated with elevated rates of HIV infection (Chaisson et al., 1988, 1989; Des Jarlais and Friedman, 1988b; Friedman et al., 1989; Novick et al., 1989). This association is thought to be the result of high frequencies of injection and decreased needle hygiene over the course of an injection session (Friedman et al., 1989). Further studies in New York (Friedman et al., 1988) and San Francisco (Fullilove et al., 1989, in press) have found that smoking crack cocaine, which in itself presents no direct risk of HIV transmission, is nonetheless associated with risky sexual behavior. Indeed, cocaine use has been associated with a higher incidence of syphilis (Minkoff et al., 1989). Such findings suggest that an outbreak of HIV infection among cocaine-using adolescents and adults is a possibility.

---

[48]L. Thompson, "Ice: New smokable form of speed," *Washington Post,* November 21, 1989, A-11.

Accuracy of Self-Reports of Drug Use Behaviors

Huang, Watters, and Case (1988) point out that the lack of standardized measures, combined with the heterogeneity of the population of drug users and the impaired cognitive functioning that may result from extensive drug use, tends to make survey research in this population a difficult task. A drug user who is inebriated, for example, cannot be expected to recall needle-sharing episodes accurately. Furthermore, the wording of key questions in past AIDS research has sometimes been ambiguous. Consider, for example, the following hypothetical experience of an injection drug user:[49]

> Bill selected the syringe that looked least-used from among four in a half-filled water glass. Its action was a little stiff, so he took it apart. He swished the plunger around in the foil packet of a lubricated condom and then dipped the metal needle into a small vial of bleach. Putting the "works" back together, he tested it by drawing up water from the glass. Very smooth now. Then he, his wife, and their friend cooked up the heroin. Bill used the syringe first, then his wife used it, but they wouldn't share with the friend, who had his own set. The next morning at the detoxification clinic Bill agreed to be interviewed for a research project. The AIDS researcher asked how often does he use condoms, clean his needles with bleach, what percent of the time does he share needles?

The drug user in this vignette could report that he uses condoms frequently (to lubricate his syringes), that he "never" shares needles (only doing so with his wife), and that he cleans his needles "every time" (even though he may subsequently contaminate a clean needle with water shared with other syringes). Furthermore, a survey question about how often Bill shared needles could be answered accurately only if it clarified that "sharing" included using needles with his wife.

Similarly, most questionnaires about the use of needle-cleaning regimens are not sensitive enough to distinguish between disinfection that is thought to provide some protection and disinfection that is clearly ineffective. (Wermuth and Ham [1989], for example, report that some drug users disinfect their syringes by using bleach before and after sessions of sharing them with others but not between use by different persons.) Clarifying some of the ambiguities in survey measurements of these behaviors may eventually explain why longitudinal studies have failed to demonstrate a relationship between needle cleaning and rates of seroconversion among injection drug users (see, for example, Moss et al., 1989).

---

[49]The term *injection user* is used to include both those who inject drugs, like heroin, intravenously and those who insert drugs intramuscularly.

Measurement Bias

As with sexual behaviors, a major problem in measuring the risk behaviors of injection drug users is that researchers usually cannot observe the behaviors of interest directly. Occasionally, outreach workers may unobtrusively observe behaviors in such sites as "shooting galleries" (places in which drug users inject drugs together), but in general, drug use is not open to observation by research workers. Consequently, most AIDS research on drug use behaviors has relied heavily on the self-reports of persons who use IV drugs. Response bias, however, is a serious problem in such research.

Because of such potential biases, there has been ongoing concern among drug use researchers about the accuracy of injection drug users' self-reports. The most frequently asked validity question has been whether subjects underreport their drug use. Several studies have investigated the accuracy of injection drug users' self-reports of their drug use. The results of these studies are quite varied. Amsel and colleagues (1976), for example, followed 865 criminally involved drug users and employed various methods to assess the reliability and validity of self-reports of criminal and drug-taking behavior. Overall, their results indicated that, although the self-reports tended to have a downward bias, 74 percent of respondents accurately reported their drug use during the previous four weeks. That is, their self-reports were consistent with urinalysis findings. (In another 9 percent of cases, a validity check could not be made owing to incomplete data.) In 14 percent of cases, however, respondents reported no drug use, whereas tests of their urine indicated the presence of drugs.

Although these findings are encouraging, it should be noted that urine specimens were provided by only 267 (of a total of 865) respondents. The rates of drug use reported by those who did and did not provide specimens showed little difference,[50] but it is possible that, in many cases a respondent's prior inaccurate reporting on the questionnaire may have prompted him or her to refuse to provide a urine sample. If this were, indeed, true, the high rates of consistency observed in this study would not be a good indicator of the overall validity of the self-report data.

In addition to using urinalysis as a validity check, Amsel and coworkers obtained evidence of reliability in two ways. First, they examined questionnaire responses to detect inconsistent reporting of patterns of drug use. In only 7 percent of cases were inconsistencies detected in

---

[50]Of those providing urine specimens, 41 percent reported no drug use, versus 45 percent of those who did not provide specimens for testing.

reports of the frequency of drug use and the reported cost of the habit. Inconsistency in the reporting of illegal activities was found in somewhat more cases (13 percent). The investigators also assessed the reliability of their measurements by readministering a small number of questions in a separate questionnaire two to six weeks later. They found that 97 percent of respondents gave consistent responses over time to the two questions asked about drug use in this second measurement. In a similarly designed study, Bale and colleagues (1981) interviewed 272 male veterans who were heroin users about their heroin use and compared their statements with a urine sample. The investigators found self-reports to be reasonably accurate in that 84 percent of those denying heroin use in the previous three months and 78 percent of those claiming no use in the previous week had urine samples that were negative for opiates.

Table 6-6 summarizes the results of 17 other studies reviewed by Magura and colleagues (1987) in which self-reports of drug use were validated by urinalysis. Several studies obtained reports of drug use that were as consistent with urinalysis findings as the studies of the Amsel (1976) and Bale (1981) research teams. Yet the findings summarized in Table 6-6 also show great variability in the results achieved by different investigators and in the results achieved by the same investigator when obtaining reports of the use of different drugs. Use of heroin and other opiates, for example, is consistently reported with greater accuracy than is the use of other illicit drugs. Yet even for heroin use, the range of validity results is quite broad ($.26 \leq K \leq .78$),[51] and the median level of agreement between urinalysis results and self-reports is relatively modest ($K \approx .5$). The range of results improves, however, if the comparison is restricted to studies that assessed heroin or opiate use within seven days of the urinalysis ($.59 \leq K \leq .78$).

Although the direction of the reporting bias in most studies is toward underreporting of drug use, the results are not entirely consistent with that interpretation. Focusing on those surveys (marked with an asterisk in Table 6-6) that asked about drug use within the period (seven days) for which urinalysis can reliably detect it, one finds instances of major studies in which underreporting biases of up to 13 percentage points were found (McGlothlin, Anglin, and Wilson, 1977; $N = 497$). On the other hand, one major study (W. F. Page et al., 1977; $N = 896$) and one small-scale study (Wish et al., 1983, $N = 26$) found small biases in the opposite direction (i.e., more respondents reported drug use than were

---

[51] Coefficient reported is kappa (see Bishop et al., 1975:395).

detected in urinalysis). (Such divergences might be attributable to the fallibility of the urinalysis itself.)[52]

Although the results shown in Table 6-6 are "usually interpreted as supporting the validity of addicts' self-reports,"[53] they also provide clear evidence of the errors that can affect these measurements. Furthermore, although the studies are not unanimous in their findings, it does appear that a bias toward underreporting of drug use is quite common.

In considering the implications of these results for AIDS research, there are further reasons to constrain one's optimism about the overall validity of drug use measurements. First, the committee notes that one statistic of considerable interest is the *prevalence* of drug use in broadly defined populations. Chapter 3, for example, discussed surveys that attempted to assess the prevalence of drug use among high school students using the students' self-reports. It is quite possible that surveys of such general populations may be subject to a rather different pattern of bias and errors than that afflicting the surveys included in Table 6-6.[54] The populations sampled in Table 6-6 were all drawn from groups who were publicly identified as drug users. Because these respondents were already labeled as users of illicit drugs, not only by researchers but by treatment personnel and the criminal justice system, they may have been less motivated to conceal drug use. Furthermore, the routine use

---

[52] It should be recognized that the validity criterion in these studies is also subject to error. In blinded testing of the proficiencies of 50 laboratories performing urinalysis for opiates, cocaine, and other illicit drugs, Davis, Hawks, and Blanke (1988) found that, of 389 urine specimens known to be negative for particular drugs, the laboratories reported five false-positive readings (a false-positive error rate of 1.3 percent). The majority of these false-positive results involved identification of the wrong drug in urine specimens that were positive for some drug; however, two false-positives were given for cannabis and for methadone in samples that were actually drug free. In 350 tests involving urine specimens known to be positive for particular drugs, the laboratory tests had a 31 percent false-negative rate (109 of 350). The substances most often missed were phenylcyclidine (51 percent), morphine (47 percent), cocaine (38 percent), and methamphetamine (28 percent). The false-positive and false-negative rates obtained in such testing are, of course, a function of analytic method and the cutoff values that are used. Although the above findings provide some indication of the error rates obtained by standard practices in contemporary drug testing by commercial laboratories, it is possible that the procedures used in the validity studies reported in Table 6-6 may be different.

[53] This characterization is offered by Magura and colleagues (1987), who cite the writings of Aiken and LoSciuto (1985) and Harrell (1985) as examples of such interpretations.

[54] Some surveys of adolescents have attempted to test for overreporting of drug use by asking teenage respondents how often they had used a fictitious drug (e.g., bindro, adrenochromes/wagon wheels, etc.). Negligible percentages (0 to 4 percent) of respondents in these surveys reported using these fictitious drugs (see Haberman et al., 1972; Whitehead and Smart, 1972; Petzel, Johnson, and McKillip, 1973; Single, Kandel, and Johnson, 1975; Needle et al., 1983). Yet although this result is encouraging, it does not speak to the more likely bias, that is, underreporting of drug use.

Table 6-6 Summary of Studies on Validity of Self-Reported Drug Use in High-Risk Populations[a] (from Magura et al., 1987 and other sources)

Investigators	Subjects	Drugs	N	Percent Using Drugs by		
				Self-report	Criterion[b]	Kappa
*Ball (1967)[n]	Noninstitutionalized narcotics addicts	Opiates	25	20	28	.78
*W.F. Page et al. (1977)[o]	Arrestees	Opiates	896	16	15	.69
		Stimulants	896	9	7	.29
		Sedatives	896	16	18	.38
*McGlothlin, Anglin, and Wilson (1977)[h]	Drug treatment admissions	Opiates Last 5 days	497	27	40[i]	.59
*Bale et al. (1981)[p]	Former VA detox and drug treatment clients	Heroin All subjects	272	35	45	.61
*Wish et al. (1983)[q]	Drug users criminals	Heroin	26	58	50	.69
		Cocaine	26	58	46	.77
		Methadone	31	52	52	.61
Eckerman et al. (1971)[c]	Arrestees	Heroin	1,693	19	15	.48
		Barbiturates	1,693	7	11	.12
		Amphetamines	878	6	3	.10
		Methadone	1,693	3	2	.16

continued

Table 6-6 *Continued*

				Percent Using Drugs by		
Investigators	Subjects	Drugs	N	Self-report	Criterion[b]	Kappa
Cisin and Parry (1979)[d]	Drug treatment clients	Heroin	85	13	27	.29
		Barbiturates	85	35	41	.23
		Tranquilizers	85	25	31	-.08
		Amphetamines	85	39	34	.04
		Cocaine	85	39	32	.23
Cox and Longwell (1974)[e]	Methadone patients	Heroin[f]	175	23	20	.57
Amsel et al. (1976)[g]	Civil commitment applicants	12 drugs	267	59	70	.60
McGlothlin, Anglin, and Wilson (1977)[h]	Drug treatment admissions	Opiates Last 4 weeks	497	38	40[i]	.56
Bale (1979)[j]	Former VA detox and drug treatment patients	Heroin By questionnaire	55	51	38	.53
		By interview	55	36	38	.65
Ben-Yehuda (1980)[k]	Methadone patients	All illicit drugs	47	47	72	.34
Hubbard, Marsden, and Allison (1984)[l]	Drug treatment clients	Heroin	767	10	20	.26
		Other opiates	767	29	22	-.08
		Cocaine	767	10	5	.18
		Minor tranquilizers	767	30	7	.10
		Barbiturates	767	13	3	.07
		Amphetamines	767	21	2	.03

Aiken and LoSciuto (1985)[m]	Methadone and drug-free outpatients	Heroin	291	21	23	.54
		Other opiates	287	4	14	.22
		Cocaine	282	11	7	.31
		Barbiturates	281	8	8	.33
		Sedatives/tranquilizers	274	20	14	.17
Zuckerman et al. (1985)[r]	Pregnant women	Marijuana	75	15	24	.62

NOTES: TLC: thin-layer chromatography; EMIT: enzyme multiplied immunoassay technique.

[a]Excludes general population and student surveys. [b]Urinalysis, clinic records, etc. [c]Subjects: Arrestees at central booking; Los Angeles, Chicago, New York City, San Antonio, St. Louis, New Orleans. Procedures: Drug use within last month from interview vs. single research TLC urinalysis. [d]Subjects: Drug treatment clients in 1974; San Francisco Bay area. Procedures: Self-administered questionnaire vs. clinic records; data grouped as "ever used" and "never used." [e]Subjects: Methadone patients (N = 106) admitted for at least 3 months; Tucson clinic. Procedures: Drug use over 3 months by period interviews vs. clinic's weekly TLC urinalysis over same 3 months; data grouped as "low" and "high use." [f]N and % refer to interviews. [g]Subjects: Applicants to NIMH civil commitment between 1967 and 1971 (follow-up); PHS hospital at Lexington and Ft. Worth. Procedures: Drug use over 4-week period by interview vs. single research TLC urinalysis. [h]Subjects: Admissions to civil commitment in 1962–63, 1964, 1970 (follow-up of nonincarcerated sample); California, statewide. Procedures: Drug use by interview (last 5 days and last 4 weeks) vs. single research urinalysis (quantitative immunoassay). [i]"Positive" and "probable positive" classed as positive. [j]Subjects: Former VA detox and drug treatment patients (1-year follow-up); Palo Alto/Stanford area. Procedures: Mailed questionnaire (drug use during past month) and subsequent interview (drug use during past week) vs. clinic's TLC urinalysis confirmed by radioimmunoassay). [k]Subjects: Methadone patients; Chicago clinic. Procedures: Self-administered questionnaire (drugs taken "now") vs. clinic's TLC urinalysis over 6 months (grouped as 0–3 and 4+ urine positives). [l]Subjects: Methadone clients admitted 1 month (outpatient detox; drug-free and methadone outpatient; and residential); numerous programs in 10 cities in 1979, 1980, 1981. Procedures: Interview (drug use during last month) vs. clinic's TLC urinalysis during that month. [m]Subjects: Methadone and drug-free outpatient; 16 programs in New York, Washington, Chicago, Los Angeles, San Francisco in 1977. Procedures: Client (N=300) vs. counselor (N = 85) interviews (drug use in past 30 days). [n]Subjects: Noninstitutionalized narcotics addicts; former federal inmates at Lexington and Ft. Worth. Procedures: Current drug use by interview vs. single research analysis (apparently TLC). [o]Subjects: Arrestees booked for felony in 1973; Dade County, Florida. Procedures: Drug use in last 48 hours by interview vs. single research urinalysis by spectrofluorometry and/or EMIT and/or TLC. [p]Subjects: Former VA detox and drug treatment clients (2-year follow-up); Palo Alto/Stanford area. Procedures: Interview (drug use during past week) vs. single research urinalysis (TLC confirmed by radioimmunoassay). [q]Subjects: Drug users recruited off street; New York City. Procedures: Interview (drug use during past 36 hours) vs. single research urinalysis (TLC and EMIT). [r]Subjects: Women registering at prenatal clinic; Boston. Procedures: Personal interview (marijuana use in previous week) vs. urinalysis (EMIT). (This study was not discussed in Magura et al. [1987].)

* Study measured drug use during time period of 7 days or less prior to urinalysis.

of urinalysis in research and in monitoring of treatment may further discourage attempts by this population to hide drug use.

Generalizations from these findings to AIDS research are further limited by the subject matter covered in the survey questions. As Rounsaville and coworkers pointed out in 1981, investigators in the drug use field traditionally examined a relatively restricted range of factual data. In AIDS research, however, the knowledge required is somewhat more extensive. Questions of particular interest include not just whether subjects use drugs but how they use them. How often do they use needles? share needles? clean needles? Little is known about the accuracy of responses to more fine-grained questions such as these, although the accuracy of self-reports of drug use has been studied extensively. A recent study by McLaws and coworkers (1988) found rates of infection with hepatitis B virus that suggested that respondents were actually sharing needles at a rate higher than that reported to researchers.

As with self-reports of sexual behaviors, differential reporting bias is a danger in the use of self-reports of drug use behaviors. In evaluation studies, for example, subjects assigned to an intervention (versus a control) group might tend to underreport such behaviors as needle sharing after having gone through an intervention that stressed the importance of stopping these risky behaviors.[55] There is some evidence that reporting biases may sometimes work in the opposite direction. Worth and colleagues (1989), for example, found that women drug users tried to be "good survey takers." After participating in an AIDS prevention group they tended to give responses indicating more frequent risk taking. The authors attribute this finding to the subjects' greater degree of honesty, reflecting increased comfort with the questions and the interviewers. Such a differential reporting bias would tend to mask the effects of interventions.

SUMMARY OF FINDINGS

Although there is ample evidence of error and bias in extant surveys of AIDS risk behaviors, and such evidence should be of concern to investigators, some important conclusions can nevertheless be drawn from this body of work.

Feasibility

First, based on the empirical evidence presented in the first section of this chapter, there appears to be little question that such surveys can enlist

---

[55] Some of the potential for bias might be eliminated by using research interviewers who are independent of the staff who deliver the intervention. This tactic, however, should not be expected to eliminate completely the potential for bias.

the cooperation of the vast majority of the American public. Carefully designed surveys inquiring about sexual matters, for example, appear to be capable of obtaining response rates that rival those of commercial and academic surveys on less sensitive topics. Of course, special efforts may be needed to ensure high levels of cooperation, and, as always, careful collection of evidence of response bias is necessary. There appears to be little question, however, that such surveys are feasible as scientific enterprises.

Replicability

Second, the recent literature contains two demonstrations that independently conducted national surveys of aspects of sexual behavior (age at first intercourse and number of sexual partners in past year) produced reassuringly similar estimates. This similarity was achieved despite variations in survey methodology. These results, if repeated across a wider range of measurements, provide salutary evidence that surveys of AIDS risk behaviors can, indeed, provide replicable measurements—that is, different investigators using roughly similar methods to survey the same population can obtain equivalent results.

Validity

In most sex surveys, it will be difficult (if not impossible) to obtain convincing evidence of measurement validity. The committee finds nonetheless that the research literature contains several important demonstrations of the validity of sexual and drug use behavior measures. When couples report independently on factual aspects of their own sexual interactions, for example, there is considerable agreement between the survey reports that are obtained. Similarly, in one instance in which physical evidence could be obtained, it was found that, when questioned in an interview, a very high proportion of married women for whom there was physical evidence of intercourse reported that they had, indeed, had intercourse. Furthermore, studies that have validated self-reported drug use with urinalysis have found moderate levels of agreement. These results are certainly encouraging, but there is also a variety of other evidence that suggests that some sexual and drug-using behaviors may be considerably underreported in surveys. Although the evidence is limited, it appears that male-male sexual contacts may be massively underreported (at least by college student populations).

Reliability

There is a fairly large body of research reporting on the consistency of responses over short periods of time in survey reports on various AIDS risk behaviors. These studies have generally demonstrated moderate levels of response consistency over time. It is possible, however, that some of the inconsistencies observed in these studies reflect true changes in behavior over time rather than errors in reporting on behavior.

IMPROVING VALIDITY AND RELIABILITY

The above evidence leads naturally to questions concerning how the reliability and validity of self-report data on these behaviors might be improved. In this regard there are a number of tactics that should be considered.

Literacy

Literacy is an obvious concern when self-administered forms or other written materials are to be used to collect data. In designing surveys, researchers should be sure that their survey questionnaires (as well as their consent forms, information sheets, etc.) are readable and, in particular, that the difficulty of the materials does not exceed the reading level of their subjects. In cases in which there is a possibility that some of the respondents recruited for a study may be illiterate, provisions must be made for detecting this problem and providing an alternate data collection method.

In this regard the committee notes that Hochhauser analyzed the readability of AIDS educational materials in 1987 and found that, on average, they required a 14th grade (i.e., college) reading level.[56] Such a mismatch in the reading level of educational materials intended for the general public suggests that sensitivity to literacy problems is not widespread. The literacy problem may be even more complex when it is extended to include the research consent forms and information sheets required by institutional review boards. It may in fact be very difficult to make these quasi-legal documents truly readable. One study of the reading level of patient information at a psychiatric institute revealed that all brochures were written below the educational level of 85 percent of their readers but that the patient's consent form was written above the educational level of 77 percent of the patients (Sorensen and Leder, 1978).

---

[56] Wells and coworkers (1989) found somewhat lower reading levels in a random sample of brochures, cards, inserts ($N = 104$), and pamphlets, books, and monographs ($N = 41$) selected from the 1988 *AIDS Information Resources Directory*. Wells et al. reported that a preliminary analysis of 57 brochures found that 72 percent were written at the equivalent of tenth grade or above and 10 percent at a grade level beyond high school.

Alternatives to Self-Reports

In addition to adopting procedures that ensure that respondents can understand the questions they are being asked, it is desirable to supplement self-reports with alternative measures whenever possible. Such measures, which include ethnographic observations, physical evidence, skills demonstrations, and reports of "significant others," can provide important data on the biases that may affect key measurements. Ethnographic observations, which are discussed at length in the next section, can be a particularly valuable tool in understanding responses to quantitative self-report measures. Lange and colleagues (1988), for example, recently reported that, according to self-reports collected in survey interviews, only 70 percent of IV drug users in New York City had shared needles at some time in their life. Ethnographic studies provided a quick corrective to this inaccurate conclusion. These studies indicated that *essentially all* IV drug users in New York had used someone else's injection equipment at least one time in their life—when they first began to inject drugs (Des Jarlais and Friedman, 1988c). In this case, ethnographic observations helped clarify a limitation of data gathered through interview methods. Other alternative measures are discussed briefly below.

Physical Evidence

A variety of other data can supplement self-reports of drug use. Skin examinations for puncture marks and urine drug screens can be used as cross-checks against self-reports (Sorensen et al., 1989c), and low-frequency physiological surrogate markers can sometimes be useful if the population is large enough. For example, Bardoux and colleagues (1989) interpreted a declining incidence of hepatitis B among injection drug users in Amsterdam as a reflection of decreases in needle-sharing and related risk behaviors among that population. Similarly, as noted previously, some researchers have monitored prevalence rates of hepatitis B virus and used these rates as a cross-check on self-reports of needle-sharing among their respondents.

Skills Demonstrations

A further supplement to self-reports are skills demonstrations in which subjects show their ability to practice preventive behaviors. For example, a test of a prevention program with injection drug users has used demonstrations of the ability to clean needles and use condoms properly as outcome measures (Heitzman et al., 1989). Such demonstrations can provide useful cross-checks against self-reports. For example, even if a subject reported cleaning needles 100 percent of the time, the preventive value of this "cleaning" would be questionable if the subject's demonstration of needle cleaning skills revealed unfamiliarity with the basic procedures needed to prevent transmission of HIV.

Other Safeguards for Surveys

Although firm guarantees cannot be made as to the beneficial effects of any particular tactic noted here, the committee believes that there is strong presumptive evidence to indicate that a considerably larger investment of resources needs to be made in exploratory work prior to the fielding of major survey investigations.[57] (This problem is not confined to studies of sexual or drug use behaviors; inadequate investment in such exploratory work is common to surveys of other topics according to knowledgeable observers. See, for example, comments by Cannell and coworkers [1989:3].) For surveys of behaviors that risk HIV transmission, this lack of exploratory work is particularly troubling, given the underdeveloped state of research in this field. In this regard, the committee notes that some of the questionnaires it reviewed made impossible demands on the cognitive capacities of respondents, an unfortunate error that would have been detected if the questionnaires had received more thorough pilot testing. For example, one previously cited survey asked respondents to report the total number of sexual encounters they had had with particular partners during the entire length of relationships whose *median* duration was 24 months. The survey further asked respondents to report the total number of times (or percentage of encounters) during which they engaged in one or more of 13 different sexual practices.[58]

As is discussed below, there may be good reasons for collecting such data despite the frailties of respondents' recall. Empirical studies of memory for other events, however, suggest that a respondent's ability to recall such events is limited, and random and systematic errors intrude on the responses. Such studies argue for careful research conducted as

---

[57] Also needed are careful methodological investigations of the relative merits of different methods of survey administration, including use of self-administered questionnaires versus interviewer questioning in surveys of sexual behavior and telephone versus face-to-face surveys. The effects of different data collection methods have not been extensively studied by drug researchers. Magura and colleagues (1987) found with their 248 methadone patients that the age of clients and the type of interviewer directly affected the rate of underreporting. On the other hand, Skinner and Allen (1983) randomly assigned 150 drug treatment clients either to a computerized interview, face-to-face interview, or self-report format and found no important differences in reliability, level of problems, or consumption patterns of alcohol, drug, and tobacco use. Similar results were found by Needle, Jou, and Su (1989), who compared adolescents' reports of drug use when randomly assigned to report with mailed questionnaires or in-person survey interviews.

[58] For example, masturbation, insertive and receptive oral sex, insertive and receptive anal sex, and so forth.

ancillary efforts to the epidemiological undertaking that would characterize these errors. Indeed, it might be argued that (in some instances) there would be good cause for restricting recall to time periods in which accurate recall might be assumed with greater certainty. So, for example, reports on sexual encounters during the preceding one to three days place more manageable demands on respondents' memory (although, even here, perfect recall should not be assumed).

Although the arguments for use of different time frames are complicated (see below), there is little doubt that researchers' appreciation of the problems that attend key measurements can be sharpened by greater use of exploratory studies prior to the launching of major surveys. Among the techniques that can be profitably employed are ethnographic studies and focus groups whose aim is to explore the frames of reference and language that respondents use in approaching a given topic area; pretests and pilot studies that explore the respondents' understanding of preliminary versions of questionnaires; and cognitive research strategies that detail the limits of recall and the strategies respondents use in answering questions that demand recall of events that are not directly accessible (e.g., how many sexual encounters have you had with John in the past two years?). Furthermore, major surveys can embed experimental studies in their designs to assess the effects of key aspects of the research process (e.g., the nature and perceptions of confidentiality guarantees, question wording and context, and the measurement variance and bias introduced by interviewers themselves). Examples of such techniques are provided below.

Randomized Response Techniques

A widely known set of tactics for increasing cooperation and accurate reporting of sensitive information in surveys are the randomized response techniques. These techniques are intended to provide an estimate of the distribution of a sensitive characteristic in the population without requiring that individuals reveal sensitive information about themselves. They introduce a random element into the response process so that no individual respondent is *definitely* identified as admitting to the sensitive trait. One variant of this technique instructs a random half of the sample to answer "yes" regardless of the question while the other half of the sample is asked to give an accurate answer to the sensitive question. (The randomization might be performed by having the respondent flip a coin without letting the interviewer know the result of the coin toss.) Because one-half of the sample would be expected to answer "yes" as a result of the coin toss, the proportion who answered "yes" to the sensitive question can be estimated. (Variations on this basic strategy include one that requests respondents to answer one of two questions—one sensitive and one not—based upon a coin toss or other randomizing device.)

Although these techniques are attractive in theory, they do have some drawbacks (Campbell, 1987). Accordingly, researchers applying randomized response methods should recognize the need for careful pilot testing prior to embarking on a major research effort using them. One drawback is that larger sample sizes are required to obtain estimates of equal precision because the randomization procedure substantially increases the sampling error.[59] Second, although these techniques permit estimation of the univariate distribution of discrete population characteristics (e.g., proportion having same-gender sex in last year); they are not easily adapted for use in estimating continuous variables (e.g., number of sexual partners).[60] Finally, respondents may not understand or follow the instructions used in these techniques, or they may distort their responses despite the theoretical safeguards afforded by the randomization technique.

Empirical evidence on the success of these techniques is mixed. Although there have been convincing demonstrations of their ability to increase response rates and to reduce bias in some instances (Goodstadt and Gruson, 1975), the evidence from other studies has been equivocal (e.g., Bradburn et al., 1979:8-13). Boruch (1989), in reviewing the results of 23 studies using randomized response techniques, concluded that these methods appeared to increase cooperation and decrease bias in about one-half of the cases in which they had been used. Unfortunately, the available evidence does not provide clear guidance as to the conditions under which these techniques will work.

Pilot Studies

Survey researchers typically distinguish between two types of exploratory studies. Pilot studies are commonly semistructured inquiries conducted prior to the design of the final (or penultimate) version of a survey questionnaire. These studies are used to gather information that is helpful in drafting the instrument. Pretests, on the other hand, are structured tests of a survey questionnaire, one or more of which may be conducted prior to the fielding of a typical survey. Pretests provide information on the range of difficulties that may be encountered in administering

---

[59] Even where the total sample size is large, use of randomized response techniques may yield estimates for subpopulations (e.g., unmarried males, ages 21–30) that have unacceptably large standard errors.

[60] See Fox and Tracy (1986:44–48) for a discussion of the randomizing devices that have been used and the estimation procedures. See Tracy and Fox (1981) for a successful application to estimating arrest rates.

a questionnaire–for example, respondent difficulty in understanding the questions, respondent resistance to providing sensitive information, interviewer difficulty in following "skip patterns,"[61] and so forth.

Although examination of survey questionnaires used in past research on AIDS reveals some deficiencies resulting from the rush to gather data, there have also been some laudable examples of careful preparatory work. The committee notes, for example, that Britain's Social and Community Planning Research unit[62] has included provisions for a three-stage development effort prior to fielding the British survey of sexual attitudes and behavior. This program (see L. Spencer, Faulkner, and Keegan, 1988:3) includes a pilot study[63] (consisting of a series of unstructured in-depth interviews), the development of structured questionnaires and small-scale pretests, and a large-scale pretest of the final questionnaire. The pilot phase of the research included among its aims exploration of the dimensions of the topics that were to be included in the survey, clarification of appropriate language to be used in posing questions, identification of sensitive issues and ways of gathering data on these topics, and preliminary examination of the impact of interviewer characteristics (e.g., gender, sexual orientation) on the willingness of respondents to discuss their sexual behaviors.

These British investigators learned several valuable lessons from their pilot work, which used semistructured interviews with 40 respondents. Three of these lessons are reported here, not because they will necessarily generalize to other samples but rather to indicate the important design considerations that can be missed without careful preparatory work. As a result of debriefing respondents about their reactions to the interviewers to whom they were assigned, the investigators learned the following:

- Women expressed a strong preference for women interviewers;[64] some women indicated that they would not consent to

---

[61] Skip patterns are instructions to skip blocks of questions that depend on responses to prior questions. For example, a series of questions on *first* sexual experiences would be skipped for respondents who indicated that they were inexperienced.

[62] Under contract to the British Health Education Authority.

[63] The work by L. Spencer, Faulkner, and Keegan (1988) testifies to the inconsistent use of the terms *pilot study* and *pretest* among survey researchers. In their publication, *pilot study* includes testing of structured questionnaires, and the large-scale test of the final questionnaire is called a large-scale pilot study or feasibility test. The preliminary unstructured research is termed an "investigative study" (p. 3).

[64] The evidence reported in this study was based entirely on respondents' statements to female interviewers. In the pilot study, male interviewers were never assigned to female respondents.

an interview with a male interviewer, whereas other women said that "they would not have been as open and might have refused to answer some of the more personal questions" (L. Spencer, Faulkner, and Keegan, 1988:10).

- There was a strong preference among respondents for use of formal rather than street language in discussing sexual behaviors. Furthermore, although terms such as penis and vagina were well understood, some of the terminology that has become standard in the epidemiological literature was quite foreign to respondents (e.g., vaginal sex), and there was considerable variation in what was inferred from the terms homosexual and bisexual.[65] Other terms (e.g., anal sex, oral sex) were widely understood.

- Masturbation, surprisingly, seemed to cause respondents more embarrassment than oral or anal sex. Furthermore, there was considerable variability in the use of this term depending on the respondent's sexual orientation. Among respondents with predominantly heterosexual histories, masturbation was usually understood to refer to self-stimulation to orgasm in the absence of a partner. Among gay-identified men, mutual masturbation was a readily acknowledged behavior. For women who identified themselves as lesbians, masturbation referred exclusively to self-stimulation; stimulation by a partner's hands or fingers was "making love" or "having sex."

One cannot, of course, assume that such findings with 40 British adults will generalize to other samples—or, indeed, that one such study fully canvasses the problems involved in surveying the British population. The study does, however, alert researchers to important aspects of the way in which these individuals perceive and talk about their sexual lives and the factors that may impede collection of accurate survey data.

---

[65]Thus, the authors (L. Spencer, Faulkner, and Keegan, 1988:24-25) write: "Some people are clear that [homosexual] refers to both men and women who are attracted to and have sex with their own sex. There are, however, a number of people of different ages and social classes who associate the word exclusively with men: 'Homo equals men.' (Woman, 37 years, married) For these people, women who have sex with each other are lesbians, not homosexuals."

The Spencer group also reported that although most respondents identified bisexuals as persons who had sex with both sexes and heterosexuals as persons who had sex with persons of the opposite sex, there were a few notable confusions. One 31-year-old single man, for example, thought bisexual meant "kinky sex, 3 in bed, that sort of thing" (p. 25); some respondents seemed confused by "ordinary people" being labeled at all with regard to sexual orientation and defined heterosexuals as persons who "liked either sex" or their own sex.

Pretests

Usually, pretests are dress rehearsals for the final survey. As such, they can have great value in allowing field staff and investigators to identify any procedural problems inherent in a questionnaire. Similarly, selective debriefing of interviewers and a subset of survey respondents can help identify aspects of the survey that were difficult to administer or understand. Indeed, simple tactics, such as asking respondents to restate in their own words what was meant by an individual survey question, can be tremendously useful in identifying survey questions that do not have equivalent meanings for all respondents (or, equally important, do not have the same meaning for respondents and the investigator).

Although much can be done using these procedures, some investigators have introduced more systematic data gathering into the pretest process. Cannell and colleagues (1989), for example, implemented ancillary data-gathering activities during pretests to provide additional information on interviewer problems with asking the questions as worded, respondent problems of comprehension, and respondent problems with knowing or providing the required information. In brief, three types of supplemental data were collected during the pretests:

- Coding of behaviors of interviewer and respondent: survey interviews were recorded, and relevant aspects of the survey interview were coded to indicate whether the interviewer asked the question as written, whether the respondent asked for clarification, and so forth. Systematic coding of the pretest interviews provides useful data for identifying questions that pose special difficulties for the interviewer or the respondent, or both, and that may need to be redesigned.

- Probes: follow-up questions are used to determine whether the respondents understood the question in the manner that the investigator intended.

- Rating of questions by interviewers: after completing their interviews (and after completing training on the nature of questionnaire problems), interviewers were asked to rate individual questions and to identify the different types of problems they encountered in asking the question.

These data, which go beyond those usually collected in pretests, can provide important ancillary information on the extent to which the survey interview is "standardized": that is, whether questions are asked in identical fashion and have the same meaning across respondents.

Cognitive Research Strategies

A further preliminary strategy to be considered involves the use of the findings and techniques of cognitive research. These strategies are particularly appropriate when the task at hand is likely to make substantial demands on a respondent's memory.

In that regard the committee notes that two examples used previously may be atypical of the types of information in which AIDS researchers are most interested. Questions regarding chronological age and sexual activity during the past day (or week) solicit information that is easily remembered. Most individuals can readily recall their sexual experiences of the previous day, and chronological age is such an important variable in this culture that the inability to recall it is considered an almost certain sign of dementia.

In contrast, many survey researchers ask for information involving matters to which respondents do not have direct and immediate access—for example, the average number of times per week they have had intercourse over the past six months or year. A mistaken estimate in this case may not be the result of "distortion"—either conscious or unconscious—but may simply be due to the relative unavailability to immediate memory of the information that has been requested.

When such information cannot be directly and easily recalled, two factors must be considered. The first factor is the recall strategy used by the respondent. For example, in estimating frequency of sexual activity over a prolonged period, the respondent may concentrate on a particular short time interval (e.g., the last week or two) and then multiply. Alternatively, the subject may rely on a recent conversation with someone else about the issue or even on some external benchmark (e.g., "I have always had intercourse at a rate twice the averages I've heard reported so therefore my rate must be . . . "). There are a number of such strategies, and each results in different types of systematic biases. A "free scan" may yield events or a period that is particularly memorable—for reasons unrelated to the purposes of the question. For example, researchers working on other topics have found that events (e.g., victimization) that have led to some subsequent actions on the part of the respondent (reporting to the police, collecting insurance) are recalled more clearly than those that have not (Wagennar, 1986). (See Bradburn, Rips, and Shevell [1987] for a more detailed discussion of such strategies.)

The second factor, as noted by Bartlett in 1932, is that memory is basically a reconstructive process and hence is amenable to influences that are described in the memory literature by such terms as "schemata," "scripts," "good stories," and so on. The reason such effects occur is simply that respondents carry out recall on the basis of the information currently available to them, and just as current expectations and preconceptions can affect perception, they can also affect memory—only often more so (see Neisser, 1981; Pearson, Ross, and Dawes, 1989).

The effects of these recall factors may not always constitute a disadvantage from the perspective of the researcher, but they certainly present problems often enough that they must be considered in designing research protocols and questionnaires. Two studies illustrate this conclusion. In the first, by Smith, Jobe, and Mingay (in press), subjects kept a diary of what they ate over a four-week period and were then asked to recall their food intake from the most recent two weeks and from the more remote two weeks. The recall for the most recent two-week period more closely matched the actual items eaten during those two weeks (i.e., those in the diary) than the recall for the items eaten during the more remote two weeks. In contrast, the recall for the more remote period matched the previous two weeks and the remote two weeks equally well. The authors concluded that recall for food intake prior to the previous two weeks produced a "generic" result (based on foods that were commonly eaten by the person recalling) whereas people had a more direct recall of the previous two weeks. Even though personal recall may be subject to social scripts and schemata, such distortions may be unimportant to the researcher. Indeed, for many purposes, the "generic" result may be of equal or greater interest.[66]

During the last decade, a number of promising examples of the use of cognitive research techniques in survey development have been proposed (Biderman and Moore, 1980; Jabine et al., 1985). The last year in particular has witnessed publication of several studies that used such techniques to evaluate and improve survey measurements of health-related and other events (Brewer, Dull, and Jobe, 1989; Lessler, Tourangeau, and Salter, 1989; Means et al., 1989; Tucker et al., 1989). Yet, although these techniques offer researchers new possibilities to "take account" of the effect of the recall strategy and belief factors in assessing responses, such a task is difficult and may present problems for which there are no easy solutions. Clearly, if the phenomena of interest can be restricted to time frames that do not make impossible demands on the accuracy of the respondent's memory, then there is much to be gained by ensuring that the phrasing of questions appropriately restricts the time frame, although this kind of restriction may be impossible in some situations.

---

[66]Neisser (1981), for example, found (by comparing John Dean's testimony before the discovery of Nixon's White House tapes to the evidence of the tapes) that the "gist" of what happened was maintained, even though the recall was wrong in almost every detail.

In other situations, there may be no alternative. Some epidemiological research, for example, requires information on patterns of behavior that are sufficiently removed in time to make severe demands on memory. If the information is needed for distant time periods, then researchers have no alternative but to buttress their survey measurements with carefully conducted studies that probe the character of the memory processes that underlie subjects' reports (and misreports).

A final strategy that can be used profitably in developing more accurate survey instruments involves the use of ethnographic research techniques. Not only can these techniques be helpful in preliminary investigations to develop better questionnaires and research designs, but they also provide an important research strategy in their own right for studying questions and populations that may be inaccessible using other research techniques. This chapter concludes with a brief overview of current AIDS research using these techniques.

ETHNOGRAPHIC STUDIES

Anthropologists often deal with phenomena for which other scientific methods are unsuitable. For example, a description of the day's events in a drug shooting gallery or the attempt to understand the meaning of condom use for certain individuals and groups are problems of quite different dimensions than determining the HIV status of those same individuals and populations. The anthropologist's task is one of observation and interpretation rather than statistical evaluation or prediction and thus depends more on human powers to learn, understand, and communicate. Although anthropologists consider an understanding and interpretation of the unique aspects of social life to be an important part of their research, they also analyze their data for patterns and systematic relationships that can lead to generalizations and theory building.

Ethnographic data gathered in the course of fieldwork requires intimate participation in a community and observation of ways of life that often differ from one's own. Long-term participation in the everyday events of a community, neighborhood, or group provides access to detailed information on behaviors, the contexts in which they are enacted, and the vocabulary used to describe them. Participant observation can thus help to identify contradictions between what people say they do and what they actually do. The recording and interpretation of another people's way of life (ethnography) is a process that reveals alternative conceptual frameworks, modes of being, forms of property, and ways of organizing domestic, religious, or political affairs. An appreciation of the diversity of social and cultural forms challenges the aura of naturalness that surrounds the institutions and conventions of life at home and allows one to rethink the basic categories and assumptions of one's own society.

Ethnographic research methods provide particularly useful tools for gathering information about hard-to-reach populations, for acquainting investigators with the diversity of conceptual frameworks and social forms used to organize and interpret events, and for refining and assessing the appropriateness of questionnaires and other research instruments.

Examples of Studies Related to HIV Transmission

Male-Male Sexual Contacts

Anthropological research among Mexicans and Mexican Americans in southern California[67] provides a telling example of the benefits of an ethnographic approach to data gathering. Studies of sexual behavior in Mexico indicate that Mexican men who engage in same-gender sex have a strong preference for anal intercourse over fellatio. Conceptually, the male playing the receptive role is considered homosexual (by societal standards), but the one playing the insertive role is not, a view that is not shared by men in the Anglo community. Because many Mexicans who engage in same-gender sex may not consider themselves to be homosexual or bisexual, AIDS education programs designed for Anglo gay men may not seem relevant to them (Carrier, 1989; Carrier and Magana, n.d.). Alonso and Koreck (1989) confirmed these findings among rural workers in northern Mexico, adding that similar patterns of sexual behavior may be found among other Latino groups, such as Cubans, in the United States. These researchers caution, however, that other important differences will become apparent once such variables as class and geographic location are considered.

Carrier and Magana (n.d.) similarly note the variability of same-gender sexual behaviors among immigrant Mexican men. Although most immigrant Mexican men continue to engage in behaviors patterned on their prior sexual experiences in Mexico, some adopt mainstream Anglo behaviors. The major determinant of the change appears to be the extent to which their socialization in adolescence was with Mexican or Anglo-American sex partners. The development of appropriate AIDS

---

[67] By August 1989, 1,151 cases of AIDS had been recorded in Orange County, mainly among homosexual (67.8 percent) or bisexual (18.3 percent) men. Although most cases so far have occurred in the Anglo community, in the past two years the number of Latino cases has grown more rapidly than the number of cases in the Anglo community. Mexicans (sojourners who move back and forth across the border) and Mexican Americans (those born in the United States) constitute the largest proportion of the Latino male population in California (Carrier and Magana, n.d.).

intervention strategies thus depends on an appreciation of the range, context, meaning, and distribution of sexual practices among different ethnic groups within the United States. Targeted educational interventions may also be required for people who are less educated or for those who are preliterate (Carrier, 1989; Carrier and Magana, n.d.).

Variation in Drug Use Patterns

A second example of how ethnographic research may broaden and enhance the knowledge base on hard-to-reach populations concerns stereotypical views of IV drug users. Anthropological descriptions of the diversity of behaviors, social networks, and self-distinctions that exist in different drug-using communities discount the widely held image of the "dope fiend" as a person who devotes his life to acquiring and using drugs. Although IV drug users in a black community in Baltimore (Mason, 1988) can certainly identify "dope fiends among their numbers," they also recognize and distinguish several other types of drug users:

- "addicts" who pursue drugs constantly but who often have families and jobs and thus participate to some extent in the "straight" world;
- "hope fiends" who are either unable or unwilling to pursue money to support their habit but who hang around drug areas waiting for an opportunity to get drugs by hustling or through cunning;
- casual users or "chippers" who use IV drugs recreationally on the weekends; and
- people who at various points in their drug-using careers move between these categories.

Seen in this light, IV drug users are a diverse and shifting population, and consequently, prevention and outreach services must be tailored to meet a variety of needs and objectives (Mason, 1988).[68]

Ethnographic Methods

Anthropologists thus investigate, interpret, and attempt to explain cultural difference and its changing nature. By emphasizing the diversity of beliefs, practices, and social conditions in different communities, anthropologists counter the tendency to see Hispanics, blacks, whites, Asians,

---

[68]Koester's (1989b) study of black IV drug users in Denver also challenges the common stereotype of the drug addict. In Denver, Koester found heroin habits that rarely required more than a $50 a day to sustain, and the petty thefts that supported the drug user's habits were often directed at other addicts.

Native Americans, men, women, or adolescents in the United States as undifferentiated monocultures. Such an appreciation, however, requires a foundation of quantitative data for better interpretation of the illustrative case. Demographic data, usually gathered by the ethnographer using techniques of mapping and census-taking in the study of small-scale societies, are supplemented by census or epidemiological survey data in larger, more complex settings.

In recent years, anthropologists have become more sensitive to sampling issues as greater theoretical attention has been given to variations in the ideologies and beliefs of different individuals in tribal societies. The question of sampling becomes more acute in large populations in which cultural diversity, social stratification, and rapid change raise greater concern regarding methodological precision and the validity and reliability of ethnographic data (see Pelto and Pelto, 1978; Bernard, 1988). The task of ethnographic analysis is further complicated by an awareness that, like data in all the sciences, anthropological data are not acquired through a pristine encounter with the world. Rather, observation, recording, and measurement are directed by concepts and theories, and these concepts and ideas are subject to modification and change. Unless ethnographers take what they suppose to be a purely empirical approach to the world, they often have a "double sense" of the way they go about their work: they assume that their ideas are suitable for interpreting other peoples' beliefs but that these ideas, like the beliefs they are intended to interpret, are also the products of particular historical and social circumstances.[69]

The methods used to gather ethnographic data fall into five main categories:

- direct observation of daily life on mundane and ceremonial occasions, description of the observed environment (sometimes with detailed accounts of commerce or household economies), and the recording of spontaneous conversations in which the ethnographer may or may not be a participant (careful records of speech events provide important material for linguistic analysis);
- relatively open-ended interviews and discussions with key informants, as well as the recording of life histories;
- gathering of information from existing records, "native"

---

[69] Analysis of anthropological data is tempered by an awareness that knowledge in various societies is distributed and controlled in different ways. Anthropologists thus see cultures not as fixed entities but rather as the products of continual processes of creation and contest.

texts, songs, visual material, government records, and historical archives;

- surveys using structured interviews and involving large numbers of respondents; and

- an important type of learning that receives little attention and involves knowledge not reported in notebooks or on filecards comes from long-term residence in the study community. Memories of experiences, as well as perhaps unconscious recollections and understandings (associated with certain sights, sounds, and smells) often form the backdrop for the patterns and connections that are made during interpretations and analysis of field data.

Much ethnographic data collection depends on developing relationships of trust with those whose lives are the subject of study. Such relationships may develop over an extended period of time, and to some degree they determine the accuracy, sensitivity, and complexity of the data. The researcher has an ethical responsibility to ensure that identities are protected and that the study causes no harm, an objective that the subjects of the study often monitor and probe.

AIDS research presents a special methodological challenge as anthropologists investigate the worlds of men and women who have bisexual and same-gender sexual relations or who may be IV drug users and their sex partners, prostitutes and their clients, male hustlers, prison inmates, and undocumented laborers. Some ethnographic studies have looked at health care workers, insurance companies, or students and staff in schools, but most research concerns populations that are seen as "marginalized"— outside the mainstream, often impoverished, and involved in activities that are illegal or that are seen as deviant. Methods of ethnographic or anthropological fieldwork developed in other contexts may not be well suited to studies of sexual behaviors and IV drug use, the behaviors that need to be understood and changed in order to stem the epidemic. Both of these areas of study thus present a challenge to accepted notions of participant observation.

Ethnographic Methods in AIDS Research

The difficulties encountered in AIDS research have elicited a variety of methodological responses from the anthropological community. Some ethnographers continue to undertake something close to what is thought of as classical fieldwork. Working alone, they establish rapport and trust with the subjects of study and observe incidents in natural settings. Outside the United States, in Haiti and Brazil, for example, the researcher "lives" in the field, participating extensively in community affairs (Parker, 1987; Farmer and Kleinman, 1989; Farmer, 1990). In the United States, on the other hand, investigators tend to follow an approach often used in urban fieldwork, that is, "visiting the field" more or less on a daily basis (Leonard, 1990; Connors, 1989; Sterk, 1989).

To overcome the difficulties of research with contemporary drug users, for example, the ethnographer may belong to a team that includes former drug users as outreach workers. As a participant observer, the ethnographer documents the kinds of questions, attitudes, and theories the former drug users express, training them to do the same in their own daily reports. In turn, the ethnographer learns about drug use from these outreach workers, and their presence facilitates his or her acceptance as an outsider asking questions on sensitive issues (Mason, 1988; Weibel, in press). The use of a field station storefront appears to provide a context in which surprisingly sensitive information can be gathered. The protocol of an AIDS intervention project for the sex partners of IV drug users in the predominantly black south side of Chicago, for example, began with a preliminary questionnaire (to gather sociodemographic and epidemiological data), followed by a longer, open-ended conversation that reconstructed the routines of everyday life and some aspects of the respondent's life history. This latter session was designed to alert the sexual partners to the dangers of their day-to-day behavior and offered the chance for a discussion of more subtle issues and personal concerns that were not elicited by the questionnaire (Kane, 1989a,b).

"Captive" populations are also the subject of anthropological study. Hospital clinics, county health departments, and bars provide settings for personal interviews, focus group discussions, or the distribution of questionnaires to be filled in and returned to the investigator (McCombie, 1986, 1990; Marshall et al., in press; K. Kennedy, personal communication).[70] Although this approach is constrained by its inability to compare self-reported and observed behaviors, it can provide information on sexual behavior and drug use that is otherwise difficult to obtain.

Adaptation of the traditional methods of kinship charting to construct a visual image of concrete social relations is an ethnographic method that has been used to elicit information from male and female black and Puerto Rican patients at a methadone clinic in the Bronx. Patients and an anthropologist worked together to create a visual chart of the patient's kin and friends, to which were added color-coded records of his or her drug-using and non-drug-using associates, the particular drugs chosen, sexual

---

[70] K. Kennedy, Montefiore Family Health Center, Bronx, N.Y., personal communication, August 1989.

and social intimates, those who were aware of the patient's HIV status, those who were informed about their own HIV status, and the patient's household composition as well as that of his or her children (who often lived separately). From an anthropological point of view, the chart is only a starting point for more extended enquiries about various aspects of social life. For an epidemiologist, however, the chart provides an index of the number of people at risk for HIV infection because it records the frequency of sexual intercourse, the categories of sexual partners (those who live together, those who are lovers or more casual partners, and those involved in prostitution), and whether contraceptives are used.[71]

Regional comparisons, which are commonly used in ethnographic research, have been rare in the anthropology of HIV infection. A comparison of two ethnically distinct neighborhoods in Baltimore, however, provides some insight into the different drug choices and the motivations for and meanings of multiple drug use among African Americans and European Americans, as well as the relative risks of HIV infection (Mason, in press). Similarly, an ethnographic study of the social contexts of injection equipment sharing conducted in New York City and San Francisco revealed that, in the "shooting galleries" of New York, several sets of injection equipment might be shared by more than 100 individuals in a single day. In San Francisco, however, smaller circles of friends shared injection equipment. Given New York's much higher seroprevalence among IV drug users, documentation of these widely varying conditions of injection equipment use provides some contextual understanding of the spread of the virus and the differing character of the epidemic in each location (Watters, 1989).

Although most social research on AIDS has concerned the behaviors that put people at risk for HIV infection, a recent review of the ethnographic literature on sexual behaviors (Cassidy and Porter, 1989) attempted to identify "safer" (nonpenetrative) sexual practices that might form a core of culturally sensitive interventions to control the spread of the virus (keeping in mind that the concept of "safer" sex is a peculiarly Western medical notion). As the review shows, low-risk nonpenetrative

---

[71] A. Pivnik, Montefiore Hospital, Bronx, N.Y., personal communication, October 1989. A different kind of creative mapping plots the distribution of circumcision practices in Africa with areas of high and low AIDS prevalence, an association that has provided significant results, as it suggests that uncircumcised men run a greater risk of becoming infected during sexual intercourse than do those who are circumcised (Reining, 1989). In response to the uncritical use of ethnographic data that marked the early years of the AIDS epidemic, a computer-assisted data base is also being designed to collate cultural information from a variety of sources to complement local, national, and international data bases on HIV seroprevalence (Conant, 1989).

behaviors (interfemoral intercourse, masturbation, mutual grooming, sexual joking, and so on) occur commonly throughout the world. A mere listing of sexual behaviors that appear to be universal—including coitus, other forms of intercourse, masturbation, same-sex relations—is not very informative, however, and may even be misleading because the contexts in which the behaviors occur, the attitudes people express about these behaviors, and the meanings of the behaviors vary enormously from locale to locale. Sexual behavior cannot be understood apart from its cultural context, which includes historical, economic, and political aspects. As the example of Mexican American and Anglo sexual behavior in Orange County illustrates, "homosexual" and "bisexual" relations may have a different meaning and expression for different ethnic groups living in the same community. Thus, to communicate effectively with people at risk, AIDS research and interventions must be sensitive to the variability of sexual meaning and experience within and among cultural groups (Cassidy and Porter, 1989).

Findings of Ethnographic Research on AIDS

Ethnographic research on the spread of HIV infection is still in the preliminary phases of data gathering. Nevertheless, some suggestive patterns appear to be emerging. First, prostitutes' use of condoms for professional but not personal sex has been widely observed in Europe and in some parts of the United States (Kane, 1989b; Worth, 1989), the West Indies (McCombie, 1990), and Africa (Bledsoe, 1990). That a similar pattern does not currently exist among prostitutes in Orange County, southern California (Carrier, 1989; Carrier and Magana, n.d.) or among church women in Zaire (Schoepf et al., in press) is a salutary reminder that cultural data should always be examined for its internal variability and in appropriate historical context.

Second, studies of the perceptions of some segments of the scientific community in the United States suggest that scientists—like people everywhere—may hold local views of the world that are at variance with statistical or scientific understanding. Thus health care professionals sometimes fail to adopt precautions when they are at risk, although they show excessive caution in less risky situations. The perception of whether an individual is considered "safe" or "unsafe," for example, depends on a combination of social, economic, and visual criteria (McCombie, 1989).

Third, despite the hazards of attempting to compare heterogeneous data from several countries, some consistent cultural themes can be identified. A comparison of data from Central and East Africa (Zaire, Zambia, Tanzania, and Uganda) and West Africa (Nigeria and Sierra Leone), for example, indicates that condom use poses problems for populations that stress fertility in heterosexual relations; in addition, condoms are associated with promiscuity. Moreover, polygyny is an accepted cultural behavior among men in all three regions, and women may also have multiple sexual partners, often as a result of economic pressures (Bledsoe, 1990).

Finally, several studies indicate that educational messages concerning the dangers of unprotected sex reach some audiences but have actually increased the dangers of HIV infection for other segments of the population. In response to public education about AIDS, men in some parts of Africa continue to pursue an active sexual life but have turned from high-risk groups (e.g., prostitutes) to low-risk pools (e.g., schoolgirls, who may be willing to exchange sex for money to finance their education) (Bledsoe, 1990). Similarly, as a result of educational campaigns in the United States, the clients of street prostitutes in New Jersey report choosing novices and apparently inexperienced young girls in hopes of avoiding long-term drug users who may be infected with HIV (Leonard, 1990).

Gaps and Deficiencies in Current Ethnographic Research

The current flurry of anthropological research on sexual behavior and drug use suffers from the absence of a sustained scholarly tradition in both fields. Although there is more research on sexual behavior than on drug use, the study of sexuality has focused for several decades on sexual meanings and beliefs and has tended to ignore sexual behaviors. The usefulness of such data for HIV research thus is limited. When sexual behaviors were reported, normative behaviors were highlighted rather than the varied ways in which people often choose to lead their sexual lives. Moreover, this earlier literature provides little information concerning the substantial changes that have now altered behaviors in once-isolated regions.

Studies of drug use have provided information on patterns of behavior in homes and shooting galleries (Koester, 1989a,b; Watters, 1989; B.P. Page et al., 1990), on the meaning and practices of injection equipment use (Connors, 1989), and on different patterns of multiple drug use and high-risk behaviors in different ethnic communities (Mason, in press). Attention is now beginning to turn to the broader determinants of high-risk drug behaviors—such as the history and political economy of drug use and drug marketing (Hamid, 1990; Mason, in press) and the way in which laws that make carrying a syringe a crime increase the probability that drug users will adopt risky behaviors (Koester, 1989a,b). Much more information is needed, however, on such social determinants, as well as on individual perceptions of the risky behaviors associated with drug use.

Anthropologists and epidemiologists have had some success in identifying and investigating "risky" behaviors in many locations. Yet intervention strategies have sometimes been directed too narrowly at behaviors rather than at people in context. Effective intervention may require a broader understanding of both the personal and social determinants of risk behaviors (cf. O'Reilly, 1989). A further area in which much ethnographic work deserves to be conducted involves the relationship between belief and behavior. In this regard, there is a distinction to be drawn between constructs that constitute a public language and constructs that guide individual choices in specific situations. Recent studies point to the way in which individuals personalize the rules of behavior to fit their own wishes and the limited options from which they might choose (Eyre, 1989; Kane, 1989a,b; Cassidy and Porter, 1989). The ability of impoverished women to practice "safer" sexual behaviors, for example, may be particularly circumscribed. Furthermore, very little is known about the interaction between private worlds of erotic behavior and the public domain of shared meanings recently explored by Parker (1989). It has been suggested that rules regulating sexual behavior may be particularly prone to individual negotiation and improvisation (Cassidy and Porter, 1989). All of these factors emphasize the continuing valuable role to be played by ethnographic research and the discipline of anthropology.

RECOMMENDATIONS

Given the evidence reviewed in the foregoing pages, the committee concludes that there is good reason to believe that accurate measurements of AIDS risk behaviors can be obtained. The committee notes, however, that there is substantial room for improvement in current efforts. This potential is not surprising given the immaturity of many of the relevant research fields.

The committee believes that appropriate investments to create a better foundation of relevant methodological knowledge can lead to more certain scientific understanding about the behaviors that transmit HIV and the factors that motivate and shape these behaviors. Toward this end the committee makes the following recommendations.

The committee recommends that the Public Health Service and other organizations supporting AIDS research provide increased support for methodological research on the measurement of behaviors

that transmit HIV. Such research should consider inferential problems introduced by nonresponse and by nonsampling factors, including (but not limited to) the effects of question wording and question context, the time periods and events that respondents are asked to recall, and the effects of anonymity guarantees on survey responses.

The committee recommends that researchers who conduct behavioral surveys on HIV transmission make increased use of ethnographic studies, pretests, pilot studies, cognitive laboratory investigations, and other similar developmental strategies to aid in the design of large-scale surveys.

The committee recommends that, where appropriate, researchers embed experimental studies within behavioral surveys on HIV transmission to assess the effects of key aspects of the survey measurement process.

The committee recommends that, whenever feasible, researchers supplement self-reports in behavioral surveys on HIV transmission with other indicators of these behaviors that do not rely on respondent reports.

REFERENCES

Aiken, L. S. (1986) Retrospective self-reports by clients differ from original reports: Implications for the evaluation of drug treatment programs. *International Journal of the Addictions* 21:767–788.

Aiken, L. S., and LoSciuto, L. A. (1985) Ex-addict versus nonaddict counselors' knowledge of clients' drug use. *International Journal of the Addictions* 20:417–433.

Allen, R. M., and Haupt, T. D. (1966) The sex inventory: Test-retest reliability of scale scores and items. *Journal of Clinical Psychology* 22:375–378.

Alonso, A. M., and Koreck, M. T. (1989) Silences: Hispanics, AIDS, and sexual practices. *Differences* 1:101–124.

Amsel, Z., Mandell, W., Matthias, L., Mason, C., and Hocherman, I. (1976) Reliability and validity of self-reported illegal activities and drug use collected from narcotic addicts. *International Journal of the Addictions* 11:325–336.

Anastasi, A. (1976) *Psychological Testing.* 4th ed. New York: Macmillan.

Andersen, B. L., and Broffitt, B. (1988) Is there a reliable and valid self-report measure of sexual behavior? *Archives of Sexual Behavior* 17:509–525.

Andersen, R., Kasper, J., Frankel, M. R., and Associates. (1979) *Total Survey Error.* San Francisco: Jossey-Bass.

Anderson, R. M., and May, R. M. (1988) Epidemiological parameters of HIV transmission. *Nature* 333:514–519.

Aral, S. O., Magder, L. S., and Bowen, G. S. (1989) HIV risk behavior screening: Concordance between assessments through interviews and questionnaires. Presented at the Fifth International Conference on AIDS, Montreal, June 4–9.

Axinn, W. G. (n.d.) The influence of interviewer gender on responses to sensitive questions in less developed settings: Evidence from Nepal. Population Studies Center, Institute for Social Research and Department of Sociology, University of Michigan, Ann Arbor, Mich.

Baddeley, A. D. (1979) The limitations of human memory: Implications for the design of retrospective surveys. In L. Moss and H. Goldstein, eds., *The Recall Method in Social Surveys.* London: University of London Institute of Education.

Bailar, B. (1975) The effects of rotation group bias on estimates from panel surveys. *Journal of the American Statistical Association* 70:23–30.

Bailar, B., Bailey, L., and Stevens, J. (1977) Measures of interviewer bias and variance. *Journal of Marketing Research* 14:337–343.

Bailey, L., Moore, T., and Bailar, B. (1978) An interviewer variance study for the eight impact cities of the National Crime Survey cities sample. *Journal of the American Statistical Association* 73:16–23.

Bale, R. N. (1979) The validity and reliability of self-reported data from heroin addicts: Mailed questionnaires compared with face-to-face interviews. *International Journal of the Addictions* 14:993–1000.

Bale, R. N., Van Stone, W. W., Engelsing, T. M. J., Zarcone, V. P., and Kuldau, J. M. (1981) The validity of self-reported heroin use. *International Journal of the Addictions* 16:1387–1398.

Ball, J. C. (1967) The reliability and validity of interview data obtained from 59 narcotic drug addicts. *American Journal of Sociology* 72:650–654.

Ball, J. C., Lange, W. R., Myers, C. P., and Friedman, S. R. (1988) Reducing the risk of AIDS through methadone maintenance treatment. *Journal of Health and Social Behavior* 29:214–226.

Bardoux, C., Buning, E., Leentvaar-Kuijpers, A., Verster, A., and Coutinho, R. A. (1989) Declining incidence of acute hepatitis B among drug users in Amsterdam may indicate a change in risk behavior. Presented at the Fifth International Conference on AIDS, Montreal, June 4–9.

Bartlett, F. C. (1932) *Remembering: A Study in Experimental Social Psychology.* Cambridge University Press: Cambridge, Great Britain.

Batki, S. L., Sorensen, J. L., Coates, C., and Gibson, D. R. (1989) Methadone maintenance for AIDS-affected IV drug users: Psychiatric factors and outcome three months into treatment (abstract). In L. S. Harris, ed., *Problems of Drug Dependence 1988: Proceedings of the Committee on the Problems of Drug Dependence.* Washington, D.C.: U.S. Government Printing Office.

Bauman, L. J., and Adair, E. G. (1989) Use of ethnographic interviewing to inform questionnaire construction. Presented at the Annual Meeting of the American Association for Public Opinion Research, St. Petersburg, Fla., May.

Beck, C., Ward, C., Mendelson, M., Mock, J., and Erbaugh, J. (1961) An inventory measuring depression. *Archives of General Psychiatry* 4:561–571.

Beniger, J. R. (1984) Mass media, contraceptive behavior, and attitudes on abortion: Toward a comprehensive model of subjective social change. In C. F. Turner and E. Martin, eds., *Surveying Subjective Phenomena.* Vol. 2. New York: Russell Sage.

Benney, M., Riesman, D., and Star, S. A. (1956) Age and sex in the interview. *American Journal of Sociology* 62:143–152.

Bentler, P. M. (1968a) Heterosexual behaviour assessment. I. Males. *Behaviour Research and Therapy* 6:21–25.

Bentler, P. M. (1968b) Heterosexual behaviour assessment. II. Females. *Behaviour Research and Therapy* 6:27–30.

Benus, J., and Ackerman, J. C. (1971) The problem of nonresponse in sample surveys. In J. B. Lansing, S. B. Withey, A. C. Wolfe et al., eds., *Working Papers on Survey Research in Poverty Areas,* Ann Arbor: Survey Research Center, Institute for Social Research, University of Michigan.

Ben-Yehuda, N. (1980) Are addicts' self-reports to be trusted? *International Journal of the Addictions* 15:1265–1270.

Bernard, H. R. (1988) *Research Methods in Cultural Anthropology.* Newbury Park, Calif.: Sage.

Biderman, A. D., and Lynch, J. P. (1981) Recency bias in data on self-reported victimization. *Proceedings of the American Statistical Association (Social Statistics Section)* 1981:31–40.

Biderman, A. D., and Moore, J. C. (1980) Report of the workshop on applying cognitive psychology to recall problems of the National Crime Survey. Unpublished manuscript. Bureau of Social Science Research, Washington, D.C.

Bihari, B., and Ottomanelli, G. (1989) Defense mechanisms and HIV risk related behaviors in substance abusers. Presented at the Fifth International Conference on AIDS, Montreal, June 4–9.

Billy, J. O. G., and Udry, J. R. (1985) Patterns of adolescent friendship and effects on sexual behavior. *Social Psychology Quarterly* 48:27–41.

Bishop, Y. M. M., Fienberg, S., and Holland, P. W. (1975) *Discrete Multivariate Analysis.* Cambridge, Mass.: Massachusetts Institute of Technology Press.

Bledsoe, C. (1990) The politics of AIDS and condoms for stable heterosexual relations in Africa: Recent evidence from the local print media. In W. P. Handwerker, ed., *Births and Power: The Politics of Reproduction.* Boulder, Colo.: Westview Press.

Blumstein, P., and Schwartz, P. (1977) Bisexuality: Some social psychological issues. *Journal of Social Issues* 33:30–45.

Blumstein, P. W., and Schwartz, P. (1983) *American Couples: Money, Work, and Sex.* New York: Morrow.

Bonito, A. J., Nurco, D. N., and Shaffer, J. W. (1976) The veridicality of addicts' self-reports in social research. *International Journal of the Addictions* 11:719–724.

Borgatta, E. F., Blumstein, P., and Schwartz, P. (1987) Research Methodologies for Sensitive Data Collection: Final Report submitted to the Centers for Disease Control. Department of Sociology, University of Washington, Seattle.

Boruch, R. F. (1989) Resolving privacy problems in AIDS research: A primer. In L. Sechrest, H. Freeman, and A. Mulley, eds., *Health Services Research Methodology: A Focus on AIDS.* Conference Proceedings. Rockville, Md.: National Center for Health Services Research and Health Care Technology Assessment.

Bradburn, N. W., Rips, L. J., and Shevell, S. K. (1987) Answering autobiographical questions: The impact of memeory and inference on surveys. *Science* 236:157–161.

Bradburn, N. M., Sudman, S., and Associates. (1979) *Improving Interview Method and Questionnaire Design.* San Francisco: Jossey Bass.

Brady, J. P., and Levitt, E. E. (1965) The scalability of sexual experiences. *Psychological Record* 15:275–279.

Brewer, M. B., Dull, V. T., and Jobe, J. B. (1989) Social cognition approach to reporting chronic health conditions. *Vital and Health Statistics,* Series 6, Whole No. 3.

Brooks, C. A., and Bailar, B. (1978) *An Error Profile: Employment as Measured by the Current Population Survey.* Statistical Policy Working Paper 3. Washington, D.C.: U.S. Department of Commerce.

Brown, L. S., Phillips, R., Ajulchukwu, D., Battjes, R., Primm, B. J., and Nemoto, T. (1989) Demographic and behavioral features of HIV infection in intravenous drug users in New York City drug treatment programs: 1985–1988. Presented at the Fifth International Conference on AIDS, Montreal, June 4–9.

Cain, V. S., and Baldwin, W. (1989) The national study of health and sexual behavior. Presented at the Fifth International Conference on AIDS, Montreal, June 4–9.

Campbell, A. A. (1987) Randomized response technique (letter). *Science* 236:1049.

Cannell, C. F., Fisher, G., and Bakker, T. (1965) Reporting of hospitalization in the Health Interview Survey. *Vital and Health Statistics,* Series 2, Whole No. 6.

Cannell, C. F., Marquis, K. H., and Laurent, A. (1977) A summary of studies of interviewing methodology. *Vital and Health Statistics,* Series 2, Whole No. 69.

Cannell, C. F., Miller, P. V., and Oksenberg, L. (1981) Research on interviewing techniques. In S. Leinhardt, ed., *Sociological Methodology 1981.* San Francisco: Jossey-Bass.

Cannell, C., Oksenberg, L., Kalton, G., Bischoping, K., and Fowler, F. J. (1989) New techniques for pretesting survey questions. Final Report to the National Center for Health Services Research and Health Care Technology Assessment. Survey Research Center, University of Michigan, Ann Arbor, Mich.

Carrier, J. M. (1989) Sexual behavior and the spread of AIDS in Mexico. *Medical Anthropology* 10:129–142.

Carrier, J. M., and Magana, J. R. (n.d.) Applied anthropology and AIDS in a health care agency. Unpublished manuscript. Orange County Health Care Agency, Orange County, Calif.

Cassidy, C. M., and Porter, R. W. (1989) *Ethnographic Perspectives on Nonpenetrative Sexual Behavior.* Research Triangle Park, N.C.: AIDSCOM, Family Health International.

Castro, K. G., Lieb, S., Jaffe, H. W., Narkonas, J. P., Calisher, C. H., et al. (1988) Transmission of HIV in Belle Glade, Florida: Lessons for other communities in the United States. *Science* 239:193–197.

Catania, J. A., McDermott, L. J., and Pollack, L. M. (1986) Questionnaire response bias and face-to-face interview sample bias in sexuality research. *Journal of Sex Research* 22:52–72.

Catania, J. A., Gibson, D. R., Chitwood, D. D., and Coates, T. J. (In press,a) Methodological problems in AIDS behavioral research: Influences of measurement error and participation bias in studies of sexual behavior. *Psychological Bulletin.*

Catania, J. A., Gibson, D. R., Marin, B., Coates, T. J., and Greenblatt, R. M. (In press,b) Response bias in assessing sexual behaviors relevant to HIV transmission. *Evaluation and Program Planning.*

Centers for Disease Control (CDC). (1988) HIV-related beliefs, knowledge, and behaviors among high school students. *Morbidity and Mortality Weekly Report* 37:717–721.

Chaisson, R. E., Osmond, D., Moss, A. R., Feldman, H. W., and Bernacki, P. (1987) HIV, bleach, and needle sharing. *Lancet* 20 June:1430.

Chaisson, R. E., Osmond, D., Bacchetti, P., Brodie, B., Sande, M. A., and Moss, A. R. (1988) Cocaine, race and HIV infection in IV drug users. Presented at the Fourth International Conference on AIDS, Stockholm, June 12–16.

Chaisson, R. E., Bacchetti, P., Osmond, D., Brodie, B., Sande, M. A., and Moss, A. R. (1989) Cocaine use and HIV infection in intravenous drug users. *Journal of the American Medical Association* 261:561–609.

Cisin, I. H., and Parry, H. L. (1979) Sensitivity of survey techniques in measuring illicit drug use. In J. D. Rittenhouse, ed., *Developmental Papers: Attempts to Improve the Measurement of Heroin Use in the National Survey.* Washington, D.C.: National Institute on Drug Abuse.

Citro, C. F., and Cohen, M. L. (1985) *The Bicentennial Census: New Directions for Methodology in 1990.* Report of the National Research Council Panel on Decennial Census Methodology. Washington, D.C.: National Academy Press.

Clark, A. L. and Wallin, P. (1964) The accuracy of husbands' and wives' reports of the frequency of marital coitus. *Population Studies* 18:165–173.

Clark, J. P., and Tifft, L. L. (1966) Polygraph and interview validation of self-reported deviant behavior. *American Sociological Review* 31:516–523.

Coates, R. A., Soskolne, C. L., Calzavara, L., Read, S. E., Fanning, M. M., et al. (1986) The reliability of sexual histories in AIDS-related research: Evaluation of an interview-administered questionnaire. *Canadian Journal of Public Health* 77:343–348.

Coates, R. A., Calzavara, L. M., Soskolne, C. L., Read, S. E., Fanning, M. M., et al. (1988) Validity of sexual histories in a prospective study of male sexual contacts of men with AIDS or an AIDS-related condition. *American Journal of Epidemiology* 128:719–728.

Cochran, W. G., Mosteller, F., and Tukey, J. W. (1953) Statistical problems of the Kinsey report. *Journal of the American Statistical Association* 48:673–716.

Communication Technologies, Inc. (1987) *A Report on Designing an Effective AIDS Prevention Campaign Strategy for San Francisco: Results from the Fourth Probability Sample of an Urban Gay Male Community.* San Francisco: Communication Technologies, Inc., July 31, 1987.

Communication Technologies, Inc. (1988) *A Report on Planning for the AIDS Epidemic in California: A Population-Based Assessment of Knowledge, Attitudes, and Behavior.* San Francisco: Communication Technologies, Inc., June 30, 1988.

Conant, F. P. (1989) AIDS and beyond: The need, and a design, for a targeted cultural information management system. Unpublished manuscript. Department of Anthropology, Hunter College, City University of New York.

Connors, M. (1989) Perception of risk and HIV infection among intravenous drug users (IVDUs) in Worcester, Mass. Unpublished manuscript. Department of Anthropology, University of Massachusetts, Amherst.

Conte, H. R. (1983) Development and use of self-report techniques for assessing sexual functioning: A review and critique. *Archives of Sexual Behavior* 12:555–576.

Converse, J. M., and Schuman, H. (1974) *Conversations at Random: Survey Research as Interviewers See It.* New York: Wiley.

Coombs, L. C. (1977) Levels of reliability in fertility survey data. *Studies in Family Planning* 8:218–232.

Council of American Survey Research Organizations (CASRO). (1982) *On the Definition of Response Rates. A Special Report of the CASRO Task Force on Completion Rates.* Port Jefferson, N.Y.

Cox, T. J., and Longwell, B. (1974) Reliability of interview data concerning current heroin use from heroin addicts on methadone. *International Journal of the Addictions* 9:161–165.

Coxon, A. P. M. (1986) Report of a Pilot Study: Project on Sexual Lifestyles of Non-Heterosexual Males. Unpublished manuscript. Social Research Unit, University College, Cardiff, Wales.

Coxon, A. P. M. (1988) Something sensational: The sexual diary as a tool for mapping detailed sexual behavior. *Sociological Review* 35:353–367.

Coxon, A. P. M., and Carballo M. (1989) Editorial Review: Research on AIDS: Behavioral perspectives. *AIDS* 3:191–197.

Coxon, A. P. M., and Davies, P. M. (1989) Using structured sexual diaries data to estimate rates, predictors and context of high-risk sexual behaviour. Presented at the Fifth International Conference on AIDS, Montreal, June 4–9.

Coyle, S. L., Boruch, R. F., and Turner, C. F., eds. (1990) *Evaluating AIDS Prevention Programs, Expanded Edition.* Washington, D.C.: National Academy Press.

Crider, R. A. (1985) Heroin incidence: A trend comparison between National Household Survey data and indicator data. In B. A. Rouse, N. J. Kozel, and L. G. Richards, eds., *Self-Report Methods of Estimating Drug Use: Meeting Current Challenges to Validity.* DHHS Publication No. (ADM) 85–1402. National Institute on Drug Abuse Research Monograph No. 57. Washington, D.C.: U.S. Government Printing Office.

Criqui, M. H. (1979) Response bias and risk ratios in epidemiologic studies. *American Journal of Epidemiology* 109:394–399.

Cronbach, L. J., and Gleser, G. C. (1965) *Psychological Tests and Personnel Decisions.* 2nd ed. Urbana: University of Illinois Press.

Cynamon, M. L. (1989) The national survey of health and sexual behavior: The pretest experience. Presented at the Fifth International Conference on AIDS, Montreal, June 4–9.

Czaja, R. (1987–88) Asking sensitive behavioral questions in telephone surveys. *Applied Research and Evaluation* 8:23–32.

Daniel, W. W. (1975) Nonresponse in sociological surveys. *Sociological Methods and Research* 3:291–307.

Darrow, W. W., Jaffe, H. W., Thomas, P. A., Haverkos, H. W., Rogers, M. F., et al. (1986) Sex of interviewer, place of interview, and responses of homosexual men to sensitive questions. *Archives of Sexual Behavior* 15:79–88.

Davies, P. M. (1986) Some problems in defining and sampling non-heterosexual males. Working Paper No. 21. Social Research Unit, University College, Cardiff, Wales.

Davis, K. H., Hawks, R. L., and Blanke, R. V. (1988) Assessment of laboratory quality in urine drug testing. *Journal of the American Medical Association* 260:1749–1754.

Day, N., Houston-Hamilton, A., Taylor, D., Lemp, G., and Rutherford, G. (1989) Tracking survey of AIDS knowledge, attitudes and behaviors in San Francisco's Black communities. Presented at the Fifth International Conference on AIDS, Montreal, June 4–9.

De Gruttola, V., and Fineberg, H. V. (1989) Estimating prevalence of HIV infection. Considerations in the design and analysis of a national seroprevalence survey. *Journal of Acquired Immune Deficiency Syndromes* 2:472–480.

DeLamater, J. D. (1974) Methodological issues in the study of premarital sexuality. *Sociological Methods and Research* 3:30–61. DeLamater, J., and MacCorquodale, P. (1975) The effects of interview schedule variations on reported sexual behavior. *Sociological Methods and Research* 4:215–236.

DeLamater, J., and MacCorquodale, P. (1979) *Premarital Sexuality: Attitudes, Relationships, Behavior.* Madison, Wisc.: University of Wisconsin Press.

DeMaio, T. J., ed. (1984) *Approaches to Developing Questionnaires.* Statistical Policy Working Paper No. 10. Washington, D.C.: Office of Management and Budget.

DeMaio, T. J. (1984) Social desirability and survey measurement: A review. In C. F. Turner and E. Martin, eds., *Surveying Subjective Phenomena.* Vol. 2. New York: Russell Sage.

Derogatis, L. R. (1980) Psychological assessment of psychosexual functioning. *Psychiatric Clinics of North America* 3:113–131.

Derogatis, L. R., and Melisaratos, N. (1979) The DSFI: A multidimensional measure of sexual functioning. *Journal of Sex and Marital Therapy* 5:244–281.

Des Jarlais, D. C., and Friedman, S. R. (1988a) Intravenous cocaine, crack, and HIV infection. *Journal of the American Medical Association* 259:1945–1946.

Des Jarlais, D. C., and Friedman, S. R. (1988b) Needle sharing among IVDUs at risk for AIDS. *American Journal of Public Health* 78:1498.

Des Jarlais, D. C., and Friedman, S. R. (1988c) The psychology of preventing AIDS among intravenous drug users: A social learning conceptualization. *American Psychologist* 43:865–870.

Des Jarlais, D. C., Friedman, S. R., and Stoneburner, R. L. (1988) HIV infection and intravenous drug use: Critical issues in transmission dynamics, infection outcomes, and prevention. *Reviews of Infectious Diseases* 10:151–158.

Des Jarlais, D. C., Friedman, S. R., Sotheran, J. L., and Stoneburner, R. (1988) The sharing of drug injection equipment and the AIDS epidemic in New York City: The first decade. In R. J. Battjes and R. W. Pickens, eds., *Needle Sharing Among Intravenous Drug Abusers: National and International Perspectives.* National Institute on Drug Abuse Research Monograph 80. Washington, D.C.: U.S. Government Printing Office.

Des Jarlais, D. C., Tross, S., Abdul-Quader, A., Kouzi, A., and Friedman, S. R. (1989a) Intravenous drug users and maintenance of behavior change. Presented at the Fifth International Conference on AIDS, Montreal, June 4–9.

Des Jarlais, D. C., Hagen, H., Purchase, D., Reid, T., and Friedman, S. R. (1989b) Safer injection among participants in the first North American syringe exchange program. Presented at the Fifth International Conference on AIDS, Montreal, June 4–9.

Dougherty, J. A. (1988) Prevention of HIV transmission in IV drug users. Presented at the IV International Conference on AIDS, Stockholm, June 12–16.

Drug Enforcement Administration (DEA). (1988) *Crack cocaine availability and trafficking in the United States.* Washington, D.C.: U.S. Department of Justice. January.

Eckerman, W. C., Bates, J. D., Rachal, J. V., and Poole, W. K. (1971) *Drug Usage and Arrest Charges.* Washington, D.C.: Bureau of Narcotics and Dangerous Drugs.

Eisenberg, D. (1981) A scientific gold rush. *Science* 213:1104–1105.

Ericsson, K. A., and Simon, H. A. (1980) Verbal reports as data. *Psychological Review* 87:215–251.

Exner, T. M., Meyer-Bahlburg, H. F. L., Gruen, R. S., Ehrhardt, A. A., and Gorman, J. M. (1989) Peer norms for safer sex as a predictor of sexual risk behaviors in a cohort of gay men. Presented at the Fifth International Conference on AIDS, Montreal, June 4–9.

Eyre, S. L. (1989) Metaphors of AIDS: Social and existential function. Presented at the Annual Meeting of the American Anthropological Association, Washington, D.C., November 16–19.

Farmer, P. (1990) Sending sickness: Sorcery, politics, and changing concepts of AIDS in rural Haiti. *Medical Anthropology Quarterly* 4:6–27.

Farmer, P., and Kleinman, A. (1989) AIDS as human suffering. *Daedalus* 118:135–160.

Fay, R. E., Turner, C. F., Klassen, A. D., and Gagnon, J. H. (1989) Prevalence and patterns of same-gender sexual contact among men. *Science* 243:338–348.

Feldman, H. F., and Biernacki, P. (1988) The ethnography of needle sharing among intravenous drug users and implications for public policies and intervention strategies. In R. J. Battjes and R. W. Pickens, eds., *Needle Sharing Among Intravenous Drug Abusers: National and International Perspectives.* DHHS Publication No. (ADM) 88–1567. National Institute on Drug Abuse Research Monograph 80. Washington, D.C.: U.S. Government Printing Office.

Ferber, R. (1966) *The Reliability of Consumer Reports of Financial Assets and Debts.* Bureau of Economic and Business Research, University of Illinois, Urbana.

Fineberg, H. (1988) Education to prevent AIDS: Prospects and obstacles. *Science* 239:592–596.

Flaskerud, J. H., and Nyamathi, A. M. (1989) An AIDS education program for black and Latina women. Presented at the Fifth International AIDS Conference, Montreal, June 4–9.

Fowler, F. J., and Mangione, T. W. (1990) *Standardized Survey Interviewing.* Newbury Park, Calif: Sage.

Fox, J. A., and Tracy, P. E. (1986) *Randomized Response: A Method for Sensitive Surveys.* Beverly Hills, Calif: Sage Publications.

Franks, F. (1981) *Polywater.* Cambridge, Mass.: Massachusetts Institute of Technology Press.

Friedman, S. R., and Des Jarlais, D. C. (1989) *Measurement of Intravenous Drug Use Behaviors that Risk HIV Transmission.* Unpublished manuscript. Narcotic and Drug Research, Inc., New York.

Friedman, S. R., Sotheran, J. L., Abdul-Quader, A., Primm, B. J., Des Jarlais, D. C., et al. (1987a) The AIDS epidemic among blacks and Hispanics. *The Milbank Quarterly* 65:455–499.

Friedman, S. R., Des Jarlais, D. C., Sotheran, J. L., Garber, J., Cohen, H., and Smith, D. (1987b) AIDS and self-organization among intravenous drug users. *International Journal of the Addictions* 22:201–219.

Friedman, S. R., Dozier, C., Sterk, C., Williams, T., Sotheran, J. L., et al. (1988) Crack use puts women at risk for heterosexual transmission of HIV from intravenous drug users. Presented at the Fourth International Conference on AIDS, Stockholm, June 12–16.

Friedman, S. R., Rosenblum, A., Goldsmith, D., Des Jarlais, D. C., Sufian, M. , et al. (1989) Risk factors for HIV-1 infection among street-recruited intravenous drug users in New York City. Presented at the Fifth International Conference on AIDS, Montreal, June 4–9.

Fullilove, R. E. III, Fullilove, M. T., Bowser, B., and Gross, S. A. (1989) Crack use and risk for AIDS among black adolescents. Presented at the Fifth International Conference on AIDS, Montreal, June 4–9.

Fullilove, R. E., Fullilove, M. T., Bowser, B., and Gross, S. (In press) Crack users: The new AIDS risk group? *Journal of Cancer Prevention and Detection.*

Gagnon, J. H. (1988) Sex research and sexual conduct in the era of AIDS. *Journal on AIDS* 1:593–601.

Gawin, F. H., and Ellinwood, E. H., Jr. (1988) Cocaine and other stimulants: Actions, abuse, and treatment. *New England Journal of Medicine* 318:1173–1182.

Gebhard, P. H. (1972) Incidence of overt homosexuality in the United States and Western Europe. In National Institute of Mental Health Task Force on Homosexuality, *Final Report and Background Papers.* Washington, D.C.: U.S. Government Printing Office.

Gebhard, P. H., and Johnson, A. B. (1979) *The Kinsey Data: Marginal Tabulations of 1938–1963 Interviews Conducted by the Institute for Sex Research.* Philadelphia: W. B. Saunders.

Gelmon, K., Schechter, M. T., Sheps, S. B., Hershler, R., and Craib, K. J. P. (1989) Recall bias and memory failure: An empiric demonstration in persons with acquired immune deficiency syndrome. Presented at the Fifth International Conference on AIDS, Montreal, June 4–9.

Gibson, D., Wermuth, L., Sorensen, J. L., Menicucci, L., and Bernal, G. (1987) Approval need in self-reports of addicts and family members. *International Journal of the Addictions* 22:895–903.

Gibson, D. R., Sorensen, J. L., Lovelle-Drache, J., Catania, J., Kegeles, S., and Young, M. (1988) Psychosocial predictors of AIDS high risk behavior among intravenous drug users and their sexual partners. Presented at the Fourth International Conference on AIDS, Stockholm, June 12–16.

Gibson, D. R., Lovelle-Drache, J., Derby, S., Garcia-Soto, M., Sorensen, J. L., and Melese-d'Hospital, I. (1989) Brief counseling to reduce AIDS risk in IV drug users: Update. Presented at the Fifth International Conference on AIDS, Montreal, June 4–9.

Gonzalez, M., Ogus, J., Shapiro, G., and Tepping, B. (1975) Standards for discussion and presentation of errors in survey and census data. *Journal of the American Statistical Association* 70(351, whole pt. 2).

Goodstadt, M. S., and Gruson, V. (1975) The randomized response technique: A test on drug use. *Journal of the American Statistical Association* 70:814–818.

Goodstadt, M. S., Cook, G., and Gruson, V. (1978) The validity of reported drug use: The randomized response technique. *International Journal of the Addictions* 13:359–367.

Goyder, J. (1987) *The Silent Minority: Nonrespondents on Sample Surveys.* Cambridge, U.K.: Polity Press.

Groves, R. M., and Kahn, R. L. (1979) *Surveys by Telephone: A National Comparison with Personal Interviews.* New York: Academic Press.

Gulliksen, H. (1950) *Theory of Mental Tests.* New York: Wiley.

Haberman, P. W., Josephson, E., Zanes, A., and Ellinson, J. (1972) High school drug behavior: A methodological report on pilot studies. In S. Einstein and S. Allen, eds., *Proceedings of First International Conference on Student Drug Surveys.* New York: Baywood Publishing.

Hamid, A. (1990) The political economy of crack-related violence. *Contemporary Drug Problems* Spring 1990.

Hamilton, M. (1960) A rating scale for depression. *Journal of Neurological and Neurosurgical Psychiatry* 23:56–61.

Harbison, J. J. M., Graham, P. J., Quinn, J. T., McAllister, H., and Woodward, R. (1974) A questionnaire measure of sexual interest. *Archives of Sexual Behavior* 3:357–366.

Harrell, A. V. (1985) Validation of self-report: The research record. In B. A. Rouse, N. J. Kozel, and L. G. Richards, eds., *Self-Report Methods of Estimating Drug Use: Meeting Current Challenges to Validity.* National Institute on Drug Abuse Research Monograph No. 57. Washington, D.C.: U.S. Government Printing Office.

Heckert, K., Shultz, J., and Salem, N. (1989) The Minnesota general public AIDS survey: A behavioral risk factor survey supplement. Presented at the Fifth International Conference on AIDS, Montreal, June 4–9.

Heitzman, C. A., Sorensen, J. L., Gibson, D. R., Morales, E. R., Costantin, M., et al. (1989) AIDS prevention among IV drug users: Behaviors changes. Presented at the Annual Meeting of the Society of Behavioral Medicine, San Franciso, Calif.

Henson, R., Cannell, C. F., and Lawson, S. (1973) *Effects of Interviewer Style and Question Form on Reporting of Automobile Accidents.* Ann Arbor: Survey Research Center, University of Michigan.

Herb, F., Watters, J. K., Case, P., and Petitti, D. (1989) Endocarditis, subcutaneous abscesses, and other bacterial infections in intravenous drug users and their association with skin-cleaning at drug injection sites. Presented at the Fifth International Conference on AIDS, Montreal, June 4–9.

Herold, E. S., and Way, L. (1988) Sexual self-disclosure among university women. *Journal of Sex Research* 24:1–14.

Hesselbrock, M., Babor, T. F., Hesselbrock, V., Meyer, R. E., and Workman, K. (1983) Never believe an alcoholic? On the validity of self-report measures of alcohol dependence and related constructs. *International Journal of the Addictions* 18:593–609.

Himmelweit, H. T., and Turner, C. F. (1982) Social and psychological antecedents of depression. In P. Baltes and O. Brim, eds. *Life-span Development and Behavior.* New York: Academic Press.

Hingson, R. W., Strunin, L., Berlin, B. M., and Heeren, T. (1990) Beliefs about AIDS, use of alcohol, drugs and unprotected sex among Massachusetts adolescents. *American Journal of Public Health* 80:295-299.

Hingson, R. W., Strunin, L., Craven, D. E., Mofenson, L., Mangione, T., et al. (In press) Survey of AIDS knowledge and behavior changes among Massachusetts adults. *Preventive Medicine.*

Ho, C. Y., Powell, R. W., and Liley, P. E. (1974) Thermal conductivity of the elements: A comprehensive review. *Journal of Physical and Chemical Reference Data* 3:1–244.

Hochhauser, M. (1987) Readability of AIDS educational materials. Presented at the Annual Meeting of the American Psychological Association, New York, August.

Hofferth, S. L., Kahn, J. R., and Baldwin, W. (1987) Premarital sexual activity among U.S. teenage women over the past three decades. *Family Planning Perspectives* 19:46–53.

Hoon, E. F., Hoon P. W., and Wincze, J. P. (1976) An inventory for the measurement of female sexual arousability: The SAI. *Archives of Sexual Behavior* 5:291–300.

Huang, K. H. C., Watters, J. K., and Case, P. (1988) Psychological assessment and AIDS research with intravenous drug users: Challenges in measurement. *Journal of Psychoactive Drugs* 20:191–195.

Huang, K. H. C., Watters, J., and Case, P. (1989) Compliance with AIDS prevention measures among intravenous drug users: Health beliefs or social/environmental factors? Presented at the Fifth International Conference on AIDS, Montreal, June 4–9.

Hubbard, R. L, Marsden, M. E., and Allison, M. (1984) *Reliability and Validity of TOPS Data.* Research Triangle Park, N.C.: Research Triangle Institute.

Hubbard, R. L., Eckerman, W. C., Rachal, J. V. and Williams, J. R. (1977) Factors affecting the validity of self-reports of drug use: An overview. *Proceedings of the American Statistical Association (Social Statistics Section)* 1977:360–365. Chicago, Ill., August 15–18.

Hunter, J. S. (1977) Quality assessment of measurement methods. In National Research Council, *Environmental Monitoring,* Vol. 4a. Washington, D.C.: National Academy of Sciences.

Hunter, J. S. (1980) The national system of scientific measurement. *Science* 210:869–874.

Hyman, H. H., Cobb, W. J., Feldman, J. J., Hart, C. W., and Stember, C. H. (1954) *Interviewing in Social Research.* Chicago: University of Chicago Press.

Jabine, T. B., Straf, M. L., Tanur, J. M., Tourangeau, R., eds. (1985) *Cognitive Aspects of Survey Methodology.* Washington, D.C.: National Academy Press.

Jackson, D. D., Lee, W. B., and Liu, C. (1980) Aseismic uplift in southern California: An alternative interpretation. *Science* 210:534–536.

Jacobson, N. S., and Moore, D. (1981) Spouses as observers of the events in their relationship. *Consulting and Clinical Psychology* 49:269–277.

Johnson, A., Wadsworth, J., Elliot, P., Prior, L., Wallace, P., et al. (1989) A pilot study of sexual lifestyle in a random sample of the population of Great Britain. *AIDS* 3:135–141.

Johnston, L. D., and O'Malley, P. M. (1985) Issues of validity and population coverage in student surveys of drug use. In B. A. Rouse, N. J. Kozel, and L. G. Richards, eds., *Self-report methods of estimating drug use: Meeting current challenges to validity.* DHHS Publication No. (ADM) 85–1402. National Institute on Drug Abuse Research Monograph No. 57. Washington, D.C.: U.S. Government Printing Office.

Josephson, E. (1970) Resistance to community surveys. *Social Problems* 18:117–129.

Kahn, J. R., Kalsbeek, W. D., and Hofferth, S. L. (1988) National estimates of teenage sexual activity: Evaluating the comparability of three national surveys. *Demography* 25:189–204.

Kahn, R. L., and Cannell, C. F. (1957) *The Dynamics of Interviewing.* New York: Wiley.

Kane, S. (1989a) Heterosexuals, AIDS and the heroin subculture. Unpublished manuscript. Kane Agency, New York, N.Y.

Kane, S. (1989b) Interviews with two women: AIDS, addiction and hetero-sex on Chicago's south side. Unpublished manuscript. Kane Agency, New York, N.Y.

Kann, L., Nelson, G. D., Jones, J. T., and Kolbe, L. J. (1989) Establishing a system of complementary school-based surveys to annually assess HIV-related knowledge, beliefs, and behaviors among adolescents. *Journal of School Health* 59:55–58.

Kann, L., Nelson, G., Jones, J., and Kolbe, L. (1989) HIV-related knowledge, beliefs and behaviors among high school students in the United States. Presented at the Fifth International Conference on AIDS, Montreal, June 4–9.

Kaplan, H. B. (1989) Methodological problems in the study of psychosocial influences in the AIDS process. *Social Science and Medicine* 29:277–292.

Kaplan, H. B., Johnson, R. J., Bailey, C. A., and Simon, W. (1987) The sociological study of AIDS: A critical review of the literature and suggested research agenda. *Journal of Health and Social Behavior* 28:140–157.

Keeter, S., and Bradford, J. B. (1988) Knowledge of AIDS and related behavior change among unmarried adults in a low-prevalence city. *American Journal of Preventive Medicine* 4:146–152.

Kelly, J. A., St. Lawrence, J. S., Hood, H. V., and Brasfield, T. L. (1989) Behavioral intervention to reduce AIDS risk activities. *Journal of Consulting and Clinical Psychology* 57:60–67.

King, F. W. (1970) Psychology in action: Anonymous versus identifiable questionnaires in drug usage surveys. *American Psychologist* 25:982–985.

Kinsey, A. C., Pomeroy, W. B., and Martin, C. E. (1948) *Sexual Behavior in the Human Male.* Philadelphia: W. B. Saunders.

Kinsey, A. C., Pomeroy, W. B., Martin, C. E., and Gebhard, P. H. (1953) *Sexual Behavior in the Human Female.* Philadelphia: W. B. Saunders.

Kipke, M. D., and Drucker, E. (1988) A method for assessing needle-sharing behavior in intravenous drug users. Presented at the Fourth International Conference on AIDS, Stockholm, June 12–16.

Klassen, A. D., Williams, C. J., and Levitt, E. E. (1989) *Sex and Morality in the U.S.,* edited by H. J. O'Gorman. Middletown, Conn.: Wesleyan University Press.

Klassen, A. D., Williams, C. J., Levitt, E. E., Miniot-Rudkin L., Miller H., and Gunjal, S. (1989) Trends in premarital sexual behavior. In C. F. Turner, H. G. Miller, and L. E. Moses, eds., *AIDS, Sexual Behavior, and Intravenous Drug Use.* Washington, D.C.: National Academy Press.

Koblin, B., McCusker, J., Lewis, B., Sullivan, J., Birch, F., and Hagen, H. (1988) Racial differences in HIV infection in IVDUs. Presented at the Fourth International Conference on AIDS, Stockholm, June 12–16.

Koester, S. (1989a) The risk of HIV transmission from sharing water, drug-mixing containers and cotton filters among intravenous drug users. Unpublished manuscript. University of Colorado School of Medicine, Boulder, Colo.

Koester, S. (1989b) When push comes to shove: Poverty, law enforcement and high risk behavior. Unpublished manuscript. University of Colorado School of Medicine, Boulder, Colo.

Koss, M. P., and Gidycz, C. A. (1985) Sexual experiences survey: Reliability and validity. *Journal of Consulting and Clinical Psychology* 53:422–423.

Lange, W. R., Snyder, F. R., Lozovsky, E., Kaistha, V., Jaffe, J. H., et al. (1988) Geographic distribution of human immunodeficiency virus markers in parenteral drug abusers. *American Journal of Public Health* 78:443–446.

Leach, C., Viker, S., Kuhls, T., Parris, N., Cherry, J., and Christenson, P. (1989) Changes in sexual behavior of a cohort of female health care workers during the AIDS era. Presented at the Fifth International Conference on AIDS, Montreal, June 4–9.

Leonard, T. L. (1990) Male clients of female street prostitutes: Unseen partners in sexual disease transmission. *Medical Anthropology Quarterly* 4:41–55.

Lessler, J., Tourangeau, R., and Salter, W. (1989) Questionnaire design in the cognitive research laboratory. *Vital and Health Statistics* Series 6, Whole No. 1.

Lever, J., Rogers, W. H., Carson, S., Hertz, R., and Kanouse, D. E. (1989) Behavioral patterns of bisexual males in the U.S., 1982. Presented at the Fifth International Conference on AIDS, Montreal, June 4–9.

Levinger, G. (1966) Systematic distortion in spouses' reports of preferred and actual sexual behavior. *Sociometry* 29:291–299.

Lide, D. R., Jr. (1981) Critical data for critical needs. *Science* 212:1343–1349.

Loftus, E. F. (1975) Leading questions and the eyewitness report. *Cognitive Psychology* 7:560–572.

Loftus, E. F., and Marburger, W. (1983) Since the eruption of Mt. St. Helens, has anyone beaten you up? Improving the accuracy of retrospective reports with landmark events. *Memory and Cognition* 11:114–120.

Loftus, E. F., and Palmer, J. C. (1974) Reconstruction of automobile destruction: An example of the interaction between language and memory. *Journal of Verbal Learning and Verbal Behavior* 13:585–589.

LoPiccolo, J., and Steger, J. C. (1974) The sexual interaction inventory: A new instrument for assessment of sexual dysfunction. *Archives of Sexual Behavior* 3:585–595.

Luetgert, M. J., and Armstrong, A. H. (1973) Methodological issues in drug usage surveys: Anonymity, recency, and frequency. *International Journal of the Addictions* 8:683–689.

MacKuen, M. B. (1981) Social communication and the mass policy agenda. In M. B. MacKuen and S. L. Coombs, eds., *More than News: Media Power in Public Affairs.* Beverly Hills, Calif.: Sage.

MacKuen, M. B. (1984) Reality, the press, and citizens' political agendas. In C. F. Turner and E. Martin, eds., *Surveying Subjective Phenomena.* Vol. 2. New York: Russell Sage.

MacKuen, M. B. and Turner, C. F. (1984) The popularity of presidents: 1963–80. In C. F. Turner and E. Martin, eds., *Surveying Subjective Phenomena.* Vol. 2. New York: Russell Sage..

Maddux, J., and Desmond, D. (1975) Reliability and validity of information from chronic heroin users. *Journal of Psychiatric Research* 12:87–95.

Madow, W. G., Nisselson, H., and Olkin, I., eds. (1983) *Incomplete Data in Sample Surveys. Vol. 1, Report and Case Studies; Vol. 2, Theory and Bibliographies; Vol. 3, Proceedings of the Symposium.* New York: Academic Press.

Magura, S., Goldsmith, D., Casriel, C., Goldstein, P. J., and Lipton, D. S. (1987) The validity of methadone clients' self-reported drug use. *International Journal of the Addictions* 22:727–749.

Maisto, S. A., and O'Farrell, T. J. (1985) Comment on the validity of Watson et al.'s "Do alcoholics give valid self-reports?" *Journal of Studies on Alcohol* 46:447–453.

Maisto, S. A., Sobell, L. C., and Sobell, M. B. (1982–83) Corroboration of drug abusers' self-reports through the use of multiple data sources. *American Journal of Drug and Alcohol Abuse* 9:301–308.

Marasca, G., D'Arcangelo, E., De Candido, D., Della Giusta, G., Liseo, B., et al. (1989) Sexual behaviour and HIV related knowledge among a random sample of young population of Italy. Presented at the Fifth International Conference on AIDS, Montreal, June 4–9.

Marks, I. M., and Sartorius, N. H. (1968) A contribution to the measurement of sexual attitude. *Journal of Nervous and Mental Disease* 145:441–451.

Marshall, P., O'Keefe, J. P., Fisher, S. G., Caruso, A. J., and Surdukowski, J. (In press) Patients' fear of contracting AIDS from physicians. *Medical Anthropology Quarterly.*

Martin, J. L., and Vance, C. S. (1984) Behavioral and psychosocial factors in AIDS: Methodological and substantive issues. *American Psychologist* 39:1303–1308.

Mason, T. (1988) AIDS prevention among black IV drug users and their sexual partners in a Baltimore public housing project. Presented at the First International Symposium on Information and Education on AIDS, Ixtapa, Mexico, October 18.

Mason, T. (1989) The politics of culture: Drug users, professionals, and the meaning of needle sharing. Presented at the Annual Meeting of the Society for Applied Anthropology, Santa Fe, April.

Mason, T. (In press) A preliminary look at social and economic dynamics influencing drug markets, drug use patterns, and HIV risk behaviors among injecting drug users in two Baltimore networks. In *Proceedings of the Community Epidemiology Work Group: Chicago, Illinois, June 1989.* National Institute on Drug Abuse, Division of Epidemiology and Statistical Analysis, Rockville, Md.

May, R. M., and Anderson, R. M. (1987) Transmission dynamics of HIV infection. *Nature* 326:137–142.

May, R. M., Anderson, R. M., and Blower, S. M. (1989) The epidemiology and transmission dynamics of HIV-AIDS. *Daedalus* 118:163–201.

McCombie, S. C. (1986) The cultural impact of the AIDS test: The American experience. *Social Science and Medicine* 23:455–459.

McCombie, S. C. (1989) Rituals of infection control among health care workers. Unpublished manuscript. Annenberg School of Communications, University of Pennsylvania.

McCombie, S. C. (1990) Patterns of condom use in Trinidad and Tobago. Unpublished manuscript. Annenberg School of Communications, University of Pennsylvania.

McGlothlin, W. H., Anglin, M. D., and Wilson, B. D. (1977) *An Evaluation of the California Civil Addict Program.* Rockville, Md.: National Institute on Drug Abuse.

McLaws, M. L., McGirr, J., Croker, W., and Cooper, D. A. (1988) Risk factors for HIV and HBV infections in intravenous drug users. Presented at the Fourth International Conference on AIDS, Stockholm, June 12–16.

McNemar, Q. (1946) Opinion-attitude methodology. *Psychological Bulletin* 43:289–374.

Means, B., Nigam, A. Zarrow, M., Loftus, E. F., and Donaldson, M. S. (1989) Autobigraphical Memory for health related events. *Vital and Health Statistics* Series 6, Whole No. 1.

Michael, R. T., Laumann, E. O., Gagnon, J. H., and Smith, T. W. (1988) Number of sex partners and potential risk of sexual exposure to human immunodeficiency virus. *Mortality and Morbidity Weekly Report* 37:565–568.

Millstein, S., and Irwin, C. (1983) Acceptability of computer-acquired sexual histories in adolescent girls. *Journal of Pediatrics* 103:815–819.

Minkoff, H., McCalla, S., Delke, I., Feldman, J., Stevens, R., and Salwen, M. (1989) Cocaine use and sexually transmitted diseases including HIV. Presented at the Fifth International Conference on AIDS, Montreal, June 4–9.

Moatti, J. P., Tavares, J., Durbec, J. P., Bajos, N., Menard, C., and Serrand, C. (1989) Modifications of sexual behavior due to AIDS in French heterosexual "at risk" population. Presented at the Fifth International Conference on AIDS, Montreal, June 4–9.

Mooney, H. W., Pollack, B. R., and Corsa, L. (1968) Use of telephone interviewing to study human reproduction. *Public Health Reports* 83:1049–1060.

Moser, C. A., and Kalton, G. (1972) *Survey Methods in Social Investigation.* 2d ed. New York: Basic.

Moss, A. R., Bacchetti, P., Osmond, D., Meakin, R., Keffelew, A., and Gorter, R. (1989) Seroconversion for HIV in intravenous drug users in San Francisco. Presented at the Fifth International Conference on AIDS, Montreal, June 4–9.

Mukherjee, B. N. (1975) Reliability estimates of some survey data on family planning. *Population Studies* 29:127–142.

Myers, V. (1977a) Survey methods for minority populations. *The Journal of Social Issues* 33:11–19.

Myers, V. (1977b) Toward a synthesis of ethnographic and survey methods. *Human Organization* 36:244–251.

National Research Council (NRC). (1979) *Privacy and Confidentiality as Factors in Survey Response.* Washington, D.C.: National Academy of Sciences.

Needle, R. H., Jou, S., and Su, S. S. (1989) The impact of changing methods of data collection on the reliability of self-reported drug use of adolescents. *American Journal of Drug and Alcohol Abuse* 15:275–289.

Needle, R., McCubbin, H., Lorence, J., and Hochhauser, M. (1983) Reliability and validity of adolescent self-reported drug use in a family-based study: A methodological report. *International Journal of the Addictions* 18:901–912.

Neisser, U. (1981) John Dean's memory: A case study. *Cognition* 9:1–22.

Newcomer, S., and Udry, J. R. (1988) Adolescents' honesty in a survey of sexual behavior. *Journal of Adolescent Research* 3:419–423.

Newman, R. G., Cates, M., Tytun A., and Werbell, B. (1976) Reliability of self-reported age of first drug use: Analysis of New York City narcotics register data. *International Journal of the Addictions* 11:611–618.

Newmeyer, J. A. (1988) Why bleach? Development of a strategy to combat HIV contagion among San Francisco intravenous drug users. In R. J. Battjes, and R. W. Pickens, eds., *Needle Sharing Among Intravenous Drug Abusers: National and International Perspectives.* DHHS Publication No. (ADM) 88–1567. National Institute on Drug Abuse Research Monograph 80. Washington, D.C.: U.S. Government Printing Office.

Nisbett, R. E., and Wilson, T. D. (1977) Telling more than we can know: Verbal reports on mental processes. *Psychological Review* 84:231–259.

Novick, D. M., Trigg, H. L., Des Jarlais, D. C., Friedman, S. R., Vlahov, D., et al. (1989) Drug abuse patterns and ethnicity in IVDA during the early years of the HIV epidemic. Presented at the Fifth International Conference on AIDS, Montreal, June 4–9.

Nurco, D. N. (1985) A discussion of validity. In B. A. Rouse, N. J. Kozel, and L. G. Richards, eds., *Self-Report Methods of Estimating Drug Use: Meeting Current Challenges to Validity.* DHHS Publication No. (ADM) 85–1402. National Institute on Drug Abuse Research Monograph No. 57. Washington, D.C.: U.S. Government Printing Office.

Oetting, E. R., Edwards, R., and Beauvais, F. (1985) Reliability and discriminant validity of the children's drug-use survey. *Psychological Reports* 56:751–756.

O'Reilly, K. R. (1989) Risk behaviors and their determinants. In R. Kulstad, ed., *AIDS 1988: American Association for the Advancement of Science Symposia Papers.* Washington, D. C.: American Association for the Advancement of Science.

Page, B. P., Chitwood, D. D., Smith, P. C., Kane, N., and McBride, D. C. (1990) Intravenous drug use and HIV infection in Miami. *Medical Anthropology Quarterly* 4:56–71.

Page, W. F., Davies, J. E., Ladner, R. A., Alfassa, J., and Tennis, H. (1977) Urinalysis screened versus verbally reported drug use: The identification of discrepant groups. *International Journal of the Addictions* 12:439–450.

Parker, R. (1987) Acquired immunodeficiency syndrome in urban Brazil. *Medical Anthropology Quarterly* 1:155–175.

Parker, R. (1989) Bodies and pleasures. Erotic meanings in contemporary Brazil. *Anthropology and Humanism Quarterly* 14:58–64.

Pearson, R. W., Ross, M., and Dawes, R. (1989) A theory of personal recall and the limits of retrospection in surveys. Unpublished manuscript. Social Science Research Council, August 1, 1989.

Pelto, P., and Pelto, G. (1978) *Anthropological Research: The Structure of Enquiry.* London: Cambridge University Press.

Peterson, J. L., and Bakeman, R. (1989) AIDS and IV drug use among ethnic minorities. *Journal of Drug Issues* 19:27–37.

Petzel, T. P., Johnson, J. E., and McKillip, J. (1973) Response bias in drug surveys. *Journal of Consulting and Clinical Psychology* 40:437–439.

Podell, L., and Perkins, J. C. (1957) A Guttman scale for sexual experience—A methodological note. *Journal of Abnormal and Social Psychology* 54:420-422.

Poti, S. J., Chakraborti, B., and Malaker, C. R. (1960) Reliability of data relating to contraceptive practices. In C. V. Kiser, ed., *Research In Family Planning*. Princeton: Princeton University Press.

Public Health Service (PHS). (1988) Report of the Second Public Health Service AIDS Prevention and Control Conference. *Public Health Reports* 103, Supplement No. 1.

Quart, A. M., Small, C. B., and Klein, R. S. (1989) Local destruction of labial surface of mandibular teeth by direct application of cocaine in drug users with AIDS. Presented at the Fifth International Conference on AIDS, Montreal, June 4–9.

Reining, P. (1989) Male circumcision status in relationship to seroprevalence data in Africa: A review of method. Unpublished manuscript. Department of Anthropology Catholic University.

Research Triangle Institute (RTI). (1989) *National Household Seroprevalence Survey: Pilot Study Report*. Research Triangle Park, N.C.: Research Triangle Institute.

Robertson, J. R., Skidmore, C. A., and Roberts, J. J. K (1988) HIV infection in intravenous drug users: A follow-up study indicating changes in risk-taking behaviour. *British Journal of Addiction* 83:387–391.

Robinson, T. W., Davies, P., and Beveridge, S. (1989) Sexual practices and condom use amongst male prostitutes in London: Differences between streetworking and non-streetworking prostitutes. Presented at the Fifth International Conference on AIDS, Montreal, June 4–9.

Rodgers, J. L., Billy, J. O. G., and Udry, J. R. (1982) The rescission of behaviors: Inconsistent responses in adolescent sexuality data. *Social Science Research* 11:280–296.

Rolnick, S. J., Gross, C. R., Garrard, J., and Gibson, R. W. (1989) A comparison of response rate, data quality, and cost in the collection of data on sexual history and personal behaviors. *American Journal of Epidemiology* 129:1052–1061.

Rossi, P. H., Wright, J. D., and Anderson, A. B., eds. (1983) *Handbook of Survey Research*. New York: Academic Press.

Rounsaville, B., Kleber, H. D., Wilber, C., Rosenberger, D., and Rosenberger, P. (1981) Comparisons of opiate addicts' reports of psychiatric history with reports of significant-other informants'. *American Journal of Drug and Alcohol Abuse* 8:51–69.

Rouse, B. A., Kozel, N. J., and Richards, L. G., eds. (1985) *Self-Report Methods of Estimating Drug Use: Meeting Current Challenges to Validity*. National Institute on Drug Abuse Research Monograph No. 57. Washington, D.C.: U.S. Government Printing Office.

Saltzman, S. P., Stoddard, A. M., McCusker, J., Moon, M. W., and Mayer, K. H. (1987) Reliability of self-reported sexual behavior risk factors for HIV infection in homosexual men. *Public Health Reports* 102:692–697.

Schaeffer, N. C. and Thomson, E. (1989) The discovery of grounded uncertainty: Developing standardized questions about strength of fertility motivation. Center for Demography and Ecology Working paper No. 88–19. Madison, Wisc.: Center for Demography and Ecology, University of Wisconsin.

Schiavi, R. C., Derogatis, L. R., Kuriansky, J., O'Connor, D., and Sharpe, L. (1979) The assessment of sexual function and marital interaction. *Journal of Sex and Marital Therapy* 5:169–224.

Schilling, R. F., Schinke, S. P., Nichols, S. E., Zayas, L. H., Miller, S. O., et al. (1989) Developing strategies for AIDS prevention research with black and Hispanic drug users. *Public Health Reports* 104:2–11.

Schmidt, K. W., Krasnik, A., Brendstrup, E., Zoffman, H., and Larsen, S. O. (1988) Occurrence of sexual behaviour related to the risk of HIV-infection. *Danish Medical Bulletin* 36:84–88.

Schoepf, B. G., Walu, E., Rukarangira, Wn., Payanzo, N., and Schoepf, C. (In press) Action research on AIDS with women in Central Africa. *Social Science and Medicine.*

Schofield, M. (1965) *The Sexual Behavior of Young People.* Boston: Little, Brown, and Co.

Schuman, H. and Presser, S. (1981) *Questions and Answers in Attitude Surveys: Experiments in Question Form, Wording, and Context.* New York: Academic Press.

Seage, G. R., III, Mayer, K. H., Horsburgh, C. R., Cai, B., and Lamb, G. A. (1989) Validation of sexual histories of homosexual male couples. Presented at the Fifth International Conference on AIDS, Montreal, June 4–9.

Siegel, K., and Bauman, L. J. (1986) Methodological issues in AIDS-related research. In D. A. Feldman and T. M. Johnson, eds., *The Social Dimensions of AIDS: Method and Theory.* New York: Praeger. Single, E., Kandel, D. B., and Johnson, B. D. (1975) The reliability and validity of drug use responses in a large scale longitudinal survey. *Journal of Drug Issues* 5:426–443.

Skinner, H. A., and Allen, B. A. (1983) Does the computer make a difference? Computerized versus face-to-face self-report assessment of alcohol, drug, and tobacco use. *Journal of Consulting and Clinical Psychology* 51:267–275.

Smith, A. F., Jobe, J. B., and Mingay, D. J. (In press) Retrieval from memory of dietary information. *Applied Cognitive Psychology.*

Smith, T. W. (1988) *A Methodological Review of the Sexual Behavior Questions on the 1988 General Social Survey (GSS).* GSS Methodological Report No. 58, National Opinion Research Center: University of Chicago.

Sorensen, J. L., and Leder, D. (1978) Measuring the readability of written information for clients. In G. Landsberg, W. D. Neigher, R. J. Hammer, C. Windle, and J. R. Woy, eds., *Evaluation in Practice: A Sourcebook of Program Evaluation Studies from Mental Health Care Systems in the United States.* DHEW Publication No. (ADM) 78–763. Washington, D.C.: U.S. Government Printing Office.

Sorensen, J. L., Gibson, D., Heitzmann, C., Calvillo, A., Dumontet, R., et al. (1988) Pilot trial of small group AIDS education with IV drug abusers (abstract). In L. S. Harris, ed., *Problems of Drug Dependence 1988: Proceedings of the 50th Annual Scientific Meeting, Committee on the Problems of Drug Dependence.* National Institute on Drug Abuse, Research Monograph 90. Washington, D.C.: U.S. Government Printing Office.

Sorensen, J. L., Gibson, D. R. , Heitzmann, C., Dumontet, R., London, J., et al. (1989a) AIDS prevention: Behavioral outcomes with outpatient drug abusers. Presented at the Annual Meeting of the American Psychological Association, New Orleans, La.

Sorensen, J. L., Guydish, J., Costantini, M., and Batki, S. L. (1989b) Changes in needle sharing and syringe cleaning among San Francisco Drug Abusers. *New England Journal of Medicine* 320:807.

Sorensen, J. L., Batki, S. L., Gibson, D. R., Dumontet, R., and Purnell, S. (1989c) Methadone maintenance and behavior change in seropositive drug abusers: The San Francisco General Hospital Program for AIDS Counseling and Education (PACE). Presented at the Fifth International Conference on AIDS, Montreal, June 4–9.

Spencer, B. D. (1989) On the accuracy of current estimates of the numbers of intravenous drug users. In C. F. Turner, H. G. Miller, and L. E. Moses, eds., *AIDS, Sexual Behavior, and Intravenous Drug Use.* Washington, D.C.: National Academy Press.

Spencer, L., Faulkner, A., and Keegan, J. (1988) *Talking About Sex.* (Publication P.5997), London: Social and Community Planning Research.

Steger, K., Comella, B., Forbes, J., McLoughlin, R., Hoff, R. A., and Craven, D. E. (1989) Use of a fingerstick paper-absorbed blood sample for HIV serosurveys in intravenous drug users. Presented at the Fifth International Conference on AIDS, Montreal, June 4–9.

Stephens, R. (1972) The truthfulness of addict respondents in research projects. *International Journal of the Addictions* 7:549–558.

Sterk, C. (1989) Fieldwork among prostitutes in the AIDS era. In C. Smith and W. Kornblum, eds., *In the Field: Readings on the Field Research Experience.* New York: Praeger.

Stimson, G. V., Donoghoe, M., Alldritt, L., and Dolan, K. (1988a) HIV transmission risk behaviours of clients attending syringe-exchange schemes in England and Scotland. *British Journal of Addiction* 83:1449–1455.

Stimson, G. V., Alldritt, L. J., Dolan, K. A., Donoghoe, M. C., and Lart, R. A. (1988b) *Injecting Equipment Exchange Schemes: Final Report.* London: Monitoring Research Group, Goldsmiths' College.

Strunin, L., and Hingson, R. (1987) Acquired immunodeficiency syndrome and adolescents: Knowledge, beliefs, attitudes, and behaviors. *Pediatrics* 79:825–828.

Sudman, S., and Bradburn, N. M. (1974) *Response Effects in Surveys.* Chicago: Aldine.

Sundet, J. M., Kvalem, I. L., Magnus, P., Grommesby, J.K., Stigum, H., and Bakketeig, L. S. (1989) The relationship between condom use and sexual behavior. Presented at the Fifth International Conference on AIDS, Montreal, June 4–9.

Tracy, P. E., and Fox, J. A. (1981) The validity of randomized response for sensitive measurements. *American Sociological Review* 46:187–200.

Traeen, B., Rise, J., and Kraft, P. (1989) Condom behavior in 17, 18 and 19 year-old Norwegians. Presented at the Fifth International Conference on AIDS, Montreal, June 4–9.

Tross, S., Abdul-Quader, A., Des Jarlais, D. C., Kouzi, A., and Friedman, S. R. (1989) Determinants of sexual risk reduction in female IV drug users recruited from the street. Presented at the Fifth International Conference on AIDS, Montreal, June 4–9.

Tucker, C., Vitrano, F., Miller, L., and Doddy, J. (1989) Cognitive issues and research on the consumer expenditure diary survey. Presented at the 1989 Annual Meetings of the American Association for Public Opinion Research, St. Petersburg, Fla., May.

Turner, C. F. (1978) Fallible indicators of the subjective state of the nation. *American Psychologist* 33:456–470.

Turner, C. F. (1984) Why do surveys disagree? Some preliminary hypotheses and some disagreeable examples. In C. F. Turner and E. Martin, eds., *Surveying Subjective Phenomena*. Vol. 2. New York: Russell Sage.

Turner, C. F. (1989) Research on sexual behaviors that transmit HIV: Progress and problems. *AIDS* 3:563–569.

Turner, C. F., and Fay, R. E. (1987/1989) Monitoring the spread of HIV infection. Background paper for ad hoc advisory group, Centers for Disease Control. Atlanta, Ga., July 7, 1987. Reprinted in C. F. Turner, H. G. Miller, and L. E. Moses, eds., (1989) *AIDS, Sexual Behavior, and Intravenous Drug Use*. Washington, D.C.: National Academy Press.

Turner, C. F., and Martin, E., eds. (1984) *Surveying Subjective Phenomena*. Two volumes. New York: Russell Sage.

Turner, C. F., Miller, H. G., and Barker, L. F. (1989) AIDS research and the behavioral and social sciences. In R. Kulsad, ed., *AIDS, 1988: AAAS Symposium Papers*. Washington, D.C.: American Association for the Advancement of Science.

Turner, C. F., Miller, H. G., and Moses, L. E., eds. (1989) *AIDS, Sexual Behavior, and Intravenous Drug Use*. Washington, D.C.: National Academy Press.

Udry, J. R., and Morris, N. M. (1967) A method for validation of reported sexual data. *Journal of Marriage and the Family* 29:442–446.

Vessey, M. P., Johnson, B., and Donnelly, J. (1974) Reliability of reporting by women taking part in a prospective contraceptive study. *British Journal of Preventive and Social Medicine* 28:104–107.

Vinokur, A., Oksenberg, L., and Cannell, C. F. (1977) Effects of feedback and reinforcement on the report of health information. In C. F. Cannell, L. Oksenberg, and J. M. Converse, eds., *Experiments in Interviewing Techniques*. Washington, D.C.: National Center for Health Surveys Research.

Wagennar, W. A. (1986) My memory: A study of autobiographical memory over six years. *Cognitive Psychology* 18:225–252.

Waterton, J. J., and Duffy, J. C. (1984) A comparison of computer interviewing techniques and traditional methods in the collection of self-report alcohol consumption data in a field survey. *International Statistical Review* 52:173–182.

Watson, C. G. (1985) More reasons for a moratorium: A reply to Maisto and O'Farrell. *Journal of Studies on Alcohol* 46:450–453.

Watters, J. K. (1989) Observations on the importance of social context in HIV transmission among intravenous drug users. *Journal of Drug Issues* 19:9–26.

Webb, E. J., Campbell, D. T., Schwartz, R. D., and Sechrest, L. (1966) *Unobtrusive Measures: Nonreactive Research in the Social Sciences*. Chicago: Rand McNally.

Weibel, W. W. (In press) Combining ethnographic and epidemiologic methods in targeted AIDS interventions: The Chicago model. In *Needle Sharing Among Intravenous Drug Abusers: National and International Perspectives*. National Institute on Drug Abuse Monograph 80. Washington, D.C.: U.S. Government Printing Office.

Wells, J. A., Wilensky, G. R., Valleron, A. J., Bond, G., Sell, R. L., and DeFilippes, P. (1989a) Population prevalence of AIDS high risk behaviors in France, the United Kingdom and the United States. Presented at the Fifth International Conference on AIDS, Montreal, June 4–9.

Wells, J. A., Sell, R. L., Will, A., and DeFilippes, P. (1989b) Readability analysis of AIDS brochures and pamphlets from the United States. Presented at the Fifth International Conference on AIDS, Montreal, June 4–9.

Wermuth, L., and Ham, J. (1989) Women don't wear condoms: Coping with AIDS risk among women partners of intravenous drug users. Presented at the Annual Meeting of the American Sociological Association, San Francisco, Calif.

Whitehead, P. C., and Smart, R. G. (1972) Validity and reliability of self-reported drug use. *Canadian Journal of Criminology and Corrections* 14:83–89.

Wigdor, A. K., and Garner, W. R., eds. (1982) *Ability Testing*. Two vols. Washington, D.C.: National Academy Press.

Wiley, J. (1989) *Studying Nonreponse in the AMEN Cohort Survey* (unpublished notes). Survey Research Center, University of California at Berkeley, July.

Winkelstein, W., Jr., Samuel, M., Padian, N. S., Wiley, J. A., Lang, W., et al. (1987a) The San Francisco Men's Health Study. III. Reduction in human immunodeficiency virus transmission among homosexual/bisexual men, 1982–1986. *American Journal of Public Health* 77:685–689.

Winkelstein, W., Jr., Samuel, M., Padian, N. S., and Wiley, J. A. (1987b) Selected sexual practices of San Francisco heterosexual men and risk of infection by the human immunodeficiency virus. *Journal of the American Medical Association* 257:1470–1471.

Winkelstein, W., Jr., Lyman, D. M., and Padian, N. S. (1987c) Sexual practices and risk of infection by the AIDS-associated retrovirus: The San Francisco Men's Health Study. *Journal of the American Medical Association* 257:321–325.

Wish, E., Johnson, B., Strug, D., Chedekel, M., and Lipton, D. (1983) *Are Urine Tests Good Indicators of the Validity of Self-Reports of Drug Use? It Depends on the Test.* New York: Narcotic and Drug Research, Inc.

Wolk, J. S., Wodak, A., and Guinan, J. (1989) The effect of a needle and syringe exchange on a methadone maintenance unit. Presented at the Fifth International Conference on AIDS, Montreal, June 4–9.

Wolk, J. S., Wodak, A., Guinan, J. J., Morlet, A., Gold, J., et al. (1988) HIV seroprevalence in syringes of intravenous drug users using syringe exchanges in Sydney, Australia, 1987. Presented at the Fourth International Conference on AIDS, Stockholm, June 12–16.

Woodward, J. A., Retka, R. L., and Nig, L. (1984) Construct validity of heroin abuse estimators. *International Journal of Addictions* 19:93–117.

World Health Organization: Global Programme on AIDS (1988) *Progress Report No. 4.* Geneva: World Health Organization.

Worth, D. (1989) Sexual decisionmaking and AIDS: Why condom promotion among vulnerable women is likely to fail. Presented at the Population Council, New York. March 7.

Wyatt, G. E., and Peters, S. D. (1986) Methodological considerations in research on the prevalence of child sexual abuse. *Child Abuse and Neglect* 10:241–251.

Youden, W. (1961) How to evaluate accuracy. *Materials Research and Standards* 1:268–271.

Youden, W., and Steiner, E., eds. (1975) *Statistical Manual of the Association of Official Analytical Chemists.* Washington, D.C.: Association of Official Analytical Chemists.

Zelnik, M., and Kantner, J. F. (1980) Sexual activity, contraceptive use and pregnancy among metropolitan-area teenagers: 1971–1979. *Family Planning Perspectives* 12:230–237.

Zeugin, P., Dubois-Arber, F., Hausser, D., and Lehmann, P. H. (1989) Sexual behaviour of young adults and the effects of AIDS-prevention campaigns in Switzerland. Presented at the Fifth International Conference on AIDS, Montreal, June 4–9 .

Zich, J., and Temoshok, L. (1986) Applied methodology: A primer of pitfalls and opportunities in AIDS research. In D. A. Feldman and T. M. Johnson, eds., *The Social Dimensions of AIDS: Method and Theory.* New York: Praeger.

Zuckerman, M. (1973) Scales for sex experience for males and females. *Journal of Consulting and Clinical Psychology* 41:27–29.

Zuckerman, M., Tushup, R., and Finner, S. (1976) Sexual attitudes and experience: Attitude and personality correlates and changes produced by a course in sexuality. *Journal of Consulting and Clinical Psychology* 44:7–19.

Zuckerman, B. S., Hingson, R. W., Morelock, S., Amaro, H., Frank, D., et al. (1985) A pilot study assessing maternal marijuana use by urine assay during pregnancy. In B. A. Rouse, N. J. Kozel, and L. G. Richards, eds., *Self-Report Methods of Estimating Drug Use: Meeting Current Challenges to Validity.* DHHS Publication No. (ADM) 85–1402. National Institute on Drug Abuse Research Monograph No. 57. Washington, D.C.: U.S. Government Printing Office.

Appendix

TABLE A Number of Sexual Partners in the Last Year by Gender, Marital Status, and Age from the 1987 Telephone Survey Conducted by the *Los Angeles Times* (LAT) and the 1988 Personal Interview Survey Conducted by the National Opinion Research Center (NORC). (From Turner, Miller, and Moses [1989]:106-107].)

| | | Number of Sexual Partners in Last Year | | | | | |
		None	1	2	3 +	Total	(N)
Unmarried men							
18–24	LAT	14.1%	38.6%	8.7%	38.6%	100%	(83)
	NORC	19.6	24.0	12.8	43.6	100	(68)
	Comb. fit	16.5	32.3	10.5	40.7	100	(151)
	(s.e.)	(4.8)	(5.9)	(3.5)	(5.8)		
25–34	LAT	8.1	61.3	8.1	22.5	100	(99)
	NORC	17.9	41.9	7.7	32.5	100	(63)
	Comb. fit	12.4	52.9	7.9	26.9	100	(162)
	(s.e.)	(3.7)	(6.4)	(2.3)	(4.5)		
35–49	LAT	3.7	34.3	22.2	39.9	100	(64)
	NORC	20.3	44.3	15.2	20.3	100	(59)
	Comb. fit	13.5	39.7	18.2	28.5	100	(123)
	(s.e.)	(4.8)	(6.3)	(4.0)	(5.4)		
50–64	LAT	13.9	44.4	6.3	35.4	100	(43)
	NORC	50.0	30.8	11.5	7.7	100	(21)
	Comb. fit	22.3	41.3	7.5	29.0	100	(64)
	(s.e.)	(5.8)	(11.3)	(3.6)	(9.0)		
65 +	LAT	80.0	12.2	5.5	2.3	100	(37)
	NORC	61.1	27.8	2.8	8.3	100	(30)
	Comb. fit	74.0	17.2	4.6	4.2	100	(67)
	(s.e.)	(6.4)	(5.3)	(3.0)	(2.1)		
Unmarried women							
18–24	LAT	16.3	56.1	10.4	17.3	100	(112)
	NORC	23.5	47.9	16.8	11.8	100	(50)
	Comb. fit	19.0	52.8	12.7	15.5	100	(162)
	(s.e.)	(3.9)	(5.9)	(4.1)	(5.1)		
25–34	LAT	17.7	69.2	10.6	2.5	100	(108)
	NORC	9.1	62.2	16.1	12.6	100	(90)
	Comb. fit	13.2	65.3	13.6	7.9	100	(198)
	(s.e.)	(3.2)	(4.8)	(3.1)	(2.4)		
35–49	LAT	23.5	57.9	12.0	6.6	100	(107)
	NORC	27.5	51.9	12.2	8.4	100	(94)
	Comb. fit	25.5	54.9	12.1	7.5	100	(201)
	(s.e.)	(4.3)	(4.8)	(3.7)	(2.4)		
50–64	LAT	52.8	32.5	12.8	1.9	100	(85)
	NORC	69.0	25.0	6.0	0.0	100	(60)
	Comb. fit	60.2	29.9	8.8	1.2	100	(145)
	(s.e.)	(5.6)	(5.5)	(3.8)	(0.8)		
65 +	LAT	92.7	7.3	0.0	0.0	100	(114)
	NORC	95.0	5.0	0.0	0.0	100	(114)
	Comb. fit	93.7	6.3	0.0	0.0	100	(228)
	(s.e.)	(1.7)	(1.7)	(0.0)	(0.0)		

NOTE: Percentage distributions for the *Los Angeles Times* data set were calculated using weights encoded in the data set by the survey organization. Sample sizes shown are unweighted Ns. NORC percentages are calculated from weighted tabulations. Combined fit estimates and standard errors were derived using procedures of Fay (1982) to take account of complex sample design and sample weighting. (Weights in each survey were normalized so that the weighted N for each survey equaled the unweighted case count.)

Continued

| | | \multicolumn{4}{c|}{Number of Sexual Partners in Last Year} | | |
		None	1	2	3 +	Total	(N)
Married men							
18–24	LAT	0.0%	84.3%	3.2%	12.5%	100%	(22)
	NORC	0.0	80.8	0.0	19.2	100	(13)
	Comb. fit	0.0	83.6	2.5	13.9	100	(35)
	(s.e.)	(0.0)	(9.1)	(2.5)	(9.2)		
25–34	LAT	0.1	92.6	2.1	5.2	100	(127)
	NORC	2.8	93.1	2.8	1.4	100	(72)
	Comb. fit	1.0	92.7	2.3	4.0	100	(199)
	(s.e.)	(0.6)	(2.9)	(1.2)	(2.4)		
35–49	LAT	4.1	92.0	0.0	3.8	100	(190)
	NORC	5.1	89.1	3.6	2.2	100	(129)
	Comb. fit	4.6	90.7	1.7	3.1	100	(319)
	(s.e.)	(1.7)	(2.0)	(0.7)	(1.2)		
50–64	LAT	3.4	94.9	0.6	1.1	100	(91)
	NORC	10.9	85.5	1.2	2.4	100	(74)
	Comb. fit	5.9	91.7	0.9	1.6	100	(165)
	(s.e.)	(2.0)	(2.3)	(0.6)	(0.8)		
65 +	LAT	11.4	83.4	4.0	1.2	100	(64)
	NORC	25.5	71.5	0.0	2.9	100	(68)
	Comb. fit	17.3	78.4	2.3	1.9	100	(132)
	(s.e.)	(3.0)	(4.8)	(2.3)	(1.0)		
Married women							
18–24	LAT	2.6	97.4	0.0	0.0	100	(44)
	NORC	0.0	86.6	10.4	3.0	100	(32)
	Comb. fit	1.7	93.6	3.7	1.0	100	(76)
	(s.e.)	(1.7)	(2.9)	(2.1)	(1.1)		
25–34	LAT	0.1	97.9	2.0	0.1	100	(156)
	NORC	1.1	97.8	0.0	1.1	100	(87)
	Comb. fit	0.5	97.8	1.2	0.5	100	(243)
	(s.e.)	(0.5)	(1.2)	(0.9)	(0.5)		
35–49	LAT	3.4	92.6	0.7	3.3	100	(235)
	NORC	3.5	96.5	0.0	0.0	100	(125)
	Comb. fit	3.5	94.2	0.4	1.9	100	(360)
	(s.e.)	(1.5)	(1.8)	(0.2)	(1.1)		
50–64	LAT	17.5	82.5	0.0	0.0	100	(125)
	NORC	14.5	83.7	0.6	1.2	100	(78)
	Comb. fit	16.3	83.0	0.2	0.5	100	(203)
	(s.e.)	(5.2)	(5.2)	(0.2)	(0.5)		
65 +	LAT	15.9	84.0	0.1	0.0	100	(66)
	NORC	29.0	69.4	0.0	1.6	100	(61)
	Comb. fit	21.7	77.5	0.1	0.7	100	(127)
	(s.e.)	(4.2)	(4.2)	(0.1)	(0.7)		

Question Wordings. Los Angeles Times: "About how many sexual partners would you say you have had in the last year?" NORC: "How many sex partners have you had in the last 12 months?"

Index

A

Abstinence
  by adolescents, 14, 173, 174, 177 n.42, 204
  predictors of, 173, 174
  promotion of, 14, 203–204, 206, 207
Acute normovolemic hemodilution, 338
Adolescents
  abortions by, 205 n.86
  abstinence by, 173
  AIDS cases, 141, 151–152, 157–160
  anal intercourse by heterosexuals, 179–180
  awareness about AIDS, 15–16, 182–183, 208–213, 216–217
  blood donation by, 314–315
  childbearing, 155–156, 161, 166
  clustering of risky behaviors, 194–197
  community norms and behavior modification among, 218–219
  contraception and condom use, 12–13, 177–179
  data sources on, 11–12, 150, 168–170, 184–185
  delinquents, 173, 174, 185, 197–199, 216 n.98, 223, 230
  delivery of programs to, 221–231
  drug use and users, 13, 183–194, 199, 200, 202–203, 227–231
  environmental factors in risk of AIDS, 13
  epidemiology of AIDS and HIV infection among, 148–167
  fear of AIDS, 213–215
  frequency of intercourse, 174–175
  gender differences in AIDS and HIV prevalence, 56–57, 157–160
  gender differences in drug use, 189–190
  geographic distribution of AIDS and HIV prevalence, 161–166
  goals of intervention programs for, 202–208
  HIV seroprevalence, 4, 11, 56, 147, 153–167, 200
  hotlines for, 220, 222, 227
  incubation period for AIDS in, 149–150
  initiation of drug use, 13, 185–186
  injection practices among, 186–187
  knowledge levels and risky behavior, 216–217
  number in U.S., 157 n.14, 233 n.117
  number of sexual partners, 12, 175–177
  in other studies, 156–157
  out-of-school youth, 16, 197, 226–227
  personal vulnerability messages in prevention, 215–216
  pregnancy rates, 13, 205, 207
  prevalence of AIDS, 141, 151–152, 157–160
  prevalence of drug use, 187–190
  prevalence of HIV, 4, 11, 56, 147, 153–167, 200
  prevention programs, 11, 13–15, 17, 35, 201–232
  prostitution by, 15, 17, 199–200, 270

477

C

N